Hip Fractures

Springer
*New York
Berlin
Heidelberg
Barcelona
Hong Kong
London
Milan
Paris
Singapore
Tokyo*

Kenneth J. Koval
Chief, Fracture Service
Department of Orthopaedic Surgery
NYU – Hospital for Joint Diseases
Associate Professor, Orthopaedic Surgery
NYU School of Medicine

Joseph D. Zuckerman
Chairman
NYU – Hospital for Joint Diseases
Department of Orthopaedic Surgery
Walter A. L. Thompson Professor, Orthopaedic Surgery
NYU School of Medicine

Hip Fractures

A Practical Guide to Management

Foreword by Charles A. Rockwood, Jr.
With 403 Figures, in 628 Parts
Illustrations by Hugh Nachamie and Martin Finch

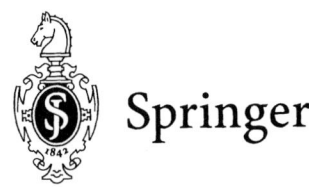

Kenneth J. Koval, MD
Joseph D. Zuckerman, MD
Hospital for Joint Diseases
301 East 17th Street
New York, NY 10003
USA

Library of Congress Cataloging-in-Publication Data
Koval, Kenneth J.
   Hip fractures: a practical guide to management / Kenneth J.
Koval, Joseph D. Zuckerman
      p.   cm.
      Includes bibliographical references and index.
      ISBN 0-387-98387-2 (hardcover : alk. cover)
      1. Hip joint—Fractures—Treatment.   2. Hip joint—Fractures—
Patients—Rehabilitation.   I. Zuckerman, Joseph D. (Joseph David),
1952– . II. Title.
      [DNLM: 1. Hip Fractures—therapy.   2. Hip Fractures—diagnosis.
WE 855 K88h 1999]
RD549.K68   1999
617.1′58—dc21
DNLM/DLC
for Library of Congress   99-11424

Printed on acid-free paper.

© 2000 Springer-Verlag New York, Inc.
All rights reserved. This work may not be translated or copied in whole or in part without the written permission of the publisher (Springer-Verlag New York, Inc., 175 Fifth Avenue, New York, NY 10010, USA), except for brief excerpts in connection with reviews or scholarly analysis. Use in connection with any form of information storage and retrieval, electronic adaptation, computer software, or by similar or dissimilar methodology now known or hereafter developed is forbidden.
The use of general descriptive names, trade names, trademarks, etc., in this publication, even if the former are not especially identified, is not to be taken as a sign that such names, as understood by the Trade Marks and Merchandise Marks Act, may accordingly be used freely by anyone.
While the advice and information in this book are believed to be true and accurate at the date of going to press, neither the authors nor the editors nor the publisher can accept any legal responsibility for any errors or omissions that may be made. The publisher makes no warranty, express or implied, with respect to the material contained herein.

Production coordinated by Impressions Book and Journal Services, Inc., and managed by Steven Pisano; manufacturing supervised by Joe Quatela.
Typeset by Impressions Book and Journal Services, Inc., Madison, WI.
Printed and bound by Maple-Vail Book Manufacturing Group, York, PA.
Printed in the United States of America.

9 8 7 6 5 4 3 2 1

ISBN 0-387-98387-2   Springer-Verlag New York Berlin Heidelberg   SPIN 10656803

This book is dedicated to my role models in Orthopaedics: (1) my father, a dedicated physician who showed me the value of hard work; (2) Arsen Pankovich, who was my first experience with a true traumatologist; (3) Roy Sanders, who taught me how to perform surgery and research; and (4) Joseph D. Zuckerman, my friend and partner who showed me how to deal with people.

—Kenneth J. Koval

To Victor H. Frankel, M.D., Ph.D., KNO, who, in 1985, said to me, "Joe, you should study hip fractures in the elderly." And that is how it started . . .

—Joseph D. Zuckerman

Foreword

I was delighted when I received the invitation from Drs. Zuckerman and Koval to write the foreword for this text. I appreciate the invitation to be a part of this text. Both authors are good friends and because of their help with our textbook on fractures, I know that they generate excellent educational material.

Fractures of the hip are a very common problem in orthopaedics, and the authors have presented an overview of this problem in a very clear and concise manner. They have broken the subject down into 12 individual chapters. Following the anatomy chapter, the authors present a detailed description of how the reader should manage treatment of various types of hip fractures. They follow this with essential chapters on how to avoid problems, various types of rehabilitation, how to assess outcome, the economics of hip fracture, and, finally, prevention.

Dr. Koval is a respected orthopedist who, following his residency in New York, served several orthopaedic trauma fellowships. He currently serves as the chief of the fracture service at the Hospital for Joint Diseases and New York University Medical Center in New York City. Joe Zuckerman is an internationally known expert in the care of hip fractures, and I don't know how he found the time to serve as a coauthor with Dr. Koval for this text. I have always admired the way Joe can present his material in a lively, entertaining, and lucid manner. Dr. Zuckerman is surgeon in chief at the Hospital for Joint Diseases and New York University Medical Center in New York City. Both authors are superb teachers, writers, lecturers, and researchers. I congratulate them for this text, and on behalf of orthopaedic surgeons around the world, I thank them for this contribution.

Charles A. Rockwood, Jr, MD
University of Texas Health Science Center
San Antonio, Texas

Preface

This book represents the cumulative knowledge and experience of the many surgeons who have practiced and taught at the Hospital for Joint Diseases. Founded in 1906, the Hospital for Joint Diseases has had a long history of excellence in the evaluation and treatment of fractures of the proximal femur. David Telson, in 1933, pioneered the use of threaded Steinmen pins to stabilize femoral neck fractures. He performed surgery either in the hospital or at the patient's home, on the kitchen table, using a blowtorch to sterilize the implants. Joseph Buchman was one of the first surgeons to advocate use of open reduction under direct visualization to treat displaced femoral neck fractures; he recognized that the ability to perform an open reduction distinguished the orthopaedic surgeon from the general surgeon. Drs. Emanuel Kaplan and Herman Robbins both had a love for anatomic dissections and lectured on the anatomy of the proximal femur.

Victor H. Frankel, MD, PhD, former chairman of the Department of Orthopaedic Surgery at the Hospital for Joint Diseases, has dedicated his life's work to the prevention and treatment of fractures of the proximal femur. His doctoral thesis, published in 1960, focused on the forces required to create a femoral neck fracture, as well as the optimum implant configuration for fracture stabilization. Later in his career, he developed and implanted a telemetrized hip nail into femoral neck fractures to determine the forces across the hip during activities of daily living. This work was the basis for our belief that all hip fracture patients should be allowed to bear weight as tolerated after surgery.

In 1985, upon the advice and support of Victor H. Frankel, the Hospital for Joint Diseases planned and initiated the geriatric hip fracture program, an interdisciplinary research group comprising orthopaedic surgeons, geriatricians, anesthesiologists, nursing staff, physical therapists, social workers, nutritionists, and epidemiologists. This program was designed for both patient care and research. Many aspects of patient care are collected prospectively and entered into our database. This registry now includes information on more than 1000 patients and has served as the basis for many clinical studies.

In conjunction with the initiation of the geriatric hip fracture program, the hospital established a musculoskeletal research center staffed by bioengineers and other basic scientists. Equipped with state-of-the-art testing equipment, the laboratory has initiated and completed numerous biomechanical studies, including evaluation of different types of hip fracture fixation techniques.

This comprehensive text on fractures of the proximal femur incorporates many of the teachings and philosophies of hip fracture management at the Hospital for Joint Diseases, including anatomy, diagnosis, preoperative evaluation, nonoperative and operative treatment, rehabilitation, and outcome assessment. We are deeply grateful for the contribution of all the physicians and scientists on whose hard work and experience this book was conceived and written. We recognize that this book would not have been possible without the wealth of experience in hip fracture management and research gained at the Hospital for Joint Diseases.

Kenneth J. Koval, MD
Joseph D. Zuckerman, MD

Acknowledgments

We would like to thank all the people who made the writing of this book possible. In particular, we would like to acknowledge the work of Frank Martucci and Dwayne Harris whose photographic skills are evident throughout the book, William Green for his editorial insight, and the people of Springer who gave us the opportunity to produce this manuscript.

Contents

Foreword by Charles A. Rockwood, Jr.	**vii**
Preface	**ix**
Acknowledgments	**xi**

Chapter One
Anatomy — **1**

Chapter Two
Epidemiology and Mechanism of Injury — **9**

Chapter Three
Diagnosis — **27**

Chapter Four
Treatment Principles — **37**

Chapter Five
Femoral Neck Fractures — **49**

Chapter Six
Intertrochanteric Fractures — **129**

Chapter Seven
Subtrochanteric Fractures — **191**

Chapter Eight
Pitfalls and Their Avoidance — **253**

Chapter Nine
Rehabilitation — **287**

Chapter Ten
Outcome Assessment **295**

Chapter Eleven
Economics of Hip Fracture Treatment **303**

Chapter Twelve
Prevention **313**

Index **323**

Chapter One

Anatomy

The hip is a ball-and-socket joint formed by the femoral head and the acetabulum. The *femoral head,* an imperfect sphere of cancellous bone sheathed in articular cartilage, is characterized by a relatively dense meshwork of trabecular bone that facilitates the absorption and distribution of weight-bearing stresses to the dense cortical bone of the femoral neck and proximal femur. The size of the femoral head varies more or less in proportion to body mass, ranging from roughly 40 to 60 mm in diameter.[1] The thickness of the articular cartilage covering the femoral head averages 4 mm superiorly and tapers to 3 mm at the periphery.[2]

The *femoral neck* comprises the region between the base of the femoral head and the intertrochanteric line anteriorly and the intertrochanteric crest posteriorly (Figure 1.1). The femoral neck forms an angle with the femoral shaft ranging from 125° to 140° in the anteroposterior plane and 10° to 15° (anteversion) in the lateral plane[3] (Figure 1.2). The cancellous bone of the femoral neck is characterized by trabeculae organized into medial and lateral systems[4] (Figure 1.3). The medial trabecular system forms in response to the joint reaction force on the femoral head; the epiphyseal plates are perpendicular to the medial trabecular system. The lateral trabecular system resists the compressive force on the femoral head resulting from contraction of the abductor muscles.

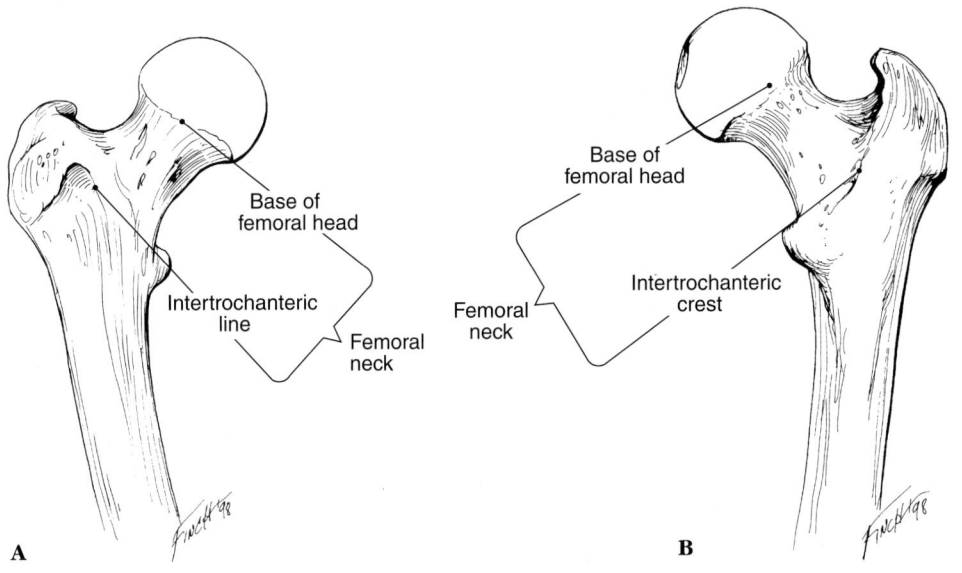

Figure 1.1. Anterior (**A**) and posterior (**B**) views of the proximal femur.

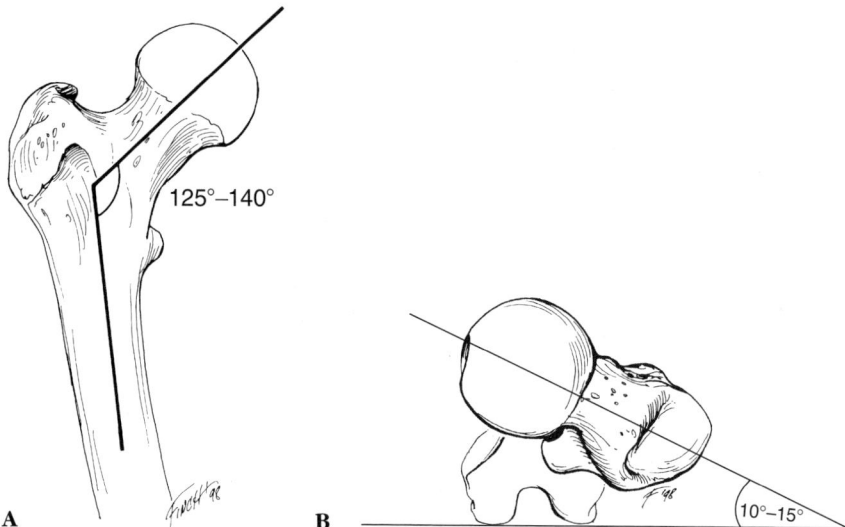

Figure 1.2. The femoral neck forms an angle with the femoral shaft ranging from 125° to 140° in the anteroposterior plane (**A**) and 10° to 15° (anteversion) in the lateral plane (**B**).

The *intertrochanteric region* of the hip, consisting of the greater and lesser trochanters, represents a zone of transition from the femoral neck to the femoral shaft. This area is characterized primarily by dense trabecular bone that serves to transmit and distribute stress, similar to the cancellous bone of the femoral neck. The greater and lesser trochanters are the sites of insertion of the major muscles of the gluteal region (Figure 1.4): the gluteus medius and gluteus minimus, the iliopsoas, and the short external rotators. The calcar femorale, a vertical wall of dense bone extending from the posteromedial aspect of the femoral shaft to the posterior portion of the femoral neck, forms an internal trabecular strut within

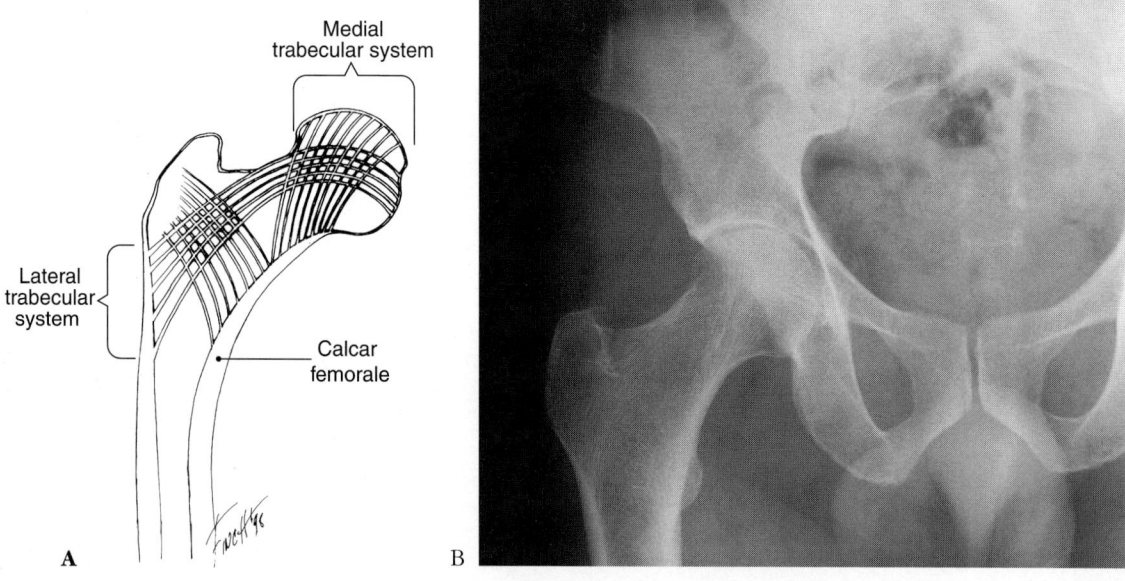

Figure 1.3. Diagram (**A**) and radiograph (**B**) depicting the cancellous bone of the femoral neck.

1. Anatomy

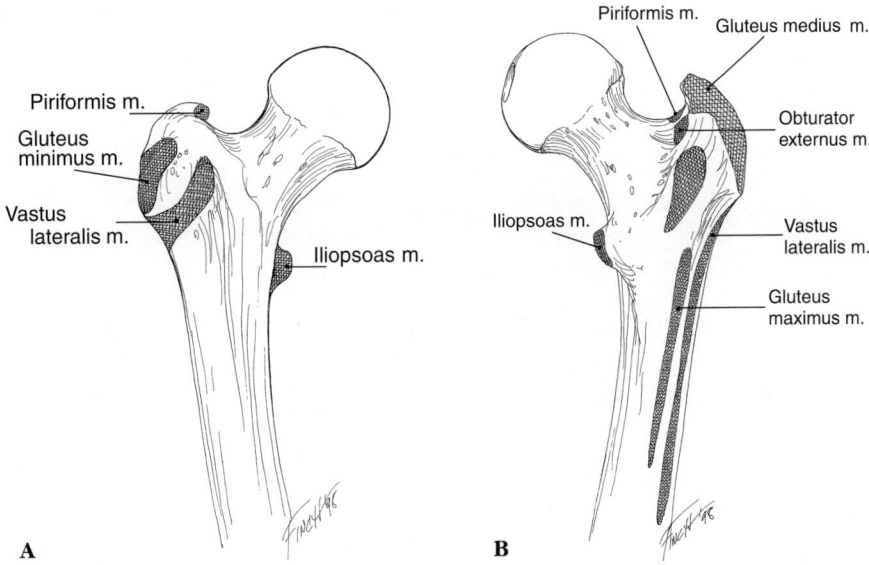

Figure 1.4. Anterior (**A**) and posterior (**B**) views of the proximal femur demonstrating the muscle insertion regions.

the inferior portion of the femoral neck and intertrochanteric region and acts as a strong conduit for stress transfer[5,6] (Figure 1.5).

The *subtrochanteric region,* which extends from the lesser trochanter to an area 5 cm distal, consists primarily of thick, dense cortical bone (Figure 1.6). This is an area of high stress concentration, with large compressive forces medially and tensile forces laterally (Figure 1.7). The dense cortical bone permits efficient transmission of both axial and torsional loads.

The *acetabulum* is formed by the confluence of the ilial, ischial, and pubic ossification centers, which are joined at the triradiate cartilage (Figure 1.8). The cavity of the acetabulum faces obliquely forward, outward, and downward; it is extended and deepened by the fibrocartilaginous *labrum,* which forms an outer rim of tissue (Figure 1.9). The acetabular labrum extends across the acetabular notch as the transverse acetabular ligament.

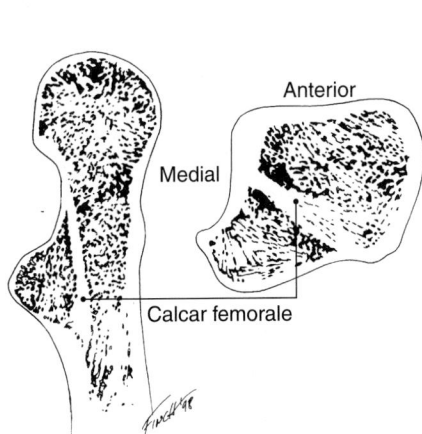

Figure 1.5. The calcar femorale is a vertical wall of dense bone extending from the posteromedial aspect of the femoral shaft to the posterior portion of the femoral neck.

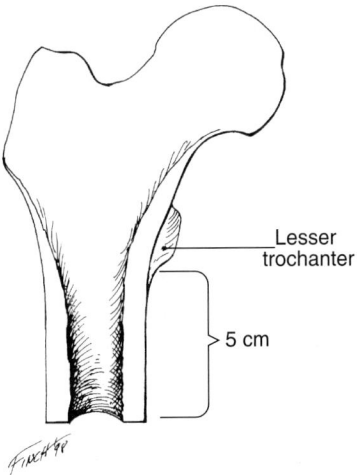

Figure 1.6. The subtrochanteric region, which extends from the lesser trochanter to an area 5 cm distal, consists primarily of thick, dense cortical bone.

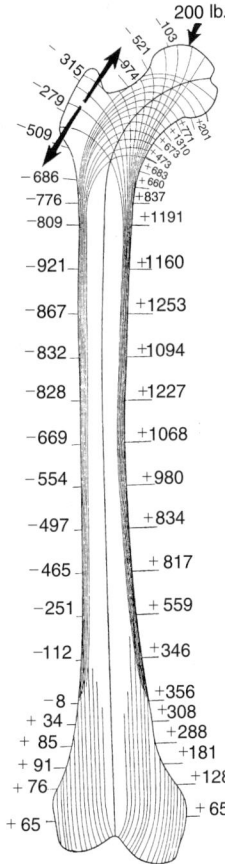

Figure 1.7. The subtrochanteric region is an area of high stress concentration, with large compressive forces medially and tensile forces laterally.

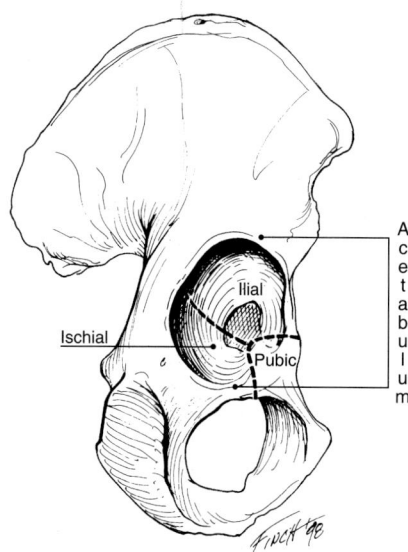

Figure 1.8. The acetabulum is formed by the confluence of the ilial, ischial, and pubic ossification centers, which are joined at the triradiate cartilage.

The *hip capsule* is attached to the labrum and the transverse acetabular ligament of the acetabulum, the medial side of the greater trochanter, the intertrochanteric line anteriorly, a site immediately superior and medial to the lesser trochanter, and the femoral neck posteriorly.[7] The entire anterior aspect of the femoral neck and the proximal half of its posterior portion lie within the capsule of the hip joint. Fractures within this area are thus termed *intracapsular*.

Three prominent ligaments (the iliofemoral, ischiofemoral, and pubofemoral) and one minor ligament (the zona orbicularis) conjoin with the hip joint capsule[7] (Figure 1.10). Of these, the *iliofemoral ligament* (the Y-shaped ligament of Bigelow) is the largest and most important, extending from the anterior inferior iliac spine to the anterior aspect of the greater trochanter and intertrochanteric line as an inverted Y. The *ischiofemoral ligament* extends from the ischium to the base of the posterosuperior femoral neck. The *pubofemoral ligament*, originating from the body of the pubis, crosses anterior to the hip joint to insert onto

Figure 1.9. The cavity of the acetabulum is extended and deepened by the fibrocartilaginous labrum, which forms an outer rim of tissue. The acetabular labrum extends across the acetabular notch as the transverse acetabular ligament.

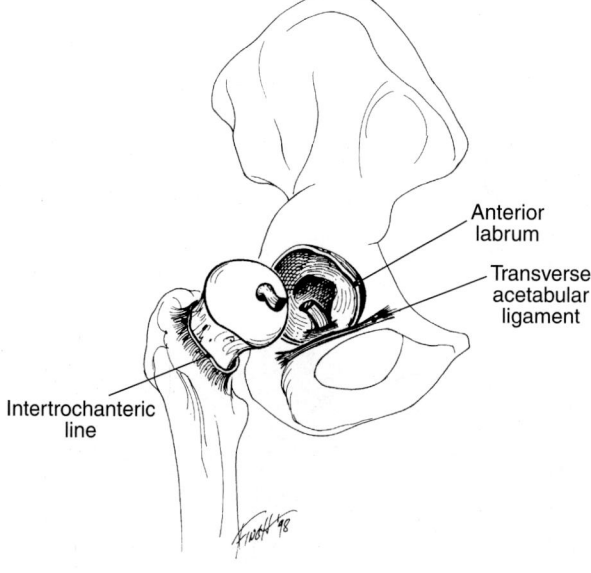

1. Anatomy

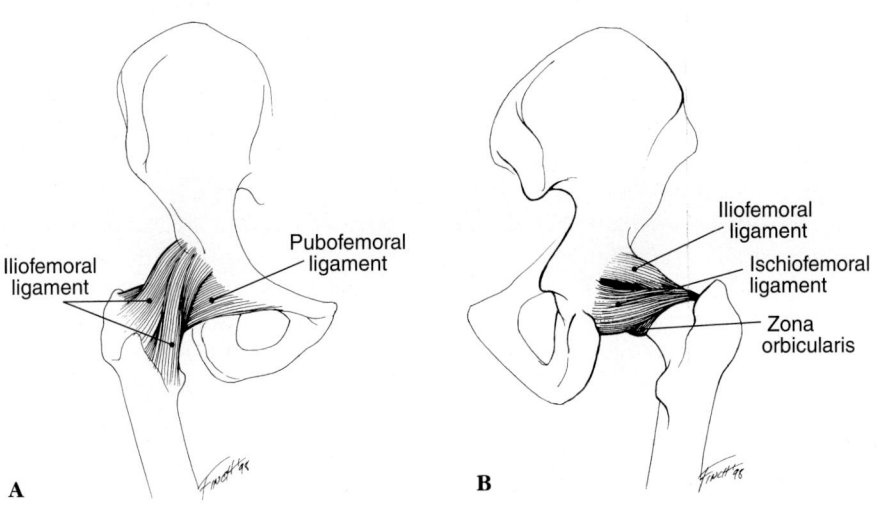

Figure 1.10. Anterior (**A**) and posterior (**B**) views of the hip. Three prominent ligaments (the iliofemoral, ischiofemoral, and pubofemoral) and one minor ligament (the zona orbicularis) conjoin with the hip joint capsule.

the lower aspect of the femoral neck and the lower limb of the iliofemoral ligament. The *zona orbicularis,* the least prominent of the four (it is in fact covered by the other three), consists of fibers that encircle the capsule at the femoral neck. Inside the hip capsule, extending from the acetabular fossa and transverse acetabular ligament to the fovea of the femoral head and surrounded by synovium, is the ligament of the femoral head, the *ligamentum teres.*

Innervation of the hip joint varies from individual to individual and may include branches of the *femoral nerve* (anteriorly), anterior-inferior branches of the *obturator nerve* (and sometimes an *accessory obturator nerve*), and a branch from either the nerve to the quadratus femoris or the superior gluteal nerve posteriorly.

The musculature of the hip region can be grouped according to function and location[7] (Figure 1.11). The abductors of the gluteal region, the *gluteus*

Figure 1.11. Anterior (**A**) and posterior (**B**) views of the gluteal region and thigh, demonstrating the muscle groups.

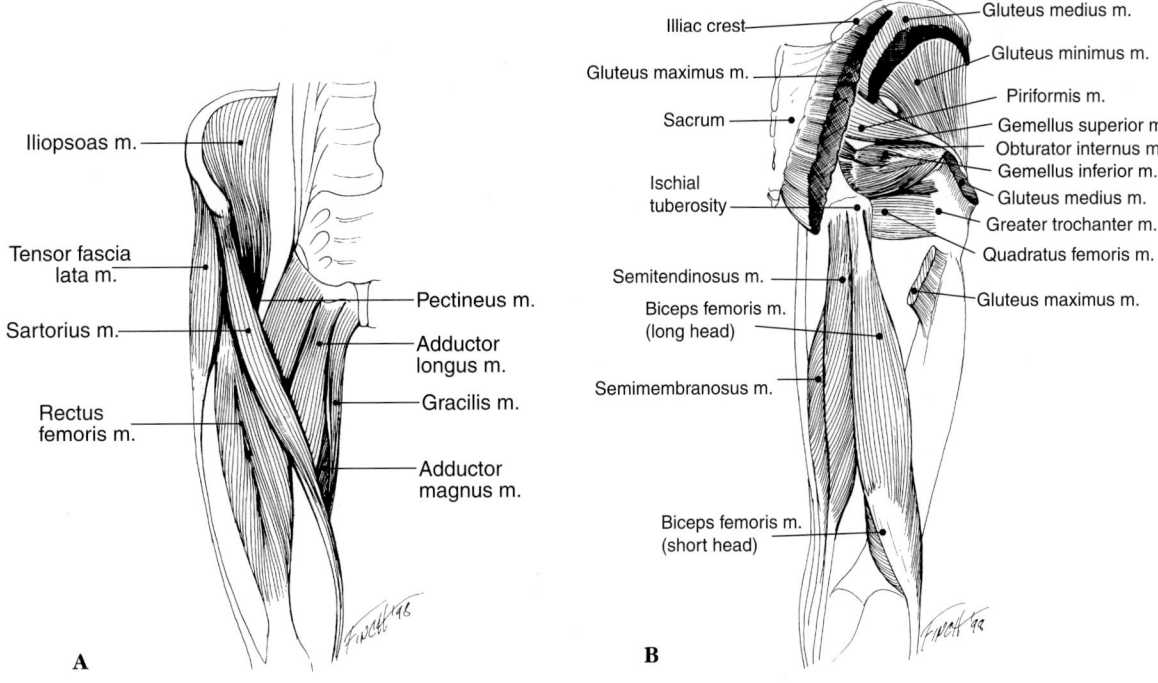

medius and *gluteus minimus muscles*, which originate from the outer table of the ilium and insert onto the greater trochanter, function to control pelvic tilt in the frontal plane. The gluteus medius and gluteus minimus muscles, along with the *tensor fascia lata muscle,* are also internal rotators of the hip. The hip flexors are located in the anterior aspect of the thigh and include the sartorius, pectineus, iliopsoas, and rectus femoris muscles. The *iliopsoas muscle* inserts onto the lesser trochanter. The *gracilis muscle* and the *adductor* muscles (longus, brevis, and magnus) are located in the medial aspect of the thigh. The short external rotators—the *piriformis, obturator internus, obturator externus, superior* and *inferior gemelli,* and *quadratus femoris muscles*—all insert onto the posterior aspect of the greater trochanter. The *gluteus maximus muscle,* originating from the ilium, sacrum, and coccyx, inserts onto the gluteal tuberosity along the linea aspera in the subtrochanteric region of the femur and the iliotibial tract. The gluteus maximus muscle serves as an extensor and external rotator of the hip. The *semitendinosus, semimembranosus,* and *biceps femoris muscles,* which originate from the ischium to form the hamstring muscles of the thigh, are responsible for knee flexion as well as hip extension.

The *femoral triangle,* located in the anterior proximal thigh, is formed by the inguinal ligament proximally, the sartorius muscle laterally, and the medial border of the adductor longus muscle medially[7] (Figure 1.12). The iliopsoas and pectineus muscles constitute the floor. Contained within the femoral triangle from lateral to medial are the femoral nerve, artery, and vein, which all enter the femoral triangle deep to the inguinal ligament and exit distally deep to the sartorius muscle. Within this region, the *femoral artery* gives off the *profunda femoris artery* from its posterolateral side. The two largest tributaries of the profunda femoris artery are the *medial* and *lateral femoral circumflex arteries.* The latter originates from the lateral aspect of the profunda femoris artery and proceeds laterally across the iliopsoas muscle and then deep to the sartorius and rectus femoris muscles, where it divides into ascending, descending, and transverse branches. The *medial femoral circumflex artery,* which originates from the medial or posteromedial side of the profunda femoris artery, runs posteriorly between the iliopsoas and pectineus muscles. The *cruciate* or *crucial anastomosis,* located at the inferior margin of the quadratus femoris muscle, is formed by a descending branch of the inferior gluteal artery, the first perforating branch of the profunda femoris artery, and

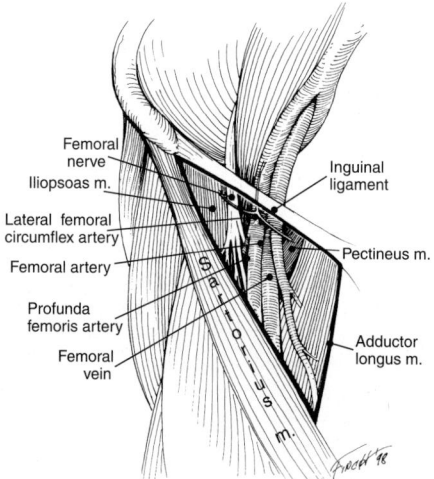

Figure 1.12. Diagram illustrating the boundaries and floor of the femoral triangle.

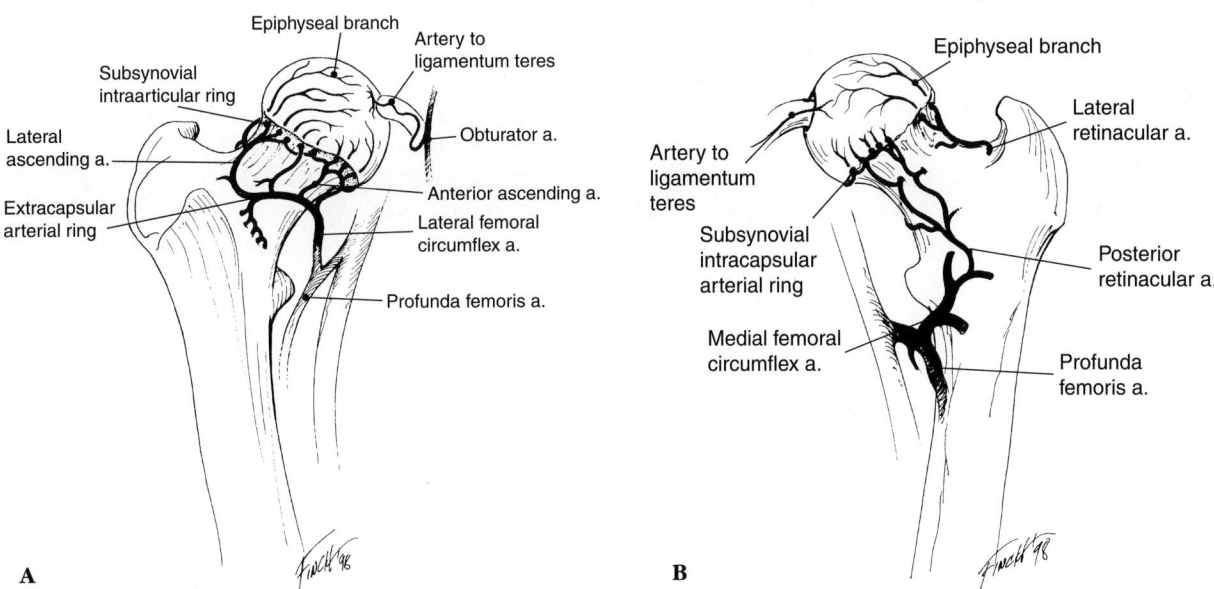

Figure 1.13. Anterior (**A**) and posterior (**B**) views of the proximal femur demonstrating the blood supply to the femoral head and neck.

the medial and lateral circumflex arteries. The *superficial femoral artery* continues in the thigh within the adductor canal, separated from the profunda femoris vessel by the adductor longus muscle. The femoral artery then passes from medial to posterior in the thigh through a tendinous hiatus in the adductor magnus muscle *(Hunter's canal),* becoming the *popliteal artery.*

The blood supply to the femoral head and neck is complex and has important orthopaedic implications[8–10] (Figure 1.13). The medial and lateral circumflex arteries send branches that anastomose to form an extracapsular arterial ring at the base of the femoral neck. Coming off this arterial ring are the ascending cervical arteries, also known as the *capsular* or *retinacular arteries,* which pierce the joint capsule and traverse the neck of the femur deep to the synovial membrane. There are four major retinacular arteries—*anterior, medial, posterior,* and *lateral*—named for their position relative to the femoral neck. The lateral retinacular artery is the most important blood supply to the femoral head and neck. The retinacular vessels anastomose at the base of the femoral head to form the subsynovial intraarticular ring. Small epiphyseal arterial branches then pierce and supply blood to the femoral head. The artery of the ligamentum teres is either a branch of the posterior division of the obturator artery or a branch from the medial circumflex artery. This artery, which supplies blood to a small area of bone adjacent to the fovea of the femoral head, is clinically important only in children.

References

1. Cathcart RF. The shape of the femoral head and preliminary results of clinical use of a non-spherical hip prosthesis. *J Bone Joint Surg Am* 1971; 53:397.
2. Hoaglund FT, Low WD. Anatomy of the femoral neck and head, with comparative data from Caucasians and Hong Kong Chinese. *Clin Orthop* 1980; 152:10–16.
3. Noble PC, Alexander JW, Lindahl LJ. The anatomic basis of femoral component design. *Clin Orthop* 1988; 235:148–165.
4. Ward FO. *Human Anatomy.* London: Renshaw, 1838.

5. Harty M. The calcar femorale and the femoral neck. *J Bone Joint Surg Am* 1957; 39:625–630.
6. Griffin JB. The calcar femorale redefined. *Clin Orthop* 1982; 164:211–214.
7. Williams PL, Warwick R, Dyson M, Bannister LH, eds. *Gray's Anatomy,* Vol 37. New York: Churchill Livingstone, 1989:267–635.
8. Trueta J, Harrison MHM. The normal vascular anatomy of the femoral head in adult man. *J Bone Joint Surg Br* 1953; 35:442–461.
9. Trueta J. The normal vascular anatomy of the human femoral head during growth. *J Bone Joint Surg Br* 1957; 39:358–393.
10. Howe WW, Lacey T, Schwartz RP. A study of the gross anatomy of the arteries supplying the proximal portion of the femur and acetabulum. *J Bone Joint Surg Am* 1950; 32:856–866.

Chapter Two

Epidemiology and Mechanism of Injury

Incidence

The incidence of hip fracture varies substantially from country to country. Table 2.1 summarizes hip fracture incidence by age, sex, and region. The lowest incidence, 5.6 per 100,000, has been documented among the South African Bantus.[1] A study in Spain reported an incidence of 27 per 100,000,[2] whereas an incidence of 31.5 cases per 100,000 has been reported in Hong Kong.[3] The incidence in England has been reported as 43 per 100,000.[4] In Sweden, the incidence of hip fractures is 69.6 per 100,000,[5] while in the United States, it is approximately 80 per 100,000.[6]

The incidence of hip fractures worldwide is increasing. Between 1966 and 1985, the incidence of hip fractures among the elderly in Hong Kong more than doubled.[7] Between 1985 and 1989, there was a 20% increase in the incidence of hip fractures in Japan.[8] In Finland, the incidence of hip fractures increased by almost 300% during the period from 1970 to 1991.[9] Between 1973 and 1984, there was a 32% increase in hip fracture incidence in northern Sweden that was not exclusively attributable to the increase in the proportion of elderly individuals.[10]

Estimates of the incidence of hip fracture in the future also differ. Cummings et al. predicted that the annual number of hip fractures in the United States will rise from 238,000 in 1986 to 512,000 by the year 2040.[11] Another study predicted that the number of hip fractures in the elderly will double or triple

Table 2.1. Incidence of hip fracture, 1990, by age, sex, and region (fractures per 100,000 population)

Region	Men (age in years)							Women (age in years)						
	50–54	55–59	60–64	65–69	70–74	75–79	80+	50–54	55–59	60–64	65–69	70–74	75–79	80+
W. Europe	28	33	67	103	203	331	880	33	54	115	184	362	657	1808
S. Europe	10	16	34	55	81	190	534	11	21	47	100	170	380	1075
E. Europe	38	38	88	88	194	194	475	58	58	155	155	426	426	1251
N. Europe	58	66	97	198	382	682	1864	74	78	190	327	612	1294	2997
N. America	33	33	81	123	119	338	1230	60	60	117	252	437	850	2296
Oceania	20	34	63	92	180	445	1157	31	63	112	204	358	899	2476
Asia	20	20	37	47	102	150	364	14	14	38	75	156	252	563
Africa	6	10	14	27	8	0	116	4	12	17	12	16	50	80
Latin America	25	40	40	106	106	327	327	19.5	50	50	162.5	162.5	622	622
World	23	25	47	69	119	219	630	24	28	69	122	240	458	1289

Adapted from Gullberg et. al.[15]

within 20 years.[12–14] Gullberg et al. projected that the total number of hip fractures worldwide (1.66 million in 1990) will reach 2.6 million by the year 2025 and 4.5 million by 2050.[15]

Risk Factors

Numerous factors may affect the risk of hip fracture, including gender, race, age, ethnicity, hip axis length, bone mass, nutrition, height and weight, maternal history of hip fracture, prior fracture, use of psychotropic drugs and antihypertensive medications, place of residence, fluoridation of public water supplies, institutionalization, season of the year, and climate. Certain ethnic groups may have a unique combination of different risk factors that may place them at greater risk for sustaining a hip fracture. This may explain the significant international variations of hip fracture incidence that have been reported.

Age

Virtually every study of hip fracture incidence cites age as an important risk factor; only 2% to 3% of hip fractures are sustained by patients younger than 50 years,[16] although evidence from workers in U.S. trauma centers indicates a rise in the numbers of young, active adults with hip fractures resulting from vehicular trauma. This may be a result of the increasingly popular smaller automobiles with lower dashboards that tend to place the rider in a position that, in the event of a collision, results in forces that cause a proximal femur fracture.[17]

Gallagher et al. observed that hip fracture incidence doubles for each decade of life after age 50.[6] Hedlund et al. reported that this figure doubles every 7 to 8 years in women and every 5 to 6 years in men after age 50.[18] Lauritzen et al. found that 80% of hip fractures occur in women over age 70 years.[19] It has been postulated that the association of increased hip fracture incidence with advancing age is related to the greater likelihood in the elderly of defective vision, impaired walking capability, lack of balancing or protective responses, medications that impair balance and gait, and decreased bone strength and mass.

Gender

Women sustain the majority of hip fractures. Cooper et al. reported that 72% of the 1.66 million hip fractures in 1990 occurred in women.[20] Most investigators have found a female-to-male ratio of 2:1 in patients over 65 years of age.[15,18] In black populations in the United States and South Africa, as well as in Chinese in Hong Kong, however, this ratio is 1:1.[1,3,21] In Singapore, Wong reported a female-to-male ratio of 0.6:1.[22] Utilizing a different approach, Cummings et al. in 1985 calculated a 15% lifetime risk of hip fracture for white women who live in the United States and live to an age of 80 years, and a 5% lifetime risk for men who live to an age of 75 years.[11] Melton attributed the disparity in hip fracture risk to women's lower bone mass, lower bone density, and higher frequency of falling.[23]

Race

As suggested in the preceding section, the incidence of hip fractures varies with race. In general, the age-specific rates for hip fracture among black women are approximately 50% of those among white women.[21,24] Cummings et al. in 1989 determined that among persons 50 years of age and older in the United States, the lifetime risk of a hip fracture was approximately 17% for white women versus 6% for black women, and 5.6% for white men versus 2.8% for black men.[25] Several authors have attributed this difference to greater bone mass in blacks than in whites.[26] It has also been observed that black women have a lower risk of falling than white women.[27] Bauer reported that Mexican Americans had a significantly lower risk of hip fracture than whites, but the authors could offer no reason for this.[28]

The incidence of hip fractures among Asian Americans is 61% that of age-matched whites.[29] This finding was confirmed by Ross et al., who found that older Japanese immigrants in the United States had a lower incidence of hip fracture than age-matched whites.[30] These results are nevertheless surprising in light of studies demonstrating that Asians have lower bone mineral density than white Americans at all skeletal sites.[31] Other factors may therefore play a role in determining susceptibility to hip fracture—such as factors that vary by racial groupings (e.g., geometric characteristics of the femoral neck and distance of impact as measured from the hip to the surface below).

Institutionalization and Hospitalization

Several studies have reported that the risk of hip fracture in elderly persons living in institutions is greater than for elderly persons living in private homes.[32,33] Ooms et al. reported that the relative risk of hip fracture in the age group 70 to 74 years is 5.8 times greater for institutionalized individuals than for community-dwelling elderly persons.[32] These findings were confirmed by Rudman and Rudman, who found a higher incidence of hip fracture among men living in nursing homes than in age-matched community-dwelling men.[33]

In analyzing institutionalization as a risk factor for hip fracture, one must first factor out the characteristics of elderly institutionalized individuals that distinguish them from the noninstitutionalized elderly. A likely explanation for the increased incidence of hip fracture among the institutionalized elderly is that they already exhibit more risk factors, particularly those associated with an increased risk of falling, such as poor visual acuity, poor depth perception, and use of antipsychotic or antidepressant agents. In a study of risk factors for hip fracture in a hospital for elderly psychiatric patients, Vieweg et al. reported that the risk for hip fracture among institutionalized patients is several times greater than that of age- and sex-matched control subjects and that the use of drugs causing sedation and hypotension contributed significantly to this heightened risk.[34] Cumming reported that living in a skilled nursing facility was not an independent risk factor for hip fracture[35]; he proposed that the observed increase in hip fracture rates in such facilities was not the result of residence there, but rather because of attributes—in particular, cognitive impairment—common in this population.

Medical Comorbidities

Medical comorbidities—especially those affecting mental status, sensory perception, balance, and locomotion—are associated with an increased risk of hip fracture.[11,36] Any condition that predisposes the individual to syncope or falling represents an important risk factor. Cerebrovascular diseases such as stroke have been associated with an increased risk of hip fracture in black women.[37] Occlusion of cerebrovascular vessels supplying the motor and/or sensory cortex of the brain can cause disturbances in gait, coordination, sensory perception, and balance. Cardiac disease may also play a role in the incidence of hip fracture. Disturbances in cardiac rhythms can cause dizziness and syncope, which in turn can lead to a fall.

There is frequently a history of mild illness prior to a fall, which may have resulted in dehydration, electrolyte imbalance, confusion, and/or impaired coordination. Dehydration can affect drug metabolism and consequently increase the risk of falling. Any condition that affects mobility and balance increases the risk of falling and subsequent hip fracture. Greater incidences of Parkinson's disease, diabetes, and epilepsy have been noted in hip fracture patients.[38,39] Patients with arthritis are at increased risk for falling because of the immobility and gait disturbance that typically accompany this condition.

Any medical condition that results in accelerated bone loss, such as diabetes mellitus, hyperthyroidism, hyperparathyroidism, and Cushing's disease, increases the risk for hip fracture; bilateral ovariectomy has been shown to increase the risk of hip fracture anywhere from 2- to 7-fold.[40] Several studies have cited mental confusion and dementia as risk factors for hip fracture.[34,41] Vieweg et al. reported a 75% incidence of dementia in patients who sustained a hip fracture,[34] whereas Buchner reported that patients with Alzheimer's disease have three times the risk of hip fracture compared with age- and sex-matched control subjects, with most hip fractures traceable to wandering episodes, drug reactions, and associated comorbidities.[41]

Visual impairment has been implicated as a risk factor for hip fracture in many studies.[42,43] Felson et al. reported that even low levels of visual impairment increased the risk of hip fracture.[42] Cummings et al. demonstrated that both poor depth perception and reduced contrast perception increased the risk for hip fracture.[43]

Individuals who have previously sustained a fragility fracture (a vertebral compression fracture or a distal radius fracture) are likewise at increased risk for hip fracture. An individual who has sustained a prior hip fracture is 1.6 times more likely than others to sustain a second, contralateral hip fracture, which in the majority of cases is of the same fracture type.[44] Cummings et al. demonstrated that women with a maternal history of hip fracture had twice the risk for hip fracture, possibly because of genetic factors that influence femoral bone mass.[43] Both Arden et al. and Slemenda et al. concluded that genetic factors influence such characteristics as bone mineral density and hip axis length.[45,46]

Hip Geometry

One factor that has been suggested in explanation for the differences in hip fracture incidence among countries and races is the difference in osseous geometry among these populations. Specifically, hip axis length—the distance along the femoral neck axis from the base of the greater trochanter to the inner pelvic brim—has been positively correlated with increased fracture risk.[47] Hip axis length is shorter in Japanese women than in white American women, and Japanese women experience a lower hip fracture rate[48]; similarly, among Chinese, who experience a lower hip fracture rate than white Americans, hip axis length was found to be 1.2 standard deviations shorter than in whites.[49] Since a longer hip axis length contributes to a larger bending moment during a fall, hip fracture is more likely to occur during a fall in a person with a longer hip axis length. Villa et al. also demonstrated an association between shorter hip axis length and a lower incidence of hip fracture.[50]

Medication

Cummings et al. demonstrated an increased risk of hip fracture in women taking long-acting benzodiazepines, whose side effects include confusion, ataxia, dizziness, and impaired motor coordination.[43] According to Ray et al., one serious side effect of benzodiazepines is an increased risk of falling and fall-induced fractures.[51] Long-term use of anticonvulsants can induce production of hepatic enzymes and increase the metabolism of vitamin D_3, resulting in osteomalacia.[52] Use of corticosteroids has also been associated with reduction in bone density and has been identified as a risk factor for hip fracture.[53] Thyroxine, which increases the turnover rate of bone and may cause osteoporosis, has been associated with hip fracture.[52]

The use of antihypertensives, which have been shown to cause a higher frequency of fainting and dizziness in the elderly than in younger individuals, may increase the risk of hip fracture in this population.[54] Furthermore, in patients with medical conditions that compromise drug metabolism and clearance, antihypertensive agents and sedatives may accumulate and can compound preexisting motor dysfunction, which may result in a fall. Antipsychotic and antidepressant agents cause sedation and hypotension, thereby increasing the risk for hip fracture.

Bone Density and Body Habitus

Bone density exhibits a strong negative correlation with fracture risk; bone strength and density decrease with advancing age, resulting in an increased risk of fracture.[55,56] According to Cummings et al., hip fracture risk increases 2.4 to 3.0 times for each standard deviation reduction in bone mineral density.[55] Furthermore, physical activity also generally decreases with advancing age, which accelerates the rate of bone loss. Lack of physical activity could be a risk factor for hip fracture since it results in a lowered bone density, reduced muscle mass, and reduced muscle strength.

Height and body mass as risk factors for hip fracture have recently been the subject of several studies. Some have demonstrated a positive correlation between patient height and hip fracture.[43,57,58] In the event of a fall, taller stature results in a greater impact velocity and a corresponding increase in force at the site of impact. Hayes et al. calculated that an increase in fall height of 3.5 inches increases the odds of a hip fracture by almost 50%.[59] In a study of

50,000 American men, Hemenway et al. showed that men 6 ft or taller were more than twice as likely to sustain a hip fracture than those under 5 ft 9 in.[60] In a cohort study of 90,000 women, Hemenway et al. concluded that taller stature also increased the risk of hip fracture in women; women 5 ft 8 in or taller were more than twice as likely than women under 5 ft 2 in to sustain a hip fracture.[61] Height can also be used as an indirect measure of geometric features of the hip such as hip axis length and femoral neck length.

The body mass index is a ratio of weight in kilograms divided by height in meters. Low body mass index is positively correlated with low bone mass.[62] Similarly, several authors have shown that low body mass index (a reflection of amount of fat mass, lean mass, and body build) is a risk factor for both osteoporosis and hip fracture.[62,63] Meyer et al. reported that the increased incidence of hip fracture in Oslo, Norway, relative to neighboring European countries may be due to the population's taller stature and lean body stature as reflected in a reduced body mass index.[64] Maitland et al. established that reduced trochanteric soft tissue thickness is correlated with a low body mass index.[65] Leanness as reflected by a reduced body mass index may influence the risk of hip fracture by reducing the thickness of the soft protective subcutaneous tissue surrounding the hip.

Diet

There is good evidence that inadequate dietary calcium intake increases the risk of hip fracture. Matkovic et al., studying two regions of Yugoslavia that were ethnically, physically, and socially similar but whose populations consumed different levels of calcium, found that in the region with the high-calcium diet (which was also characterized by higher amounts of fat, protein, and phosphorus as well as higher caloric intake overall) the incidence of hip fracture was approximately half that in the region with the lower-calcium diet.[66] Holbrook et al., in a well-controlled prospective study, found that the age-adjusted risk of hip fracture was inversely associated with calcium intake, a relationship that persisted after adjustment for other possible covariants.[67]

The association between weight change and hip fracture risk was studied in 3683 community-dwelling white women age 67 years and older by Langlois et al.[68] Weight loss greater than 10% or more beginning at 50 years of age was associated with a significantly increased risk of hip fracture, greatest among women in the lowest and middle terciles of body mass index at age 50. Weight gain of 10% or more provided borderline protection.

At the extreme of dietary circumstances stands malnutrition, which is much more prevalent in the elderly than is commonly thought and appears to be a risk factor for hip fracture. Malnutrition magnifies the risk of hip fracture in several ways. To begin with, it results in impaired muscular coordination and reduced strength, both of which increase the likelihood of a fall.[69] Malnutrition can also result in a reduction in the thickness of subcutaneous tissue covering the hip area, thus reducing the force required to cause a hip fracture and increasing the likelihood that a fall will result in a hip fracture. Among the micronutrients that are negatively affected by malnutrition and that may play a role in affecting the risk for hip fracture is vitamin K, which plays a key role in bone formation and has been implicated in the modulation of the proliferation and function of osteoblast-like cells.

Smoking

The role of smoking as a risk factor for hip fracture is somewhat controversial. Several studies have identified smoking as a risk factor for hip fracture. Law and Hackshaw showed that long-term smokers had significantly reduced bone density compared with nonsmokers.[70] Their study estimated that the average bone density loss is 0.2% per year for postmenopausal women smokers; cumulative bone loss spanning several years increased the lifetime risk of hip fracture in women from 12% in nonsmokers to 19% in smokers. By age 90, this risk increased from 22% in nonsmokers to 37% in smokers. Other studies, however, have been unable to demonstrate that smoking is an independent risk factor for hip fracture. In a case-control study of hip fractures among the Japanese elderly, Suzuki et al. failed to identify smoking as a risk factor for hip fracture,[71] while in an evaluation of risk factors for hip fractures in white American women, Cummings et al., using multivariate analysis, showed that smoking was not a significant risk factor.[43]

Alcohol Consumption

Consumption of alcohol as a risk factor for hip fracture, as in the case of tobacco use, is somewhat controversial. Various studies have shown that alcohol consumption is not an independent risk factor. Grisso et al. reported that even heavy alcohol use (14 or more drinks per week) did not increase the risk for hip fracture among men.[72] Johnell et al. were also unable to demonstrate an association between overall alcohol consumption and increased incidence of hip fracture.[73] At the extreme, Suzuki et al. reported that moderate consumption of alcohol was associated with a significantly decreased risk of hip fracture.[71] Several authors nevertheless cite alcohol consumption as a risk factor for hip fracture. Fujiwara et al. showed that regular alcohol consumption nearly doubled the risk of hip fracture in his Japanese study population.[74] Heavy alcohol intake may lower bone mass and thus increase the risk of hip fracture. Felson et al. proposed that alcohol causes osteoporosis as a result of its toxicity to bone or by affecting bone cell metabolism or vitamin D levels.[75] Alcohol abuse may also increase the risk for hip fracture by compromising balance, impairing gait, increasing risk-taking behavior, and contributing to malnutrition.

Fluoridated Water

The effects of fluoridation of the public water supply on the incidence of hip fracture have been investigated, with conflicting results. In the past 50 years, many communities have fluoridated public drinking water supplies in an attempt to prevent tooth decay. Several studies have reported that fluoride affects bone mineralization and may influence the risk of fracture. Simonen et al. reported lower incidence of hip fracture in a Finnish city with a fluoridated water supply than in a city with low fluoride levels.[76] Other authors, however, have been able to detect neither a positive nor a negative effect of fluoridation on hip fracture risk.[77] Furthermore, several studies have reported an increased risk of hip fracture associated with fluoridation of the public water supply.[78]

Urban Versus Rural Residence

Several authors have reported a greater incidence of hip fracture in urban than in rural areas.[10,79] One possible explanation is that urban dwellers have lower bone mass and density due to a less active lifestyle. Swanson and Murdoch, on the other hand, reported hip fracture incidence to be 22% higher in the vicinity of rural Dundee (Scotland) than in urban Dundee itself,[80] and Luthje et al. reported no difference in incidence of hip fracture between urban and rural populations in Finland.[81]

Climate

There is extensive literature regarding the relationship between climate and hip fracture, with little consensus. Lizaur-Utrilla et al. and Gallagher et al. reported no seasonal variation in Alicante, Spain, and Minneapolis, respectively.[2,6] Several studies, however, both in the United States and abroad, have reported a seasonal variation in the incidence of hip fractures. Jacobsen et al. conducted the largest study, evaluating more than 600,000 hip fractures in the United States, and found a distinctive pattern of seasonal periodicity, with an increased incidence of hip fractures during the winter in both men and women across all age groups.[82] Similar seasonal trends have been reported in the United Kingdom,[69] Sweden,[83] Australia,[84] and Italy.[85] The purported explanation for this midwinter peak in hip fracture incidence is the increase in falls due to ice and snow conditions. Jacobsen et al., however, in a study of the influence of the weather on hip fracture occurrence during a 38-year period in Rochester, Minnesota, found that on days with snow or freezing rain, the risk of hip fracture was greater among women age 45 to 74 years than on other days, but neither greater nor less among women 75 years or older.[82] This lack of association between ice or snow and hip fracture in the elderly are supported by reports of increased risk of hip fracture during winter in the southern United States, where winters are typically mild and snow and ice are exceedingly rare. Several authors have postulated that seasonal differences in sunlight might be responsible for the seasonal variation in hip fracture incidence.[86-88] In the winter, there are fewer hours of sunlight and the sun is lower on the horizon, resulting in decreased visual acuity and an increased likelihood of a fall. Others investigators postulate that reduced exposure to sunlight leads to a decrease in active vitamin D synthesis and an increased incidence of osteomalacia.[89]

Lower winter temperatures have also been implicated in seasonal differences in hip fracture incidence. Collins et al. noted that a significant percentage of elderly people live in particularly cold indoor conditions, at temperatures well below the comfort zone of sedentary adults.[90] Additionally, an age-related decline in patient thermoregulatory capacity has been reported, with a state of transient hypothermia existing in the elderly during the winter.[90] As a result of this hypothermic state, coordination, judgment, and orthostasis may be impaired, leading to an increase in falls and fractures. This seasonal pattern of hip fracture incidence is quite complicated and is most likely multifactorial in nature, with decreased sunlight, hypothermia, malnutrition, and perhaps other factors all playing a role.

Osteopenia, Osteoporosis, and Osteomalacia

Osteopenia is a nonspecific decrease in bone density. Osteopenia has many different etiologies, including osteoporosis (a decrease in bone mineral density with normal bone mineralization) and osteomalacia (a decrease in bone matrix mineralization with or without a change in bone density).

Osteoporosis is divided into two types: type I or postmenopausal osteoporosis (natural or surgical), associated with decreased estrogen production, and type II or senile osteoporosis, which occurs as a result of decreased formation and increased resorption of bone mass. Type I is associated with vertebral body and distal radius fractures, whereas type II is associated with proximal femur and proximal humerus fractures.[91] Many contend that the decrease in bone mass beginning in early adulthood in both sexes is responsible, in part, for the increased incidence of hip fracture in the elderly.[18,92] Women achieve a lower peak bone mass and subsequently lose bone mass at a higher rate than men.[92] Nevertheless, although postmenopausal women are frequently osteoporotic, only 20% to 25% are prone to fracture.[93]

Other factors associated with osteoporosis may contribute to the incidence of hip fracture. These factors include a low percentage of body fat, low calcium intake, alcohol ingestion, smoking, and inactivity.[92] Various medical conditions (e.g., diabetes mellitus, hyperthyroidism, hyperparathyroidism, Cushing's disease, rheumatoid arthritis, postgastrectomy syndrome) and medications (especially corticosteroids) predispose to osteoporosis and may increase the incidence of hip fracture.

The presence of osteomalacia in hip fracture specimens has been confirmed histologically by several investigators, with reported rates as high as 20% to 30%.[94–96] Wilton et al., however, identified osteomalacia in only 2% of over 1000 iliac crest biopsies taken from elderly patients who sustained a femoral neck fracture.[97] Further studies are needed to define the importance of osteomalacia as a risk factor for hip fracture.

Epidemiology of Specific Fracture Types

The incidence of femoral neck and intertrochanteric fractures is gender and race dependent and varies from country to country. In the United States, the annual rate among elderly women of both femoral neck and intertrochanteric fractures is about 63 per 100,000; among men the rates are about 28 per 100,000 for femoral neck fractures and 34 per 100,000 for intertrochanteric fractures.[16] Baudoin et al. in a meta-analysis of 16 reports involving 36,451 hip fractures, reported that in women over age 60 years, the femoral neck/intertrochanteric fracture ratio decreased with age and reached unity in patients over age 90[98]; in men, this ratio hovered around unity and rose to 1.7 after age 90. In a review of 27,370 hip fracture patients age 65 years or older in Maryland, Hinton and Smith reported that the ratio of femoral neck to intertrochanteric fracture showed a statistically significant linear age-proportional decrease in both white and black women.[99] This ratio stayed at slightly less than 1.0 for white men and at slightly greater than 1.0 for black men.

Investigators have tried to identify patient characteristics that could be used to predict whether one might sustain a femoral neck or intertrochanteric fracture. Several studies have documented an increasing incidence of intertrochanteric fractures with advancing age.[5,6,100] Gallagher et al. reported an eightfold increase in intertrochanteric fracture incidence in males over 80 years of age and a fivefold increase in women this age.[6] In a series of 710 hip fractures, Alffram reported that the average age of female patients with intertrochanteric fractures was significantly higher than those with femoral neck fractures, although men exhibited no such significant difference.[5] Mannius et al. reported a similar association between patient age and fracture type in a series of 3030 hip fracture patients, with older female patients being significantly more likely to sustain an intertrochanteric fracture.[100] In an analysis of 20,538 hip fractures, however, Hedlund et al. found no effect of age on the likelihood of a patient of either sex sustaining a femoral neck or intertrochanteric hip fracture.[18] (The studies cited included all hip fracture patients, including those who were institutionalized, nonambulatory, or mentally incompetent.)

The relationship between health status—including number of comorbidities and activity level—and hip fracture type is similarly controversial. Lawton et al. reported that intertrochanteric hip fracture patients are biologically older than those who sustain a femoral neck fracture[101]; they had lower hemoglobin levels at hospital admission, poorer prefracture ambulatory ability, and a higher number of associated medical conditions that altered fracture management. Similarly, Jarnlo and Thorngren reported that patients who sustained an intertrochanteric fracture seemed to be less active than patients who had a femoral neck fracture[102]; men with intertrochanteric fractures had visited the doctor more frequently and had consumed more hospital care during the year prior to fracture. Sernbo and Johnell found that women who sustained an intertrochanteric hip fracture were significantly more likely to have required a prefracture walking aid and to have been dependent in activities of daily living[103]; these relationships, however, were not statistically significant when controlling for age. In a series of 216 hip fracture patients, Dias et al. reported no significant differences in prefracture patient mobility, medication use, or associated comorbidities in patients who sustained a femoral neck or an intertrochanteric fracture.[104] The series reported by Lawton et al. and Dias et al. were nonexclusionary and considered the total hip fracture population; Sernbo and Johnell excluded patients with pathologic hip fractures, while Jarnlo and Thorngren excluded patients with pathologic fractures as well as those admitted from psychiatric hospitals.

There appears to be an association between prior vertebral, proximal humerus, or distal radius fracture and type of hip fracture. Gallagher et al. reported a significantly higher prevalence of prior vertebral fractures in patients who sustained an intertrochanteric fracture than in those who sustained a femoral neck fracture.[6] Sernbo and Johnell, in an age-matched study, reported that patients who sustained an intertrochanteric fracture were more likely to have previously sustained other osteoporosis-related ("fragility") fractures, such as a vertebral compression, proximal humerus, or distal radius fracture.[103] Furthermore, a previous contralateral femoral neck or intertrochanteric fracture has been shown to be predictive of sustaining a similar type of hip fracture. Boston noted that patients sustaining a second contralateral hip fracture had an 83% chance of having the same type of fracture.[105]

Degree of osteoporosis may influence fracture type. Aitken reported that intertrochanteric fractures were more common in severely osteoporotic women, whereas femoral neck fractures predominated in those who were not osteoporotic.[106] Using a diagnosis based on lateral radiographs of the spine, Pogrund et al. reported that osteoporotic female patients who fractured their proximal femur as a result of a fall were more likely to sustain an intertrochanteric fracture than a femoral neck fracture.[107] Using measurements obtained by single-photon absorptiometry, Eriksson and Wilde reported that women who sustained an intertrochanteric fracture had lower bone mineral density in the femoral neck and intertrochanteric region than those who had a femoral neck fracture[108]; furthermore, bone mineral distribution was essentially the same in women who sustained a femoral neck fracture and a control group of healthy women. Advancing patient age is associated with progression of osteoporosis, particularly in women; decreased patient activity level also results in lower bone mass. These factors may explain the association found between older age, home ambulatory ability, dependency in activities of daily living, and intertrochanteric hip fracture.

Osteoarthritis is "protective" against femoral neck fracture. Patients with osteoarthritis of the hip have sclerosis of the femoral head associated with the formation of osteophytes that afford the femoral neck substantial protection in this regard; these patients are more likely to sustain an intertrochanteric or subtrochanteric fracture.

We reported on a prospective series of 680 elderly hip fracture patients treated at the Hospital for Joint Diseases to compare the demographic profile of patients who sustained a femoral neck fracture with that of patients who had an intertrochanteric fracture.[109] All patients were community-dwelling, cognitively intact, previously ambulatory elderly persons with a diagnosis of femoral neck or intertrochanteric fracture. Three hundred fifty-eight patients (52.6%) sustained a femoral neck fracture and 322 patients (47.4%) an intertrochanteric fracture. Patients who sustained an intertrochanteric fracture were significantly older, more likely to be limited to home ambulation, and more dependent in basic and instrumental activities of daily living. After stratifying by sex and adjusting for age, these differences remained significant in women only. There were no differences in age, prefracture ambulatory ability, or dependence in activities of daily living in men who sustained either fracture type.

Mechanism of Injury

Most hip fractures occur at home. A prospective analysis involving 832 patients was performed at the Hospital for Joint Diseases to determine the circumstances surrounding the falls leading to hip fracture in a homogenous elderly urban population.[110] All patients were community-dwelling, cognitively intact, previously ambulatory elderly persons who had sustained a femoral neck or intertrochanteric fracture. Most of these hip fractures occurred at home, particularly in patients age 85 and older. More than 75% of fractures resulted from a fall while the patient was walking or standing. Most falls occurred during daylight hours, with a peak noted in the afternoon. No seasonal variation in the incidence of hip fractures was observed.

According to the literature, 90% of hip fractures in the elderly result from a fall. On the basis of interviews with women who sustained a fracture of the hip, Nevitt and Cummings reported that 92% of the women attributed their fracture to a fall.[111] In a more recent study, Cumming found that 89% of patients who fractured their hip reported a fall as the cause of fracture.[112] Another study found that among 260 patients who sustained a hip fracture, 96% of fractures were due to falls that resulted in direct impact on the hip.[113]

The tendency to fall increases with patient age and is dependent on many factors, including poor vision, decreased muscle power, labile blood pressure, decreased reflexes, vascular disease, and coexisting musculoskeletal abnormality. Based on laboratory research, falls from a standing height in a typical elderly individual generate at least 16 times the energy necessary to fracture the proximal femur.[114] Although these data suggest that such falls should cause fracture almost every time they occur, only 5% to 10% of falls in older white women result in a fracture and fewer than 2% in a hip fracture.[115] The fact that the overwhelming majority of falls do not result in a hip fracture implies that the mechanics of the fall are important in determining whether a fracture will occur.

Cummings hypothesized that four factors are important in determining whether a particular fall will result in a fracture of the hip[115]: (1) the fall must be oriented so the person lands on or near the hip; (2) protective reflexes must be inadequate to reduce the energy of the fall below the critical threshold; (3) local shock absorbers such as muscle and fat around the hip must be inadequate; and (4) bone strength at the hip must be insufficient.

One must land on or near the hip for the energy of the fall to be transmitted to the proximal femur; falling onto the lateral thigh or buttock near the greater trochanter is much more likely to cause hip fracture than an impact elsewhere.[59] Such falls are also much more likely when there is little or no forward momentum, as when the person is standing still or walking slowly—another factor that helps explain why the elderly sustain a greater proportion of fractures in these incidents. Furthermore, because their reaction times are longer and muscle strength less, the older person's protective responses tend to be too little and too late.

Skin, fat, and muscles surrounding the hip can absorb large amounts of energy from an impact. The abductors of the hip are the largest muscle group attached to the proximal femur; the age-related decline in muscle mass around the hip may account for some of the increased incidence of hip fractures with aging.[116] Lauritzen and Askegaard reported that women who had sustained a hip fracture had on average 22 mm of soft tissue coverage over the trochanter area compared with 32 mm in healthy women with the same body mass index.[117] The same study found that when a weight was dropped from various heights onto porcine soft tissue, a layer of 29 mm could absorb 60% more energy than a 20-mm-thick layer.

Although the muscles surrounding the hip may serve a protective function, contraction of these muscles during a fall may actually lead to increased rates of hip fracture. In a laboratory study, Hayes et al. found that muscle-relaxed falls resulted in a significant (7%) decrease in hip impact velocity compared with muscle-active falls.[118] Their study also found that muscle activation caused a 100% increase in predicted average peak force of the fall. These findings reflect two phenomena that arise from contraction of the trunk muscles at impact: (1) increased effective mass as more of the trunk and lower extremities participate in the impact; (2) increased rigidity of the muscular connection between the trunk, pelvis, and lower limbs, which increases the risk of fracture.

Cyclic mechanical stresses can also result in a hip fracture; such a fracture (stress fracture) that occurs in normal bone in a healthy young or middle-aged individual secondary to repetitive mechanical stress is defined as a fatigue fracture; repetitive loading results in a decrease in the bone's failure strength. In elderly persons, whose bone fatigue strength has been lowered secondary to osteoporosis, osteomalacia or other diseases states, lower loads (e.g., normal activities) or fewer loading cycles can result in osseous failure. This type of stress fracture is considered to be an insufficiency fracture.

Stress fractures involving the hip region result from alterations of the normal stress and strain patterns of the proximal femur secondary to either increased mechanical loads or muscle fatigue. The level and distribution of stress and strain in the femoral neck is controlled both by gravitational and muscle forces.[119] If gravitational forces are increased, such as with use of a knapsack, the tensile stress in the femoral neck will increase. If the abductor muscles fatigue and are unable to provide normal tension, the tensile stress in the femoral neck will also increase. Muscle fatigue secondary to repetitive exercise can decrease its shock-absorbing capacity so that higher peak stresses and strains occur in the femoral neck. Muscle fatigue also results in gait alterations that affect the position of the body's center of mass and alter the stress and strain patterns within the femoral neck.

Fractures caused by intrinsic factors such as muscle contraction or cyclic mechanical stresses and not preceded by a fall tend to be predominantly femoral neck fractures. Sloan and Holloway found that 25% of the patients they studied attributed their falls to their hip having given way, and 67% of this group gave a clear history of hip pain that preceded the fall.[120] These authors proposed that a fatigue fracture became displaced in this group of patients and ultimately led to the fall; 77% in this group sustained a femoral neck fracture. By contrast, among the 29 patients who directly attributed their hip fracture to a fall, only 41% sustained a femoral neck fracture.

In conclusion, fractures of the proximal femur can result from either external trauma, intrinsic factors (i.e., muscle contraction), or cyclic mechanical stress. External trauma, as typified by the fall, should not be considered the sole cause of hip fracture. Although a fall undoubtedly causes fracture of the proximal femur in a significant proportion of cases, the traditional order of events in the pathogenesis of hip fractures may be reversed (fracture precedes the fall) in a much greater frequency than was previously realized.

References

1. Soloman L. Osteoporosis and fracture of the femoral neck in South African Bantu. *J Bone Joint Surg Br* 1968; 50:2–13.
2. Lizaur-Utrilla A, Orts AP, Del Campo FS, et al. Epidemiology of trochanteric fractures of the femur in Alicante, Spain 1974–1982. *Clin Orthop* 1987; 218:24–31.
3. Chalmers J, Ho KC. Geographical variations in senile osteoporosis. *J Bone Joint Surg Br* 1970; 52:667–675.
4. Knowelden J, Buhr AJ, Dunbar O. Incidence of fractures in persons over 35 years of age. *Br J Prev Soc Med* 1964; 18:130–141.
5. Alffram PA. An epidemiologic study of cervical and trochanteric fractures of the femur in an urban population: Analysis of 1,664 cases with special reference to etiologic factors. *Acta Orthop Scand* 1964; 65:9–109.
6. Gallagher JC, Melton LJ, Riggs BL, Bergtrath E. Epidemiology of fractures of the proximal femur in Rochester, Minnesota. *Clin Orthop* 1980; 150:163–171.
7. Lau E, Donnan D, Barker D, Cooper C. Physical activity and calcium intake in fractures of the proximal femur in Hong Kong. *BMJ* 1988; 296:1441–1443.
8. Orimo H. Epidemiology of fractures in Asia. In: Christiansen C, Overgaard K, eds. *Proceedings of the Third International Symposium on Osteoporosis*. Copenhagen: Osteopress, 1990:66–70.
9. Parkkari J, Kannus P, Niemi S, et al. Increasing age adjusted incidence of hip fracture in Finland: the number and incidence of fractures in 1970–1991 and predictions for the future. *Calcif Tissue Int* 1994; 55:342–345.

10. Larsson S, Elrasson P, Hansson L. Hip fractures in Northern Sweden 1973–1984: a comparison of rural and urban populations. *Acta Orthop Scand* 1989; 60:567–571.
11. Cummings SR, Rubin SM, Black D. The future of hip fractures in the Untied States: numbers, costs, and potential effects of postmenopausal estrogen. *Clin Orthop* 1990; 252:163–166.
12. Zein Elabdien B, Olerud S, Karlstrom G, Smedby B. Rising incidence of hip fracture in Uppsala 1965–1980. *Acta Orthop Scand* 1984; 55:284–289.
13. Gerhart T. Managing and preventing hip fractures in the elderly. *Journal of Musculoskeletal Medicine* 1987; 4:60–68.
14. Luthje P. Incidence of hip fracture in Finland: A forecast for 1990. *Acta Orthop Scand* 1985; 56:223–225.
15. Gullberg B, Johnell O, Kanis J. Worldwide projection for hip fracture. *Osteoporos Int* 1997; 7:407–413.
16. Melton JL, Ilstrup DM, Riggs BL, Beckenbaugh RD. Fifty year trend in hip fracture incidence. *Clin Orthop* 1982; 162:144–149.
17. Swiontkowski MF. Intracapsular hip fractures. In: Browner BD, Levine AM, Jupiter JB, Trafton PG, eds. *Skeletal Trauma,* Vol 2. Philadelphia: WB Saunders, 1992:1751–1832.
18. Hedlund R, Lindgren U, Ahlbom A. Age- and sex- specific incidence of femoral neck and trochanteric fractures: an analysis based on 20,538 fractures in Stockholm County, Sweden 1972–1981. *Clin Orthop* 1987; 222:132–139.
19. Lauritzen J, Schwarz P, Lund B, et al. Changing incidence and residual incidence and residual lifetime risk of common osteoporosis-related fractures. *Osteoporos Int* 1993; 3:127–132.
20. Cooper C, Campion G, Melton LJ. Hip fractures in the elderly: a worldwide projection. *Osteoporos Int* 1992; 2:285–289.
21. Farmer ME, White L, Brody JA, Bailey K. Race and sex differences in hip fracture incidence. *Am J Public Health* 1984; 74:1374–1380.
22. Wong PCN. Fracture epidemiology in a mixed southeastern Asian community (Singapore). *Clin Orthop* 1966; 45:55–61.
23. Melton LJ. Hip fractures: a worldwide problem today and tomorrow. *Bone* 1993; 14:S1–S8.
24. Kellie S, Brody J. Sex specific and race specific hip fracture rates. *Am J Public Health* 1990; 80:326–328.
25. Cummings S, Black D, Rubin S. Lifetime risk of hip, Colles' or vertebral fracture and coronary artery disease among white postmenopausal women. *Arch Intern Med* 1989; 149:2445–2448.
26. Trotter M, Broman GE, Peterson RR. Densities of bones of white and Negro skeletons. *J Bone Joint Surg Am* 1960; 42:50–58.
27. Tinetti M, Speechley M, Ginter S. Risk factors for falls among elderly persons living in the community. *N Engl J Med* 1988; 319:1701–1707.
28. Bauer RL. Ethnic differences in hip fracture: a reduced incidence in Mexican Americans. *Am J Epidemiol* 1988; 127:145–149.
29. Silverman S, Madison R. Decreased incidence of hip fracture in Hispanics, Asians, and Blacks: California hospital discharge data. *Am J Public Health* 1988; 78:1482–1483.
30. Ross P, Norimatsu H, Davis J, et al. A comparison of hip fracture incidence among native Japanese, Japanese Americans, and American Caucasians. *Am J Epidemiol* 1991; 133:801–809.
31. Kin K, Kushida K, Yamazaki K, et al. Bone mineral density of the spine in normal Japanese subjects using dual-energy x-ray absorptiometry: effect of obesity and menopausal status. *Calcif Tissue Int* 1991; 49:101–106.
32. Ooms M, Vlasman P, Lip P, et al. The incidence of hip fracture in independent and institutionalized elderly people. *Osteoporos Int* 1994; 4:6–10.
33. Rudman I, Rudman D. High rate of fractures for men in nursing homes. *Am J Phys Med Rehab* 1989; 68:2–5.
34. Vieweg V, Lewis R, Dam T, et al. Dementia and other risk factors for hip fractures in a state-operated geopsychiatric hospital. *Va Med Q* 1993; Fall:210–213.
35. Cumming RG. Nursing home residence and risk of hip fracture. *Am J Epidemiol* 1996; 143:1191–1194.
36. Kelsey JL, Hoffman S. Risk factors for hip fracture. *N Engl J Med* 1987; 316:404–406.
37. Grisso JA, Kelsey JL, Strom BL, et al. Risk factors for hip fractures in black women. *N Engl J Med* 1994; 330:1555–1559.

References

38. Grisso JA, Kelsey JL, Strom BL, et al. Risk factors for falls as a cause of hip fracture in women. *N Engl J Med* 1991; 324:1326–1331.
39. Johnell O, Sernbo I. Health and social status in patients with hip fractures and controls. *Age Ageing* 1986; 15:285–291.
40. Kreiger N, Kelsey JL, Holford TR, O'Connor T. An epidemiologic study of hip fracture in post menopausal women. *Am J Epidemiol* 1982; 116:141–148.
41. Buchner DM, Larson EB. Falls and fractures in patients with Alzheimer-type dementia. *JAMA* 1987; 257:1492–1495.
42. Felson D, Anderson J, Hannan M, et al. Impaired vision and hip fractures: the Framingham study. *J Am Geriatr Soc* 1989; 37:495–500.
43. Cummings S, Nevitt M, Browner W, et al. Risk factors for hip fracture in white women. Study of Osteoporotic Fractures Research Group. *N Engl J Med* 1995; 332:767–773.
44. Melton LJ, Ilstrup MS, Beckenbaugh RD, Riggs BL. Hip fracture recurrence. A population-based study. *Clin Orthop* 1982; 167:131–138.
45. Arden N, Baker J, Hogg C, Baan K, Spector T. The heritability of bone mineral density, ultrasound of the calcaneus and hip axis length: a study of postmenopausal twins. *J Bone Miner Res* 1996; 11:530–534.
46. Slemenda C, Turner C, Peacock M. The genetics of proximal femur geometry, distribution of bone mass and bone mineral density. *Osteoporos Int* 1996; 6:178–182.
47. Faulkner KG, Cummings SR, Black D, et al. Simple measurement of femoral geometry predicts hip fracture: the study of osteoporotic fractures. *J Bone Miner Res* 1993; 8:1211–1217.
48. Nakamura T, Turner CH, Yoshikawa T, et al. Do variations in hip geometry explain differences in hip fracture risk between Japanese and white Americans? *J Bone Miner Res* 1994; 9:1071–1076.
49. Cummings S, Cauley J, Palermo L, et al. Racial differences in hip axis length might explain racial differences in rates of hip fracture. *Osteoporos Int* 1994; 4:226–229.
50. Villa M, Marcus R, Delay R, Kelsey J. Factors contributing to skeletal health of postmenopausal Mexican-American women. *J Bone Miner Res* 1995; 10:1233–1242.
51. Ray WA, Griffin MR, Downey W. Benzodiazepines of long and short elimination half-life and the risk of hip fracture. *JAMA* 1989; 262:3303–3307.
52. Muckle D. Iatrogenic factors in femoral neck fracture. *Injury* 1977; 8:98–101.
53. Cooper C, Coupland C, Mitchell M. Rheumatoid arthritis, corticosteroid therapy and hip fracture. *Ann Rheum Dis* 1995; 54:49–52.
54. Hale W, Steward R, Marks R. Central nervous system symptoms of elderly subjects using anti-hypertensive drugs. *J Am Geriatr Soc* 1984; 32:5–10.
55. Cummings S, Black D, Nevitt M. Bone density at various sites for prediction of hip fracture. *Lancet* 1993; 341:72–75.
56. Lips P. Vitamin D deficiency and osteoporosis: the role of vitamin D deficiency and treatment with vitamin D and analogues in the prevention of osteoporosis related fractures. *Eur J Clin Invest* 1996; 26:436–442.
57. Meyer H, Tverdal A, Falch J. Risk factors for hip fracture in middle-aged Norwegian women and men. *Am J Epidemiol* 1993; 137:1203–1211.
58. Ribot C, Tremollieres F, Pouilles J, et al. Risk factors for hip fracture. MEDOS study: results of the Toulouse Center. *Bone* 1993; 14:S77–S80.
59. Hayes WC, Meyers ER, Morris JN, et al. Impact near the hip dominates fracture risk in elderly nursing home residents who fall. *Calcif Tissue Int* 1993; 52:192–198.
60. Hemenway D, Azrael D, Rimm E, et al. Risk factors for hip fracture in US men aged 40 through 75 years. *Am J Public Health* 1994; 84:1843–1845.
61. Hemenway D, Feskanich D, Colditz G. Body height and hip fracture: a cohort study of 90,000 women. *Int J Epidemiol* 1995; 24:783–786.
62. Edelstein S, Barret-Connor E. Relation between body size and bone mineral density in elderly men and women. *Am J Epidemiol* 1993; 138:160–169.
63. Farmer M, Harris T, Madans J, et al. Anthropometric indicators and hip fracture. The NHANES I epidemiologic follow-up study. *J Am Geriatr Soc* 1989; 37:9–16.
64. Meyer H, Falch J, O'Neill T, et al. Height and body mass index in Oslo, Norway compared to other regions in Europe: do they explain differences in the incidence of hip fracture? *Bone* 1995; 17:347–350.
65. Maitland L, Myers E, Hipp J, et al. Ready my hips: measuring trochanteric soft tissue thickness. *Calcif Tissue Int* 1993; 52:85–89.
66. Matkovic V, Kostiac K, Simonvic I, et al. Bone status and fracture rates in two regions in Yugoslavia. *Am J Clin Nutr* 1979; 32:540–549.

67. Holbrook T, Barrett-Connor E, Wingard DL. Dietary calcium and risk of hip fracture: fourteen-year prospective population study. *Lancet* 1988; 2:1046–1049.
68. Langlois JA, Harris T, Looker AC, Madans J. Weight change between age 50 years and old age is associated with risk of hip fracture in white women aged 67 and older. *Arch Intern Med* 1996; 156:989–994.
69. Bastow MD, Rawlings J, Allison SP. Undernutrition, hypothermia, and injury in elderly women with fractured femur: an injury response to altered metabolism? *Lancet* 1983; 1:143–146.
70. Law M, Hackshaw A. A meta-analysis of cigarette smoking, bone mineral density and risk of hip fracture: recognition of a major effect. *BMJ* 1997; 315:841–846.
71. Suzuki T, Yoshida H, Hashimoto T, et al. Case-control study of risk factors for hip fractures in the Japanese elderly by a Mediterranean osteoporosis study (MEDOS) questionnaire. *Bone* 1997; 21:461–467.
72. Grisso J, Kelsey J, O'Brien L, et al. Risk factors for hip fracture in men. *Am J Epidemiol* 1997; 145:786–793.
73. Johnell O, Gullberg B, Kanis J, et al. Risk factors for hip fracture in European women: the MEDOS study. *J Bone Miner Res* 1995; 10:1802–1815.
74. Fujiwara S, Kasagi F, Yamada M, Kodama K. Risk factors for hip fracture in a Japanese cohort. *J Bone Miner Res* 1997; 12:998–1004.
75. Felson DT, Kiel DP, Anderson JJ, Kannel WB. Alcohol consumption and hip fractures: the Framingham study. *Am J Epidemiol* 1988; 128:1102–1110.
76. Simonen O, Laitinen O. Does fluoridation of drinking water prevent bone fragility and osteoporosis? *Lancet* 1985; 2:432–434.
77. Jacobsen S, O'Fallon W, Melton LI. Hip fracture incidence before and after fluoridation of the public water supply, Rochester, Minnesota. *Am J Public Health* 1993; 83:743–745.
78. Sowers M, Wallace R, Lemke J. The relationship of bone mass and fracture history to fluoride and calcium intake: a study of three communities. *Am J Clin Nutr* 1986; 44:889–898.
79. Finsen V, Benum P. Changing incidence of hip fractures in rural and urban areas of central Norway. *Clin Orthop* 1987; 218:104–110.
80. Swanson A, Murdoch G. Fractured neck of femur. Pattern of incidence and implications. *Acta Orthop Scand* 1983; 54:348–355.
81. Luthje P, Peltonen A, Nurmi I, et al. No difference in the incidence of old people's hip fractures between urban and rural populations—a comparative study in two Finnish health care regions in 1989. *Gerontology* 1995; 41:39–44.
82. Jacobsen SJ, Sargent DJ, Atkinson EJ, et al. Population-based study of the contribution of the contribution of weather to hip fracture seasonality. *Am J Epidemiol* 1995; 141:79–83.
83. Zetterberg C, Elmersson S, Andersson GB. Epidemiology of hip fractures in Goteborg, Sweden 1940–1983. *Clin Orthop* 1984; 191:43–52.
84. Lau EMC, Gillespie BG, Valenti L, O'Conell D. The seasonality of hip fracture and its relationship with weather conditions in New South Wales. *Australian Journal of Public Health* 1995; 19:76–80.
85. Caniggia M, Morreale P. Epidemiology of hip fractures in Sienna, Italy 1975–1985. *Clin Orthop* 1989; 238:131–138.
86. Jacobsen SJ, Goldberg J, Miles TP, et al. Seasonal variation in the incidence of hip fracture among white persons aged 65 years and older in the United States 1984–1987. *Am J Epidemiol* 1991; 133:996–1004.
87. Holmberg S, Thorngren KG. Statistical analysis of femoral neck fractures based on 3053 cases. *Clin Orthop* 1987; 218:32–41.
88. Campbell AJ, Spears GFS, Borrie MJ, Fitzgerald JL. Falls, elderly women and the cold. *Gerontology* 1988; 34:205–208.
89. Lund B, Sorensen OH, Christensen AB. 25-Hydroxycholecalciferol and fractures of the proximal femur. *Lancet* 1975; 2:300–302.
90. Collins KJ, Easton JC, Belfield-Smith H, et al. Effects of age on body temperature and blood pressure in cold environments. *Clin Sci* 1985; 69:465–470.
91. Riggs BL, Melton LJ. Evidence for two distinct syndromes of involutional osteoporosis. *Am J Med* 1983; 75:891–899.
92. Cummings SR, Kelsey JL, Nevitt MC, O'Dowd KJ. Epidemiology of osteoporosis and osteoporotic fractures. *Epidemiol Rev* 1985; 7:178–208.
93. Hofeldt F. Proximal femoral fractures. *Clin Orthop* 1987; 218:12–18.
94. Aaron JE, Gallagher JC, Anderson J, et al. Frequency of osteomalacia and osteoporosis in fractures of the proximal femur. *Lancet* 1974; 1:229–233.

References

95. Hoikka V, Alhava EM, Savolainen K, Parviainen M. Osteomalacia in fractures of the proximal femur. *Acta Orthop Scand* 1982; 53:255–260.
96. Lund B, Sorensen OH, Melsen F, Mosekilde L. Vitamin D metabolism and osteomalacia in patients with fractures of the proximal femur. *Acta Orthop Scand* 1982; 53:251–254.
97. Wilton TJ, Hosking DJ, Pawley E, et al. Osteomalacia and femoral neck fractures: prevalence and a method of screening. *J Bone Joint Surg Br* 1988; 70:677.
98. Baudoin C, Fardellone P, Sebert JL. Effects of sex and age on the ratio of cervical to trochanteric hip fracture. *Acta Orthop Scand* 1993; 64:647–653.
99. Hinton RY, Smith GS. The association of age, race, and sex with the location of proximal femoral fractures in the elderly. *J Bone Joint Surg Am* 1993; 75:752–759.
100. Mannius S, Mellstrom D, Oden A, et al. Incidence of hip fracture in Western Sweden 1974–1982. Comparison of rural and urban populations. *Acta Orthop Scand* 1987; 58:38–42.
101. Lawton JO, Baker MR, Dickson RA. Femoral neck fractures: two populations. *Lancet* 1983; 2:70–72.
102. Jarnlo GB, Thorngren KG. Background factors to hip fractures. *Clin Orthop* 1993; 287:41–49.
103. Sernbo I, Johnell O. Background factors in patients with hip fractures—differences between cervical and trochanteric fractures. *Compr Gerontol A* 1987; 1:109–111.
104. Dias JJ, Robbins JA, Steingold RF, Donaldson LJ. Subcapital vs intertrochanteric fracture of the neck of the femur: are there two distinct subpopulations? *J R Coll Surg Edinb* 1987; 32:303–305.
105. Boston DA. Bilateral fractures of the femoral neck. *Injury* 1982; 14:207–210.
106. Aitken JM. Relevance of osteoporosis in women with fractures of the femoral neck. *BMJ* 1984; 288:597–601.
107. Pogrund H, Makin M, Robin G, et al. Osteoporosis in patients with fractured femoral neck in Jerusalem. *Clin Orthop* 1977; 124:165–172.
108. Eriksson SAV, Wilde TL. Bone mass in women with hip fracture. *Acta Orthop Scand* 1988; 59:19–23.
109. Koval KJ, Aharonoff GB, Rokito AS, et al. Patients with femoral neck and intertrochanteric fractures. Are they the same? *Clin Orthop* 1996; 330:166–172.
110. Aharonoff GB, Dennis MG, Elshinawy A, et al. Circumstances of falls causing hip fractures in the elderly. *Clin Orthop* 1998; 348:10–14.
111. Nevitt MC, Cummings SR. Falls and fractures in older women. In: Vellas B, Toupet M, Rubenstein L, eds. *Falls, Balance and Gait Disorders in the Elderly*. Paris: Elsevier, 1992:69–80.
112. Cumming RG, Klineberg RJ. Fall frequency and characteristics and the risk of hip fractures. *J Am Geriatr Soc* 1994; 42:774–778.
113. Goh JC, Bose K, Das DS. Pattern of fall and bone mineral density measurement in hip fractures. *Ann Acad Med Singapore* 1996; 25:820–823.
114. Hayes WC. Biomechanics of falls and hip fracture in the elderly. In: Apple DF, Hayes WC, eds. *Prevention of Falls and Hip Fractures in the Elderly*. Rosemont, IL: American Academy of Orthopaedic Surgeons, 1994:41–65.
115. Cummings SR, Nevitt MC. Non-skeletal determinants of fractures: the potential importance of the mechanics of falls. *Osteoporos Int* 1994; 4 (suppl 1):67–70.
116. Cummings SR, Nevitt MC. A hypothesis: the causes of hip fractures. *J Gerontol* 1989; 44:107–111.
117. Lauritzen JB, Askegaard V. Protection against hip fractures by energy absorption. *Dan Med Bull* 1992; 39:91–93.
118. Hayes WB, Myers ER, Robinovitch SN. Etiology and prevention of age-related hip fractures. *Bone* 1996; 18 (1 suppl):77S–86S.
119. Egol K, Koval K, Kummer F, Frankel V. Stress fractures of the femoral neck. *Clin Orthop* 1998; 348:72–78.
120. Sloan J, Holloway G. Fractured neck of the femur: the cause of the fall? *Injury* 1981; 13:230–233.

Chapter Three

Diagnosis

The clinical presentation of patients who have sustained a fracture of the proximal femur can vary widely depending on the type, severity, and cause of the fracture. Displaced fractures are clearly symptomatic; such patients usually cannot stand, much less ambulate. On the other hand, there are patients with nondisplaced or impacted fractures who may be ambulatory and experience minimal pain, as well as cases in which patients complain of thigh or groin pain but have no history of antecedent trauma. In each situation, it is incumbent on the clinician to exclude the possibility of hip fracture in any individual who complains of thigh or groin pain.

History

History of Accident

As with all fractures, it is important to determine the mechanism of injury whenever possible. Most hip fractures in elderly persons are the result of a low-energy fall, whereas in young adults they are more often caused by high-energy trauma—for example, a motor vehicle accident. In the latter, one must assess for associated head, neck, chest, and abdominal injuries. Patients with a stress fracture of the proximal femur, although they usually deny specific trauma, should be questioned about any recent changes in the type, duration, or frequency of physical activity. In patients in whom trauma can reasonably be ruled out (e.g., sedentary individuals with no history of injury), pathologic fracture must be considered.

It is also important to determine, whenever possible, the timing of the injury. In elderly individuals who live alone, hospital presentation may be delayed for hours or even days, by which time the patients are often dehydrated and confused. In these patients, it may be difficult to determine the exact day or time when the fracture occurred. In addition, the potential for dehydration makes it imperative to evaluate the fluid and electrolyte status of these patients.

Previous Medical History

It is important to obtain a careful medical history, as preexisting medical co-morbidities affect both treatment and prognosis. Cardiopulmonary disease

Table 3.1. American Society of Anesthesiologists (ASA) rating of operative risk

Class	Physical status
I	Normal, healthy
II	Mild systemic disease
III	Severe systemic disease, not incapacitating
IV	Severe incapacitating systemic disease constituting a constant threat to life
V	Moribund

Reprinted with permission from American Society of Anesthesiologists. New classification of physical status. *Anesthesiology* 1963; 24:111.

(congestive heart failure, intermittent myocardial ischemia, chronic obstructive pulmonary disease) is a common preexisting medical condition that affects fracture management in the elderly. In this population, the disease affects the patient's ability to tolerate prolonged recumbency, undergo surgery, and participate in rehabilitation; it is also a major determinant of the rating system used by the American Society of Anesthesiologists (ASA) to assess operative risk[1] (Table 3.1). Injuries resulting from a fall in such patients may cause further deterioration of already compromised cardiopulmonary function.

Neurological conditions such as parkinsonism, Alzheimer's disease, and the residual effects of a previous cerebrovascular event must also be considered during treatment. Clinical manifestations in patients with parkinsonism range from mild tremors to complete incapacitation with severe contractures; well-controlled disease generally will not affect treatment decisions. Patients who have had a prior stroke are at increased risk for fracture secondary to residual balance and gait problems as well as osteopenia of the paretic limb.[2,3] Treatment of these patients may be complicated by the presence of osteopenia, spasticity, and/or contracture. The degree of involvement, as in parkinsonism, ranges from minimal to severe spasticity with contracture. For patients with Alzheimer's disease and severe cognitive dysfunction, a treatment plan requiring a high degree of patient cooperation would be inappropriate.

Medication History

Because the elderly, on average, utilize more medication than people in younger age groups, a thorough medication history is particularly important. It is not uncommon for a patient to use 10 or more different medications per day. Polypharmacy can cause serious consequences in the elderly, since they are more sensitive to drug interactions, adverse reactions, and side effects.[4] A thorough medication inventory is thus a necessary component of a comprehensive assessment of a patient who has experienced a fall. Medications most often associated with falls include antihypertensives, antidepressants, diuretics, hypnotics, narcotics, sedatives, and hypoglycemics.[4] Adverse and enhanced effects of drugs that are associated with falls include sedation, hypotension, confusion, poor coordination, respiratory depression, and increased urinary frequency.[4]

Functional Ability

To establish a reasonable management plan, one must obtain a detailed history of the patient's preinjury function. The treatment goals for an active, independent ambulator with a femoral neck fracture differ from those for an institutionalized nonambulator. The former requires surgical treatment followed by aggressive rehabilitation; the latter patient should probably be treated nonoperatively with early bed-to-wheelchair mobilization. In both cases, return to preinjury function will have been achieved utilizing radically different approaches.

Ambulatory status is best defined as one of four types:[5] (1) a *community ambulator* who walks indoors and outdoors; (2) a *household ambulator* who walks only indoors; (3) a *nonfunctional ambulator* who walks only during physical therapy sessions; and (4) a *nonambulator* who is wheelchair bound but may be able to transfer from bed to chair. The patient's living status (community or institutionalized) and social support network (living alone or with another person) both affect the patient's disposition status after hospital discharge and should be assessed during the initial evaluation.

Examination

Physical Examination

The amount of clinical deformity in patients with a proximal femur fracture reflects the degree of fracture displacement. Patients with a nondisplaced fracture may present with a virtual absence of clinical deformity, whereas those who sustain a displaced fracture exhibit the classic presentation of a shortened and externally rotated extremity (Figure 3.1). There may be tenderness to palpation in the area of the greater trochanter. Ecchymosis may be present and should be noted. Range-of-motion testing of the hip will be painful and should be avoided. Although neurovascular injury is rare after hip fracture, careful evaluation is nevertheless mandatory. Preexisting peripheral vascular disease or peripheral neuropathy mandate careful skin monitoring and avoidance of excessive pressure during reduction maneuvers. Evidence of preexisting sacral or heel decubitus ulcers should be noted and appropriate treatment measures instituted.

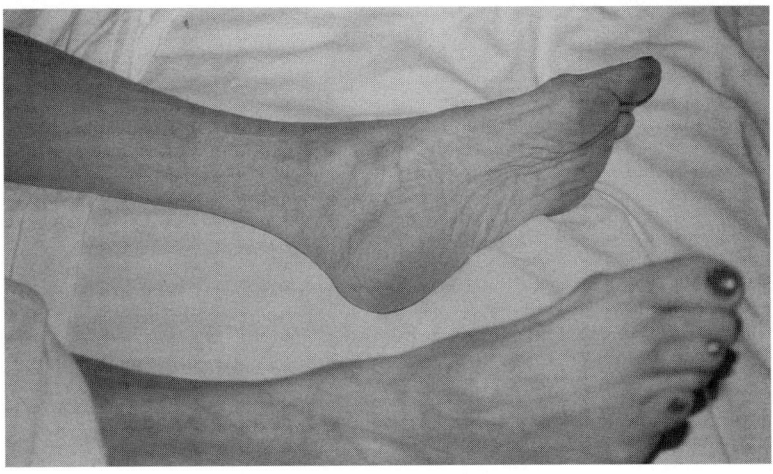

Figure 3.1. Patient with a displaced left intertrochanteric fracture; the left lower extremity is shortened and externally rotated.

Radiographic Examination

The standard radiographic examination of the hip includes an anteroposterior (AP) view of the pelvis and an AP and cross-table lateral view of the involved proximal femur (Figure 3.2). The AP pelvis radiograph allows comparison of the involved side with the contralateral side and can help to identify nondisplaced and impacted fractures. The lateral radiograph can help to assess posterior comminution of the femoral neck and proximal femur; a cross-table lateral view is preferred to a frog lateral view because the latter requires abduction, flexion, and external rotation of the affected lower extremity and involves a risk of fracture displacement. An internal rotation view of the injured hip may be helpful to identify nondisplaced or impacted fractures. Internally rotating the involved femur 10° to 15° offsets the anteversion of the femoral neck and provides a true AP view of the proximal femur (Figure 3.2). A second AP view, of the contralateral side, can be used for preoperative planning.

When a hip fracture is suspected but not apparent on standard radiographs, a technetium bone scan (Figure 3.3) or a magnetic resonance imaging (MRI) study (Figure 3.4) should be obtained. Two or three days may be required before a bone scan becomes positive in an elderly individual with a hip fracture.[6,7] Magnetic resonance imaging has been shown to be at least as accurate

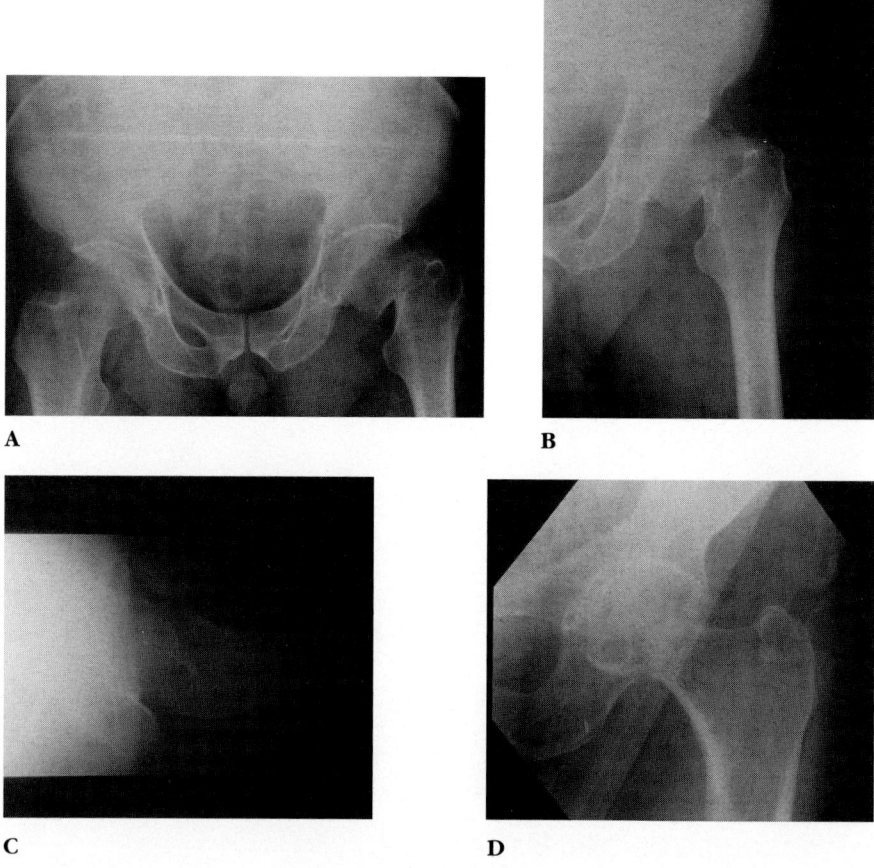

Figure 3.2. Anteroposterior (AP) view of the pelvis (**A**) and AP (**B**) and cross-table lateral (**C**) views of the hip, demonstrating a displaced left femoral neck fracture. Internal rotation of the injured extremity helped to better delineate the fracture pattern (**D**).

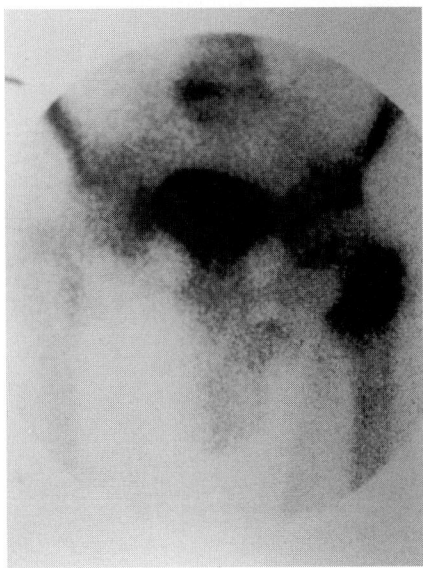

Figure 3.3. Technetium bone scan demonstrating a left intertrochanteric fracture.

as bone scanning in the identification of occult fractures of the hip and can be performed within 24 hours of the injury.[8,9] Rizzo et al. performed magnetic resonance imaging and bone scanning in 62 patients in whom a fracture about the hip was clinically suspected but not radiographically evident. MRI was performed within 24 hours of hospital admission, and bone scanning within 72 hours.[9] MRI was as accurate as bone scanning in the detection of occult hip fractures. However, it required less than 15 minutes to perform and was well tolerated by the patient—both improvements compared with bone scanning. MRI within 48 hours of fracture does not, however, appear to be useful for assessing femoral head viability or vascularity or for predicting the development of osteonecrosis or healing complications.[10,11]

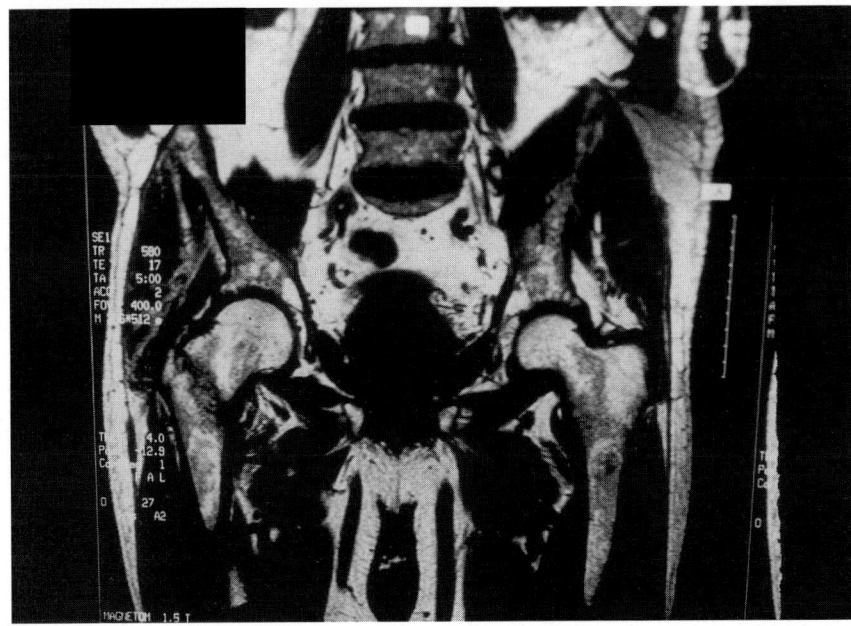

Figure 3.4. Magnetic resonance image demonstrating a right intertrochanteric fracture.

Laboratory Indices

Selective preoperative laboratory tests should be ordered in confirmed fractures of the proximal hip. In older individuals, a complete blood count, electrolyte measurement including blood urea nitrogen (BUN) and creatinine, an electrocardiogram, and a chest radiograph are probably sufficient. An arterial blood gas analysis (as a baseline) is also probably warranted in older patients as well as in any patient with a history of a pulmonary disorder. Studies have demonstrated that the yield of nonselective laboratory testing to find clinically important abnormalities is low.[12] Even though a prothrombin time or partial thromboplastin time is frequently ordered on a preoperative patient to evaluate the possibility of a coagulopathy, these tests are more likely to yield a false-positive than a true positive result and are thus not indicated.[12] Furthermore, it is unlikely that a coagulopathy will be found in an asymptomatic patient with no history of bleeding problems.[12] Additional laboratory studies should be ordered based on the medical history.

Preoperative Medical Evaluation

Most elderly patients who sustain a fracture of the proximal femur require medical evaluation to help determine whether they are sufficiently medically stable for operative treatment and to help prevent and treat medical complications in the perioperative period. Although advanced age is not by itself a risk factor for complications after surgery, older people tend to have more coexisting medical conditions that increase the surgical risk. The internist or geriatrician must evaluate these different factors to optimize the patient's outcome.

Cardiac Disease

Controversy exists over the need for perioperative cardiac evaluation of patients undergoing noncardiac surgery in patients with known or suspected coronary heart disease.[12] According to the most recent guidelines of the American College of Cardiology and the American Heart Association, the need for cardiac workup is identical whether or not the patient requires surgical intervention[13]: a preoperative stress test should be considered for patients with an unstable cardiac profile, patients who have new-onset angina, and patients whose anginal pattern has undergone a change. A patient with a fracture of the proximal femur would require a dipyridamole thallium stress test or a dobutamine echocardiogram stress test. One should also consider a cardiac stress test in those patients in whom the mechanism of injury suggests a cardiac event. In addition, an echocardiogram may be useful in patients with a history of angina.

Studies have shown that patients with poorly controlled hypertension (i.e., patients with a systolic blood pressure greater than 200 or a diastolic blood pressure greater than 105) develop larger elevations and declines in their blood pressure during surgery than do normotensive patients.[12] These patients are at increased risk for cardiac arrhythmias and myocardial ischemia. Patients who have well-controlled blood pressure prior to surgery behave similarly to normotensive patients. Patients with mildly elevated blood pressure (i.e., those with systolic blood pressure greater than 110) also behave similarly to normotensive patients. However, studies have suggested that the blood pressure measured just before or during surgery is less important than the blood pressure measured at hospital admission. This suggests that it is more important to have chronically well-controlled blood pressure than blood pressure controlled immediately before surgery. Isolated systolic blood pressure elevation is also probably associated with an increased incidence of intraoperative cardiac complications.[14]

Pulmonary Disease

Several studies suggest that the most important factors in determining the risk of pulmonary complications in the perioperative period are a prior history of smoking and a low oxygen level on arterial blood gas monitoring.[12] Incentive spirometry has not been shown to be particularly useful in the prevention of pulmonary complications. There is controversy over whether preoperative treatment and optimization of patients with chronic obstructive pulmonary disease (COPD) are useful in the prevention of postoperative pulmonary complications. Stein and Cassara reported that intensive preoperative treatment of COPD helped to prevent postoperative pulmonary complications,[15] whereas Gracey et al. reported that cessation of smoking, use of antibiotics if purulent sputum was present, administration of bronchodilators, and chest physiotherapy did not prevent such complications.[16] At the Hospital for Joint Diseases, the medical staff feel that if a patient has asymptomatic or mildly symptomatic pulmonary disease, a preoperative pulmonary workup is not warranted. For those with symptomatic pulmonary disease, a chest radiograph and arterial blood gas levels are obtained. As long as there is no radiographic evidence of an active pulmonary infiltrate and the CO_2 level is normal, the patient is cleared for surgery; if there is active pulmonary disease or a low arterial blood gas level, a pulmonologist is consulted.

Diabetes

Diabetes mellitus is a frequently associated comorbidity in elderly individuals who sustain a hip fracture. Oral hypoglycemic agents are usually stopped the morning of surgery.[12] Serum glucose levels are checked every 4 to 6 hours, and sliding-scale low-dose regular insulin is given to prevent severe hyperglycemia. Intravenous fluids should not contain glucose. Oral hypoglycemic agents are resumed when the patient is eating well. For the patient who requires insulin, a general rule of thumb is to give one-third to one-half the usual dose of long-acting insulin the morning of surgery, along with an intravenous drip containing dextrose. Sliding-scale insulin is also needed.

Anemia

Elderly patients are frequently anemic secondary to coexisting medical conditions or bleeding at the fracture site. A reasonable rule of thumb is that otherwise healthy elderly people can tolerate a hemoglobin level as low as

8.0 g/dL, whereas those with cardiac or pulmonary disease should maintain a hemoglobin level above 9 to 10 g/dL.[12,17] One should avoid the temptation to routinely transfuse elderly patients. There is evidence that allogeneic blood transfusion, in addition to introducing the risk of direct transmission of infectious diseases such as hepatitis and acquired immune deficiency syndrome (AIDS), is associated with immunosuppression. In a prospective study of 687 community-dwelling, ambulatory, operatively treated geriatric hip fracture patients, the authors found that allogeneic red blood cell transfusion was associated with an increased incidence of postoperative infections.[18] There are no studies that define an acceptable hematocrit prior to surgery; the accepted preoperative hemoglobin level should be based on the expected blood loss. If minimal blood loss is expected, the patient can undergo surgery despite a low hematocrit.

Liver Function Tests

Patients may have asymptomatic viral hepatitis B or C. As long as these patients have normal liver function with normal albumin and bilirubin levels, stable transaminases, and normal coagulation studies, they are unlikely to develop postoperative liver complications.[12] Alcoholic hepatitis, on the other hand, is associated with an increased incidence of postoperative complications, including liver failure. Although there are no studies that specifically evaluated orthopaedic patients with alcoholic hepatitis, a 50% mortality rate has been reported in patients with alcoholic hepatitis who underwent abdominal surgery.[19,20] Patients with alcoholic hepatitis and abnormal liver function should be monitored before surgery until their γ-amino transferase level falls below 100 U/L.[12] If emergency surgery is indicated, the risks of liver failure must be weighed against the benefits of surgery. In addition, these patients are at risk for delirium tremens in the perioperative period; they should therefore be observed in a monitored setting and given adequate doses of a benzodiazepine, such as lorazepam, either orally or intravenously to prevent the onset of tremors.

Renal Disease

Blood urea nitrogen (BUN) and creatinine levels should be measured as part of the preoperative laboratory evaluation. Glomerular filtration rate (GFR), the best measure of renal function, declines with advancing age, but BUN and creatinine usually remain normal because of reduced muscle mass in the elderly. The elderly also have decreased urinary concentrating ability and difficulty with water, sodium, and potassium excretion.[12] Because of a decreased glomerular filtration rate, the elderly are at increased risk for developing renal failure in the perioperative period; elderly persons with increased BUN and creatinine levels are at even higher risk for developing renal failure.

The best method to prevent renal failure is to optimize the patient medically before surgery.[12] If the patient has known renal insufficiency and the renal function is unchanged from baseline, no further workup is needed. During the operative procedure, the patient's fluid status should be carefully monitored with the use of a central venous catheter or right heart catheter, as indicated. Nephrotoxic drugs such as iodinated radiographic contrast dyes or aminoglycosides should be avoided. Tight blood pressure control is mandatory. For patients in whom new-onset renal dysfunction is suspected, a medical workup should be performed. Signs of hypovolemia, such as orthostatic hypotension, should be sought. A diagnostic renal ultrasonogram can help to detect signs of renal obstruction.[21]

Corticosteroid Use

Elderly individuals may have taken corticosteroids in the past to treat an autoimmune disease (such as lupus erythematosus or rheumatoid arthritis) or asthma, or as chemotherapy for certain malignancies. Any patient who has been using corticosteroids within the past 2 years requires preoperative stress doses of corticosteroids to prevent an addisonian crisis.[12] A reasonable routine is to give prednisone 25 mg or hydrocortisone 100 mg the night before surgery and the same dose the morning of surgery as well as on the first postoperative day.[12]

References

1. Owens WD, Felts JA, Spitznagel ELJ. ASA physical status classifications: a study of consistency ratings. *Anesthesiology* 1978; 49:239–243.
2. McClure J, Goldsborough S. Fractures neck of femur and contra-lateral intracerebral lesions. *J Clin Pathol* 1986; 39:920–922.
3. Soto-Hall R. Treatment of transcervical fractures complicated by certain common neurological conditions. *Instr Course Lect* 1960; 17:117–120.
4. Brummel-Smith K. Polypharmacy and the elderly patient. *Archives of the American Academy of Orthopaedic Surgeons* 1998; 2:39–44.
5. Hoffer MM, Feiwell E, Perry R, et al. Functional ambulation in patients with myelomeningocele. *J Bone Joint Surg Am* 1973; 55:137–148.
6. Swiontkowski MF. Intracapsular hip fractures. In: Browner BD, Levine AM, Jupiter JB, Trafton PG, eds. *Skeletal Trauma,* Vol 2. Philadelphia: WB Saunders, 1992:1751–1832.
7. Wilson MA. The effect of age on the quality of bone scans using technetium-99m pyrophosphate. *Radiology* 1981; 139:703–705.
8. Guanache CA, Kozin SH, Levy AS, Brody LA. The use of MRI in the diagnosis of occult hip fracture in the elderly: a preliminary report. *Orthopedics* 1994; 17:327–330.
9. Rizzo PF, Gould ES, Lyden JP, Asnis SE. Diagnosis of occult fractures about the hip. Magnetic resonance imaging compared with bone-scanning. *J Bone Joint Surg Am* 1993; 75:395–401.
10. Asnis SE, Gould ES, Bansal M, Rizzo PF, Bullough PG. Magnetic resonance imaging of the hip after displaced femoral neck fractures. *Clin Orthop* 1994; 298:191–198.
11. Speer KP, Spritzer CE, Harrelson JM, Nunley JA. Magnetic resonance imaging of the femoral head after acute intracapsular fracture of the femoral neck. *J Bone Joint Surg Am* 1990; 72:98–103.
12. Karp A. Preoperative medical evaluation. In: Koval K, Zuckerman J, eds. *Fractures in the Elderly.* Philadelphia: Lippincott-Raven, 1998:35–39.
13. Fleisher LA, Eagle KA. Screening for cardiac disease in patients having non-cardiac surgery. *Ann Intern Med* 1966; 24:767–772.
14. Wolfsthal S. Is blood pressure control necessary before surgery? *Med Clin North Am* 1993; 77:349–363.
15. Stein M, Cassara EL. Preoperative pulmonary evaluation and therapy for surgery patients. *JAMA* 1970; 211:787–790.
16. Gracey DR, Divertie MB, Didier EP. Preoperative pulmonary preparation of patients with chronic obstructive pulmonary disease: a prospective study. *Chest* 1979; 76:123–129.
17. Freedman ML, Sutin DG. Blood disorders and their management in old age. In: Tallis RC, Fillit HM, Brocklehurst JC, eds. *Brocklehurst's Textbook of Geriatric Medicine and Gerontology.* 5th ed. Edinburgh: Churchill Livingstone, 1998:1247–1291.

18. Koval KJ, Rosenberg AD, Zuckerman JD, et al. Does blood transfusion increase the risk of infection after hip fracture? *J Orthop Trauma* 1997; 11:260–265; discussion 265–266.
19. Greenwood SM, Leffler CT, Minkovitz S. The increased mortality rate of open liver biopsy in alcoholic hepatitis. *Surg Gynecol Obstet* 1972; 134:600–604.
20. Harville DD, Summerskill WHJ. Surgery in active hepatitis. *JAMA* 1963; 184:257–261.
21. Beck L. Perioperative renal, fluid and electrolyte management. *Clin Geriatr Med* 1990; 6:557–569.

Chapter Four

Treatment Principles

General Principles

The primary goal of fracture treatment is to return the patient to his or her prefracture level of function. There is nearly universal agreement that in patients who sustain a hip fracture, this goal can best be accomplished operatively.[1] Historically, nonoperative management has resulted in excessive rates of medical morbidity and mortality, as well as malunion and nonunion.[2] Nonoperative management is appropriate only in selected nonambulators who experience minimal discomfort from their injury.[2,3] These patients should be rapidly mobilized to avoid the complications of prolonged recumbency: decubitus ulcers, atelectasis, urinary tract infection, and thrombophlebitis.

Initial Patient Management

All patients who sustain a hip fracture should be admitted to the hospital and maintained on bed rest. In the past, we routinely placed patients in 5 lb of Buck's skin traction to prevent further fracture displacement or additional soft tissue injury that could compromise the vascular supply to the femoral head. Currently, we prefer to maintain the leg in a position of comfort—usually slight hip flexion and external rotation, supported by pillows under the knee. Several studies have shown that the extended position that results from Buck's traction increases intracapsular pressure, thereby diminishing femoral head blood flow.[4,5] Conversely, the position of external rotation and flexion allows for maximum capsular volume. Furthermore, in a prospective randomized trial conducted at the Hospital for Joint Diseases, more patients (54%) reported the placement of Buck's traction to be a painful experience than placement of a pillow under the knee (34%).

Surgical Timing

In general, hip fracture surgery should be performed as soon as possible after stabilization of all comorbid medical conditions; in this respect, particular attention must be paid to cardiopulmonary problems and fluid and electrolyte imbalances.[6] In a series of 399 hip fracture patients, Kenzora et al. reported that a surgical delay of less than 1 week to stabilize medical problems was not associated with increased mortality.[7] Interestingly, these authors found that even healthy patients who underwent surgery within 24 hours of hospital admission had a 34% mortality at 1-year follow-up compared with 5.8% for those who underwent surgery between the second and fifth days. On the other hand, Sexson and Lehner found that relatively healthy hip fracture patients (up to two comorbid conditions) who had surgery within 24 hours after admission had a higher survival rate than similar patients who had surgery after 24 hours.[8] However, patients with three or more comorbid conditions had a poorer survival rate when operated on within 24 hours than those operated on after 24 hours. In a prospectively followed series of 367 elderly hip fracture patients at the Hospital for Joint Diseases, a surgical delay of more than 2 calendar days from hospital admission approximately doubled the risk of the patient dying before the end of the first postoperative year; this relationship was significant when the factors of age, sex, and number of comorbidities were controlled.[9] When patient age, sex, and severity of comorbidities were controlled, however, there was also an increase in mortality with surgical delay, although it was not statistically significant. We therefore seek to proceed with operative management within 2 calendar days of admission in all patients. The use of "calendar" days was chosen rather than "hours" because it represents a more practical approach to the realities of patient care and the scheduling of surgery.

Anesthetic Considerations

Although much has been written on the risks and benefits of the different anesthetic techniques, no significant difference in survival rate has been found for the use of regional or general anesthesia for hip fracture surgery in elderly patients. Many anesthesiologists, internists, and surgeons believe that patients "look better" following regional anesthesia. However, studies have documented no difference in postoperative mental status in patients after regional or general anesthesia.[10,11] Studies have demonstrated the efficacy of regional anesthesia (spinal and epidural) in the prophylaxis of deep vein thrombosis and pulmonary embolus.[12] Since pulmonary embolism is a significant cause of morbidity and mortality in this population, regional anesthesia may be preferable, especially if the patient is at increased risk for thromboembolic complications and there are other medical factors that compromise the use of thromboprophylaxis.

Valentin et al. reported no effect of spinal or general anesthesia on either short-term or long-term mortality in a prospective randomized study of 578 hip fracture patients over 50 years of age.[11] Thirty days after surgery, the mortality rate was 6% after spinal and 8% after general anesthesia; 6 months to 2 years after surgery, the mortality was identical in the two groups. Davis et al. reported a prospective randomized multicenter trial of short-term and long-term mortality following general or spinal anesthesia in 538 hip fracture patients.[10] Four-week mortality was 6.6% with spinal and 5.9% with general anesthesia; this difference was not significant. The overall 1-year mortality was 20.4%, with no significant difference between the two anesthetic groups. The study by Davis et al. was nonexclusionary, whereas the study by Valentin et al. excluded patients who had significant cognitive impairment.

In a series of 642 community-dwelling, previously ambulatory elderly patients observed at the Hospital for Joint Diseases, 56% of whom received general anesthesia and 44% spinal anesthesia, no differences in the in-hospital morbidity or mortality rates or the 1-year mortality rate were found between the two groups. Koval et al. also evaluated the effect of anesthetic technique on ambulation and functional recovery after hip fracture in a series of 631 community-dwelling elderly patients.[13] When controlling for potential confounding variables, no differences were observed in the recovery of ambulatory ability or the percentage of functional recovery between the two groups at 3, 6, or 12 months after hip fracture.

Thromboprophylaxis

Patients who have sustained a fracture of the proximal femur are at increased risk for thrombophlebitis. The reported incidence of deep vein thrombosis after hip fracture is 36% to 60%,[14-21] whereas the incidence of thrombi involving the proximal venous system ranges between 17% and 36%.[18,20,21] According to the available literature, the incidence of pulmonary embolus after hip fracture ranges between 4.3% and 24%,[22] while the incidence of fatal pulmonary embolus ranges between 3.6% and 12.9%.[22] Thrombi limited to the calf veins are rarely associated with pulmonary embolus. Popliteal and more proximal venous thrombi carry a much higher embolic risk.[23] However, most above-knee deep vein thrombi represent extension of thrombi from the calf venous system.

Clinical risk factors for venous thrombosis include advanced patient age, previous venous thromboembolism, malignant disease, congestive heart failure, prolonged immobility or paralysis, obesity, and deep system venous disease.[24] In a recent prospective study of 133 hip fracture patients who had venography upon hospital admission, 13 (9.8%) had evidence of a deep vein thrombosis[25]; patients who had a delay of more than 2 days from injury to hospital presentation were at significantly increased risk for deep vein thrombosis (55% vs. 6%).

Two approaches can be taken to prevent fatal pulmonary embolism: (1) early detection of subclinical venous thrombosis by screening high-risk patients; and (2) primary prophylaxis using either drugs or physical methods that are effective for preventing deep vein thrombosis and pulmonary embolism. Several prophylactic measures have been recommended, including administration of subcutaneous heparin, low–molecular-weight heparin, intravenous dextran, warfarin sodium, or aspirin; intermittent pneumatic compression of the foot or leg; and various combined modalities.

Pathophysiology of Venous Thrombosis

Venous thrombi usually develop at sites of slow or disturbed blood flow and begin as small deposits of platelets, fibrin, and red cells in valve-cusp pockets or in the intramuscular sinuses of the veins of the lower limb.[24] As the thrombus grows, it occludes the lumen of the vein, producing venous stasis, and then extends both proximally and distally as a coagulation thrombus composed of red blood cells with interspersed fibrin. The mechanisms that are recognized to be important in the pathogenesis of venous thromboembolism are venous stasis, activation of blood coagulation, and endothelial damage. A relatively high proportion (10% to 20%) of thrombi in patients undergoing hip surgery involve the popliteal or femoral venous segments.[24,26,27]

Patients are predisposed to venous thrombosis when fulfilling the elements of Virchow's triad: venous stasis, endothelial injury, and hypercoagulability. Venous stasis occurs secondary to long periods of immobilization before or during surgery and delayed, limited, or impaired postoperative ambulation. Endothelial injury can be caused by either direct trauma to the deep veins of the lower extremity and the surrounding soft tissues or indirectly by hematoma formation and thermal injury (e.g., from electrocautery or during cement polymerization). Torsion of the deep venous system itself during extremity manipulation has also been implicated. Furthermore, a transient postoperative hypercoagulable state has been hypothesized to exist as part of the normal host response to surgical insult.

The prophylactic methods that have been evaluated have been directed at one or more of these pathogenic factors and include anticoagulants that counteract blood coagulation, drugs that suppress platelet function and the interaction of platelets with the damaged vessel wall, and mechanical devices that prevent venous stasis.

Oral Anticoagulant Prophylaxis

Oral anticoagulant prophylaxis using warfarin sodium is effective for prevention of venous thromboembolism in patients undergoing elective hip surgery and in patients who sustain a fracture of the proximal femur.[24,28,29] In patients undergoing hip fracture surgery, several studies have demonstrated a clinically and statistically significant reduction in the frequency of both venous thrombosis and pulmonary embolism. Sevitt and Gallagher found oral anticoagulant prophylaxis to be associated with a clinically and statistically significant reduction in mortality rate secondary to a decreased incidence of death from pulmonary embolism.[30] Two other studies have confirmed these findings.[28,31] Both autopsy and venographic findings indicate that administration of oral anticoagulants commencing at the time of surgery or immediately postoperatively are effective in preventing clinically significant venous thrombosis and pulmonary embolism in patients undergoing hip fracture surgery.[24] The simplest way to use this medication is to administer 10 mg orally the night before surgery followed each day by an appropriate dose to maintain an international normalizing ratio between 2 and 3. The use of warfarin sodium can be problematic, however, if there is a surgical delay. Furthermore, the risk of bleeding complications has limited the acceptance of oral anticoagulant prophylaxis.[24,28]

Heparin

Although it is effective in high-risk general surgical patients, prophylaxis with low-dose subcutaneous heparin (5000 units every 8 to 12 hours) is relatively ineffective for preventing venous thromboembolism in orthopaedic patients.[24,26,32] Definitive conclusions cannot be drawn from the published reports, but it is likely that any protection provided by low-dose heparin is incomplete in patients undergoing hip surgery. In patients undergoing surgery for a fractured hip, prophylaxis with low-dose heparin does not appear to reduce the frequency of large thrombi in the popliteal or femoral veins.

Low-Molecular-Weight Heparin

Low–molecular-weight heparins (LMWHs) represent a newer pharmacological agent for prophylaxis and treatment of venous thromboembolism. Unfractionated heparin (UFH) consists of a heterogeneous group of glycosaminoglycan polymers of various weights averaging 15,000 d.[33] By a process of depolymerization, LMWHs are produced. Heparin acts via binding to antithrombin III, a natural inhibitor of the clotting cascade, and heparin–antithrombin III complexes act to inhibit factors Xa and IIa (thrombin).[34] Although factor IIa is essential for wound hemostasis, factor Xa is believed to be more important for preventing thrombosis.[33] The lower–molecular-weight heparins have significantly higher anti-Xa than IIa activity as compared to UFH, as these smaller molecules are unable to bind IIa and antithrombin III.[35-37] Thus LMWHs provide increased protection against thromboembolism with a decreased risk of bleeding complications compared with UFH.[38-40]

The reduced nonspecific binding of LMWHs to endothelial cells and plasma proteins contribute to their superior bioavailability and to a plasma half-life four times longer than that of UFH.[41-44] There is less platelet inhibition and decreased microvascular bleeding in reaction to LMWHs than to UFH.[45] Meta-analyses and clinical trials have demonstrated the superiority of LMWHs over UFH in preventing deep vein thrombosis after orthopaedic surgery, specifically after total hip and total knee replacement, in patients with acute ischemic stroke, and after major trauma.[46-50]

Several prospective randomized trials have been performed to evaluate the efficacy of LMWHs in patients who have sustained a fracture of the proximal femur. Monreal et al., in a study of 90 patients, found that Kabi 2165 (Fragmin), given at a dose of 5000 units daily, was not as effective as conventional low-dose heparin.[51] Deep vein thrombosis occurred in 14 (30%) of 46 patients who were treated with Kabi 2165 compared with 6 (14%) of 44 patients who were treated with conventional low-dose heparin. However, Jorgensen et al., in a placebo-controlled study of 68 patients, reported that Fragmin reduced the rate of deep vein thrombosis to 30% in the treated group compared with 58% in the placebo group—a statistically significant difference.[52] Bergqvist et al. compared the use of Org 10172 with that of dextran 70 in a three-center study of 302 patients who had sustained a hip fracture.[53] Org 10172 was given as a subcutaneous dose of 750 anti-Xa units twice daily starting preoperatively and continuing for 10 to 12 days. Dextran 70 was given as an intravenous infusion of 500 mL preoperatively, immediately postoperatively, and on the first and third postoperative days. The rate of deep vein thrombosis was 10% in the Org 10172 group and 31% in the dextran 70 group ($P < .01$). Blood loss did not differ between the two groups.

Gerhart et al. performed a randomized prospective trial, comparing a LMWH to warfarin for efficacy and safety in preventing deep vein thrombosis in 263 patients who had an operatively treated fracture of the proximal femur.[54] Both drug regimens were initiated preoperatively, immediately after hospital admission. Deep vein thrombosis was detected by 125I-fibrinogen scanning and impedance plethysmography and was confirmed by phlebography and compression ultrasonography. Deep vein thrombosis was found in 9 (7%) of the 132 patients who received LMWH and in 28 (21%) of the 131 patients who received warfarin, a difference that was statistically significant. Adverse reactions were not significantly different in the two groups. The authors concluded that LMWH is a safe, convenient, effective antithrombotic agent for the prevention of venous thrombosis after hip fracture surgery.

In December 1997, the U.S. Food and Drug Administration issued a warning regarding use of LMWHs and subsequent spinal or regional anesthesia. This followed an initial report by Horlocker in 1996 of six spinal hematomas that developed after the concurrent use of Lovenox and central neuraxial anesthesia.[55] By November 1997, there were more than 30 reports of patients who had developed a spinal or epidural hematoma with concurrent use of an LMWH and spinal/epidural anesthesia; since these were isolated reports, estimates of frequency could not be made. Some of the reported hematomas caused neurological injury, including temporary and permanent paralysis. Approximately 75% of the patients were elderly women undergoing orthopaedic surgery. The following guidelines were provided by Horlocker and Heit in 1997 in relation to administration of LMWHs[56]:

- **Preoperatively:** A single-dose spinal anesthetic may be the safest neuraxial technique. Needle placement should occur 10 to 12 hours after the last dose of LMWH, with subsequent dosing delayed at least 2 hours after needle placement.
- **Postoperatively:** If continuous technique is used, the epidural catheter should be left indwelling overnight and removed the following day. The first dose of LMWH can be administered 2 hours after catheter removal.

Dextran

Dextran is a glucose polymer that was introduced as a volume expander and subsequently evaluated as an antithrombotic agent.[24] Two types of dextran polymer have been used clinically: dextran 70 (mean molecular weight 70,000) and dextran 30 (mean molecular weight 40,000). The antithrombotic properties of dextran have been attributed to a number of factors, including decreased blood viscosity, reduced platelet reactivity with the damaged vessel wall, decreased platelet aggregation, and, for fibrin clots formed in the presence of dextran, an increased susceptibility to fibrinolysis.[24]

In patients who sustain a fracture of the proximal femur, intravenous dextran has been shown to be an effective prophylactic agent that consistently reduces the frequency of postoperative venous thrombosis.[24,57] The major side effect of dextran is volume overload, which may result in cardiac failure, particularly in elderly patients who have a reduced cardiac reserve.[24] Allergic reactions have been described, particularly with dextran 70, but these are relatively uncommon.[24] Excessive oozing has been reported in some patients, but bleeding has not been a serious problem.[24]

Aspirin

It was originally hoped that the antiplatelet action of aspirin would provide protection against deep vein thrombosis in orthopaedic patients.[24] The role of aspirin prophylaxis in patients undergoing hip fracture surgery remains controversial because of the inconsistent findings of clinical trials.[24] With the exception of one randomized double-blind trial in which aspirin was effective in men, the results have been disappointingly negative.[24,32,58]

Physical Methods

Elastic stockings are inexpensive and simple to use and can be used in conjunction with other prophylactic measures. Intermittent pneumatic compression of the legs is an attractive form of prophylaxis that is effective in patients undergoing general surgery, neurosurgery, and prostatic surgery.[24] Prophylaxis with intermittent pneumatic compression is virtually free of side effects and without risk of bleeding. External pneumatic compression overcomes venous stasis by intermittently squeezing the leg to increase venous return to the heart.[24] It has also been shown to enhance fibrinolysis.[24] Thus, intermittent compression has both a physical and a pharmacological effect. At our institution, an ultrasonogram of the venous system of both lower extremities is performed prior to placement of the external pneumatic compression devices to exclude the presence of preexisting thrombi. The role of intermittent pneumatic compression in patients undergoing hip fracture surgery remains uncertain because of a lack of data concerning its effectiveness when used alone.[24] These devices may be most beneficial in patients in whom anticoagulation is contraindicated.

There has been recent interest in the use of intermittent compression of the plantar venous plexus (foot pumps) for deep vein thromboprophylaxis. The pneumatic bladder of this device straps around the patient's foot in the region of the longitudinal arch. Westrich and Sculco performed a prospective, randomized study to assess the efficacy of foot pumps for prophylaxis against deep venous thrombosis after total knee arthroplasty.[59] One hundred twenty-two patients (164 knees) were randomized to thromboprophylaxis with either aspirin alone or foot pumps in conjunction with aspirin. The prevalence of deep vein thrombosis was significantly lower ($P < 0.001$) in the foot pump group compared with patients managed with aspirin alone (27% versus 59%). No proximal thrombi were noted in any patient who used the foot pump device, whereas the prevalence of proximal thrombosis in the popliteal or femoral veins was 14% in the group treated with aspirin alone ($P < 0.01$). No adverse effects were noted in any patient who used the foot pump device. The authors concluded that the use of foot pumps in conjunction with aspirin was a safe and effective method of thromboprophylaxis after total knee arthroplasty. However, the applicability of this method for hip fracture patients remains unknown.

Recommendations

Every patient who sustains a fracture of the proximal femur should receive thromboprophylaxis while awaiting surgery. At our institution, this prophylaxis, which is initiated on the day of hospital admission, previously involved the use of LMWH. In light of the FDA warning regarding the risk for spinal hematoma when regional anesthesia is performed in patients who are receiving LMWHs, we have considered the use of intermittent pneumatic compression devices. Patients who have a delayed hospital presentation are evaluated for preexisting deep vein thrombosis; if positive, a vena cava filter is placed before surgery. All patients are also given thigh-high elastic stockings. Patients continue to receive thromboprophylaxis throughout hospitalization. Thromboprophylaxis is discontinued upon hospital discharge; however, because of the recent emphasis on early patient discharge, consideration has been given to continuing these prophylactic measures at home.

Prophylactic Antibiotics

Use of prophylactic antibiotics has lowered the incidence of superficial and deep wound infection after hip fracture surgery.[6] The duration of antibiotic treatment, however, remains controversial. Nelson et al. compared the efficacy of administration of two different antibiotics, for 24 hours and for 7 days, in conjunction with three different types of orthopaedic surgical procedures.[60] There was no difference between the postoperative rates of infection associated with the antibiotic regimens in patients who underwent prosthetic replacement of the hip or knee or internal fixation of a fracture of the proximal femur.

Studies have also been performed to evaluate the efficacy of antibiotic prophylaxis given for less than 24 hours. In a prospective, randomized study, Gatell et al. compared the results of prophylaxis administered as a single dose of cefamandole with the results of using five doses administered during a 20-hour period in patients who underwent prosthetic hip replacement or internal fixation of an upper- or lower-extremity fracture.[61] The rate of wound infection in the patients who had received a single dose of the antibiotic was 7% for those who had had prosthetic replacement of the hip and 5% for those who had had osteosynthesis. In contrast, when five doses of cefamandole were given, no patient who had undergone a prosthetic hip replacement developed an infection, compared with 1% of those who had osteosynthesis.

Kaukonen et al. compared the use of a single intravenous dose of cefuroxime during the induction of anesthesia to no antibiotic coverage in a series of 162 consecutive hip fractures.[62] The overall infection rate was 8.0% with 2.4% deep infections. There were seven infections in the prophylaxis group and six in the control group; the rate of deep infections was 3.9% and 1.4%, respectively. A single dose of antibiotics did not seem to have an effect on the infection rate.

Nungu et al. reported a prospective, randomized study in 559 patients comparing two doses of oral cefadroxil with three doses of intravenous cefuroxime as antibiotic prophylaxis for hip fracture surgery.[63] Antibiotic concentrations in the wound fluid were determined at the start and at the end of surgery. The first dose of cefadroxil was given approximately 2 hours before surgery and cefuroxime approximately 30 minutes before surgery. In 226 of 242 (93%) patients given oral cefadroxil, the mean concentration in the wound during surgery was 15 µg/mL, well above the minimum inhibitory concentration (MIC-90) for *Staphylococcus aureus*. In the cefuroxime group, antibiotic levels in the wound exceeded the MIC-90 for *S. aureus* in 204 of 210 (97%) of the patients at both the start and end of surgery. All patients were followed up for 4 months. One deep and five superficial infections occurred in the cefuroxime group and no deep but one superficial infection in the cefadroxil group. In four of seven infections, patients had adequate levels of antibiotic in the wound during surgery; in three patients, no antibiotic assay was performed. The authors concluded that administration of two doses of oral cefadroxil seems to be a practical method of antibiotic prophylaxis for hip fracture surgery and seems to be as effective as intravenously administered cefuroxime. However, the potential issues related to the ability of patients to ingest the oral medication were not considered.

Buckley et al. performed a randomized, double-blind, single-hospital clinical study to assess the effect of both antibiotic use and duration on wound infection during hip fracture surgery.[64] Wound infection rates in three groups of patients were compared: (1) those who received four doses of cefazolin (108 patients); (2) those who received one dose of cefazolin and three doses of placebo (83 patients); and (3) those who received four placebo doses (121 patients). Results showed an infection rate of 1.6% for the four-dose group, 2.4% for the one-dose group, and 3.7% for the placebo group. These differences were not statistically significant, even when both treatment groups were combined and compared with the placebo group. The authors concluded that until more patients are studied, empirical use of antibiotics should be continued in patients who undergo hip fracture surgery.

We believe that all patients should receive prophylactic antibiotics during hip fracture surgery. At our institution, it is general practice to administer a first-generation cephalosporin (Ancef 1 g) just before surgery and to continue antibiotic coverage for 24 to 48 hours after surgery. Vancomycin 1 g is administered to patients who are allergic to penicillin. Using this protocol, we reported a 0.9% wound infection rate in 687 elderly patients who sustained a fracture of the proximal femur.[65]

References

1. Zuckerman J, Schon L. Hip fractures. In: Zuckerman J, ed. *Comprehensive Care of Orthopaedic Injuries in the Elderly*. Baltimore: Urban & Schwarzenberg, 1990:23–111.
2. Koval KJ, Zuckerman JD. Hip fractures: I. Overview and evaluation and treatment of femoral neck fractures. *J Am Acad Orthop Surg* 1994; 2:141–149.
3. Winter WG. Nonoperative treatment of proximal femoral fractures in the demented nonambulatory patient. *Clin Orthop* 1987; 218:97–103.
4. Drake JK, Meyers MH. Intracapsular pressure and hemarthrosis following femoral neck fracture. *Clin Orthop* 1984; 182:172–176.
5. Melberg PE, Korner L, Lansinger O. Hip joint pressure after femoral neck fracture. *Acta Orthop Scand* 1986; 57:501–504.
6. Zuckerman JD, Schon LC. Hip fractures. In: Zuckerman J, ed. *Comprehensive Care of Orthopaedic Injuries in the Elderly*. Baltimore: Urban & Schwarzenberg, 1990:23–111.
7. Kenzora JE, McCarthy RE, Lowell JD, Sledge CB. Hip fracture mortality. Relation to age, treatment, preoperative illness, time of surgery, and complications. *Clin Orthop* 1984; 186:45–56.
8. Sexson SB, Lehner JT. Factors affecting hip fracture mortality. *J Orthop Trauma* 1988; 1:298–305.
9. Zuckerman JD, Skovron ML, Koval KJ, et al. Postoperative complications and mortality associated with operative delay in older patients who have a fracture of the hip. *J Bone Joint Surg Am* 1995; 77:1551–1556.
10. Davis FM, Laurenson VG. Spinal anaesthesia or general anaesthesia for emergency hip surgery in elderly patients. *Anaesth Intensive Care* 1981; 9:352–358.
11. Valentin N, Lomholt B, Jensen JS, et al. Spinal or general anesthesia for surgery of the fractured hip? *Br J Anaesth* 1986; 58:284–291.
12. Modig J, Borg T, Karlstrom G, et al. Thromboembolism after total hip replacement: role of epidural and general anesthesia. *Anesth Analg* 1983; 62:174–180.

13. Koval KJ, Aharonoff GB, Rosenberg AD, et al. Functional outcome after hip fracture. Effect of general versus regional anesthesia. *Clin Orthop* 1998; 348:37–41.
14. Stevens J, Fardin R, Freeark R. Lower extremity thrombophlebitis in patients with femoral neck fractures. *Trauma* 1968; 8:527–534.
15. Johnsson S, Bygdeman S, Eliasson R. Effect of dextran on postoperative thrombosis. *Acta Chir Scand* 1968; 387:80–82.
16. Ahlberg A, Nylander G, Robertson B, et al. Dextran in prophylaxis of thrombosis in fractures of the hip. *Acta Chir Scand* 1968; 387:83–85.
17. Hamilton HW, Crawford JS, Gardiner JH, Wiley AM. Venous thrombosis in patients with fractures of the upper end of the femur: a phlebographic study of the effect of prophylactic anticoagulation. *J Bone Joint Surg Br* 1970; 52:268–289.
18. Moskovitz PA, Ellenberg SS, Feffer HL, et al. Low-dose heparin for prevention of venous thromboembolism in total hip arthroplasty and surgical repair of hip fractures. *J Bone Joint Surg Am* 1978; 60:1065–1070.
19. Snook G, Chrisman O, Wilson T. Thromboembolism after surgical treatment of hip fractures. *Clin Orthop* 1981; 155:21–24.
20. Powers P, Gent M, Jay R, et al. A randomized trial of less intense postoperative warfarin or aspirin therapy in the prevention of venous thromboembolism after surgery for fractured hip. *Arch Intern Med* 1989; 149:771–774.
21. Agnelli G, Cosmi B, Fillipo D, et al. A randomized double-blind, placebo-controlled trial of dermatan sulphate for prevention of deep vein thrombosis in hip fracture. *Thromb Haemost* 1992; 67:203–208.
22. Haake D, Berkman S. Venous thromboembolic disease after hip surgery. Risk factors, prophylaxis, and diagnosis. *Clin Orthop* 1989; 242:212–231.
23. Moser K. Pulmonary thromboembolism. In: Wilson J, Braunwald E, Isselbacher KJ, et al., eds. *Harrison's Principles of Internal Medicine,* Vol 1. New York: McGraw-Hill, 1991:1090–1096.
24. Hull R, Raskob G. prophylaxis of venous thromboembolic disease following hip and knee surgery. *J Bone Joint Surg Am* 1986; 68:146–150.
25. Hefley FG Jr, Nelson CL, Puskarich-May CL. Effect of delayed admission to the hospital on the preoperative prevalence of deep-vein thrombosis associated with fractures about the hip. *J Bone Joint Surg Am* 1996; 78:581–583.
26. Harris WH, Athanasoulis C, Waltman AC, Salzman EW. Cuff-impedance phlebography and ^{125}I fibrinogen scanning versus roentgenographic phlebography for diagnosis of thrombophlebitis following hip surgery. *J Bone Joint Surg Am* 1976; 58:939–944.
27. Hull R, Hirsh J, Sackett D, et al. The value of adding impedance plethysmography to ^{125}I-fibrinogen leg scanning for the detection of deep vein thrombosis in high risk surgical patients: a comparative study between patients undergoing surgery and hip surgery. *Thromb Res* 1979; 15:227–234.
28. Eskeland C, Solheinik H, Skjorten F. Anticoagulant prophylaxis, thromboembolism and mortality in elderly patients with hip fractures. A controlled clinical trial. *Acta Chir Scand* 1966; 131:16–29.
29. Francis CW, Marder VJ, Evarts CM, Yaukoolbodi S. Two-step warfarin therapy: prevention of postoperative venous thrombosis without excessive bleeding. *JAMA* 1983; 249:374–378.
30. Sevitt S, Gallagher N. Prevention of venous thrombosis and pulmonary embolism in injured patients. A trial of anticoagulant prophylaxis and phenidine in middle-aged and elderly patients with fractured necks of femur. *Lancet* 1959; 2:981–989.
31. Morris GK, Mitchell JR. Warfarin sodium in the prevention of deep vein thrombosis and pulmonary embolism in patients with fractured neck of femur. *Lancet* 1976; 2:869–872.
32. Salzman E. Progress in preventing venous thromboembolism [letter]. *N Engl J Med* 1983; 309:980–982.
33. Tapson V, Hull R. Management of venous thromboembolic disease. The impact of low-molecular-weight heparin. *Clin Chest Med* 1995; 16:281–294.
34. Hirsh J. Heparin. *N Engl J Med* 1991; 324:1565–1574.
35. Aiach M, Michaud A, Balian J, et al. A new low molecular weight heparin derivative. In vitro and in vivo studies. *Thromb Res* 1983; 31:611–621.
36. Zimlich R, Fulbright B, Friedman R. Current status of anticoagulation therapy after total hip and total knee arthroplasty. *J Am Acad Orthop Surg* 1996; 4:54–62.
37. Danielsson A, Raub E, Lindahl U, Bjork I. Role of ternary complexes, in which heparin binds both antithrombin and proteinase, in the acceleration of the reactions between antithrombin and thrombin or factor Xa. *J Biol Chem* 1986; 261:15467–15473.

38. Cade J, Buchanan M, Boneu B, et al. A comparison of the antithrombotic and haemorrhagic effects of low molecular weight heparin fractions: the influence of the method of preparation. *Thromb Res* 1984; 35:613–625.
39. Carter C, Kelton J, Hirsh J, Cerskus A, Santos A, Gent M. The relationship between the hemorrhagic and antithrombotic properties of low molecular weight heparin in rabbits. *Blood* 1982; 59:1239–1245.
40. Bergqvist D, Nilsson B. The influence of low molecular weight heparin in combination with dihydrergotamine on experimental thrombosis and haemostasis. *Thromb Haemost* 1987; 58:893–895.
41. Blajchman M, Young E, Ofosu F. Effects of unfractionated heparin, dermatan sulfate and low molecular weight heparin on vessel wall permeability in rabbits. *Ann N Y Acad Sci* 1989; 556:245–254.
42. Bara L, Billaud E, Gramond G, Kher A, Samama M. Comparative pharmacokinetics of a low molecular weight heparin (PK 10169) and unfractionated heparin after intravenous and subcutaneous administration. *Thromb Res* 1985; 39:631–636.
43. Vinazzer H, Woler M. A new low molecular weight heparin fragment (PK 10169): in vitro and in vivo studies. *Haemostasis* 1986; 16:106–115.
44. Fernandez F, N'guyen P, Van Ryan J, et al. Hemorrhagic doses of heparin and other glycosaminoglycans induce a platelet defect. *Thromb Res* 1986; 43:491–495.
45. Brace L, Fareed J, Tomeo J, Issleib S. Biochemical and pharmacological studies on the interaction of PK 10169 and its subfractions with human platelets. *Haemostasis* 1986; 16:93–105.
46. Leclerc J, Geerts W, Desjardins L, et al. Prevention of venous thromboembolism after knee arthroplasty. A randomized, double-blind trial comparing enoxaparin with warfarin. *Ann Intern Med* 1996; 124:619–626.
47. Imperiale T, Speroff T. A meta-analysis of methods to prevent venous thromboembolism following total hip replacement. *JAMA* 1994; 271:1780–1785.
48. Nurmohamed M, Rosendaal F, Buller H, et al. Low-molecular weight heparin versus standard heparin in general and orthopaedic surgery: a meta-analysis. *Lancet* 1992; 340:152–156.
49. Turpie A. Prophylaxis of venous thromboembolism in stroke patients. *Semin Thromb Hemost* 1997; 23:155–157.
50. Colwell C, Spiro T. Efficacy and safety of enoxaparin to prevent deep vein thrombosis after hip arthroplasty. *Clin Orthop* 1995; 319:215–222.
51. Monreal M, Lafoz E, Navarro A, et al. A prospective double-blind trial of a low molecular weight heparin once daily compared with conventional low-dose heparin three times daily to prevent pulmonary embolism and venous thrombosis in patients with hip fractures. *J Trauma* 1989; 29:873–875.
52. Jorgensen PS, Knudsen JB, Broeng L, et al. The thromboprophylactic effect of a low molecular weight heparin (Fragmin) in hip fracture surgery: a placebo-controlled trial. *Ugeskr Laeger* 1993; 155:706–708.
53. Bergqvist D, Kettunen K, Fredin H, et al. Thromboprophylaxis in patients with hip fractures: a prospective randomized comparison between Org-10172 and Dextran 70. *Surgery* 1991; 109:617–622.
54. Gerhart TN, Yett HS, Robertson LK, et al. Low-molecular-weight heparinoid compared with warfarin for prophylaxis of deep-vein thrombosis in patients who are operated for fracture of the hip. *J Bone Joint Surg Am* 1991; 73:494–501.
55. Horlocker T. Low molecular weight heparin and central neuraxial anesthesia. *ASRA News* 1996:5–6.
56. Horlocker T, Heit J. Low molecular weight heparin: biochemistry, pharmacology, perioperative prophylaxis regimens, and guidelines for regional anesthetic management. *Anesth Analg* 1997; 85:874–885.
57. Evarts EM, Freil EI. Prevention of thromboembolic disease after elective surgery of the hip. *J Bone Joint Surg Am* 1971; 53:1271–1280.
58. Harris WH, Salzman EW, Athanasoulis CA, et al. Aspirin prophylaxis of venous thromboembolism after total hip replacement. *N Engl J Med* 1977; 297:1246–1249.
59. Westrich G, Sculco T. Prophylaxis against deep vein thrombosis after total knee replacement. *J Bone Joint Surg Am* 1996; 78:826–834.
60. Nelson CL, Green TG, Porter RA. One day versus seven days of preventive antibiotic therapy in orthopaedic surgery. *Clin Orthop* 1983; 176:258–263.
61. Gatell J, Garcia S, Lozano L, et al. Perioperative cefamandole prophylaxis against infections. *J Bone Joint Surg Am* 1987; 69:1189–1193.
62. Kaukonen J, Kemppainen E, Makijarvi J, Tuominen T. One dose cefuroxime prophylaxis in hip fracture surgery. *Ann Chir Gynaecol* 1995; 84:417–419.

63. Nungu K, Olerud C, Rehnberg L, et al. Prophylaxis with oral cefadroxil versus intravenous cefuroxime in trochanteric fracture surgery. A clinical multicenre study. *Arch Orthop Trauma Surg* 1995; 114:303–307.
64. Buckley R, Hughes G, Snodgrass T, Huchcroft S. Perioperative cefazolin prophylaxis in hip fracture surgery. *Can J Surg* 1990; 33:122–127.
65. Koval KJ, Rosenberg AD, Zuckerman JD, et al. Does blood transfusion increase the risk of infection after hip fracture? *J Orthop Trauma* 1997; 11:260–265; discussion 265–266.

Chapter Five
Femoral Neck Fractures

Fractures of the femoral neck are intracapsular, located in an area bounded by the femoral head and the greater and lesser trochanters (Figure 5.1). This fracture location has important implications for fracture healing and the development of osteonecrosis.

Classification

Several different systems for classifying femoral neck fractures have been proposed. One such schema, anatomically based, divides the femoral neck into three regions: subcapital, transcervical, and basicervical (Figure 5.2). The majority of femoral neck fractures are subcapital; transcervical femoral neck fractures are usually the result of repetitive stresses. Since the subcapital and transcervical regions are entirely intracapsular, fractures in these regions exhibit different characteristics than those in the basicervical region, which is extracapsular. Fractures that are entirely intracapsular are at increased risk for osteonecrosis and nonunion, sequelae that are uncommon following extracapsular fracture.

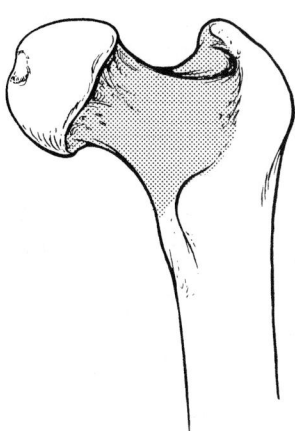

Figure 5.1. Fractures of the femoral neck are located in an area bounded by the femoral head and the greater and lesser trochanters.

The classification system proposed by Pauwels in 1935 is based on the angle of inclination of the fracture line[1] (Figure 5.3):

- Type I: Fracture line 30° from the horizontal
- Type II: Fracture line 50° from the horizontal
- Type III: Fracture line 70° from the horizontal

Pauwels maintained that the more vertical the fracture line, the greater the risk of nonunion because of increased shear stresses across the fracture[2]; subsequent investigators, however, have failed to demonstrate this relationship.[3] Furthermore, there is evidence that the inclination of the fracture line is more a reflection of radiographic technique (including positioning of the lower extremity) than of true fracture anatomy. As a result, this classification system is rarely used today.

The most popular femoral neck fracture classification system, introduced by Garden in 1961, comprises four types, based on degree of fracture displacement on the anteroposterior (AP) radiograph[4] (Figure 5.4):

- Type I: Incomplete or impacted fracture in which the bony trabeculae of the inferior portion of the femoral neck remains intact; this category includes "valgus-impacted" fractures.

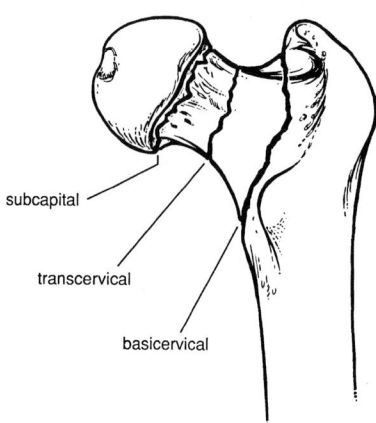

Figure 5.2. Femoral neck fractures can be classified based on anatomic location as either subcapital, transcervical, or basicervical.

- Type II: Complete fracture without displacement of the fracture fragments.
- Type III: Complete fracture with partial displacement of the fracture fragments; radiographically, in a type III fracture, the bony trabeculae of the femoral head do not line up with the trabeculae of the acetabulum, indicating that the femoral head is rotated as a result of incomplete displacement between the fracture fragments. Theoretically, there may be remaining capsular attachments to the femoral head.
- Type IV: Complete fracture with total displacement of the fracture fragments, allowing the femoral head to rotate back to an anatomical position; radiographically, the bony trabeculae of the femoral head line up with the bony trabeculae of the acetabulum.

The comprehensive classification of long bone fractures described by the AO/ASIF (Arbeitsgemeinschaft für Osteosynthesefragen/Association for the Study of Internal Fixation) group ranges from 31B1 to 31B3 (where 31 is

Figure 5.3. The classification system proposed by Pauwels is based on the angle of inclination of the fracture line[1] (**A**): type I: fracture line 30° from the horizontal; type II: fracture line 50° from the horizontal; and type III: fracture line 70° from the horizontal. Radiograph of a Pauwels type III femoral neck fracture (**B**).

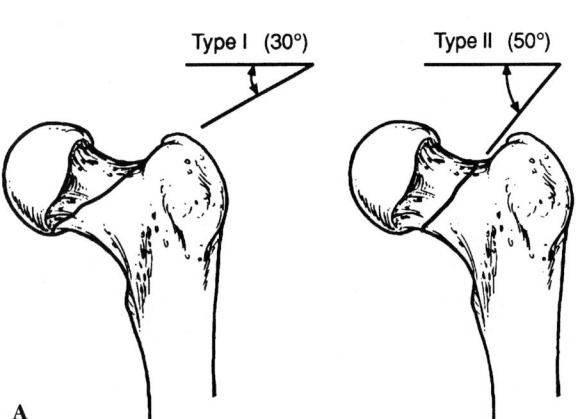
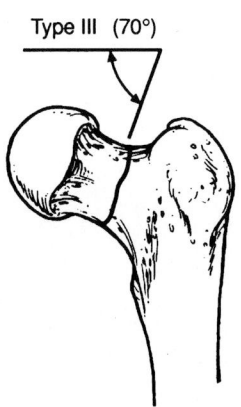
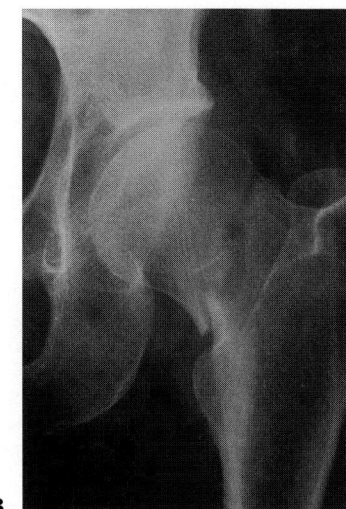

Classification

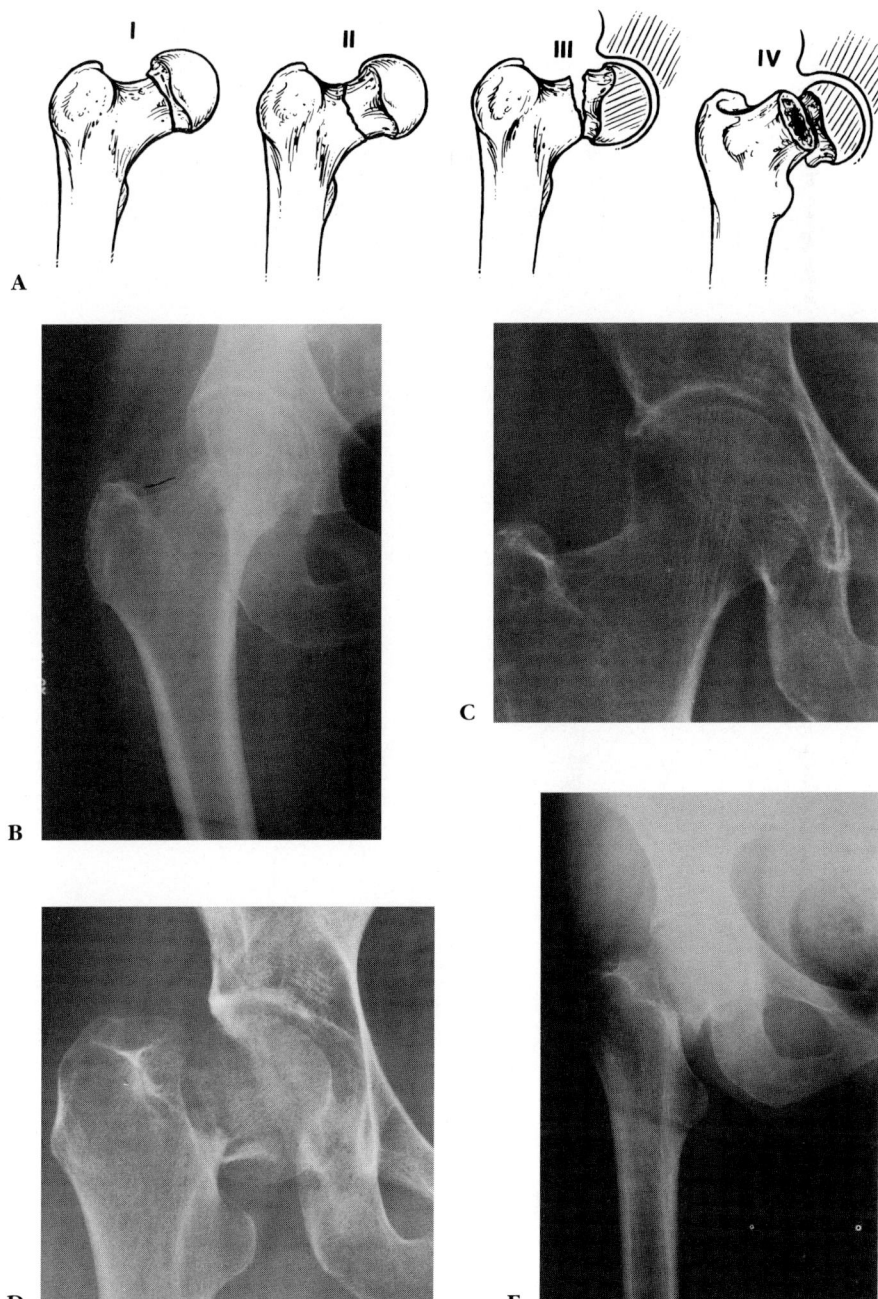

Figure 5.4. The Garden classification is based on the degree of fracture displacement on the AP radiograph[4] (**A**): Type I: incomplete or impacted fracture in which the bony trabeculae of the inferior portion of the femoral neck remains intact; this category includes "valgus-impacted" fractures. Type II: complete fracture without displacement of the fracture fragments. Type III: complete fracture with partial displacement of the fracture fragments; radiographically, in a type III fracture, the bony trabeculae of the femoral head do not line up with the trabeculae of the acetabulum. Type IV: complete fracture with total displacement of the fracture fragments, allowing the femoral head to rotate back to an anatomical position; radiographically, the bony trabeculae of the femoral head line up with the bony trabeculae of the acetabulum. Radiographs depicting a Garden I "valgus-impacted" fracture (**B**), Garden type II nondisplaced femoral neck fracture (**C**), Garden type III fracture (**D**), and Garden type IV fracture (**E**).

the proximal femur group and B the femoral neck subgroup)[5] (Figure 5.5). B1 fractures are subcapital fractures with slight displacement, B2 fractures are transcervical fractures, and B3 fractures are displaced subcapital fractures. Subcategorical codes further describe the fracture pattern and amount of fracture displacement. This schema is mainly used for research purposes.

Perhaps the simplest—and in many situations the best—approach is to classify femoral neck fractures as either nondisplaced (Garden types I and II) or displaced (Garden types III and IV). Further differentiation can be difficult to establish radiographically and has been shown to be subject to wide variability.[6]

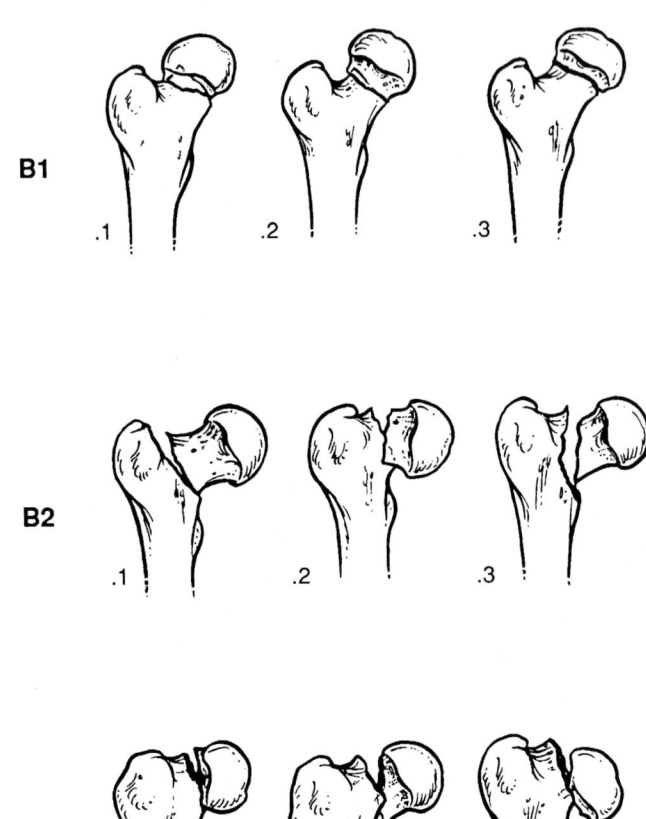

Figure 5.5. The comprehensive classification of long bone fractures described by the AO/ASIF group.[230] Femoral neck fractures comprise type 31B: B1 fractures are subcapital fractures with slight displacement, B2 fractures are transcervical fractures, and B3 fractures are displaced subcapital fractures. Subcategorical codes further describe the fracture pattern and amount of fracture displacement.

The nondisplaced/displaced schema, which has the virtue of grouping together fractures with similar treatment alternatives and similar prognoses, is our preference for classifying femoral neck fractures.

Effect of Femoral Neck Fracture on Vascular Supply

A major complication after femoral neck fracture is osteonecrosis of the femoral head, reported to occur in 9% to 35% of displaced femoral neck fractures.[7-13] Some authors have postulated that after displaced femoral neck fracture, with compromise of the retinacular vessels, the ligamentum teres system becomes the major source of blood supply for femoral head revascularization.[14] Focal mechanical failure of the femoral head during this process of revascularization and creeping substitution accounts for subsequent segmental collapse.[14]

The degree of fracture displacement determines the severity of damage to the major blood supply, the lateral epiphyseal artery system.[15] Dynamic blood flow studies in adult miniature swine have demonstrated that femoral neck fractures displaced 5 to 7 mm with an osteotome and then reduced anatomically produced a 60% decrease in femoral head blood flow.[16]

Intracapsular hematoma may elevate the capsular pressure sufficiently to occlude the venous drainage system within the capsule or even limit arteriolar flow in the retinacular reflection on the superior femoral neck. Several authors, utilizing a variety of techniques, have demonstrated experimentally that increased intracapsular pressure has an adverse effect on femoral head blood flow and may induce cellular death.[16-18] Other authors have documented increased intracapsular pressures in patients who have sustained a femoral neck fracture.[19-22] Furthermore, investigators have confirmed that extension and internal rotation of the hip elevate the intracapsular pressure by limiting capsular volume.[14] This position should therefore be avoided in the preoperative phase of treatment, and the position of flexion and external rotation, which increases capsular volume, should be encouraged.

Although the adverse effect of femoral neck fracture on femoral head blood flow has been documented with certainty, some elements of the situation remain under the surgeon's control. First, anatomic reduction of femoral neck fractures has been shown to lower the risk of femoral head osteonecrosis[8,23-26]; if some vessels of the lateral epiphyseal artery system remain intact, anatomic reduction may "unkink" them or, when reduction is performed after the acute phase, allow for rapid recanalization[14,27] (Figure 5.6). Second, stable fracture fixation allows revascularization to proceed in an optimal mechanical environment.[14] Third, although further vascular damage to the femoral head is unlikely with standard techniques of fixation, Brodetti has demonstrated that the posterior superior femoral head quadrant should be avoided because of the vicinity of the lateral epiphyseal artery system.[28]

The role of early aspiration or surgical decompression of the hemarthrosis in the management of femoral neck fractures, despite much investigation, remains controversial. Studies have shown that increased intracapsular pressure from hemarthrosis compromises femoral head vascularity and may lead to osteonecrosis in both nondisplaced and displaced fractures.[29-31] At one time it was thought that displaced fractures typically result in tearing of the capsule that would be expected to prevent accumulation of a significant hemarthrosis. Recent studies, however, have demonstrated that the capsule remains intact in as many as 60% of displaced femoral neck fractures.[19,32,33] Computed axial tomography, ultrasonography, bone scanning, and intracapsular pressure measurements have been used to quantify the effect of the hemarthrosis on femoral

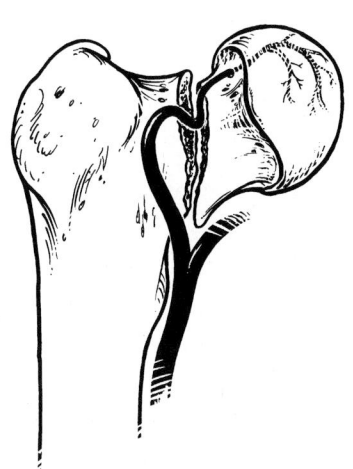

Figure 5.6. Illustration of a displaced femoral neck fracture with "kinking" of the lateral epiphyseal artery.

head blood flow. Crawford documented torn capsules and low pressures in 4 of 10 displaced fractures and 1 of 9 nondisplaced fractures[19]; in the remaining patients, the capsule was intact and distended to at least twice the size of the normal side. The highest pressures were noted in fractures with minimal or no displacement. Crawford therefore recommended early decompression of the hemarthrosis.

In a study of nondisplaced femoral neck fractures, Stromqvist et al. found elevated intracapsular pressures (>40 mm Hg) in 27 of 50 (54%) patients[34]; of the 27 patients, 16 had pressures over 80 mm Hg. A bone scan was performed on 25 patients: of 13 patients with reduced femoral blood flow, 9 showed a significant increase following hemarthrosis aspiration. Stromqvist et al. recommended avoiding preoperative traction and permitting semiflexion and external rotation of the hip. If the patient experienced hip pain at rest or with passive rotation, aspiration of the hemarthrosis was considered.

Several questions still remain regarding the clinical significance of the hemarthrosis and elevated intracapsular pressure, including the magnitude of the contribution to the development of significant long-term complications. Healing complications uncommonly occur in elderly patients with nondisplaced femoral neck fractures, even though these cases are shown to be the ones in which the intracapsular pressures are the highest. Although hip joint aspiration may indeed improve blood flow, it is likely that the hemarthrosis will reaccumulate, thus limiting the benefit of the procedure. Furthermore, the small incidence of revision surgery for healing complications in nondisplaced fractures may not justify aspirating all patients. More evidence is required before these questions are settled.

Treatment

Nonoperative Treatment

There is general agreement that surgical management is the treatment of choice for almost all hip fractures, including those involving the femoral neck. There are nevertheless exceptions to this general rule. Nonoperative management should be considered, for example, in patients whose severe medical problems place them at significant risk for perioperative mortality; on the other hand, prolonged bed rest in traction also poses a substantial risk for these patients. Therefore, if nonoperative treatment is chosen, it should include early patient mobilization with acceptance of the malunion or nonunion. Another situation in which nonoperative management may be preferred is for the demented, nonambulatory patient (Figure 5.7). The goal in treating these patients, as in treating all hip fracture patients, is return to their prefracture level of function. This may be accomplished by a few days of restricted activity followed by initiation of bed-to-chair transfers. These patients may be surprisingly comfortable, further obviating the need for surgical management.

Because impacted fractures (Garden type I) are inherently stable, some authors have recommended that patients with impacted femoral neck fractures be considered candidates for nonoperative management.[33] On the other hand, Bentley reported a disimpaction rate of 16% (7/43) in a series of impacted femoral neck fractures treated nonoperatively[35,36]; in 5 cases, fracture displacement occurred while the patient was restricted to bed rest. Holmberg et al.

Treatment

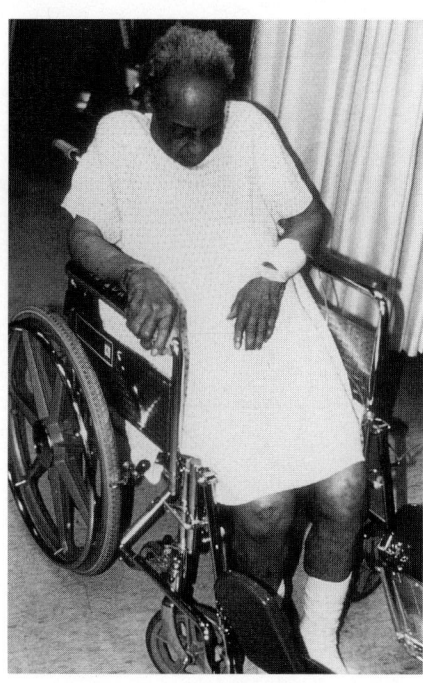

Figure 5.7. Nonoperative management was chosen for this demented, nonambulatory patient who experienced minimal discomfort after sustaining a displaced femoral neck fracture.

reported on a series of 48 impacted femoral neck fractures treated nonoperatively, of which 15 fractures (31%) had subsequent loss of reduction and required surgical treatment.[37] Recently, Peter et al. reported on a retrospective series of 124 impacted femoral neck fractures treated without surgery, 52 (42%) of which subsequently displaced; factors associated with fracture displacement included older patient age, senility, and higher amounts of valgus impaction or femoral head retroversion.[38] Nondisplaced femoral neck fractures that are not impacted (Garden type II) do not have the inherent stability of impacted fractures and are at even higher risk for fracture displacement.

Evolution of Surgical Techniques

In 1931, Smith-Petersen et al. published a report on the use of a triflanged nail for stabilization of femoral neck fractures (Figure 5.8); these authors performed an open reduction, fracture impaction, and nailing under direct visualization and reported fracture union in 15 of 20 (75%) patients.[39] Smith-Petersen subsequently became an advocate of closed reduction and insertion of the triflanged nail under roentgenographic control, arguing that closed reduction is less disruptive to the already compromised vascular supply of the femoral head.

The Smith-Petersen nail was subsequently modified by Johansson in 1932[40] and Wescott in 1934,[41] with cannulation so that the nail could be inserted over a guidewire (Figure 5.9). Henderson reported an 86% union rate in a series of 14 femoral neck fractures stabilized using this cannulated nail.[42] In a similar series, Eyre-Brook and Pridie, using a nail modified so as to make extraction easier, reported a 60% union rate after femoral neck fracture.[43]

Several major problems were associated with the Smith-Petersen nail, including its inability to maintain fracture reduction, implant backout from the proximal femur, and joint penetration through the femoral head. To secure lateral shaft fixation, Thornton added a sideplate[44] (Figure 5.10). Shortly afterward,

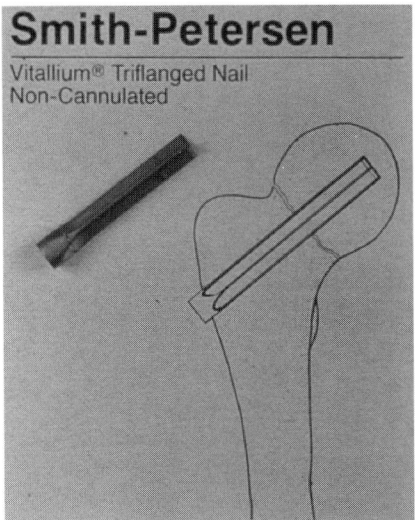

Figure 5.8. Photograph and drawing of a Smith-Petersen nail, used to stabilize a femoral neck fracture (courtesy of R. A. Calandruccio, The Campbell Clinic Foundation, Memphis TN).

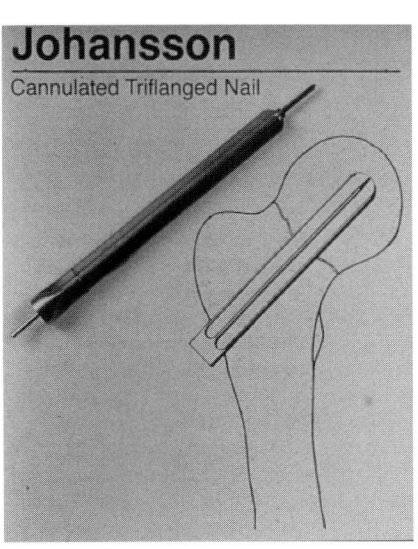

Figure 5.9. Photograph and drawing of a Johansson nail (courtesy of R. A. Calandruccio, The Campbell Clinic Foundation, Memphis TN).

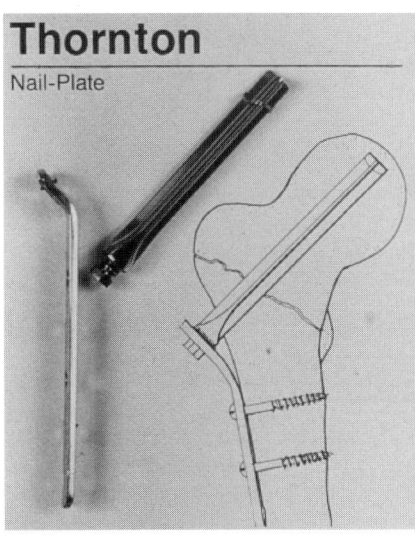

Figure 5.10. Photograph and drawing of a Thornton nail plate (courtesy of R. A. Calandruccio, The Campbell Clinic Foundation, Memphis TN).

serrations were added to the nail–plate junction to effect a more secure, interlocking design.[45] Jewett designed a one-piece nail by adding a sideplate to a triflanged nail[46] (Figure 5.11). Although he originally designed this device for use in pertrochanteric fractures, he later used it in a series of femoral neck fractures and obtained 80% good or excellent results, with a 16% nonunion rate and a 10.5% osteonecrosis rate.[47,48] Using a smaller rigid nail plate, Frangakis reported a 17% nonunion rate and a 29% osteonecrosis rate.[49] Eaton, using a similar device in 36 patients who sustained a displaced femoral neck fracture, reported 100% union, although he did not evaluate osteonecrosis.[50]

Because the one-piece nail plate did not permit fracture impaction, it was predisposed to a high incidence of nail protrusion into the hip joint. Subsequently, Charnley combined the concepts of controlled impaction and femoral shaft fixation in a compression screw: a spring-loaded screw and sleeve-plate combination designed to provide continuous fracture compression.[51] Results of series using this device to stabilize displaced femoral neck fractures, however, included a 40% nonunion rate.[52]

Sliding nail-plate devices were subsequently developed that allowed controlled fracture impaction. Pugh introduced a sliding nail consisting of a sideplate at a fixed angle of 135° with a keyed barrel to prevent rotation[53] (Figure 5.12); he reported union in 23 of 27 (85%) displaced femoral neck fractures. Jacobs, using the same device in 44 patients, obtained 73% satisfactory results, which he defined as fracture union without osteonecrosis.[54] Fielding, in a series of 256 displaced femoral neck fractures stabilized using a Pugh sliding nail, reported a 90% union rate and an osteonecrosis rate of 17%.[55,56] Massie, using a 150° sideplate with a triflanged telescoping nail (Figure 5.13), reported a 33% rate of osteonecrosis in a series of 201 displaced femoral neck fractures.[12]

The sliding nail plate for femoral neck fracture fixation next evolved into a sliding hip screw (Figure 5.14), whose advantages over the nail plate include

Treatment

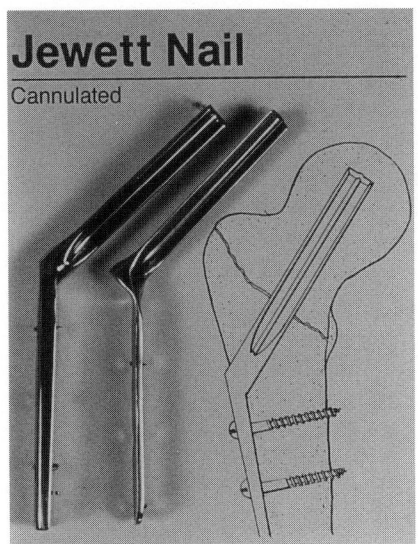

Figure 5.11. Photograph and drawing of a Jewett nail (courtesy of R. A. Calandruccio, The Campbell Clinic Foundation, Memphis TN).

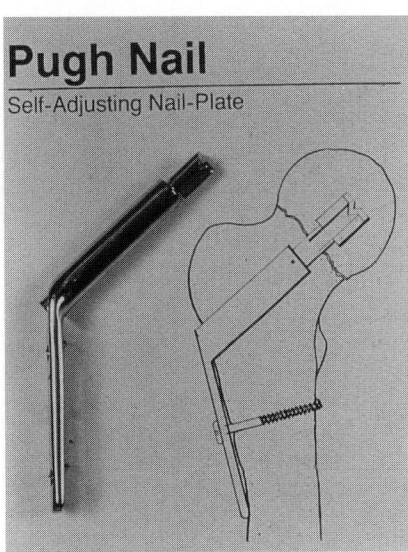

Figure 5.12. Photograph and drawing of a Pugh sliding nail (courtesy of R. A. Calandruccio, The Campbell Clinic Foundation, Memphis TN).

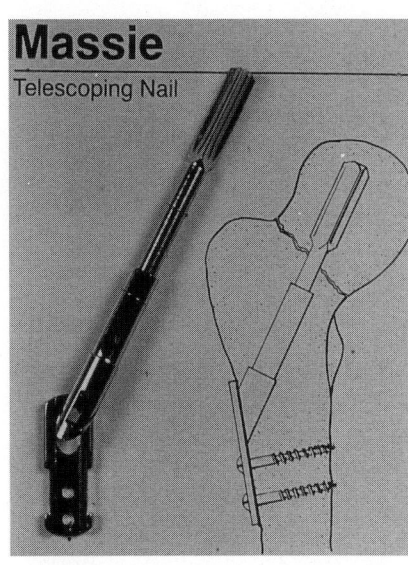

Figure 5.13. Photograph and drawing of a Massie sliding nail (courtesy of R. A. Calandruccio, The Campbell Clinic Foundation, Memphis TN).

the facts that (1) its large-diameter lag screw design may provide better fixation in osteopenic bone, and (2) lag screw insertion into the femoral head is generally less traumatic than nail impaction. When a sliding hip screw is used to stabilize an intracapsular fracture, the lag screw should be placed centrally within the femoral head to minimize the risk of femoral head rotation. Rotation of the femoral head may result in further damage to the retinacular vessels and may also occlude the vessels within the ligamentum teres. Rotation of the femoral head at surgery can also be minimized by inserting a second guidewire or antirotation screw across the fracture before insertion of the large diameter lag screw.

Svenningsen et al., in a randomized trial of 255 patients, reported results for the sliding hip screw that were superior to those for a fixed-angle plate[57]: a

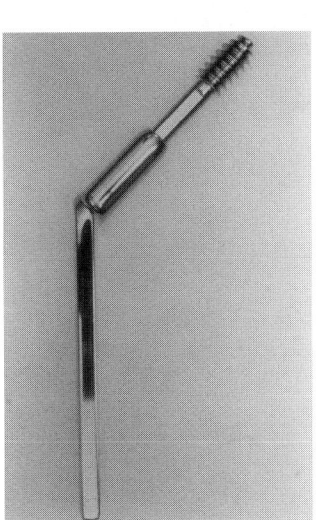

Figure 5.14. A sliding hip screw.

nonunion rate of 11% versus 25% and an osteonecrosis rate of 15% versus 21%. Nordkild et al. performed a randomized trial involving 49 patients and judged the sliding hip screw superior to the sliding nail plate, although the treatment results were not statistically significantly different.[58]

In an attempt to prevent rotation of the femoral head and minimize the trauma associated with device insertion, the use of multiple pins and screws was introduced for stabilization of femoral neck fractures. Moore designed a threaded pin with a beveled nut at its distal end to prevent pin penetration through the femoral head[59] (Figure 5.15); this implant was inserted using a multiple-pin technique. His first accounts described using four pins inserted in a crossed fashion to prevent femoral head rotation; he later recommended use of either three, four, or five parallel pins to allow fracture impaction. Using the latter technique, Moore reported union in 24 of 25 (96%) femoral neck fractures.[59] Kimbrough et al., in a series of 114 femoral neck fractures stabilized using four Moore pins, reported a 91% union and 6% osteonecrosis rate[60]; Kimbrough's group, however, did not differentiate between displaced and nondisplaced femoral neck fractures. Similar results were reported by Ackroyd[61] and by Modny and Kaiser.[62] In contrast, Green and Gay, applying the same technique to a series of 77 displaced femoral neck fractures, reported a 33% nonunion rate and a 42% osteonecrosis rate.[63]

Several other types of threaded pins have been designed (e.g., Knowles pins, Gouffon pins, Hagie pins) (Figure 5.16). Stappaerts and Broos reported that the incidence of nonunion with Knowles pins is reduced when one uses a minimum of six pins.[13] In a series of 754 displaced femoral neck fractures stabilized by percutaneous insertion of Knowles pins, Arnold et al. reported a 15% nonunion rate and a 12% osteonecrosis rate.[64] McCutchen and Carnesale reported that the union rate with Knowles pins was similar to that obtained using a Smith-Petersen nail but was inferior to that achieved by the Deyerle method of multiple-pin fixation (described later).[65]

At the Hospital for Joint Diseases, we conducted a prospective study comparing modified Knowles pins to cannulated cancellous lag screws for the treatment of nondisplaced (impacted) femoral neck fractures.[66] Forty-five such fractures were identified: 25 were stabilized with modified Knowles pins and 20 with cannulated cancellous lag screws. Patient follow-up averaged 24

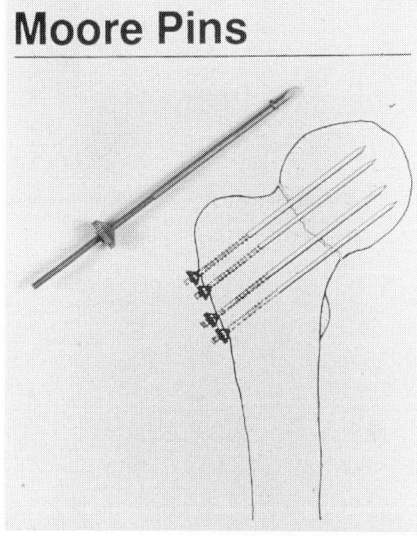

Figure 5.15. Photograph and drawing of Moore pins (courtesy of R. A. Calandruccio, The Campbell Clinic Foundation, Memphis TN).

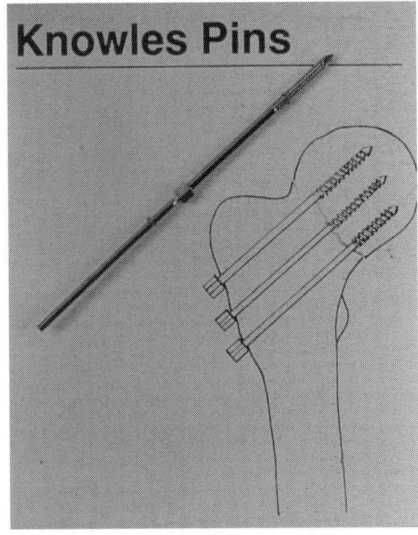 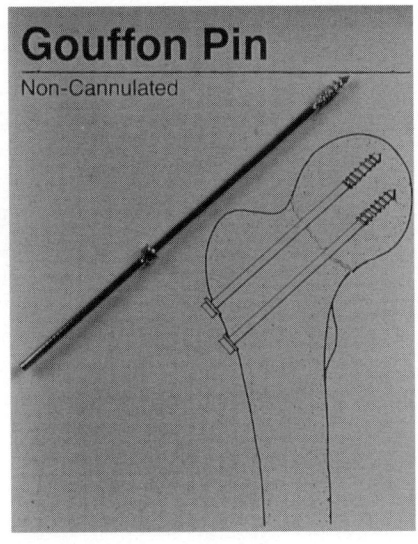 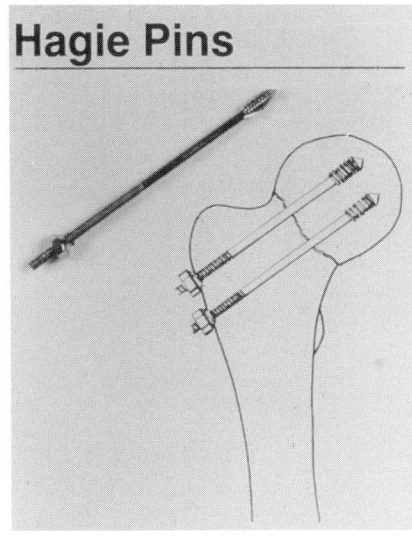

Figure 5.16. Photographs and drawings of Knowles pins (**A**), Gouffon pins (**B**), and Hagie pins (**C**) (courtesy of R. A. Calandruccio, The Campbell Clinic Foundation, Memphis TN).

months (range, 12 to 46 months). Six patients (13%) required revision surgery; these failures were evenly divided between the two groups. The remaining patients, 22 (88%) in the Knowles pin group and 17 (85%) in the cannulated screw group, were similar with respect to functional outcome.

In Sweden, Hansson hook pins have become popular for stabilization of femoral neck fractures (Figure 5.17). Initially designed to be used for stabilization of a slipped capital femoral epiphysis, these smooth, 6.5-mm-diameter

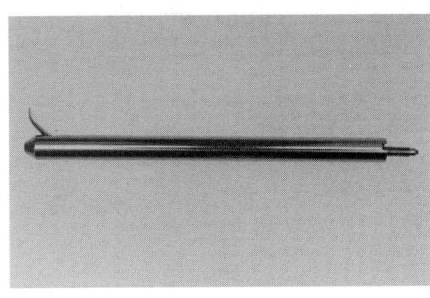

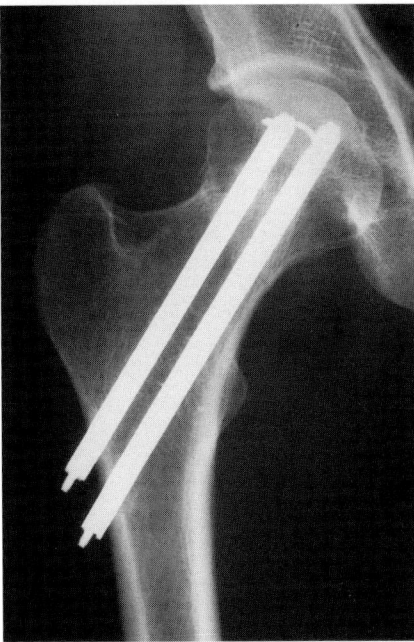

Figure 5.17. Photograph of a Hansson hook pin (**A**). AP radiograph demonstrating use of two hook pins to stabilize a femoral neck fracture (**B**).

pins have a retractable hook at the tip. Once the pins have been inserted, an extendible hook is extruded from the tip into the subchondral bone. The advantage claimed for this implant is preservation of the femoral head blood supply, since the pins are "slid" into position through prepared channels without hammering or screw rotation.

The use of Hansson hook pins for stabilization of femoral neck fractures has been described by many authors. Stromqvist et al. reported on a prospective randomized series of 152 femoral neck fractures in patients more than 50 years of age; fractures were stabilized using either two hook pins or a four-flanged nail.[67] The incidence of healing complications was significantly lower in displaced femoral neck fractures stabilized using the hook pins. The same authors also performed a prospective study to evaluate the effect of these two implants on the vascularity of the femoral head.[29] A significantly lower postoperative isotope uptake was noted in fractures stabilized with the four-flanged nail.

A subsequent study by Stromqvist and Hansson reported on a series of 300 femoral neck fractures stabilized using multiple Hansson hook pins.[68] At 2-year follow-up examination, 56 fractures (19%) had developed radiographic signs of healing complications—e.g., fracture displacement, nonunion, or segmental femoral head collapse. Three of 85 nondisplaced fractures (4%) developed segmental collapse, while among displaced fractures, there was radiographic evidence of healing complications in 53 of 215 cases (25%). For the entire series, secondary hip arthroplasty was performed in 34 cases (11%).

Deyerle, combining the concepts of multiple-pin and lateral-shaft fixation for stabilization of femoral neck fractures, inserted multiple pins into the subchondral bone of the femoral head through a plate-guide combination at a preselected angle (140°)[69] (Figure 5.18). The pins had threaded tips and smooth shafts to allow them to slide in the femoral cortex. Deyerle emphasized the need for a valgus reduction, impacted at the time of surgery, to

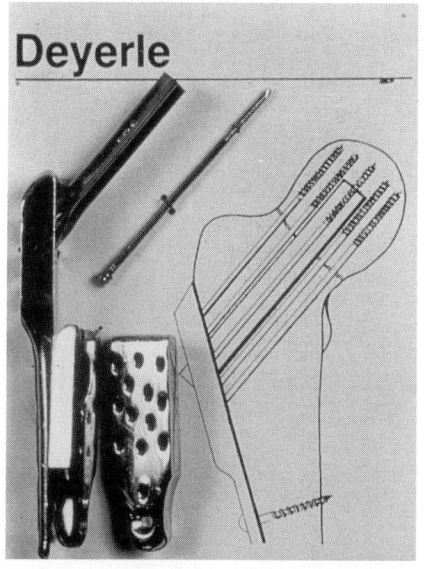
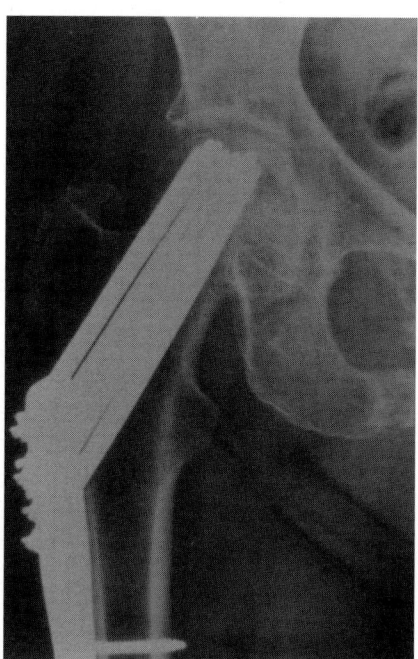

Figure 5.18. Photograph and drawing of the Deyerle pin plate (**A**) (courtesy of R. A. Calandruccio, The Campbell Clinic Foundation, Memphis TN). AP radiograph demonstrating use of the Deyerle plate to stabilize a femoral neck fracture (**B**).

optimize osseous union. He used this method of fixation in a series of 174 femoral neck fractures and reported a 1% nonunion rate and a 6% osteonecrosis rate.[69] In a subgroup of 111 displaced femoral neck fractures, these rates were 1.8% and 9%, respectively. Metz et al. reported similar results: 7% nonunion and 12% osteonecrosis in 39 patients who had sustained a femoral neck fracture.[70] Unfortunately, these excellent results could not be easily replicated. Chapman et al., reporting 18% nonunion and 31% osteonecrosis rates in 59 femoral neck fractures followed for a minimum of 2 years, cited several intraoperative technical problems as well as late postoperative complications related to pin penetration of the femoral head.[71] Similar problems were reported by Baker and Barrick in 27 of 101 (27%) patients followed up for a minimum of 2 years.[72] The eventual consensus was that although Deyerle's principles were sound, the operation itself was technically difficult and was most successful when performed by surgeons thoroughly experienced with the technique.

A cancellous lag screw is currently the most commonly used implant for stabilization of femoral neck fractures. Many different types of screws have been designed for femoral neck fixation, including Von Bahr, Uppsala, Garden, AO/ASIF, and Asnis screws (Figure 5.19). These screws are of varying diameter; some are cannulated and can be inserted over a guidewire. Use of all these implants follows common basic principles (Figure 5.20): (1) multiple screws are needed to provide fixation of the femoral head and neck (the optimal number needed is controversial); (2) the screws should be inserted in parallel; (3) screw threads should pass completely across the fracture to provide fracture compression; (4) one screw should be inserted adjacent to the cortex of the inferior femoral neck to resist varus displacement of the femoral head, and one screw should be adjacent to the cortex of the posterior femoral neck to resist posterior displacement; (5) the tips of the screws should lie within 5 mm of the subchondral bone; and (6) the screws should be spread apart to maximize fixation stability.

Madsen et at. reported a randomized trial comparing use of a sliding hip screw with a supplementary antirotation screw to stabilization by the use of four cancellous lag screws.[73] Their results showed no significant difference in

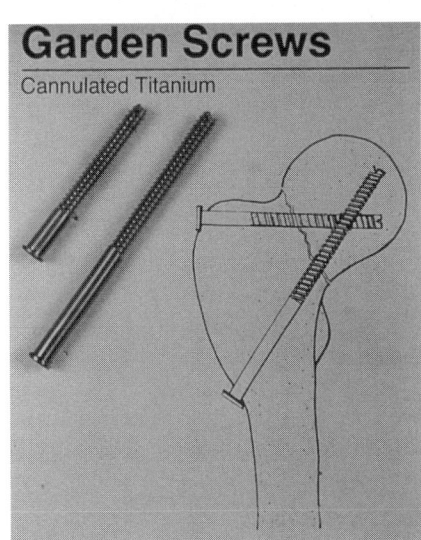
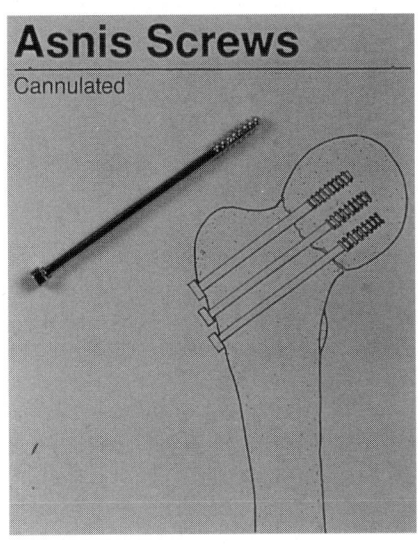
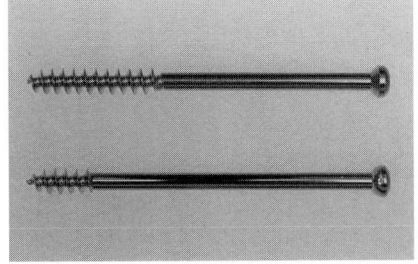

Figure 5.19. Photograph and drawing of Garden screws (**A**) (courtesy of R. A. Calandruccio, The Campbell Clinic Foundation, Memphis TN). Photograph and drawing of Asnis screws (**B**) (courtesy of R. A. Calandruccio, The Campbell Clinic Foundation, Memphis TN). Photograph of AO/ASIF 6.5-mm cancellous lag screws (**C**).

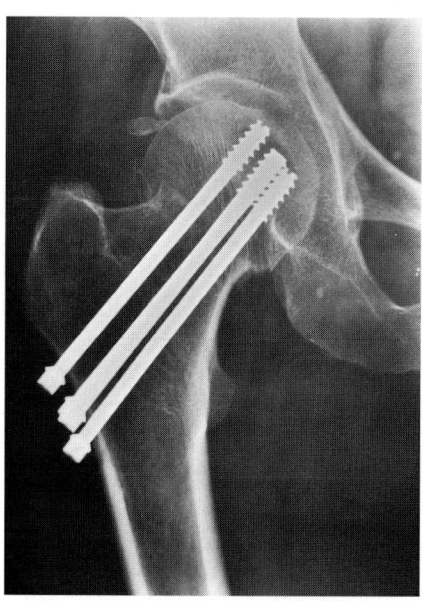

Figure 5.20. AP radiograph of a femoral neck fracture stabilized with three parallel cancellous lag screws.

the incidence of osteonecrosis. The union rate, however, was 73% for lag screws but only 49% with use of the sliding hip screw. In addition, operative time was shorter with lag screw fixation, and intraoperative blood loss was less. Technetium 99m medronate disodium scintimetry on these patients revealed a significantly greater uptake of isotope in patients treated with the parallel screws. It was suggested that damage to the vascular supply of the femoral head with use of the sliding hip screw may be caused by the reaming process or by rotation of the femoral head during insertion of the sliding hip screw.

Several biomechanical studies have demonstrated that multiple cancellous screws and pins provide fixation equal to that of a sliding hip screw in a subcapital and transcervical fracture model. Husby et al. reported comparable fixation strength of two 5-mm lag screws and a sliding hip screw in a femoral neck fracture model.[74,75] Van Audekercke et al. reported equivalent loads to failure of experimentally created femoral neck fractures stabilized with multiple Knowles pins or a sliding hip screw.[76]

Consideration of some basic concepts regarding screw design is warranted. Screw strength is exponentially related to core diameter; a 13% increase in core diameter produces a 44% increase in screw torsional strength. Cancellous screws have a relatively thin core and a wide, deep thread; this large outer thread/core diameter provides increased holding power in trabecular bone. Self-tapping screws cut their own thread during insertion, whereas non–self-tapping screws may require cutting the thread in cortical bone by using a tap before screw insertion; both types of screws have similar holding power in the femoral head. Reverse-cutting threads facilitate screw removal. A variety of thread lengths are available. A long thread is desirable to optimize fixation stability; however, the screw thread must completely cross the fracture site to provide compression. Both cannulated and noncannulated cancellous screws are commercially available; cannulated screws are easier to insert and are more commonly used for femoral neck fixation than solid screws.

The optimal number and implant pattern for the use of cancellous lag screws in femoral neck fixation have been studied in several biomechanical models. Mizrahi et al. demonstrated that three screws placed in a triangular

Treatment

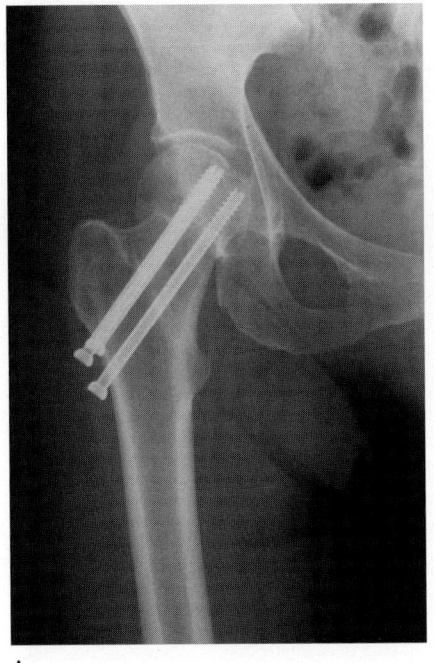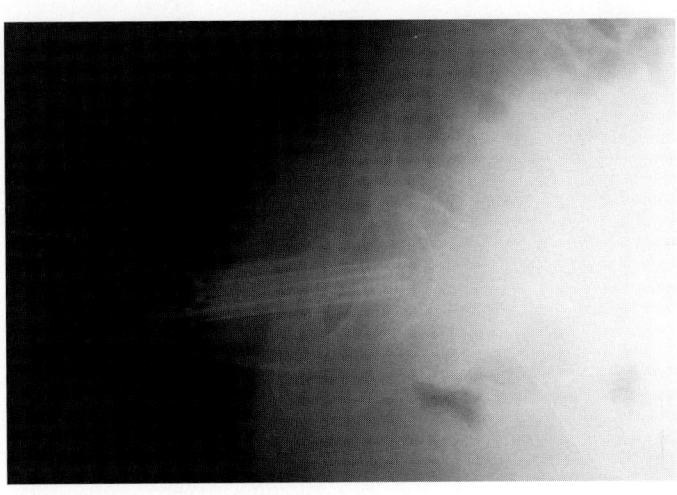

A   **B**

Figure 5.21. AP (**A**) and lateral (**B**) radiographs demonstrating use of three screws placed in a triangular pattern with two screws superior and one inferior to stabilize a femoral neck fracture.

pattern with two screws superior and one inferior constitutes the optimum screw configuration for the treatment of femoral neck fractures[77] (Figure 5.21). Swiontkowski et al., in a torsional and bending analysis of internal fixation techniques in a noncomminuted femoral neck fracture model, concluded that there was no justification for the use of more than three screws for the treatment of femoral neck fractures.[78] In a recent study performed at the Hospital for Joint Diseases, however, we demonstrated that the use of four cancellous screws provided better fixation stability than three screws in a femoral neck fracture model with posterior comminution.[79]

Operative Technique

Nondisplaced Fractures

Impacted and nondisplaced femoral neck fractures should undergo in situ internal fixation using multiple cancellous lag screws. Care must be taken to prevent fracture displacement when transferring the patient into bed or onto the operating table. The patient is positioned supine on a fracture table with both lower extremities resting in foot holders. A padded perineal post is placed in the ipsilateral groin; care must be taken that there is no impingement of the labia or scrotum. The uninvolved leg is then flexed, abducted, and externally rotated to allow positioning of the image intensifier for a lateral view (Figure 5.22). Alternatively, the contralateral extremity can be abducted with the hip and knee extended (Figure 5.23); this maneuver, however, places greater pressure from the fracture post on the perineum.[80]

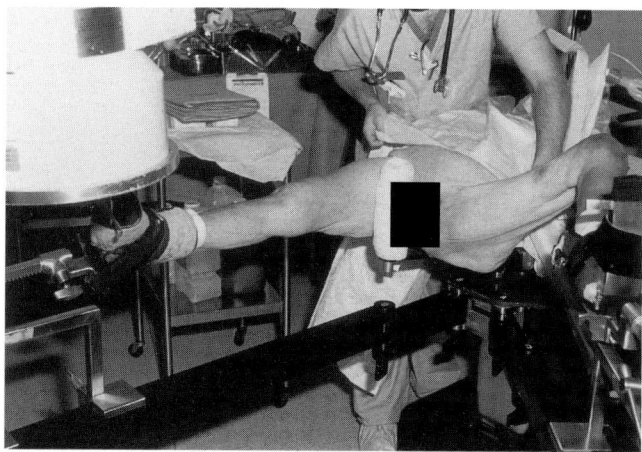

Figure 5.22. At surgery, the patient is placed on a fracture table; the uninvolved leg is then flexed, abducted, and externally rotated to allow positioning of the image intensifier for a lateral view.

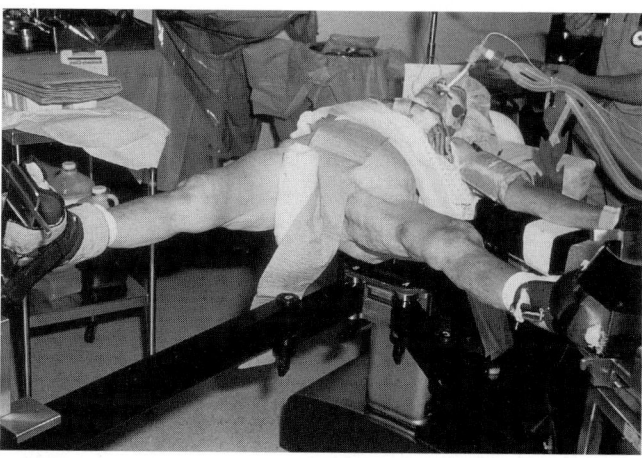

Figure 5.23. Abduction of the contralateral extremity with the hip and knee extended to allow positioning of the image intensifier for a lateral view.

Before preparing the lower extremity, the surgeon must ensure that the fracture has remained reduced and that unobstructed biplanar radiographic visualization of the entire proximal femur, including the hip joint, is obtainable (Figure 5.24). The lower extremity, from the pelvis to the lower thigh, is then prepared and draped. For this purpose, we prefer an isolation screen.

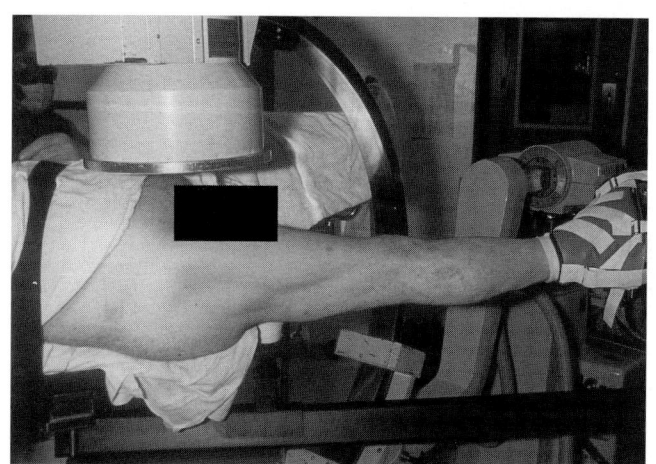

A

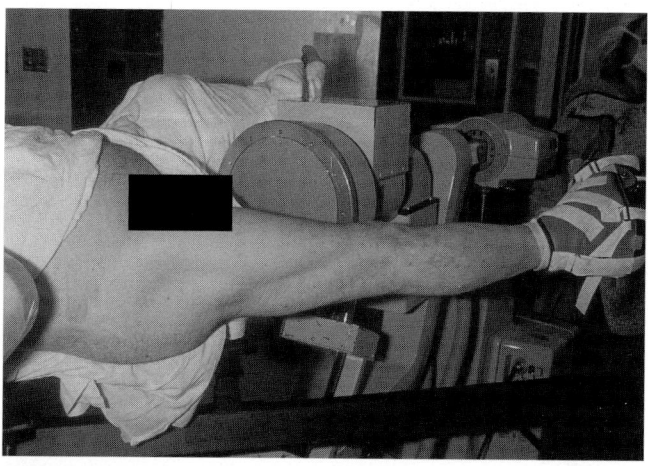

B

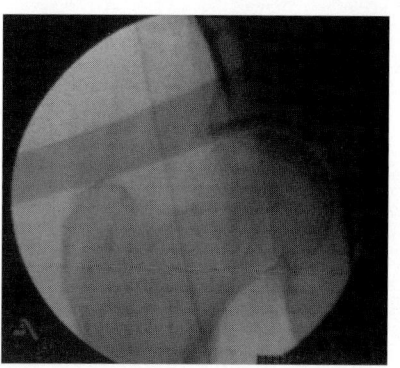

C

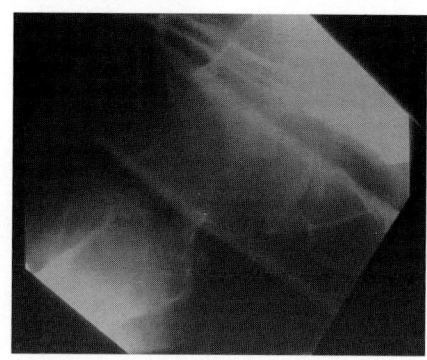

D

Figure 5.24. Positioning of the image intensifier in the AP (**A**) and lateral (**B**) planes to obtain nonobstructive biplanar radiographic visualization of the entire proximal femur (**C, D**).

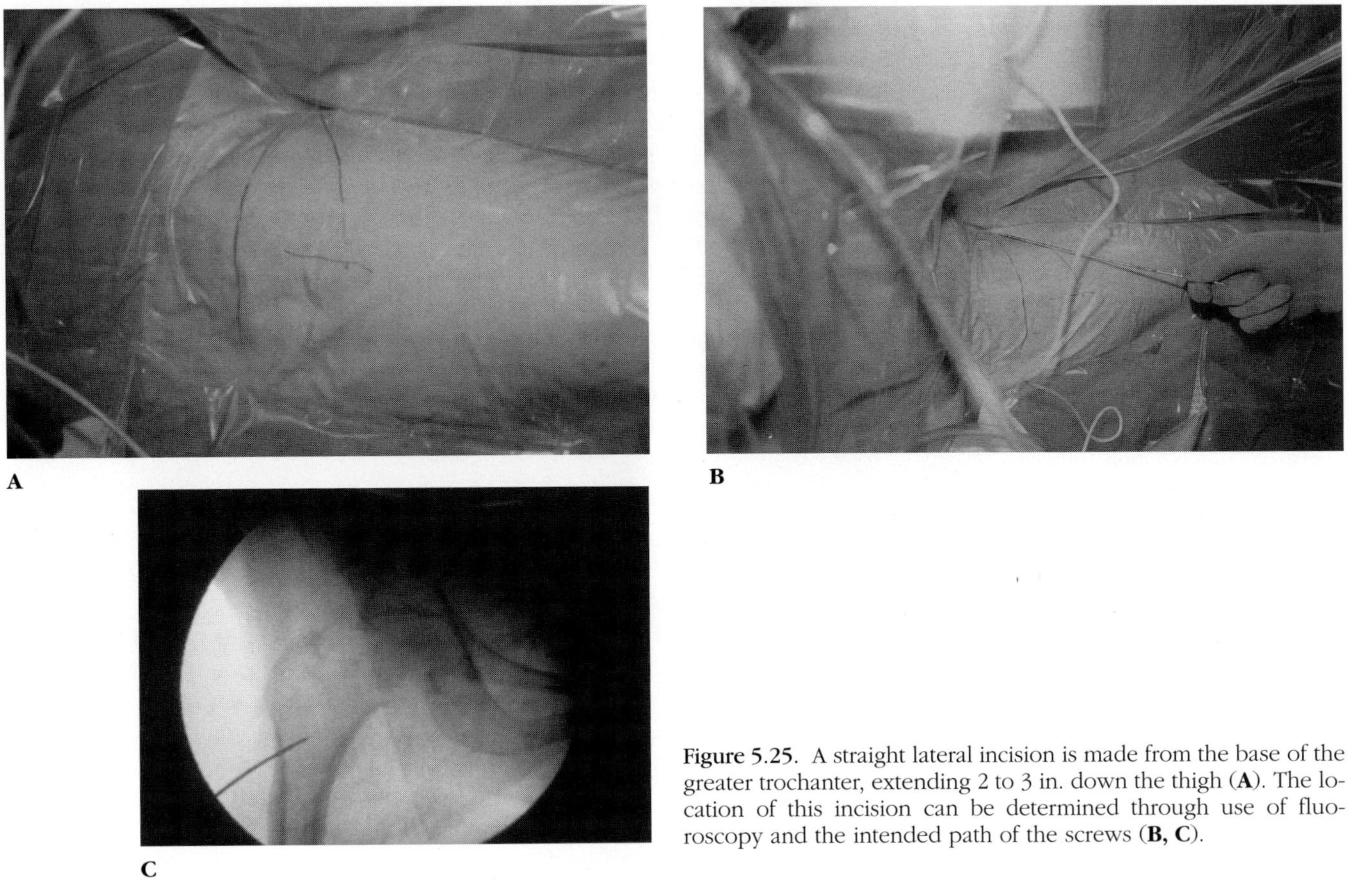

Figure 5.25. A straight lateral incision is made from the base of the greater trochanter, extending 2 to 3 in. down the thigh (**A**). The location of this incision can be determined through use of fluoroscopy and the intended path of the screws (**B, C**).

Although the screws can be inserted percutaneously, we prefer a limited open technique to facilitate screw insertion. A straight lateral incision is made from the base of the greater trochanter, extending 2 to 3 in. down the thigh (Figure 5.25). After incision of the skin and subcutaneous tissue, the iliotibial band is divided longitudinally, with care taken to ensure that the deep dissection remains posterior to the tensor fasciae latae muscle proximally (Figure 5.26). The vastus lateralis fascia is divided longitudinally to expose its muscle

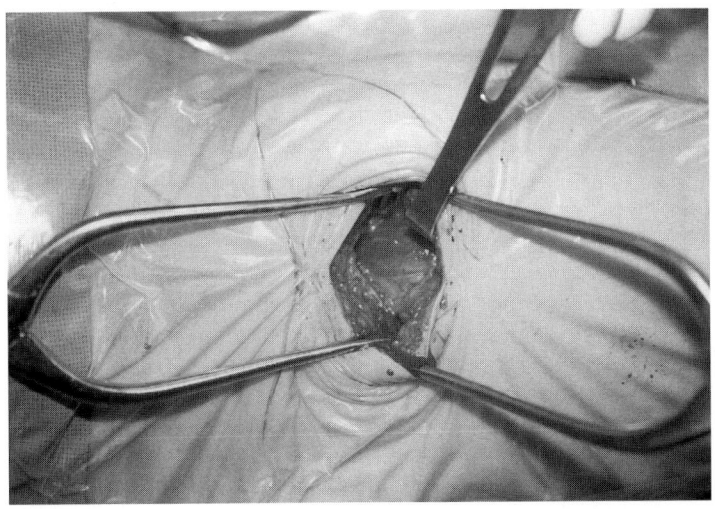

Figure 5.26. After incision of the skin and subcutaneous tissue, the iliotibial band is divided longitudinally, exposing the vastus lateralis muscle.

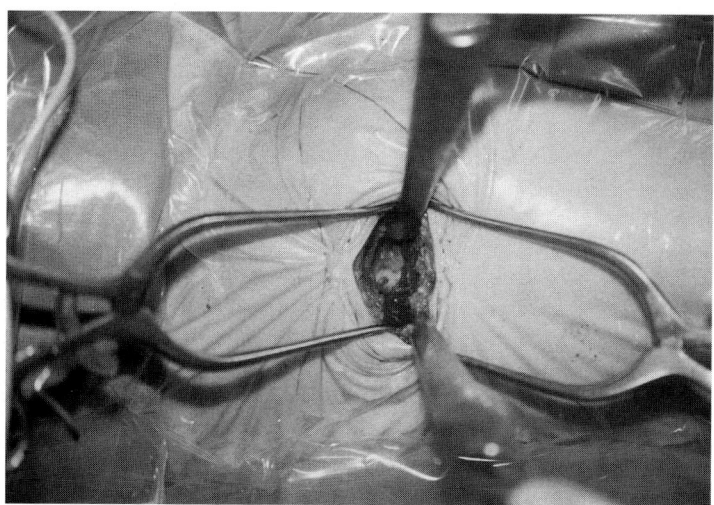

Figure 5.27. Placement of a Homan retractor under the vastus lateralis muscle, just proximal to the insertion of the gluteus maximus muscle, exposing the lateral femur.

fibers, and the posterior portion of the fascia is elevated off the underlying muscle down to the linea aspera. A Hohmann retractor is placed under the vastus lateralis muscle, just proximal to the insertion of the gluteus maximus muscle (Figure 5.27). The vastus lateralis muscle is then elevated from the lateral femur in a posterior-to-anterior direction, with care taken to identify and ligate the perforating branches of the profunda femoris artery.

Three guidewires are inserted into the femoral neck and head under image intensification. A guidewire can be placed anterior to the femoral neck to estimate femoral neck anteversion, but we find this unnecessary. The guidewires should all be parallel and oriented in an inverted triangular configuration, with one wire inferior and two wires superior; this orientation provides the most mechanically secure fracture fixation (Figure 5.28). The guidewires can be inserted using an insertion apparatus or a freehand technique; we prefer a freehand technique. The inferior wire is placed adjacent to the inferior neck cortex (to resist varus displacement), while one of the two superior wires is adjacent to the posterior femoral cortex (to resist posterior displacement). These guidewires should be spaced apart to maximize fixation stability and should be inserted into the dense subchondral bone. Once the guidewire positions have been set, the screw lengths are determined (Figure 5.29). The screws should lie in the dense subchondral bone for optimal fixation, and the threads should completely cross the fracture site. The outer cortex of the proximal femur is then reamed and the screws inserted (Figure 5.30). There is no need to ream the entire screw tract; in fact, this can result in loss of the guidewire during reamer removal. Good-quality radiographs are necessary to

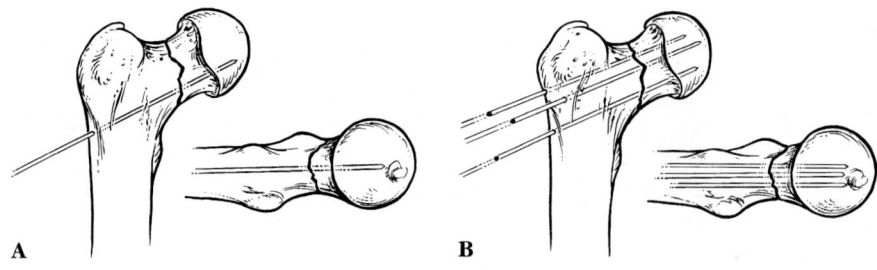

Figure 5.28. Placement of three guidewires into the femoral neck and head under image intensification. The guidewires should all be parallel and oriented in an inverted triangular configuration, with one wire inferior and two wires superior. The inferior wire is placed first, adjacent to the inferior neck cortex (**A**), followed by placement of two superior wires, one of which should lie adjacent to the posterior femoral cortex (**B**).

Treatment

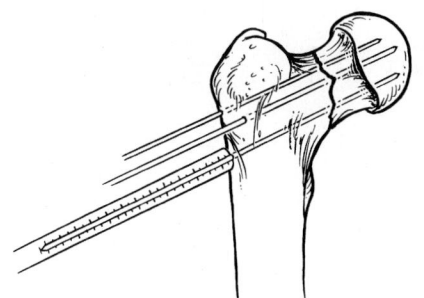

Figure 5.29. Determination of the screw lengths using a cannulated depth gauge.

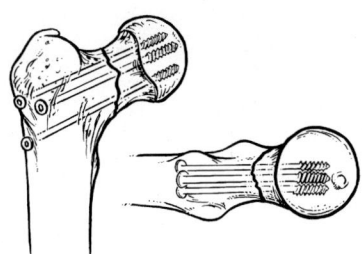

Figure 5.30. Insertion of the three cannulated cancellous lag screws.

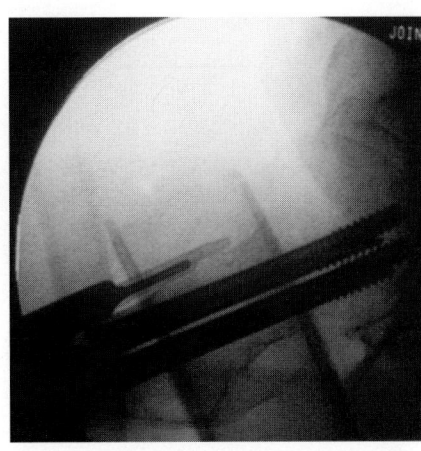

Figure 5.31. After insertion of the lag screws, a capsulotomy is performed under image intensification using a scalpel directed along the anterior femoral neck.

confirm proper placement of the screws, including rotation of the proximal femur under fluoroscopy to detect possible intraarticular screw penetration. After screw insertion, any traction is released and the screws are retightened. Because capsular distention with increased intracapsular pressure has been implicated as a possible cause of posttraumatic osteonecrosis, we usually perform a capsulotomy at surgery; the capsulotomy is performed under image intensification using a scalpel directed along the anterior femoral neck (Figure 5.31). The wound is closed in layers over suction drains.

Displaced Fractures

Whereas virtually all patients with a nondisplaced femoral neck fracture should be treated by internal fixation, this is not the case for displaced femoral neck fractures. The relatively high risk of nonunion and osteonecrosis with late segmental collapse has made primary prosthetic replacement a popular treatment option, particularly for displaced femoral neck fractures in elderly patients. Since prosthetic replacement is the treatment of choice in the elderly in cases of symptomatic nonunion and osteonecrosis following internal fixation, primary prosthetic replacement has been advocated for these high-risk fractures as a means of reducing the need for revision surgery.

The choice of internal fixation over prosthetic replacement may be difficult. Although different authors have provided indications for primary prosthetic replacement based on various criteria, we do not believe that specific indications based solely on patient care or fracture type are preferable or even possible. Rather, each clinical situation should be assessed individually, with careful consideration of patient factors (e.g., physiologic patient age, associated medical problems) and fracture factors (e.g., bone quality, amount of comminution, interval from injury to surgical treatment) to arrive at a treatment decision. If successful, fracture reduction (either closed or open) and internal fixation provide the best and most durable result after displaced femoral neck fracture. Rodriguez et al., reviewing multiple factors and concentrating on morbidity and mortality, reported internal fixation to be the most innocuous method of treatment.[81] We feel that elderly individuals who have sustained a displaced femoral neck fracture and are relatively healthy, have minimal fracture comminution, and can undergo surgery within 24 to 48 hours of injury, should have an attempt at fracture reduction and internal fixation. Fixation problems, although not always predictable, are most common in patients with osteopenic bone and posterior femoral neck comminution.

Prosthetic replacement of the proximal femur avoids the problems of nonunion and osteonecrosis but may be associated with higher perioperative morbidity than internal fixation. Additionally, it poses the potential of late problems of prosthetic loosening and acetabular erosion, either of which may require revision surgery. Furthermore, results after revision of failed hemiarthroplasty are not equivalent to those after primary total hip arthroplasty, and the procedure may be quite difficult.[14,82] Therefore, we feel that hemiarthroplasty should be restricted to older, less healthy, and low-demand individuals. Variations in arthroplasty implants and technique may increase their durability and ease of revision, although the data to support this assertion are not yet conclusive.

Factors favoring prosthetic replacement over internal fixation include pathologic bone, severe chronic illness (especially rheumatoid arthritis and chronic renal failure), and a limited life expectancy. Inactive elderly patients are candidates for modular or Austin-Moore–type unipolar hemiarthroplasty. Those with displaced femoral neck fractures who can ambulate functionally outside the home (community ambulators) and whose likelihood of success with internal fixation is low should receive a modular unipolar or bipolar hemiarthroplasty—with the awareness that revision may be required in the future because of loosening of the femoral component or acetabular degenerative changes, including protrusion. The risk of these problems is greater in younger, more active individuals.

Conscientiousness in obtaining an adequate reduction and proper use of multiple-screw or multiple-pin fixation has lowered the rate of internal fixation failure and nonunion to 10% or less in recent series.[14] Although osteonecrosis occurs in 10% to 30% of displaced femoral neck fractures, the symptoms may not be so severe as to require treatment, particularly in lower-demand individuals.[14] If they are, salvage with total hip arthroplasty is indicated.

Stromqvist et al. reported on a series of 215 consecutive displaced femoral neck fractures treated with internal fixation.[68] At 2-year follow-up, 63 patients (29%) had died. Of the survivors, 53 (25%) developed a healing complication: fracture displacement or nonunion in 39 and osteonecrosis with segmental collapse in 14 patients. These complications led to revision surgery in 36 (17%), including 31 total hip arthroplasties, 4 hardware removal procedures, and 1 osteotomy. The authors noted that 83% of patients did not require revision surgery.

At the Hospital for Joint Diseases, the strategy for treating displaced femoral neck fractures involves internal fixation, after closed or open reduction, for the majority of patients with adequate bone density. We treat this fracture as an urgent situation with rapid medical stabilization and surgical treatment within 24 hours of admission whenever possible. Prosthetic replacement is reserved for physiologically older individuals in whom internal fixation is unlikely to succeed: those with marked osteopenia and/or fracture comminution. Such patients tend to be biologically older and have lower functional demands. They may be unable to ambulate without assistive devices, and associated medical problems often limit their life expectancy.

Surgical Timing

The effect of surgical delay on the incidence of osteonecrosis and nonunion after displaced femoral neck fracture has been reviewed by several investigators. Massie demonstrated a direct relationship between delay of fracture reduction and incidence of osteonecrosis[12]; fractures reduced within 12 hours of injury had a 25% incidence of osteonecrosis, whereas for fractures reduced more than 7 days after injury, the rate was 100%. In a study by Graham, however, surgical delay for up to 3 days after injury had no effect on nonunion or late segmental collapse.[83] Barnes et al. similarly found that a surgical delay of up to 5 days had no effect on the development of osteonecrosis.[8] Similarly, results of the Orthopedic Trauma Hospital Association's series of younger patients revealed no increase in the rates of osteonecrosis or nonunion in treatment delayed up to 5 days.[84]

Focusing on shorter time spans, Manninger et al. studied the effects of reduction and internal fixation performed before and after 6 hours postinjury on the development of osteonecrosis and late segmental collapse.[85] They reported a significantly lower incidence of segmental collapse in patients treated within 6 hours. At 1-year follow-up, 1.9% of 155 fractures in the early-treatment group and 19.3% of 181 cases in the delayed-treatment group had experienced segmental collapse; follow-up at 2 years, 3 years, and 6 to 10 years revealed segmental collapse rates of 11.0%, 19.4%, and 36.8% respectively in the early-treatment group and 37.4%, 51.0%, and 63.9% in the delayed-treatment group. Furthermore, more patients in the delayed-treatment group developed nonunion. It is also interesting to note that in the early-treatment group, segmental collapse often involved only a portion of the femoral head, whereas total head involvement was much more common in the delayed-treatment group.

Taking all the data into account, we prefer to perform surgery as soon as possible following medical stabilization. Although this does not guarantee the prevention of healing complications, it probably does decrease the potential risk.

Assessment of Femoral Head Viability

Several authors have advocated the assessment of femoral head viability as a means of determining either the surgical procedure to be performed or the risk for healing complications following internal fixation.[86-88] The usefulness of preoperative and postoperative technetium bone scanning for this purpose, however, remains controversial. Advocates of the preoperative scan contend that it provides information valuable for the purpose of avoiding a second operation; advocates of postoperative scans claim that preoperative scans do not accurately predict outcome, particularly regarding the extent to which femoral head vascularity may be altered in the course of surgery.

Turner reported on a series of 30 patients who underwent preoperative technetium 99m antimony colloid scintimetry within 24 hours of femoral neck fracture.[89] Of the 12 patients with an abnormal scan, 11 (92%) developed symptomatic osteonecrosis within 2 years of injury. Normal healing occurred in 15 of 16 hips (94%) with preservation of marrow uptake in the femoral head; late segmental collapse developed in the remaining hip.

Many authors emphasize that even a nonviable femoral head that develops osteonecrosis may ultimately have a good functional result.[33] Thus, a technetium scan indicating a nonviable femoral neck is not necessarily predictive of a poor outcome. Stromqvist et al. studied 490 femoral neck fractures using technetium 99m medronate disodium scintimetry and tetracycline labeling.[90] They found that a preoperative scan was a poor predictor of outcome, particularly when considering the effects of various fixation devices and insertion techniques on femoral head vascularity.

Postoperative bone scintimetry has been used to predict healing complications after femoral neck fracture. In a series of 46 patients who sustained a femoral neck fracture and underwent postoperative bone scintimetry, healing complications were associated with decreased technetium uptake in early and 2-month scintimetry, but the specificity was only 50%.[91] With normal uptake, uncomplicated union was predicted with 90% to 100% sensitivity.

We believe that neither preoperative nor postoperative bone scanning is particularly helpful in the great majority of femoral neck fractures. Similarly, it has recently been shown that the use of magnetic resonance imaging in the first 2 weeks after femoral neck fracture is not predictive for the development of posttraumatic osteonecrosis.[92–94]

Operative Technique for Internal Fixation

The patient is positioned supine on a fracture table that can be converted into a flat operating table if closed reduction is unsuccessful and prosthetic replacement becomes necessary. A wide range of closed reduction techniques have been described.[12,43,69,95,96] Some authors advocate using forceful maneuvers to effect fracture reduction, while others recommend gentler reduction techniques. Some are proponents of reduction maneuvers in hip extension, while others argue for the importance of the same maneuvers performed with the hip flexed. Our approach is to flex the hip of the injured extremity 90° with external rotation to disengage the fracture fragments (Figure 5.32). Traction is applied as the leg is internally rotated and brought into full extension (Figure 5.33). The maximum internal rotation of the injured lower extremity is then compared to the uninjured leg (Figure 5.34); if the two do not match, then a successful reduction has most probably not been obtained. The image

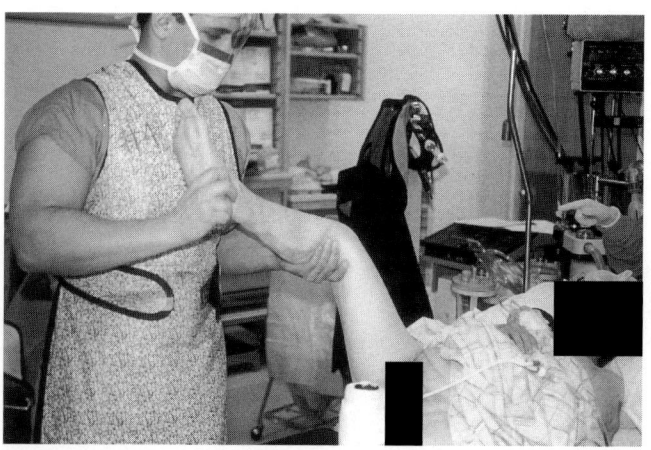

Figure 5.32. Closed reduction of a displaced femoral neck fracture involves hip flexion with external rotation to disengage the fracture fragments.

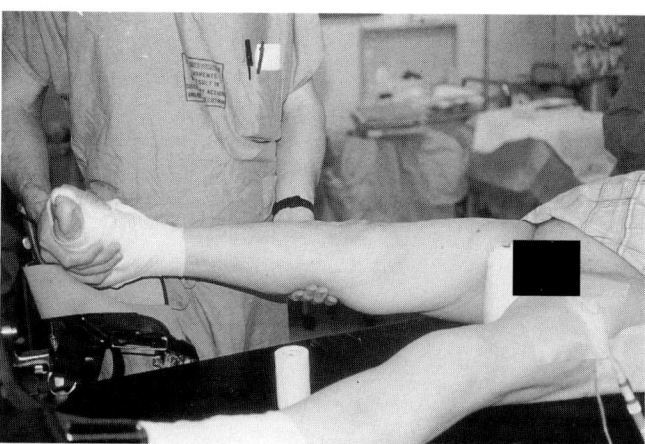

Figure 5.33. Traction is applied as the leg is internally rotated and brought into full extension.

Treatment

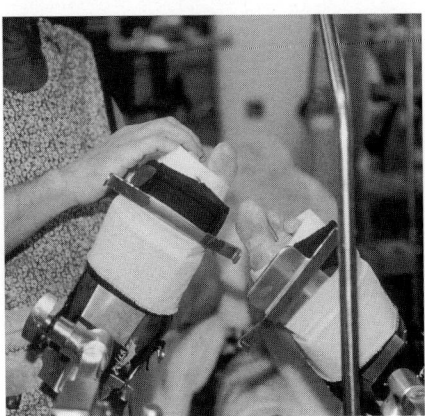

Figure 5.34. The maximum internal rotation of the injured lower extremity is compared to that of the uninjured leg; if the two do not match, then a successful reduction has probably not been obtained.

intensifier, however, should be used for AP and lateral assessment of the adequacy of the fracture reduction.

An adequate reduction is probably the most important factor affecting the incidence of nonunion and osteonecrosis.[33] Determining the adequacy of fracture reduction, however, can be difficult. In an effort to provide objective criteria for an adequate reduction, Garden proposed an "alignment index" based on postreduction AP and lateral radiographs[25] (Figure 5.35). On the AP view, the angle between the medial bony trabeculae of the femoral head and the medial cortex of the femoral shaft is measured (it is usually about 160°); on the lateral view, measurement is made of the angle formed by the central axis of the head and neck fragment and the shaft (usually 180°). Garden discovered that when either angle falls outside the range of 155° to 180°, the incidence of nonunion and osteonecrosis substantially increases. This technique of reduction assessment has limitations, however, in that postreduction radiographs of sufficient quality to accurately visualize the bony trabeculae are often difficult to obtain using the portable equipment available in the operating room.

Lowell described an assessment technique utilizing the normal radiographic convexity of the femoral head and concavity of the femoral neck[97] (Figure 5.36). In the intact proximal femur, an S-curve or reverse-S-curve outlined by the femoral head and neck can always be visualized radiographically, regardless of hip rotation. When an anatomic reduction is obtained, these opposing S-curves are present on both AP and lateral radiographs. Deviations from this appearance, which Lowell described as a C-curve, indicate a nonanatomic reduction. The C-curve is formed when the concave outline of the femoral neck

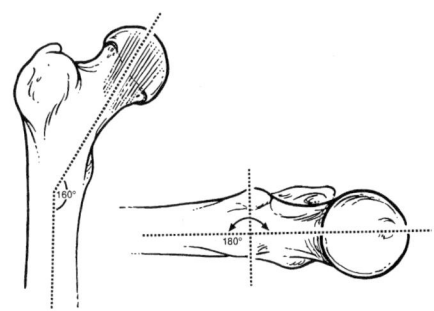

Figure 5.35. The Garden "alignment index" is based on postreduction AP and lateral radiographs.[25] On the AP view, the angle between the medial bony trabeculae of the femoral head and the medial cortex of the femoral shaft is measured (it is usually about 160°); on the lateral view, measurement is made of the angle formed by the central axis of the head and neck fragment and the shaft (usually 180°). Garden discovered that when either angle falls outside the range of 155° to 180°, the incidence of nonunion and osteonecrosis is increased.

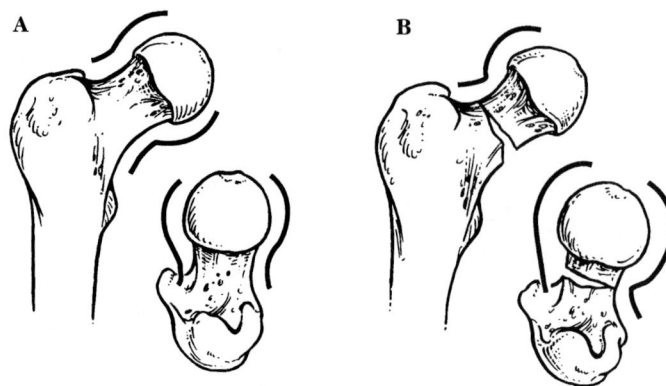

Figure 5.36. The Lowell method to assess the adequacy of reduction after femoral neck fracture.[97] In the intact proximal femur, an S-curve or reverse-S-curve outlined by the femoral head and neck can always be visualized radiographically, regardless of hip rotation (**A**). When an anatomic reduction is obtained, these opposing S-curves are present on both AP and lateral radiographs. Deviations from this appearance, which Lowell described as a C-curve, indicate a nonanatomic reduction (**B**). The C-curve is formed when the concave outline of the femoral neck appears as a tangent to the femoral head. This is usually found in conjunction with a sharply angulated cortical outline on the side of the femoral neck opposite the C-curve.

appears as a tangent to the femoral head. This is usually found in conjunction with a sharply angulated cortical outline on the side of the femoral neck opposite the C-curve.

We prefer to measure the angle of the femoral head on the true AP and cross-table lateral radiographs. An acceptable reduction may have up to 15° of valgus angulation and less than 10° of anterior or posterior angulation. Some variation is acceptable, particularly when a valgus reduction is obtained. In this situation, although the valgus reduction is nonanatomic, the risk of loss of stability posed by disimpaction of the fracture fragments probably outweighs the potential problems of a less-than-anatomic reduction.

Postreduction radiographs must also be evaluated to determine the presence and extent of posterior femoral neck comminution. Posterior comminution has been reported to range between 35% and 100% of displaced femoral neck fractures.[98] In such cases, a gap in the posterior cortex is evident on the lateral postreduction radiograph that corresponds to the area of comminution. Reduction maneuvers that maintain the leg in traction and internal rotation may exacerbate this defect and should be avoided.[33] If internal fixation is performed with a gap present in the posterior femoral neck, fixation stability may be compromised. Postoperatively, with release of traction and initiation of weight bearing, the femoral head may rotate posteriorly into the defect, with loss of fixation (Figure 5.37). Posterior comminution sufficient to compromise internal fixation is an indication for primary prosthetic replacement, discussed later.

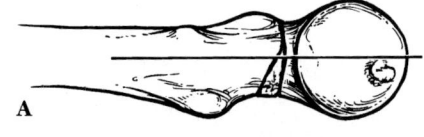

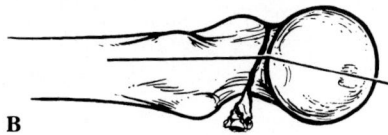

Figure 5.37. If internal fixation is performed with a gap present in the posterior femoral neck (**A**), fixation stability may be compromised. Postoperatively, with release of traction and initiation of weight bearing, the femoral head may rotate posteriorly into the defect, with loss of fixation (**B**).

Treatment

Careful evaluation of the postreduction radiographs will determine the next step in treatment. Four possibilities exist, depending on the quality of the fracture reduction and the extent of posterior femoral neck comminution. The best scenario is an acceptable reduction without posterior comminution. In this situation, internal fixation proceeds as previously described, with insertion of three or four cancellous lag screws (Figure 5.38). A capsulotomy should be performed at the time of internal fixation, as it is easily performed, adds little time to the procedure, and may help minimize the risk of osteonecrosis.

Another possibility is an unacceptable fracture reduction with minimal posterior comminution. In this situation, an open reduction is performed if the patient is active and in good health and has good-quality bone. This can be performed through either an anterior or an anterolateral approach. We prefer an anterolateral approach with the patient positioned on a fracture table, which allows use of fluoroscopy to assess fracture reduction and screw placement. The fracture site is exposed through an anterior capsulotomy, and the fracture is reduced under direct vision. Once reduced, the fracture is internally stabilized with three or four cancellous lag screws.

A third possibility is that the postreduction radiographs reveal an acceptable reduction in the presence of significant posterior comminution. In this difficult

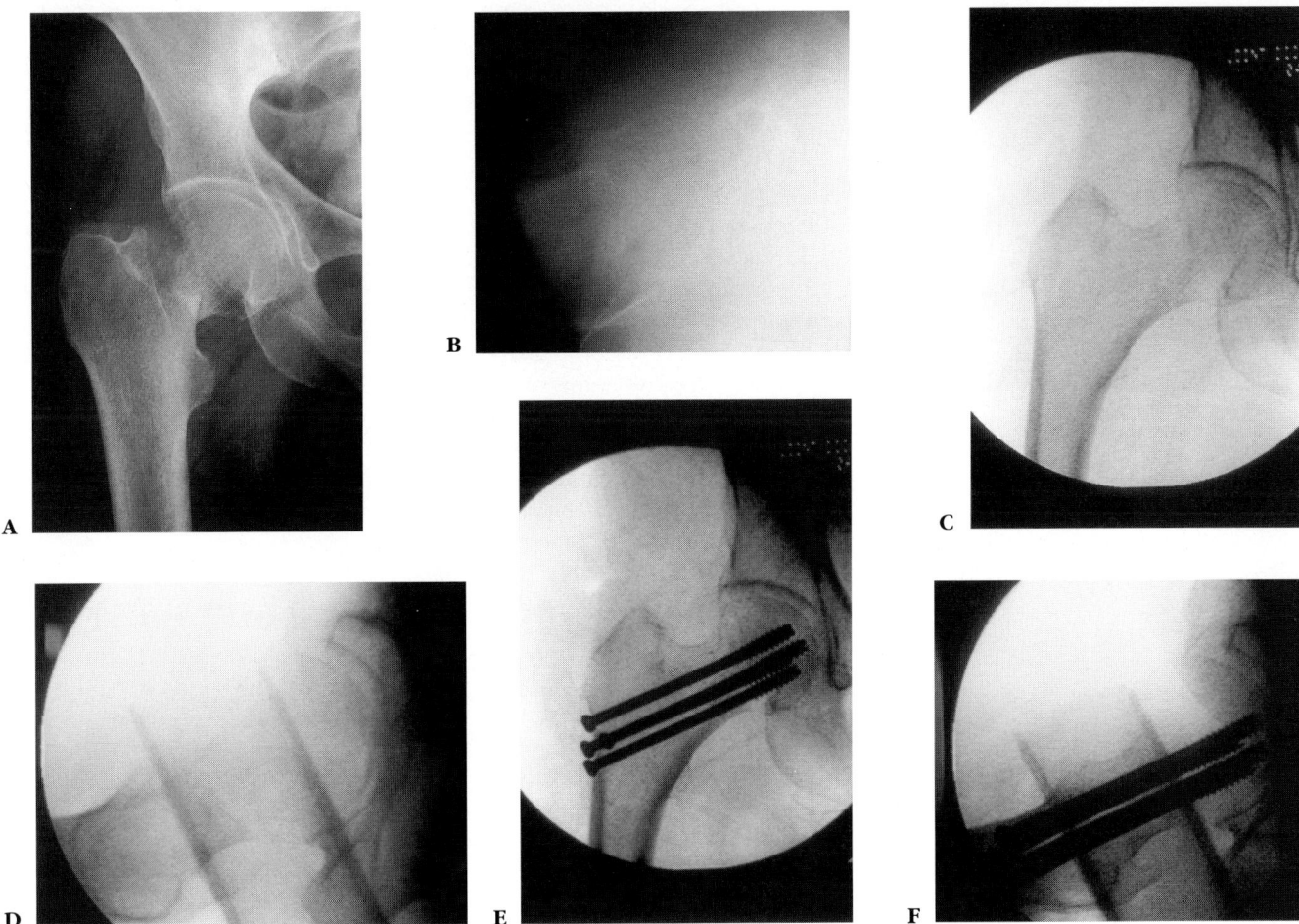

Figure 5.38. A displaced femoral neck fracture without posterior comminution (**A, B**). A closed reduction was performed (**C, D**) with placement of four cancellous lag screws (**E, F**).

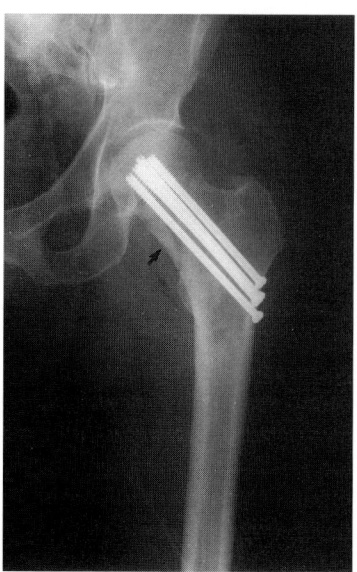

Figure 5.39. A displaced femoral fracture with posterior comminution (arrow) stabilized with four cancellous lag screws.

situation, other factors must be considered. If significant osteopenia is also present that would further compromise fracture fixation, prosthetic replacement is preferred. A variety of procedures have been proposed to compensate for posterior femoral neck comminution, including several fixation techniques, bone grafting, and the use of a muscle pedicle graft.[24,98–100] Most of these techniques, however, are of limited usefulness in the geriatric hip fracture population. If bone quality is good and the patient is reasonably healthy and active, we favor internal fixation using four cancellous lag screws (Figure 5.39), keeping in mind that the risk of healing complications is increased and that a second surgical procedure may be necessary.

The final possibility is an unacceptable reduction in the presence of significant posterior femoral neck comminution. In this situation, an open reduction would not correct the problems of stability caused by the posterior comminution. When faced with this situation in elderly patients, we elect to proceed with primary prosthetic replacement. In younger individuals, an open reduction is performed. With posterior comminution of the femoral neck, four rather than three cancellous lag screws are utilized. With significant comminution of the femoral neck, an attempt is made to reduce the fracture in a valgus position to enhance fracture stability.

Anterolateral Approach (Watson-Jones)

The anterolateral approach utilizes the intermuscular interval between the tensor fasciae latae muscle and the gluteus medius muscle; both muscles are innervated by the superior gluteal nerve. A 15-cm straight, longitudinal incision is centered over the greater trochanter and extended in both directions parallel to the femur (Figure 5.40). The deep fascia of the thigh is incised in line with the skin incision, just posterior to the border of the tensor fasciae latae muscle (Figure 5.41) to expose the vastus lateralis muscle distally and the gluteus medius muscle proximally (Figure 5.42). Using blunt dissection, the interval between the tensor fasciae latae and the gluteus medius muscle is developed (Figure 5.43). The branches of the superior gluteal artery that cross the interval between the tensor fasciae latae and the gluteus medius are ligated.

Treatment

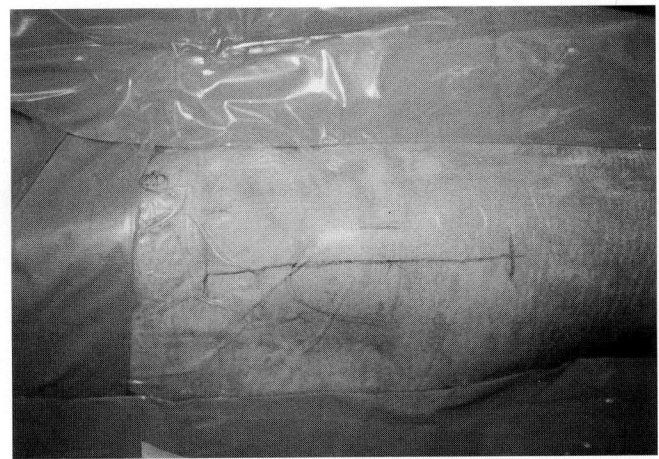

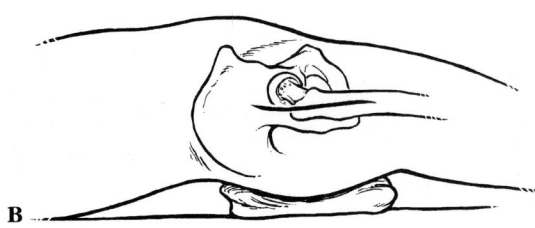

Figure 5.40. For an anterolateral approach to the hip, a 15-cm straight, longitudinal incision is made (**A**), centered over the greater trochanter and extended in both directions parallel to the femur (**B**).

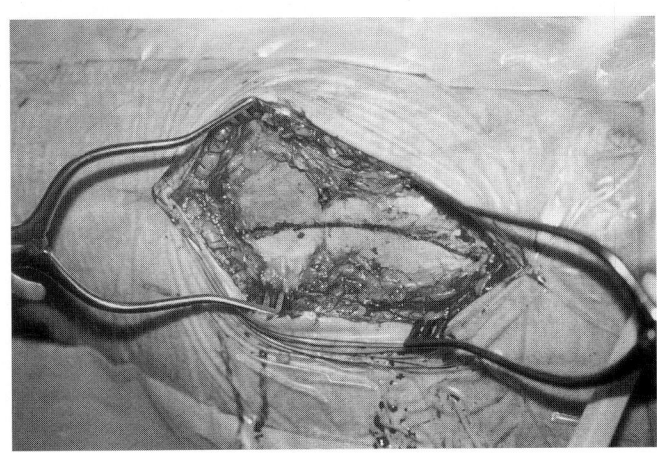

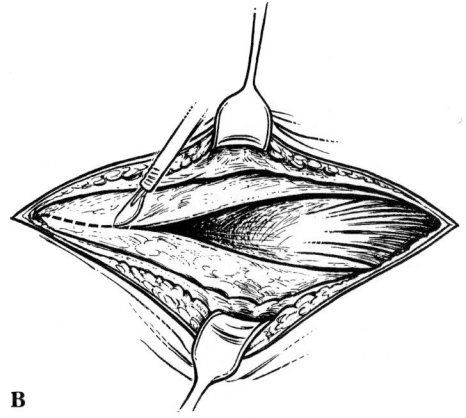

Figure 5.41. The deep fascia of the thigh is incised in line with the skin incision (**A**), just posterior to the border of the tensor fasciae latae muscle (**B**).

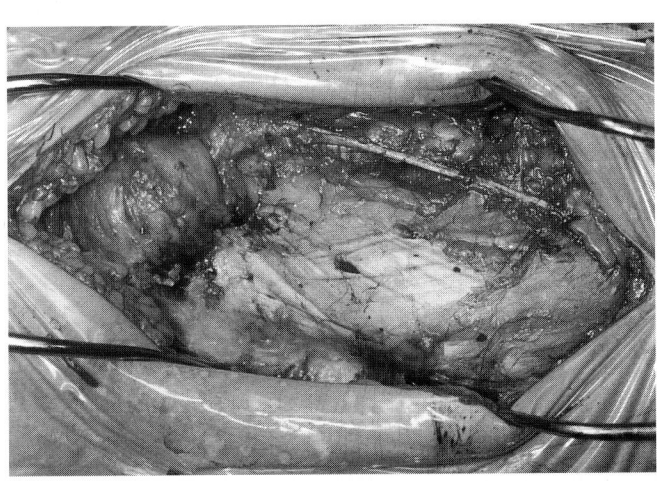

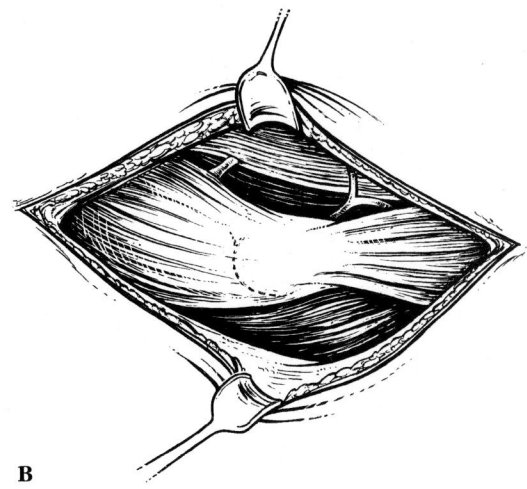

Figure 5.42. Exposure of the vastus lateralis muscle distally and the gluteus medius muscle proximally (**A, B**).

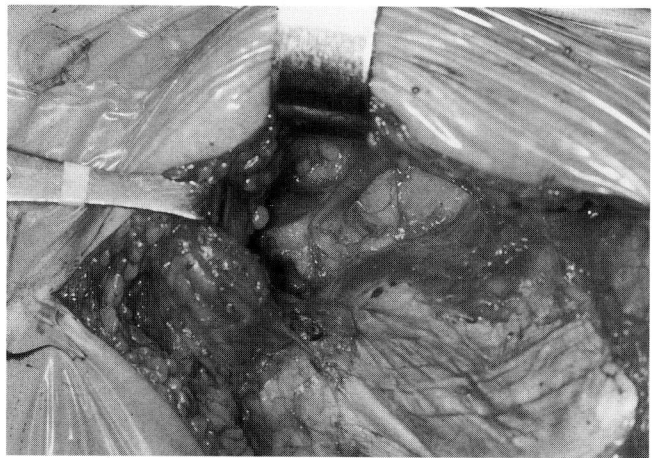

Figure 5.43. Using blunt dissection, the interval between the tensor fasciae latae and the gluteus medius muscle is developed, with exposure of the anterior hip capsule.

The vastus lateralis muscle is detached from its origin at the vastus lateralis ridge on the femur and is reflected distally (Figure 5.44). Following dissection of the reflected head of the rectus femoris muscle from its attachments on the hip joint capsule and the anterior rim of the acetabulum, the anterior capsule of the hip joint is incised in line with the femoral neck (Figure 5.45). The iliopsoas tendon may also attach to the hip joint capsule and may also need to

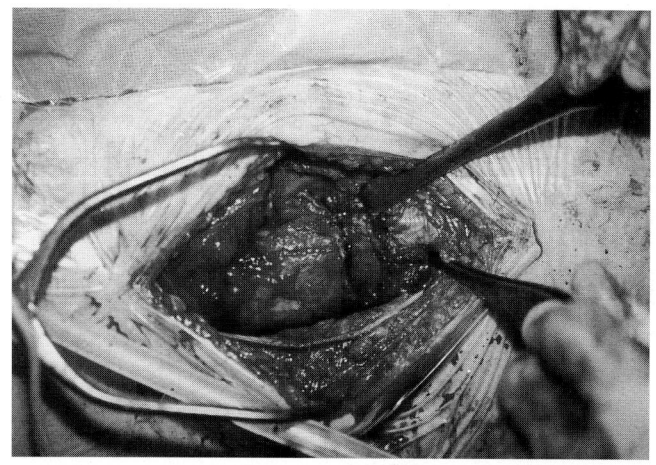
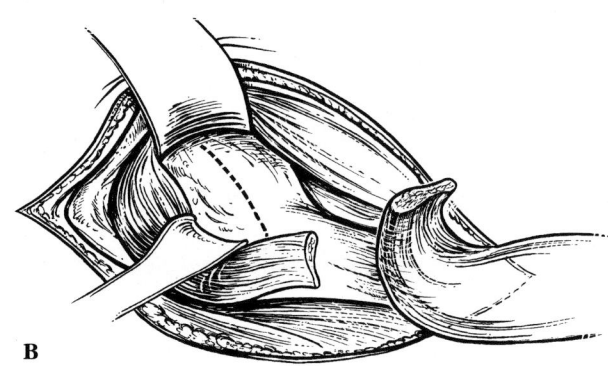

Figure 5.44. Detachment of the vastus lateralis muscle from its origin at the vastus lateralis ridge on the femur (**A, B**).

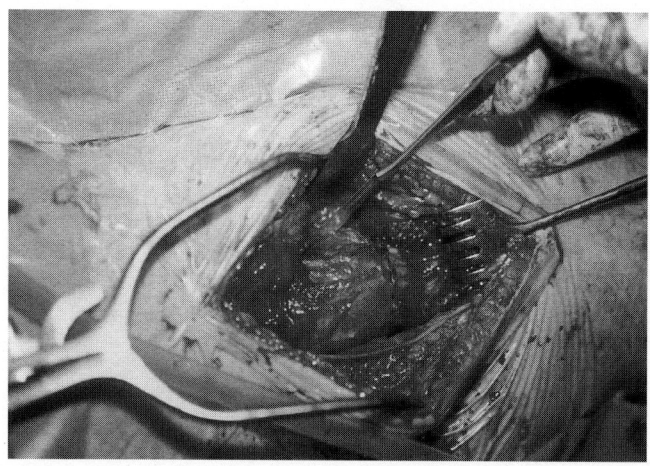
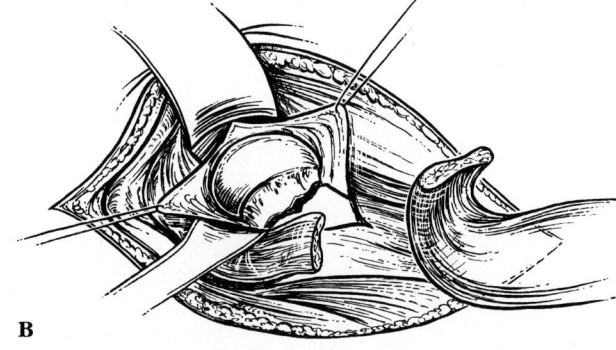

Figure 5.45. Exposure of the anterior femoral neck is performed by incising the hip capsule in line with the femoral neck (**A, B**).

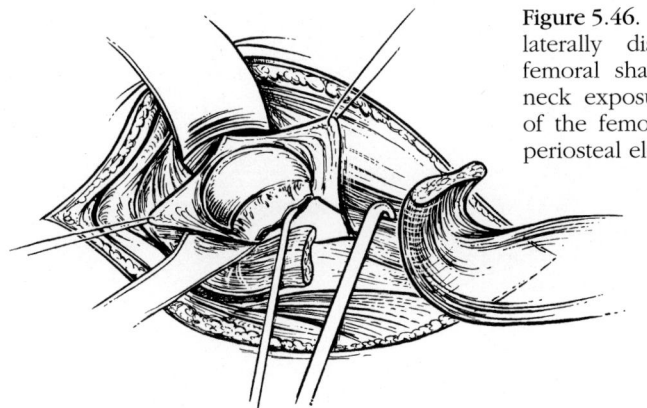

Figure 5.46. Use of a bone hook to laterally displace the proximal femoral shaft, enhancing femoral neck exposure, and manipulation of the femoral head with a small periosteal elevator.

be dissected free to improve exposure. A bone hook or clamp can be used to laterally displace the proximal femoral shaft and enhance femoral neck exposure (Figure 5.46). The femoral head can be manipulated using a periosteal elevator to assist fracture reduction. Once the fracture is reduced and verified radiographically, fracture stabilization is performed as previously described. One should avoid placement of retractors along the superior femoral neck to minimize the risk of injury to the lateral epiphyseal artery system.

Muscle Pedicle Bone Graft

Meyers et al. reported on the use of a vascularized quadratus muscle pedicle graft for treatment of displaced femoral neck fractures with posterior comminution.[101] The rationale behind the use of this graft was to improve fixation stability and local vascularity to the femoral head and thus decrease the risk of osteonecrosis. In their series of 181 fractures treated with open reduction and internal fixation in conjunction with a muscle pedicle graft, the union rate was 90%; 8 fractures (5%) developed osteonecrosis.[101] These excellent results have not been replicated, however, by other investigators. Furthermore, the extensive procedure involved may not be justified in the majority of femoral neck fracture patients; in particular, older patients who sustain a displaced femoral neck fracture with posterior comminution may be better served by prosthetic replacement.

More recently, use of a muscle pedicle graft has been described for treatment of nonunion and osteonecrosis after femoral neck fracture. Baksi reported a union rate of 75% in a series of 56 femoral neck nonunions treated with internal fixation in conjunction with a muscle pedicle graft.[102] In a separate series of 61 patients with osteonecrosis of the femoral head treated by multiple drilling of the femoral head, curettage of necrotic bone, cheilectomy of the femoral head (if necessary), and muscle pedicle grafting, Baksi reported pain relief and improved range of hip motion at 3-year minimum follow-up.[103]

The role of muscle pedicle grafting in the treatment of femoral neck fractures remains unclear. No such procedure has been performed at our institution for the treatment of femoral neck fractures. We nevertheless acknowledge that it may be appropriate, as an alternative to or in conjunction with a valgus osteotomy, in a younger individual who has either (1) sustained a displaced femoral neck fracture with posterior comminution and in whom every attempt should be made to salvage the femoral head; or (2) developed a femoral neck nonunion.

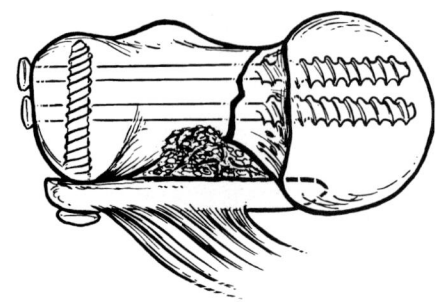

Figure 5.47. Illustration of the muscle pedicle graft to augment stabilization of a femoral neck fracture.

The surgical technique for muscle pedicle grafting to treat femoral neck fractures, as described by Meyers et al., involves positioning the patient prone on a fracture table with closed fracture reduction, if possible.[99,101] A posterior approach to the hip is performed with identification and delineation of the quadratus femoris muscle. A bone block, incorporating the tendon of the quadratus muscle, is harvested from the posterior aspect of the greater trochanter. The posterior hip capsule is incised, and after verification of the fracture reduction, the fracture is stabilized using multiple pins or screws. The defect in the posterior femoral neck is shaped to fit the bone block and then packed with cancellous bone graft. The bone block is inserted into the prepared trough and stabilized using small-diameter screws (Figure 5.47).

Primary Prosthetic Replacement

History

Since the introduction of the Austin-Moore and Thompson prostheses in the early 1950s, primary prosthetic replacement after displaced femoral neck fracture has undergone a significant evolution in terms of indications as well as prosthetic design. The Austin-Moore prosthesis (Figure 5.48) was designed for use without bone cement and was characterized by a fenestrated stem to allow "self-locking" of the prosthesis in the proximal femur.[33] The Thompson prosthesis (Figure 5.49), designed for a more extensive neck resection, had no fenestrated stem and was inserted using bone cement.[33] One problem with the use of these implants was thigh and groin pain, which was related to either prosthesis loosening within the femoral canal (thigh pain)—as a result of cementless insertion in the case of the Austin-Moore device—or progressive acetabular erosion (groin pain).[33,104–109] Protrusio acetabuli, arising from excessive erosion of the acetabulum, was reported to occur in 5% to 26% of patients using these prosthetic designs.[108,110–113] In another study, 64% of patients had acetabular erosion after 5 years, and 24% had protrusio.[109] Factors that have been found to correlate with the severity of acetabular erosion in patients with these devices are patient activity level, duration of implantation, and fixation technique (cemented versus noncemented).

Implantation of a femoral prosthesis can be accomplished through an anterior, lateral, or posterior approach, although preparation of the femoral canal is more difficult from an anterior approach unless special offset instruments are available. There are reports of increased infection risk using a posterior approach—probably because of the proximity of the incision to the perineal region and the potential for fecal contamination.[114,115] The position of instability

Treatment

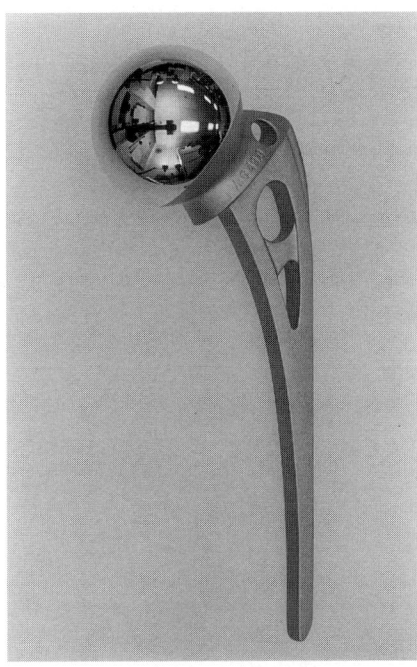

Figure 5.48. Photograph of an Austin-Moore endoprosthesis.

for the prosthesis is determined by which portion of the hip joint capsule is incised for exposure. Dislocations occur more frequently following procedures using the posterior approach, in which the prosthesis is unstable in flexion, adduction, and internal rotation—the sitting position (Figure 5.50). Anterior approaches, which preserve the posterior supporting structures, are stable in this

Figure 5.49. Photograph of a Thompson endoprosthesis.

Figure 5.50. Posterior hip dislocation following hemiarthroplasty performed through a posterior approach.

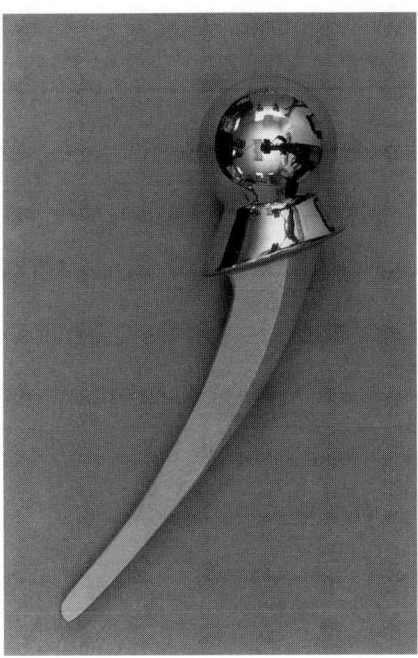

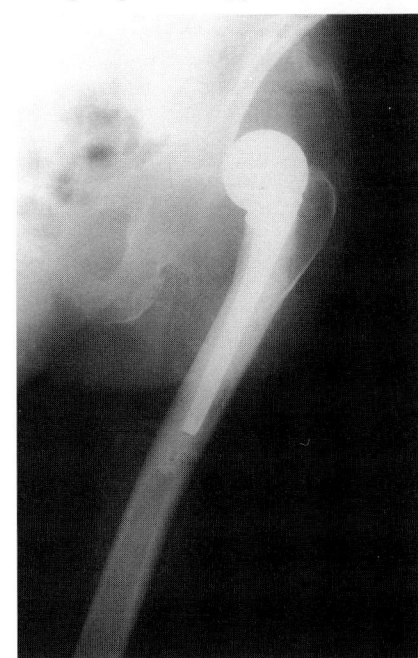

position but unstable in extension and external rotation. Lateral approaches, because they usually involve an anterior capsulotomy, are also stable in flexion, adduction, and internal rotation—the sitting position. Transtrochanteric approaches are not necessary for exposure and should be avoided because of the risk of additional complications, such as trochanteric nonunion.

The literature on prosthetic replacement after femoral neck fracture indicates a dislocation rate ranging between 0.3% and 10%, an infection rate of 2% to 20%, and a 6-month mortality rate of 1% to 39%—all higher than those for internal fixation.[116] However, Sikorski and Barrington reported that hemiarthroplasty through an anterolateral approach had a significantly lower 6-month mortality rate (20%) than did internal fixation (40%).[117] Holmberg et al. also reported lower complication rates after prosthetic replacement (15%) than after internal fixation (37%).[118]

Considerable difference of opinion exists regarding the choice of unipolar or bipolar prosthesis. The original prostheses (Austin-Moore, Thompson), one-piece, unipolar designs, were associated with an unacceptable rate of acetabular erosion, particularly when inserted using bone cement. In response to this, bipolar prostheses (with both an inner and an outer bearing) were developed, the Bateman and Gilberty designs being among the first. Bipolar prostheses (Figure 5.51) consist of an undersized femoral head that is snap-fit into the polyethylene liner (inner bearing) of a metal acetabular shell, which in turn articulates within the anatomic acetabulum (outer bearing) via suction fit. By allowing motion at the inner as well as the outer bearing surface, this device has the theoretical advantage (for which it was designed) of causing less acetabular wear. Bipolar devices can also be converted to total hip arthroplasty in the event of significant acetabular erosion. The acetabular shell can

Figure 5.51. Photograph of a bipolar endoprosthesis (**A**). Radiograph demonstrating use of a cemented bipolar endoprosthesis for treatment of a displaced femoral neck fracture (**B**).

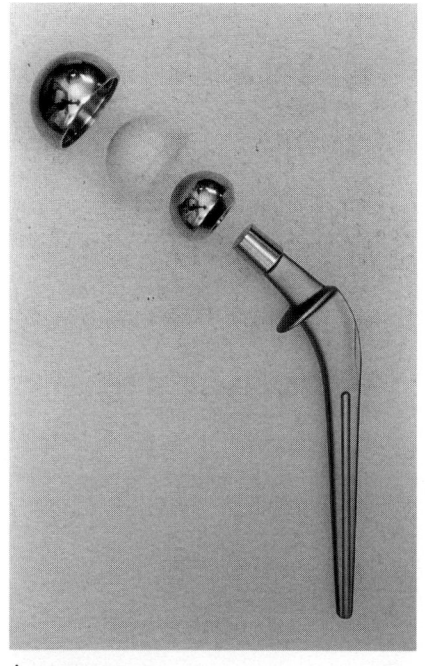
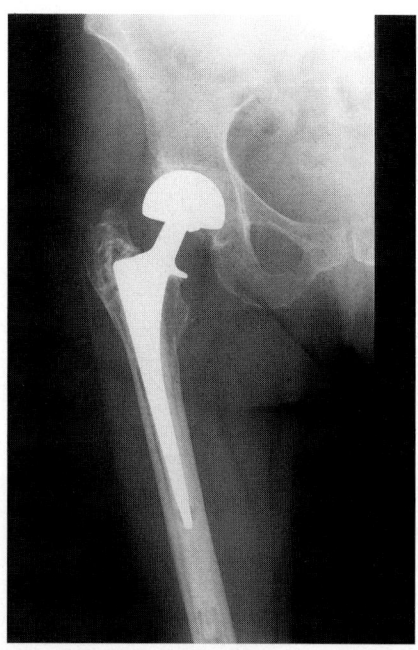

be removed and an appropriately sized acetabular component inserted to articulate with the femoral component.

Results with the bipolar prosthesis have generally been satisfactory, with early reports indicating that they were at least as good as unipolar designs.[119–122] Nevertheless, although dislocation rates were similar, the bipolar design made closed reduction much more difficult. Furthermore, with early bipolar implants, disassembly occasionally occurred during attempts at reducing a dislocation. Finally, several studies have questioned whether bipolar motion in fact occurs after insertion and suggested that inner bearing motion is at that point rapidly diminished.[123] One recent study, on the other hand, reported that bipolar motion was present for at least 2 years after surgery, with 40% of the motion occurring at the inner bearing.[119]

Yamagata et al. compared a large series of patients treated with either a unipolar or a bipolar prosthesis[124]; use of methylmethacrylate was not reported. They found that acetabular erosion occurred more often following unipolar replacement and that prosthetic loosening was more frequent following bipolar replacement. Conversion to total hip replacement was necessary in 12.5% of patients who had received a unipolar implant, compared with 7.2% of patients who had a bipolar prosthesis. A recent study of 90 cemented bipolar prostheses performed for acute femoral neck fracture and followed for at least 2 years reported excellent results[119]; 91% of the patients were free from significant thigh or groin pain, 92% had satisfactory hip motion and strength, and 83% required only a cane for ambulation. Moreover, acetabular erosion was minimal, and there were no instances of protrusio.

In reaction to the much higher cost of the bipolar prosthesis, some authors have advocated use of a cemented modular unipolar prosthesis (Figure 5.52), particularly in patients with low functional demands.[125] As with bipolar prostheses, a modular unipolar prosthesis can be converted to a total hip replacement without stem removal. We performed a prospective study at the Hospital for Joint Diseases to determine the relative efficacy of unipolar and bipolar prostheses for the treatment of displaced femoral neck fractures.[125] The study

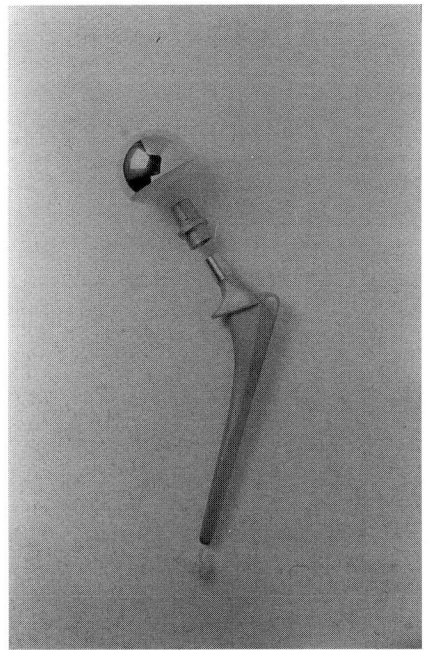

Figure 5.52. Photograph of a modular unipolar endoprosthesis.

population consisted of 179 community-dwelling patients over age 65 (mean age, 80 years) with a displaced femoral neck fracture who had undergone primary prosthetic replacement. Before 1990, a cemented bipolar prosthesis had been used for all cases ($n = 113$); after that date, cemented modular unipolar prostheses were used in all cases ($n = 66$). Because the change from bipolar to unipolar prostheses reflected a departmental policy, the indications for primary prosthetic replacement and the surgeons performing the procedure were essentially identical throughout the study. Prefracture characteristics (patient age, sex, medical comorbidities, and walking ability) were similar for the unipolar and bipolar groups. At a minimum of 1-year follow-up, there were no significant differences between the two groups with regard to postoperative medical complications, infection, dislocation, mortality, presence and severity of hip and/or groin pain, or patient function.

We performed a follow-up study to compare the effect of bipolar ($n = 47$) versus unipolar ($n = 66$) hemiarthroplasty on functional recovery 4 to 5 years after hip fracture. An in-depth functional evaluation was obtained including ambulation, basic activities of daily living (feeding, bathing, dressing, toileting) and instrumental activities of daily living (food shopping, food preparation, banking, laundry, housework, and public transportation). At 4 to 5 years' follow-up, there were no functional differences identified between the bipolar and unipolar groups. Furthermore, at latest follow-up, there were no significant differences between the two groups with regard to the rates of infection, prosthetic dislocation, or mortality. Based on the results of this study, we feel that there does not appear to be any advantage to the use of bipolar endoprostheses for the treatment of femoral neck fractures in the elderly. Furthermore, the decreased cost of modular unipolar endoprostheses compared with bipolar endoprostheses provides additional support for their use.

Three different modes of femoral stem fixation are currently available: interference fit, polymethylmethacrylate cement, and bone ingrowth. The first generation of femoral prostheses relied on an interference fit between the stem and the cancellous bone of the medullary canal (Figure 5.53), which was

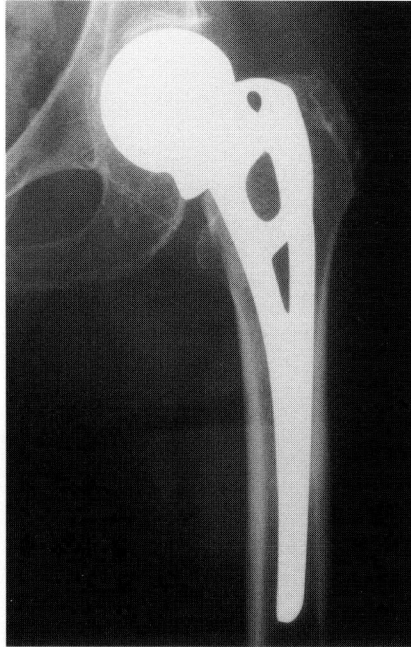

Figure 5.53. Radiograph of a Austin-Moore endoprosthesis, which relies on an interference fit between the stem and the cancellous bone of the medullary canal.

shaped by the use of broaches that matched the shape of the stem. Since many older individuals have a large medullary diameter and relatively poor-quality cancellous bone, however, a secure press fit was probably not achieved with the limited prosthetic stem diameters initially available. Newer-generation prostheses, which are available in a range of femoral stem diameters, allow an improved interference fit regardless of the femoral canal geometry. Use of the newer press-fit implants, however, is probably not warranted in the elderly in light of the cost of the implant and the exacting nature of the procedure.

Use of methylmethacrylate is of obvious value to maintain satisfactory alignment and fixation of a prosthesis that does not fill the medullary canal (Figure 5.54). It has been documented to increase patient comfort and improve clinical results in controlled trials where the same prosthesis was inserted without cement.[126–129] In active patients with early designs of unipolar prostheses, however, use of cement was associated with progressive acetabular wear, painful arthropathy, and protrusio.[126,130] The reasons for this are unclear, although cementing technique and prosthetic design—both of which have greatly improved—may have been factors. Modern techniques of cement application include (1) preliminary canal shaping to a uniformly larger size than the stem; (2) thorough cleansing of the medullary canal to remove blood and fat; (3) use of a distal plug to contain the cement; (4) injection and pressurization of semiliquid cement to fill bony interstices and increase fixation; and (5) improved mixing techniques to avoid air bubbles and lack of homogeneity.[14] We believe that, once sufficient data are available from procedures using the latest cementing techniques and implants, it may be demonstrated that acetabular erosion is not related to the use of cement.

The third approach to implant fixation is to use a prosthetic femoral stem with one of a variety of microporous surfaces at the bone–implant interface[14] (Figure 5.55). Bone ingrowth into the pores of such an implant can substantially augment the interference fit, thus providing secure fixation without resort to cement. The procedure necessitates meticulous bone tailoring to obtain intimate bone contact and a tight interference fit (with increased risk of

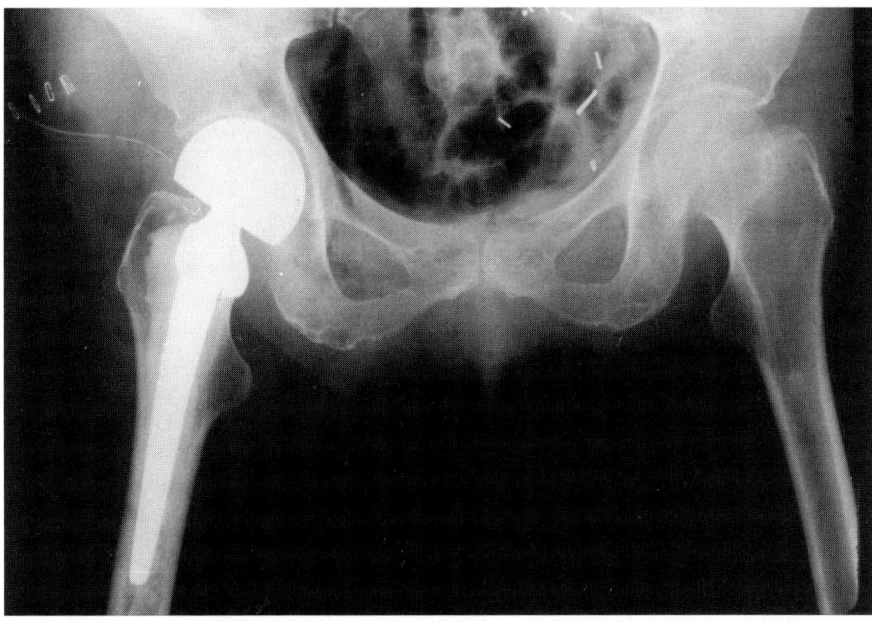

Figure 5.54. Radiograph of a cemented bipolar hemiarthroplasty.

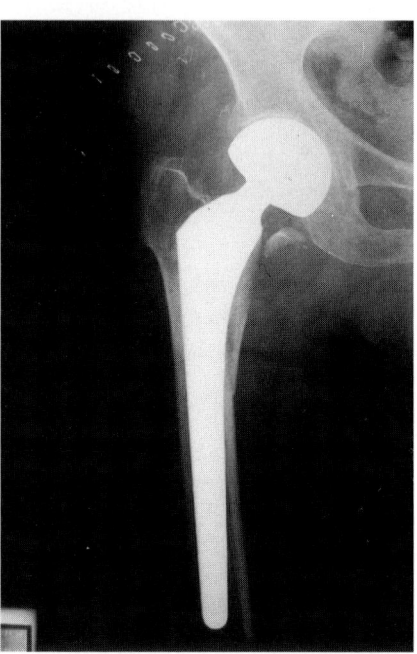

Figure 5.55. Radiograph of a porous coated endoprosthesis.

femoral shaft fracture).[14] These prostheses have an increased incidence of thigh pain and are relatively costly. Their long-term performance remains uncertain, although many surgeons favor their use in the management of younger individuals and in revision surgery. In elderly hip fracture patients with osteoporotic bone and relatively limited ingrowth potential, however, the routine use of porous coated implants for fixation cannot be justified.

Although a wide variety of hip prostheses are available from several manufacturers, almost all share certain design features[14]: (1) a system of instruments for preparing the femoral canal to the size and shape of the prosthesis; (2) modular components with Morse taper junctions that permit custom adjustment of prosthetic neck length and head size, thus permitting reduction in the inventory required to obtain optimal fit and providing the possibility for later revision of a stable femoral component to total hip arthroplasty, should acetabular problems occur after hemiarthroplasty; and (3) incorporation of high-performance alloys with appropriate strength and fatigue life so that implant failure does not occur.

Our approach to prosthetic replacement in most elderly patients is to perform a cemented unipolar hemiarthroplasty through a posterior surgical approach. This approach can be performed in the lateral decubitus position with a limited amount of blood loss. A posterior capsulotomy is performed, with care taken to preserve the acetabular labrum. Sizing of the femoral head is an important step in obtaining the proper "suction fit." An undersized component increases the probability of prosthetic dislocation and may exacerbate central acetabular wear, whereas an oversized component will limit outer bearing motion and possibly exacerbate peripheral acetabular wear. To enhance posterior stability, the capsulotomy is repaired and the short external rotators are reattached through drill holes to the posterior portion of the greater trochanter.

In patients with dementia or fecal incontinence, we use an anterior or direct lateral approach, which should also be considered for patients who are expected to be nonambulators after surgery. These approaches place the incision away from the perineal area, provide enhanced stability in patients who are unable to follow position precautions, and reduce the risk of prosthetic

Treatment

dislocation in patients whose activity will be restricted to bed-to-chair transfers by health care personnel.

One final general comment concerning the treatment of femoral neck fractures by primary prosthetic replacement is warranted: it is impossible to exaggerate the importance of meticulous technique—not only operative technique but also preoperative planning and postoperative management. Unfortunately, there has been a tendency for orthopaedic surgeons to consider these procedures as being less demanding than the reconstructive total hip replacements performed in elderly patients with degenerative hip disease. Quite the contrary: prosthetic replacement after hip fracture requires as much attention to detail as elective total hip replacement to ensure the best possibility of uneventful outcomes.

Templating

Before proceeding to hemiarthroplasty, it is important to perform preoperative templating to determine the approximate femoral stem and unipolar/bipolar head size. In most patients, the unaffected hip is used as a template to duplicate normal leg length and hip offset. Proper hip offset helps maintain proper soft tissue tension, which is critical to the stability and biomechanics of the hip.

Templating begins with an AP view of the pelvis that includes as much of the proximal femur as possible. The pelvis should not be rotated, and it is helpful if the noninjured leg is rotated internally 15° to get a true profile view of the proximal femur (this eliminates the normal anteversion). It is not necessary to obtain this view of the injured extremity.

On the AP view, the center of the head is marked on the noninjured hip (Figure 5.56). The center can be determined by using a ruler to calculate the diameter of the head and then identifying the midpoint. A line is then drawn down the center of the femoral shaft (Figure 5.57). The distance from this line to the center of the femoral head is the hip offset (Figure 5.57).

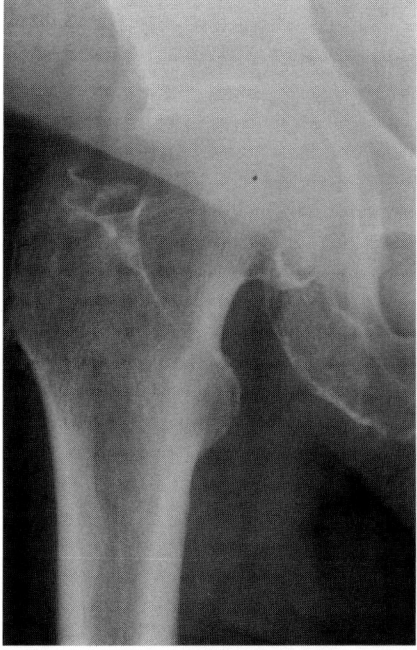

Figure 5.56. To make a preoperative template, the center of the femoral head is marked on the noninjured hip the on the AP view.

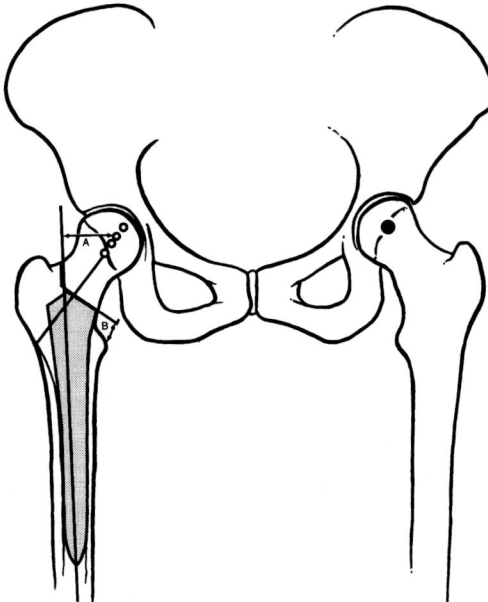

Figure 5.57. After marking the center of the femoral head, a line is drawn down the center of the femoral canal. The distance from this line to the center of the femoral head is the hip offset (line A).

Using templates, magnified to account for radiographic magnification, a stem of appropriate size is chosen (Figure 5.58). It is important to check that the stem also matches both AP and lateral views of the injured hip before templating on the normal hip. For cemented insertion, adequate space must be maintained around the stem to accommodate the cement mantle (usually 2 mm). This calls for a smaller stem than for noncemented, press-fit insertion. For noncemented press-fit insertion, the best fit is chosen to achieve intimate bone contact, which may be metaphyseal or diaphyseal depending on the type of implant chosen.

The template is placed over the AP pelvis film, directly in line with the femoral canal. It is then slid down the canal until one of the neck length mark-

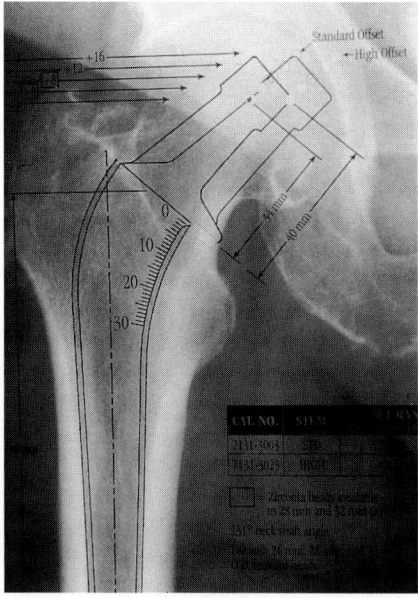

Figure 5.58. Using templates, magnified to account for radiographic magnification, a stem of appropriate size is chosen.

ings matches the offset of the normal hip. The distance from this marking down to the lesser trochanter is measured using the magnified ruler markings on the template. This distance is recorded and later measured intraoperatively to mark the level of the desired neck cut. The distance from the lesser trochanter to the center of the femoral head is also measured in order to recreate this distance intraoperatively. The neck length marking on the template that most closely matches the offset of the normal hip is the neck length that will be used first when performing an intraoperative trial and—assuming intraoperative stability—for the prosthesis itself.

Some patients have hips with a larger offset than is available on the templates. These patients will usually need a prosthesis with a high offset geometry. If a high-offset stem is not used, the soft tissue tension of the hip abductors will be subnormal; these muscles may function suboptimally and hip stability may subsequently be compromised.

Technique for a Modular Unipolar Hemiarthroplasty of the Hip

When performing hemiarthroplasty of the hip after femoral neck fracture, we most commonly utilize a posterior approach with the patient in the lateral decubitus position (Figure 5.59). A lateral positioner is used to maintain this position, and a soft axillary roll is placed under the upper thorax to protect the brachial plexus. The ankle and the knee of the noninjured leg are padded to prevent iatrogenic nerve injury (Figure 5.60), and a pillow is placed between the legs (Figure 5.61) to help abduct the operative extremity and thus facilitate the exposure. Before preparing for surgery, the hip is flexed to 90° to ensure that the lateral positioner is not blocking the range of hip motion. The entire injured extremity is then prepared and draped up to and including the iliac crest.

A slightly curved incision is made in line with the femur, centered over the greater trochanter with the hip flexed approximately 30° (Figure 5.62). The incision begins approximately 5 to 6 cm proximal to the greater trochanter and continues the same distance distal to the greater trochanter. The subcutaneous tissues are divided in line with the incision and the fascia lata is identified (Figure 5.63). A periosteal elevator is used to clear the fascia lata, which is then

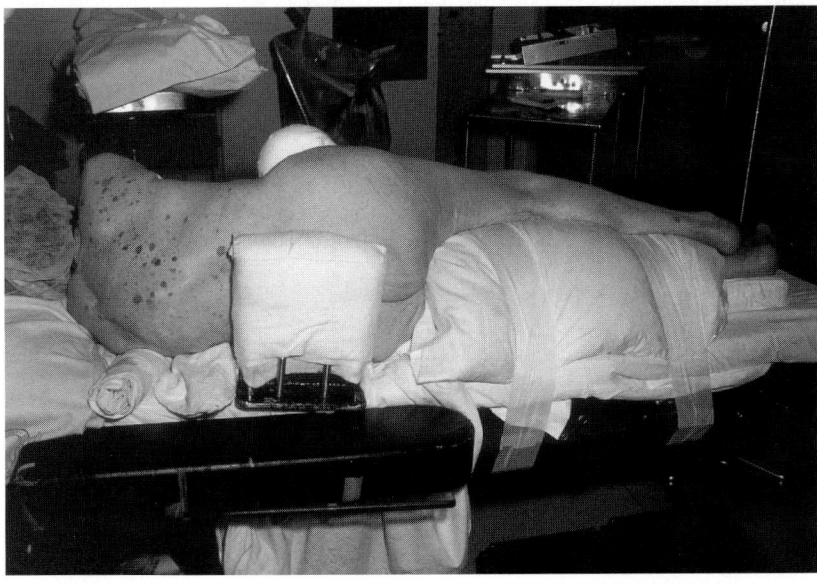

Figure 5.59. Hemiarthroplasty of the hip is performed with the patient in a lateral decubitus position. A lateral positioner is used to maintain this position, and a soft axillary roll is placed under the upper thorax to protect the brachial plexus.

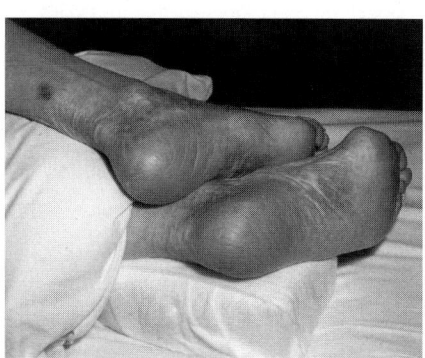

Figure 5.60. The ankle and the knee of the noninjured leg are padded to prevent iatrogenic nerve injury.

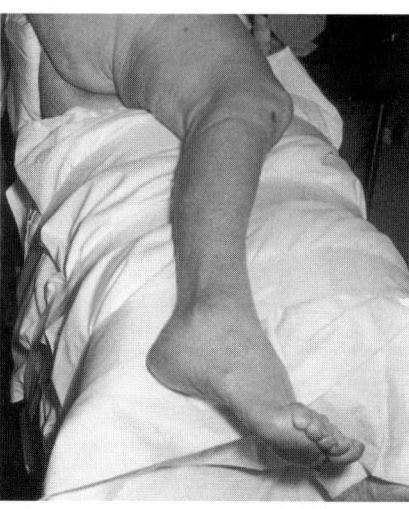

Figure 5.61. A pillow is placed between the legs to help abduct the operative extremity and facilitate the surgical exposure.

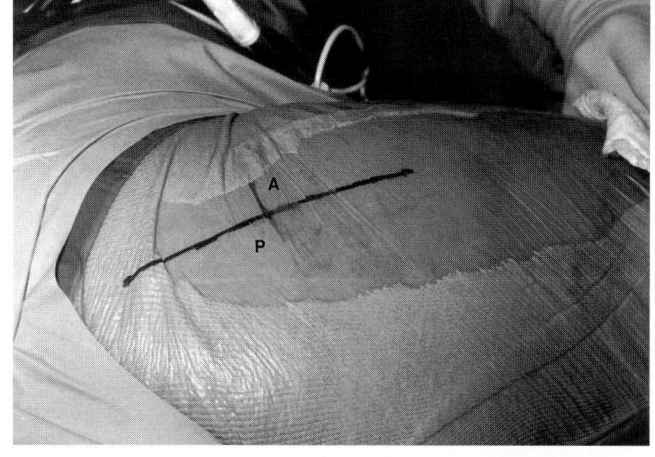

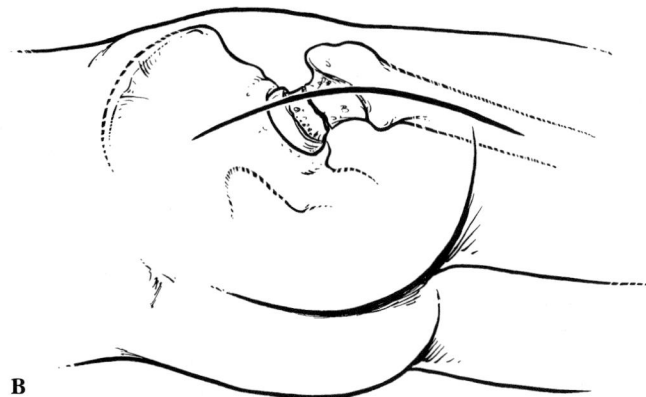

Figure 5.62. A slightly curved incision is made in line with the femur, centered over the greater trochanter with the hip flexed approximately 30° (**A**). The incision begins approximately 5 to 6 cm proximal to the greater trochanter and continues the same distance distal to the greater trochanter (**B**).

incised in line with the femur. At the proximal aspect of the incision, the muscle fibers of the gluteus maximus muscle are visible as the fascia lata thins out superficial to the gluteus maximus. The gluteus maximus fibers are bluntly split in an anterior-to-posterior direction and a Charnley retractor is inserted deep to the fascia lata for exposure (Figure 5.64). Care is taken to palpate the sciatic nerve and to ensure that it is not trapped in the blades of the retractor.

The trochanteric bursa is reflected posteriorly. The hip is maintained in extension during the posterior dissection; this relieves the sciatic nerve of any unnecessary strain and assists the exposure as the short external rotators are released. The sciatic nerve is again palpated—it is not necessary to expose it—before beginning the posterior exposure to ensure that it is not in danger of injury. A blunt retractor is passed above the superior border of the piriformis muscle, deep to the gluteus minimus muscle but superficial to the superior capsule, to assist the exposure. The hip is internally rotated to place the short external rotators under tension. Electrocautery is used to release the short rotators and the underlying capsule directly off bone along the posterior border of the proximal femur (Figure 5.65). The quadratus femoris muscle is partially released as necessary. Perforating vessels are identified and cauterized; there

Treatment

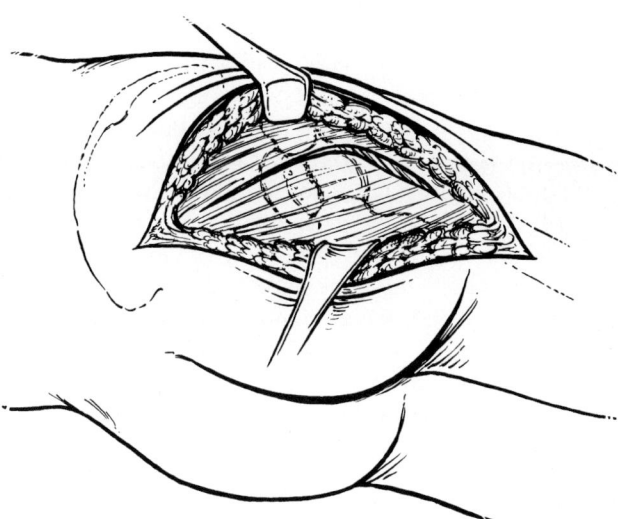

Figure 5.63. The subcutaneous tissues are divided in line with the incision, and the fascia lata and fascia overlying the gluteus maximus are identified and incised.

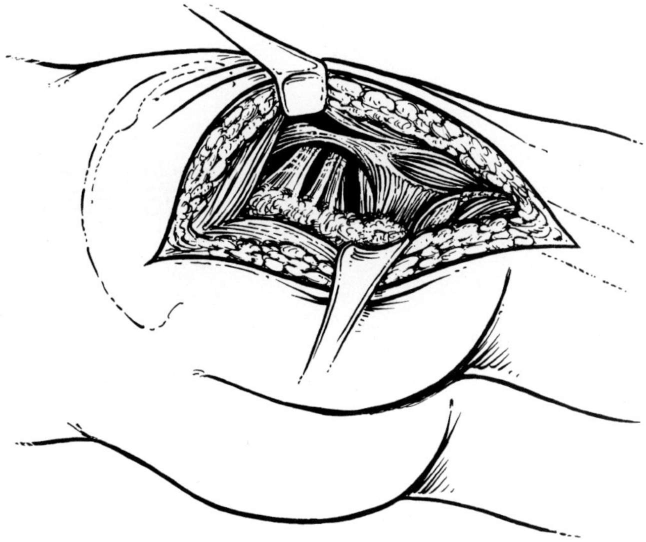

Figure 5.64. Placement of the retractors inserted deep to the fascia lata for exposure after the gluteus maximus muscle fibers are bluntly split in an anterior-to-posterior direction.

is usually a large branch of the medial femoral circumflex artery within the body of the quadratus femoris muscle. The short external rotators can be reflected separately or in conjunction with the posterior hip capsule. We prefer releasing the external rotators and capsule together. It is helpful to make a T-type incision in the capsule below the piriformis muscle so that two sleeves of tissue overlay the posterior hip joint (Figure 5.66); a suture is passed through

Figure 5.65. Use of electrocautery to release the short rotators and the underlying capsule off bone along the posterior border of the proximal femur.

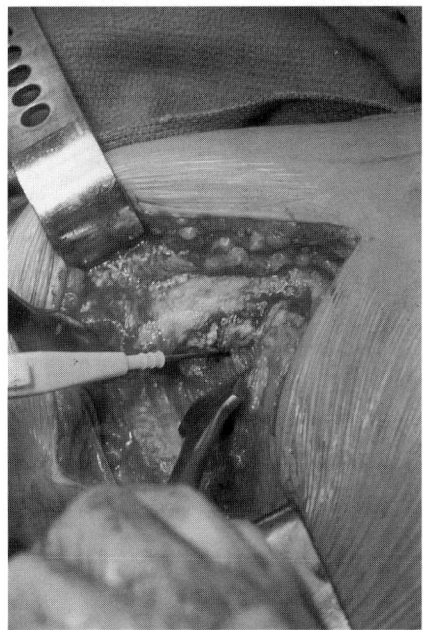

Figure 5.66. A T-type incision is made in the capsule below the piriformis so that two sleeves of tissue overlie the posterior hip joint.

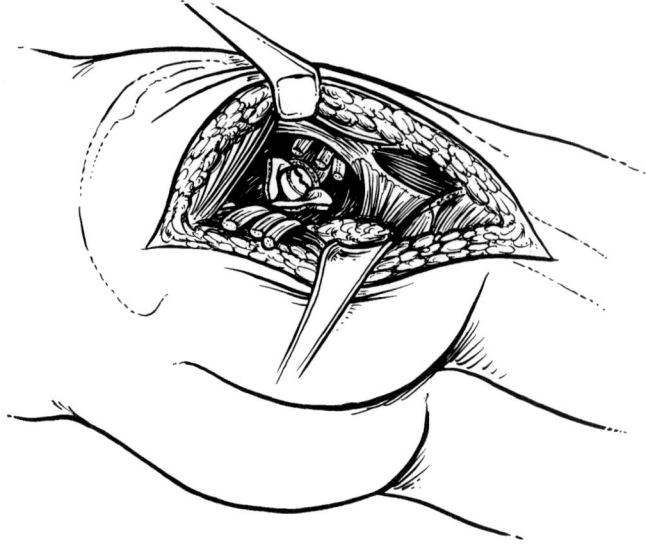

each of these sleeves. These sutures are helpful for retraction during reduction of the prosthetic hip and for later capsular reattachment. The capsulotomy is extended superiorly and inferiorly to enhance visualization of the acetabulum.

At this point the femur is flexed and internally rotated to expose the femoral neck. A femoral neck osteotomy is performed using an oscillating saw with the extremity positioned so the foot is superior, pointing toward the ceiling, and the leg perpendicular to the floor (Figure 5.67). The location of the cut with respect to the lesser trochanter is determined by preoperative templating, and the angle of the cut is matched to a trial or broach. Osteotomy of the femoral neck prior to removal of the femoral head enhances the exposure. The femoral head is extracted using a corkscrew and a skid (Figure 5.68); it may be necessary to incise the ligamentum teres. If exposure is difficult, a bone hook is passed under the femoral neck and is used to retract the femur. If exposure remains a problem and the gluteus maximus muscle is tight, the proximal portion (1 to 1.5 cm) of the gluteus maximus insertion can be released off the linea aspera of the femur using electrocautery. Care must be taken not to release too far distally to minimize bleeding from perforating vessels.

Once the femoral head is extracted, it is sized using a caliper or precut templates (Figure 5.69). The acetabulum is visually inspected to evaluate the condition of the cartilage. If the pulvinar is excessively large, it is trimmed using a cautery. Trial heads of appropriate sizes are tested in the acetabulum for a good suction fit (Figure 5.70), and the largest head that seats fully in the

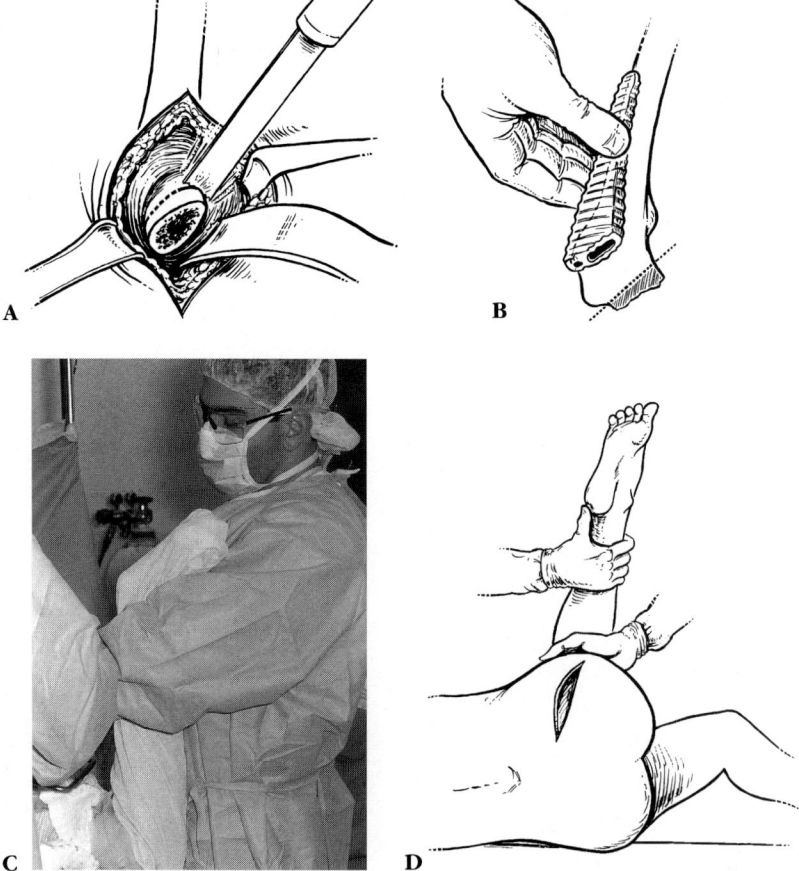

Figure 5.67. A femoral neck osteotomy is performed using an oscillating saw (**A**) using a template as a guide (**B**). The extremity is positioned with the foot superior, pointing toward the ceiling, and the leg perpendicular to the floor (**C, D**).

Treatment

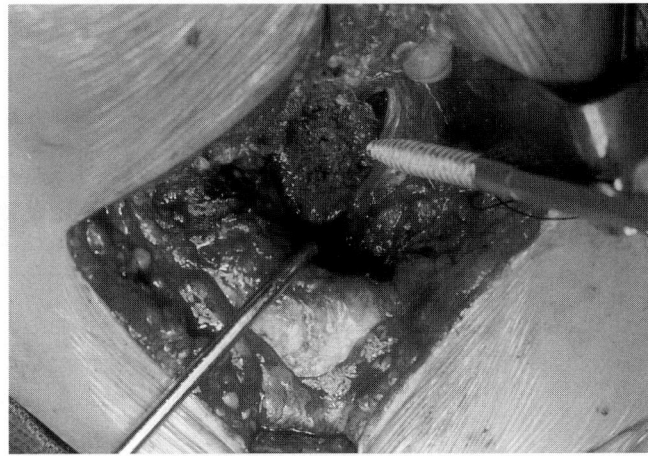

Figure 5.68. Extraction of the femoral head using a corkscrew.

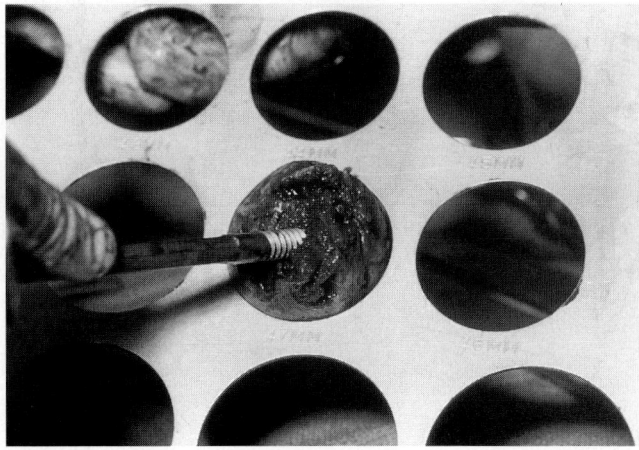

Figure 5.69. Sizing of the femoral head using precut templates.

acetabulum is selected. If the head is too small, it will hasten destruction of the acetabular cartilage.

The femoral canal is exposed by passing a broad, flat retractor under the proximal femur (Figure 5.71). Remaining soft tissue is excised from the posterior and lateral aspect of the femoral neck to the lesser trochanter. A box osteotome is used to open the proximal femur (Figure 5.72). If the greater trochanter overhangs the femoral canal, a small notch of bone is removed from the greater trochanter to prevent reaming and broaching in varus. A blunt T-handled starting reamer is placed down the femoral canal in line with femur, directed toward the knee (Figure 5.73). The femoral canal is reamed using hand or power reamers (Figure 5.74), increasing in size incrementally until the appropriately sized reamer is reached; the final reaming size depends on the size of the canal and on the type of prosthesis selected.

Broaching is then performed, using a broach at least two sizes smaller than the templated size of the femur (Figure 5.75). The broach handle is held in the appropriate amount of anteversion (approximately 15°). With the leg positioned

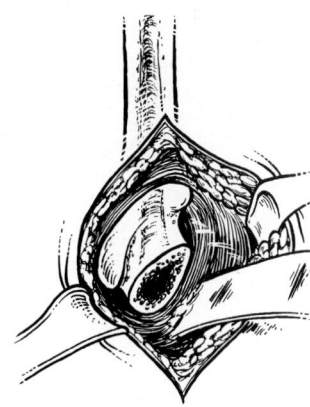

Figure 5.71. The femoral canal is exposed by passing a broad, flat retractor under the proximal femur.

Figure 5.70. Trial heads of appropriate sizes are tested in the acetabulum to determine a good suction fit.

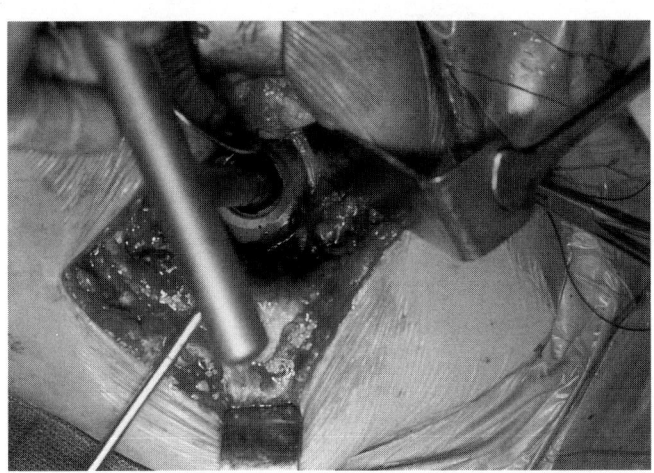

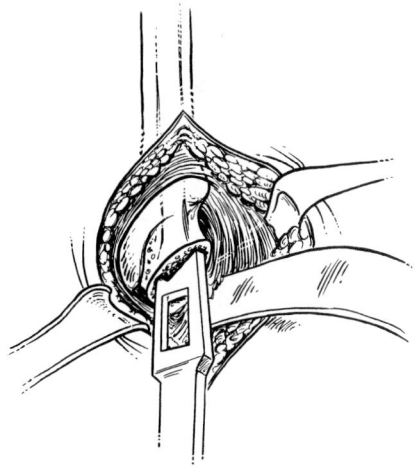

Figure 5.72. A box osteotome is used to open the proximal femur.

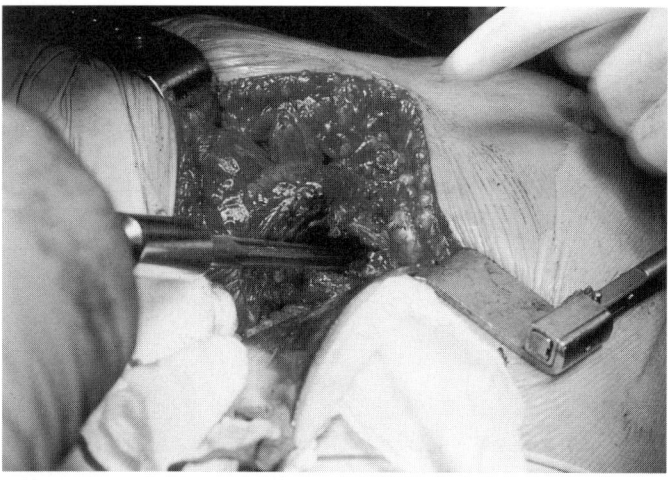

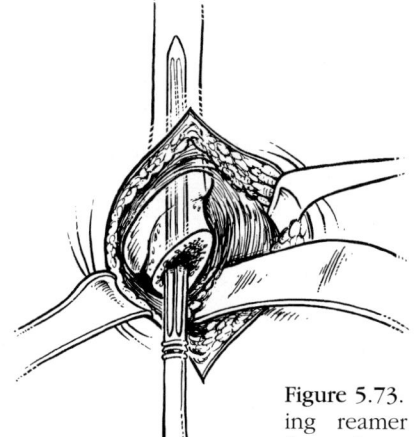

Figure 5.73. A blunt T-handled starting reamer is placed down the femoral canal in line with femur, directed toward the knee (**A, B**).

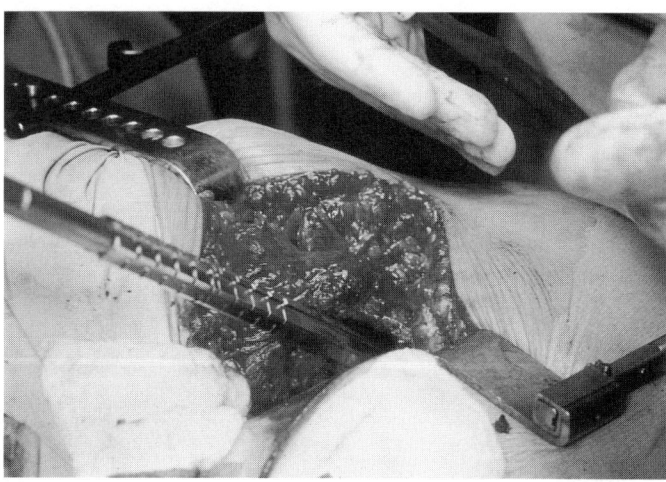

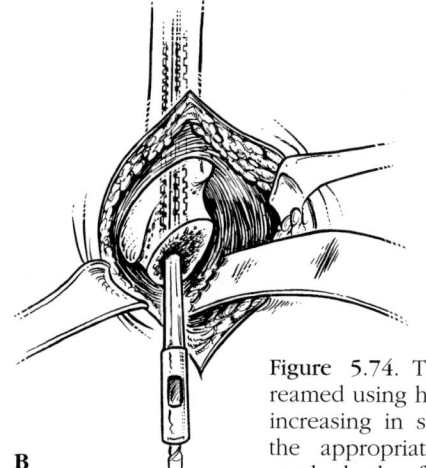

Figure 5.74. The femoral canal is reamed using hand or power reamers, increasing in size incrementally until the appropriate size of reamer is reached; the final reaming size depends on the size of the canal and on the type of prosthesis selected (**A, B**).

Figure 5.75. Broaching is performed, using a broach at least two sizes smaller than the templated size of the femur. The broach handle is held in the appropriate amount of anteversion (approximately 15°) (**A, B**).

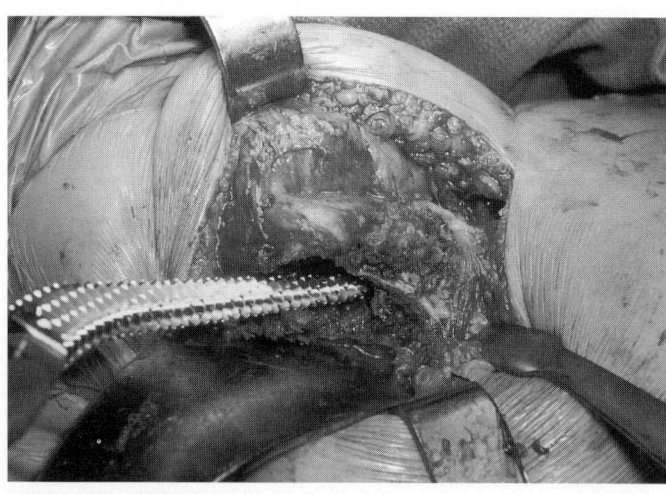

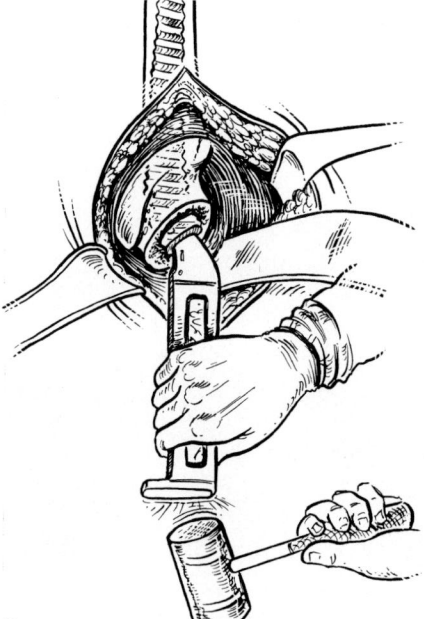

Treatment

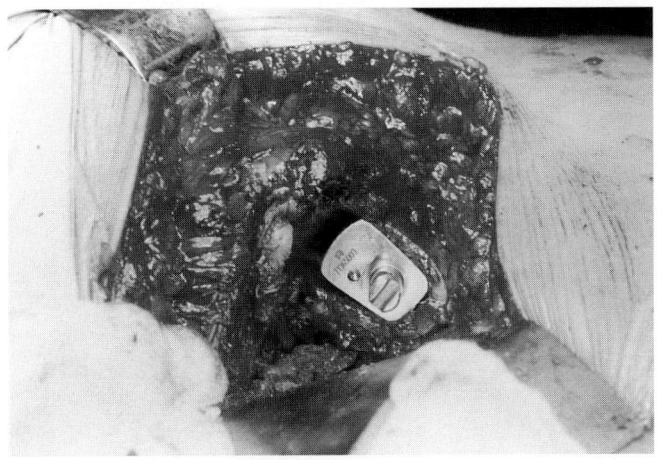
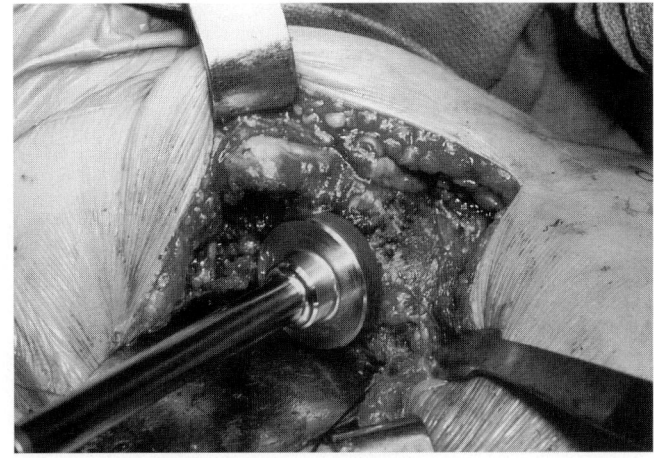

A B

perpendicular to the floor, it is easier to appreciate the amount of anteversion of the broach. When broaching and reaming, it is important to resist the tendency to fall into varus by providing a laterally directed force as the broaches and reamers are advanced. The broach is periodically advanced and removed rather than simply hammered straight down the canal; this technique reduces the risk of iatrogenic femur fracture and helps avoid incarcerating the broach in the femur. After the broach is fully seated to the level of the femoral neck cut, the next size broach is used, and the process is repeated until the appropriately sized broach is fully impacted. The final broach size is selected based on preoperative templating and, more importantly, on the ease of insertion. A broach that advances too easily is probably too small, while one that requires excessive force of insertion increases the risk of femoral fracture. In cemented applications, it is less important to achieve a tight interlock of the broach with the femur, and thus there is no need to broach with excessive force.

Once broaching is completed, a calcar planer is used to even out the femoral neck cut (Figure 5.76). With the broach in place, a trial head with the appropriate neck length can be used to assess hip stability through a range of motion (Figure 5.77). Stability in response to external rotation with the hip in full extension is assessed (Figure 5.78), as well as stability of the hip in the position of sleep (flexion and adduction) (Figure 5.79). In the flexed position, the hip should be internally rotated to determine the point at which the hip begins to lift out of the joint (an angle greater than 30° is preferred). Lastly, with the hip in neutral position, the amount of laxity to straight pulling from the foot should be tested (Figure 5.80). Although this is probably less important than other tests of stability, the push-pull laxity should be minimal if an appropriate femoral neck length and suction fit have been achieved. The distance from the level of the lesser trochanter to the center of the head is measured with a ruler and compared to the preoperative template. The center of the head should also lie at roughly the level of the top of the trochanter. Varying neck lengths should be tested until stability is achieved.

After measurements are made and stability testing completed, the hip is dislocated, the broach and trial head are removed, and the canal is brushed and irrigated (Figure 5.81). If the prosthesis is to be cemented, the canal is packed with a sponge while the cement is prepared. A cement plug is inserted to the

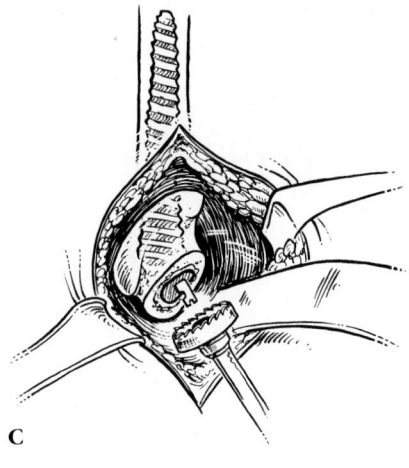

C

Figure 5.76. Once broaching is completed and the last broach has been completely seated (**A**), a calcar planer is used to even out the femoral neck cut (**B, C**).

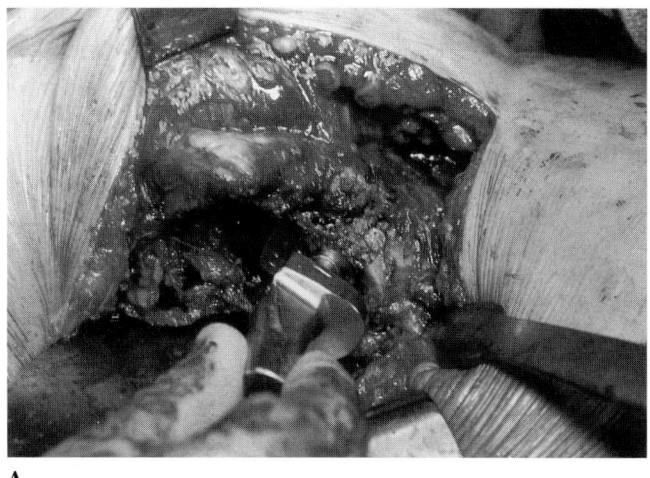 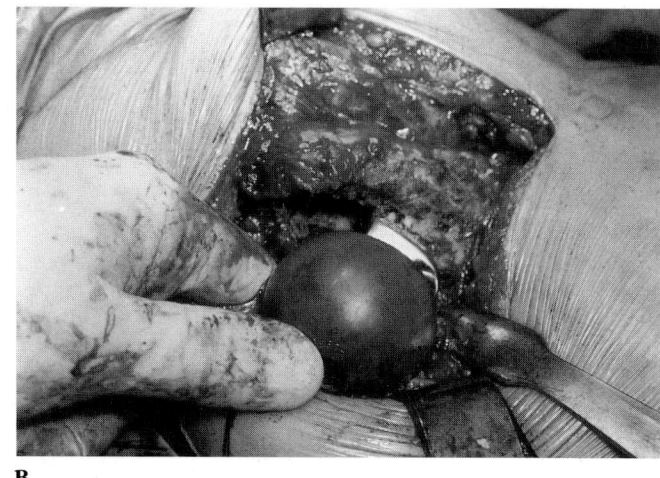

Figure 5.77. Placement of the trial neck (**A**) and head (**B**) onto the fully seated broach.

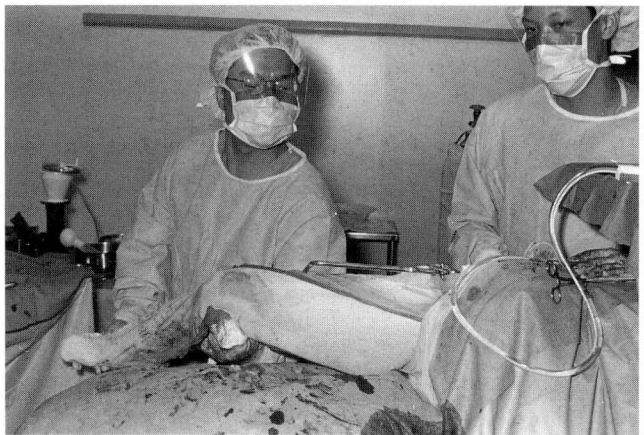

Figure 5.78. Assessment of hip stability to external rotation with the hip in full extension.

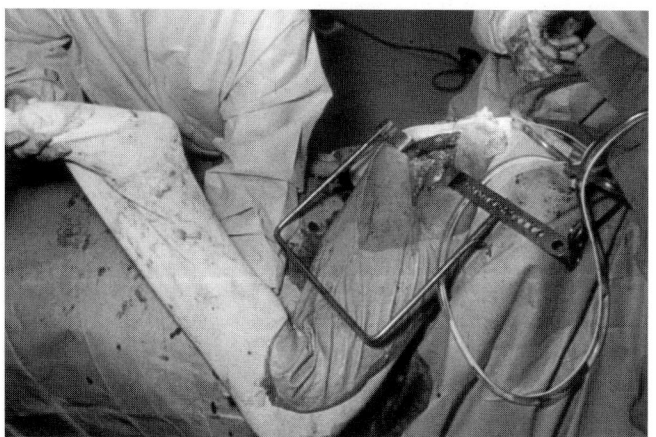

Figure 5.79. Assessment of hip stability to the position of sleep (flexion and adduction).

Figure 5.80. The amount of laxity to straight pulling from the foot is tested with the hip in neutral position.

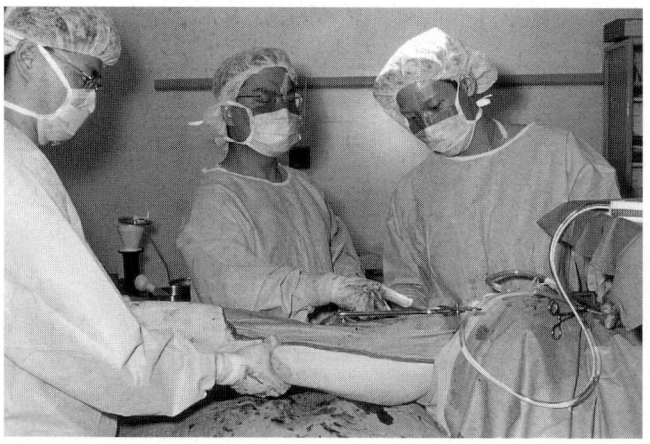

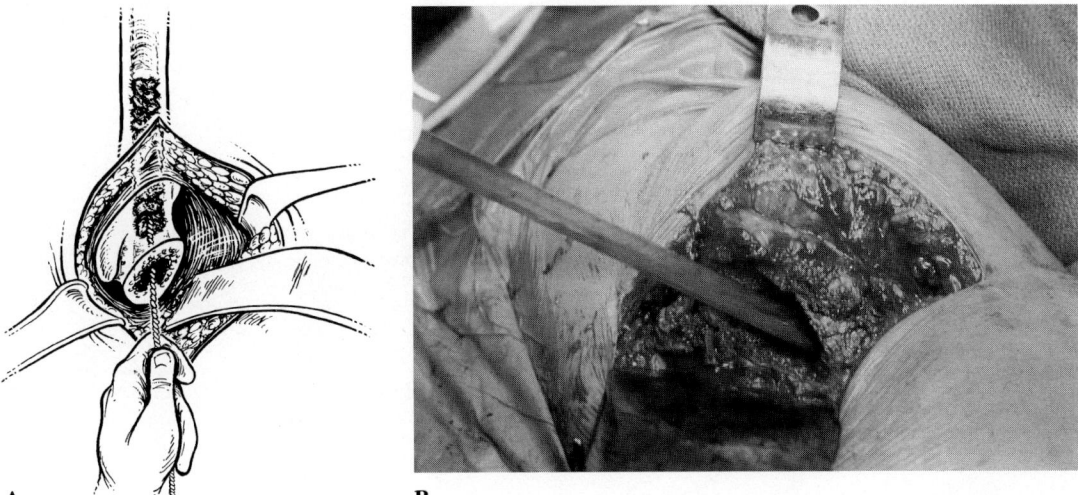

Figure 5.81. After measurements are made and stability testing completed, the hip is dislocated, the broach and trial head are removed, and the canal is brushed (**A**) and irrigated (**B**).

appropriate depth before the insertion of cement (Figure 5.82). The cement is vacuum mixed (Figure 5.83) and inserted in retrograde fashion using a cement gun and good pressurization technique (Figure 5.84). Alternatively, the cement can be hand-packed into the femoral canal. In some systems, a distal centralizer can be attached to the tip of the prosthesis before insertion, which helps to prevent varus positioning (Figure 5.85). Selection of the centralizer size is based on intraoperative measurement of canal diameter. The prosthesis is inserted using manual force and light taps with a mallet as it is fully seated to the level of the calcar cut (Figure 5.86). The position of the prosthesis should be maintained until the cement hardens (Figure 5.87); any excess cement is removed using a curette before hardening. Stability is then reassessed using head and neck trials. The final prosthetic head with the appropriate neck length is lightly impacted onto the clean and dry trunnion, and the hip is reduced after clearing all soft tissue from the opening of the acetabulum. Hip stability is once more assessed before wound closure. The short external rotators and underlying capsule are reattached through drill holes to the greater

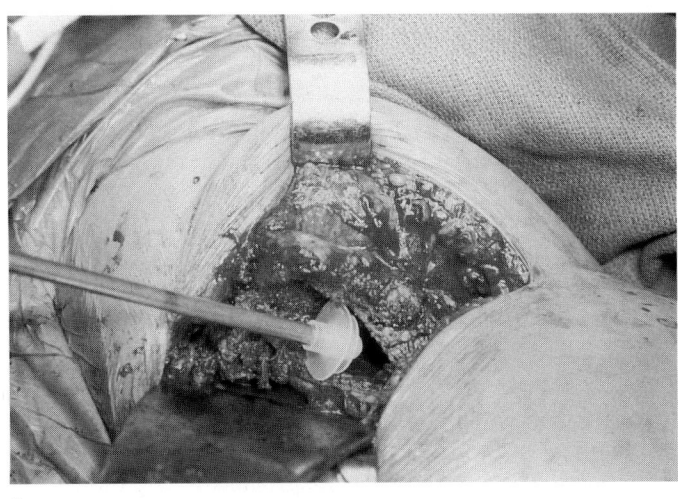
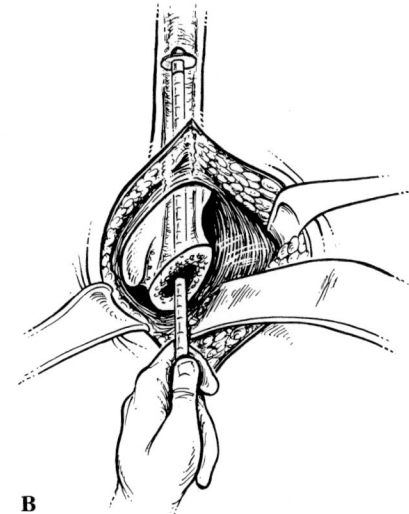

Figure 5.82. A cement plug is inserted to the appropriate depth before insertion of cement (**A, B**).

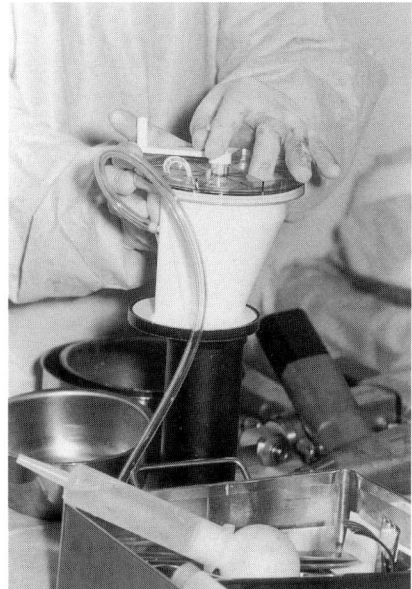

Figure 5.83. Vacuum mixing of the methylmethacrylate.

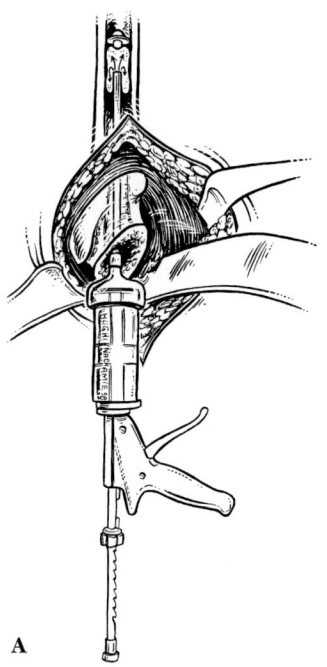

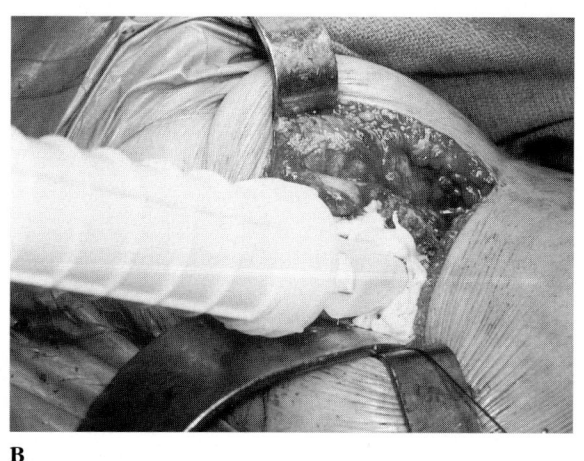

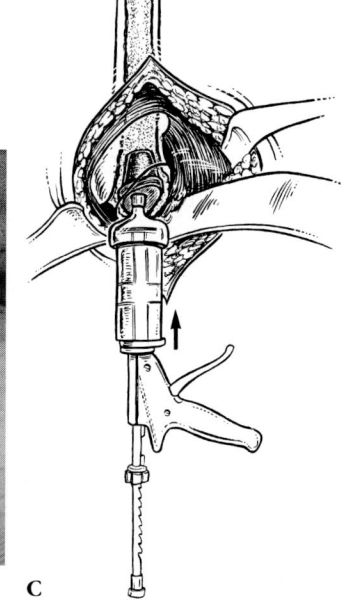

Figure 5.84. Retrograde insertion of the methylmethacrylate into the femoral canal using a cement gun (**A**), and pressurization of the cement (**B, C**).

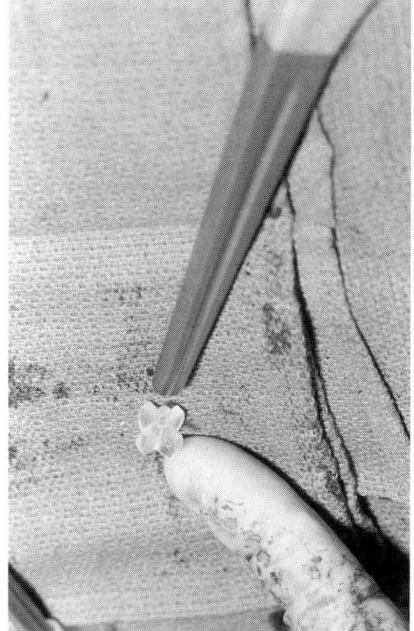

Figure 5.85. Placement of a distal centralizer to the tip of the prosthesis before insertion, which helps to prevent varus positioning.

trochanter (Figure 5.88). The fascia lata is closed using interrupted sutures, followed by skin closure. A Hemovac drain deep to the fascia lata is preferred.

Variations of this technique include use of a bipolar prosthetic head, a noncemented (press-fit) stem, and an Austin-Moore–type prosthesis. The surgical technique for the bipolar head is the same as previously described, with the addition that the bipolar head must be assembled. This technique may vary based on the system utilized. It is therefore important for the surgeon to be knowledgeable about the prosthesis being used. One should try not to use a bipolar head undersized relative to the acetabulum; a snug fit between the outer bearing of the bipolar head and the acetabulum serves to minimize motion between the two surfaces and reduces the potential for acetabular erosion.

For a noncemented press-fit or bone ingrowth prosthesis, insertion technique varies from system to system, although in most cases it is basically

Treatment

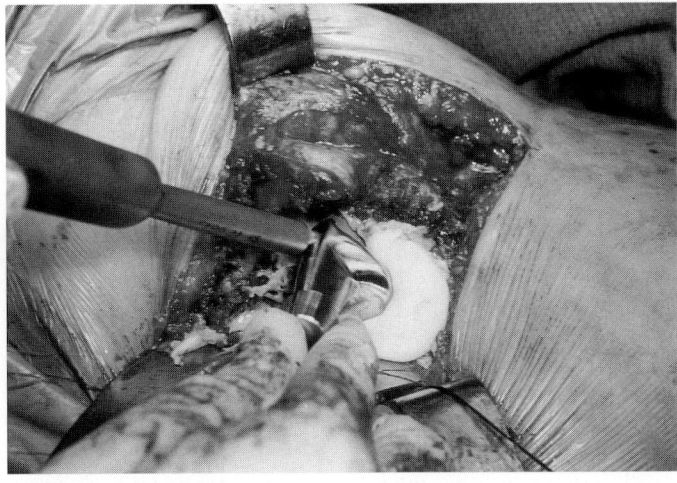

A

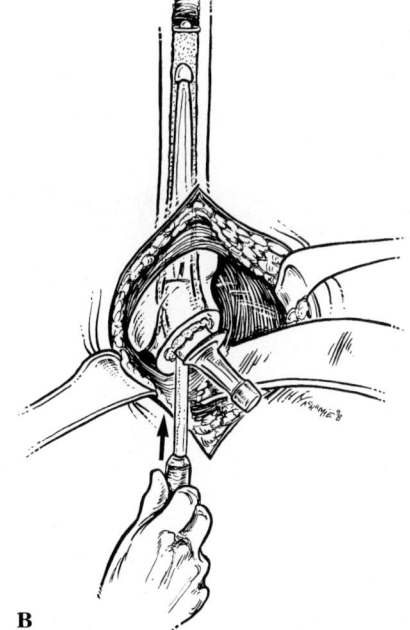

B

Figure 5.86. Insertion of the femoral prosthesis using manual force and light taps with a mallet (**A, B**).

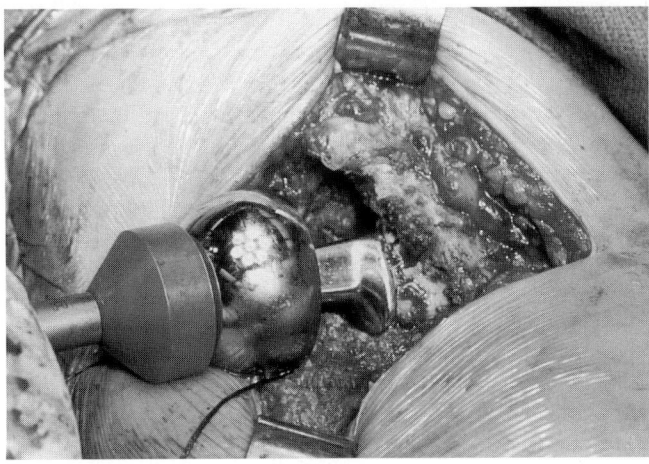

Figure 5.87. The position of the prosthesis is maintained until the cement hardens.

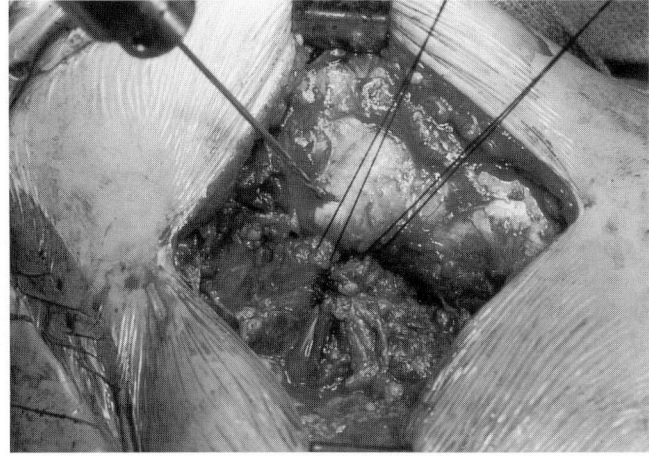

Figure 5.88. Reattachment of the short external rotators and underlying capsule to the greater trochanter.

similar to the one described previously. The most important difference with noncemented press-fit applications is that the fit of the broaches is more exacting. It is important to achieve a secure fit and fill in the metaphysis for proximally fitting stems or to achieve a secure distal fit for distally fitting stems. Because patients who undergo hemiarthroplasty secondary to hip fracture are typically osteopenic, it is important not to use excessive force during placement of the press-fit stem.

The technique for insertion of a one-piece Austin-Moore–type implant is similar to that described for a modular unipolar prosthesis. The original Austin-Moore prosthesis featured a range of femoral head sizes with a standard femoral neck and stem length. A box osteotome was used to open the proximal femur followed by a single broach. The cancellous bone removed from the box osteotome was placed within the fenestrated portion of the implant, and the prosthesis was inserted into the femoral canal. Newer-generation Austin-Moore–type implants are available as modular components; in addition, they are available as a solid-stem design for cemented application and a fenestrated-stem design for noncemented application.

Primary Total Hip Arthroplasty

Some authors have recommended total hip arthroplasty for the treatment of displaced femoral neck fractures in active patients, pointing out that such patients, when treated with a bipolar or unipolar prosthesis, are at increased risk of developing complications (e.g., acetabular erosion) that might require later revision to a total hip replacement.[131–136] A question that has important implications for this issue is whether it is reasonable to expect that the results of total hip arthroplasty after acute femoral neck fracture will be as satisfactory as those reported after elective total hip replacement. Delamarter and Moreland reported on a series of 27 patients treated with primary total hip arthroplasty after femoral neck fracture; follow-up averaged 3.8 years.[137] Eighty-two percent of patients had moderate to severe preexisting acetabular degeneration, and more than half were restricted in their activities prior to fracture because of degenerative arthritis of the hip. The results of this series were not substantially different from those reported for elective total hip arthroplasty and were better than for hemiarthroplasty. No deep infections, dislocations, or reoperations were reported.

Sim and Stauffer reported on a series of 112 patients who underwent primary total hip arthroplasty after femoral neck fracture[133,134]; only 16 (14%) had preexisting hip disease. Functional results were good: over 60% of patients regained or improved upon their prefracture level of activity. On the other hand, there was a 21% incidence of medical complications and a 22% incidence of surgical complications, including a 12% dislocation rate—much higher rates than those reported for elective total hip arthroplasty performed for degenerative arthritis. In this series, in comparison to that of Delamarter and Moreland, only 14% had preexisting acetabular degeneration.

Taine and Armour reported on a series of 160 patients treated by primary total hip arthroplasty after femoral neck fracture (average patient age, 78 years).[136] At an average follow-up of 42 months, 62% had good or excellent results; complication rates included 3.7% wound infection, 12.3% dislocation, and 30% medical problems. Pun et al. reported 94% good or excellent results after primary total hip replacement performed in a series of patients who were relatively younger (average age, 63.5 years) and more active.[132] They reported a low complication rate, with an average follow-up of 3 years.

Greenbough and Jones reported their results of primary total hip replacement after displaced femoral neck fracture in 37 patients, all less than 70 years old and none with preexisting acetabular disease.[138] At an average follow-up of 4.7 years, 49% required revision surgery and 60% had radiographic signs of loosening. Greenbough and Jones strongly recommended avoiding total hip replacement in active elderly patients without preexisting acetabular disease.

We believe that there is a place for primary total hip arthroplasty after femoral neck fracture, but that this procedure should be reserved for patients with preexisting symptomatic acetabular disease (e.g., rheumatoid arthritis, osteoarthritis, Paget's disease) (Figure 5.89). In this situation, one can expect results comparable to those reported for elective total hip arthroplasty.

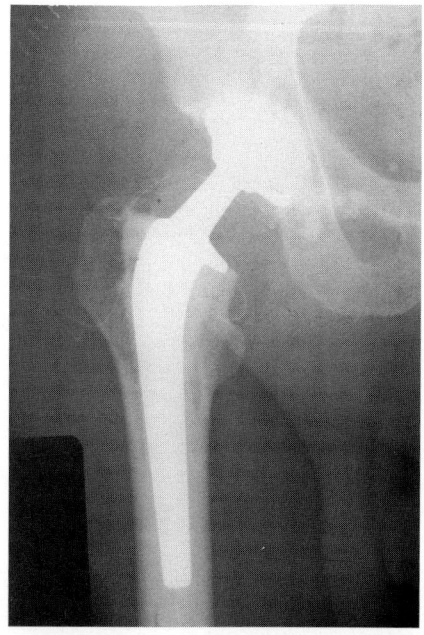

Figure 5.89. Use of a primary total hip arthroplasty after displaced femoral neck fracture in a patient who had rheumatoid arthritis and preexisting symptomatic acetabular disease.

Special Situations

Parkinson's Disease

Patients with Parkinson's disease who sustain a femoral neck fracture present a special challenge, as morbidity and mortality rates are much higher than in patients who do not have this condition.[139–141] Widely varying results have been reported for both internal fixation and prosthetic replacement, and thus no general agreement exists on how best to manage these fractures in this difficult patient population. Staehli et al., reporting the Mayo Clinic's experience with primary prosthetic replacement in 48 patients with Parkinson's disease, found that the 6-month mortality rate was 20%.[142] Over 80% of patients who were ambulatory prior to the fracture remained ambulatory after prosthetic replacement. In patients with hip contractures, an adductor tenotomy was useful to improve implant stability. The authors concluded that primary prosthetic replacement provided satisfactory results in their population of patients with Parkinson's disease.

To decide on an appropriate treatment plan, it is essential to consider the status of the disease. Parkinson's disease is a movement disorder whose clinical manifestations can range from mild tremors without significant functional limitations to severe contractures that result in complete incapacitation. Patient response to medical treatment must also be considered, since a well-controlled disease process should not affect the choice of treatment.

As in any such situation, it is essential when evaluating patients with Parkinson's disease to view cases individually rather than take an across-the-board approach. We rely on the following general guidelines: In cases of nondisplaced or impacted fracture, a patient of any age or disease severity should be treated with multiple-screw fixation and early mobilization. Patients with displaced femoral neck fractures who are relatively young and active and whose disease is well controlled should be treated by anatomic reduction and internal fixation using the approach described previously. Older patients with displaced fractures and younger patients with poorly controlled disease and significant loss of function should be treated by cemented prosthetic replacement.

Paget's Disease

Paget's disease is a metabolic bone disease, of unknown etiology, common in the elderly. Two types of fractures are encountered in patients with Paget's disease: (1) incomplete or fissure fractures, and (2) complete fractures. Specifically addressed here are complete fractures of the proximal femur, which are for the most part displaced fractures. In most series of complete proximal femur fractures in Paget's disease, the usual fracture location is in the intertrochanteric or subtrochanteric region.[143] Femoral neck fractures nevertheless do occur in this patient population, at reported frequencies from 7% to 22% of proximal femur fractures.[143–147] Thirty years ago it was thought that fracture union in Paget's disease proceeds as in normal bone, with some authors suggesting that healing occurs rapidly in the vascular phase of the disease.[146] More recently, however, it has become evident that delayed union and nonunion are common sequelae of fractures in pagetoid bone.[147–149] Treatment of femoral neck fractures in these patients has correspondingly evolved. Early reports utilizing internal fixation demonstrated high rates of delayed union and nonunion.[146] Early results with prosthetic replacement were also unacceptable, but this probably reflected, in part, problems with the available prostheses.[143,147] In a study by Dove et al., 75% of patients who had a femoral neck fracture treated with internal fixation developed a painful nonunion[144]; however, 78% of patients treated by cemented prostheses were able to ambulate without pain. Stauffer and Sim reported excellent results with total hip replacement in three patients with displaced femoral neck fractures.[149] These results support the use of primary prosthetic replacement for displaced femoral neck fractures in Paget's disease.

Our treatment of choice for displaced femoral neck fractures in Paget's disease is primary prosthetic replacement. The decision whether to opt for a prosthesis or total hip replacement is made by determining the presence and severity of prefracture hip symptoms as well as the extent of pagetoid involvement of the acetabulum. If there is no history of such symptoms and acetabular involvement is minimal, then a hemiarthroplasty should be performed; we prefer a cemented, modular unipolar prosthesis. When, however, there are significant preinjury symptoms and/or extensive acetabular involvement with secondary degenerative changes, total hip replacement is indicated. Although the technical aspects of primary prosthetic replacement in Paget's disease are beyond the scope of this text, it is worth mentioning that the surgeon must be prepared to encounter either sclerotic bone with obliteration of the canal or extremely soft bone. Preexisting deformity of the proximal femur as well as a tendency toward excessive bleeding can make this procedure quite challenging.

Spastic Hemiplegia

Patients with spastic hemiplegia following cerebrovascular accident are at increased risk for sustaining a femoral neck fracture. Soto-Hall reported that femoral neck fracture commonly occurs at the time of the cerebrovascular accident[150]; furthermore, weakness of the affected side predisposes to a later fall, usually on the affected side.[150,151] Treatment of these patients may be problematic because of osteopenia, spasticity, and/or contracture.[33] Functional prognosis is particularly compromised if the fracture occurs within 1 week of the stroke.[33] As in Parkinson's disease, the severity of symptoms varies greatly, ranging from minimal spasticity without contracture in ambulatory patients to severe spasticity and contracture in nonambulatory patients. Treatment approach thus must likewise be individualized.

Soto-Hall observed that problems arise when internal fixation is used in patients with spasticity and contracture.[150] Arguing that the imbalance of muscle forces about the hip tends to angulate the fracture and lever the internal fixation out of the femoral head, he recommended contracture release prior to internal fixation in order to restore proper muscle balance. Unfortunately, he did not report the results of internal fixation using this approach. Indeed, there is very little experience with internal fixation reported in the literature. Most authors have recommend primary prosthetic replacement for femoral neck fractures in patients with hemiplegia.[33]

We favor an approach based on the type of fracture and severity of spasticity and contracture. Nondisplaced fractures in ambulatory patients with minimal spasticity should be treated with internal fixation. Displaced fractures in ambulatory patients with minimal spasticity should be treated similar to fractures in patients without hemiplegia; that is, treatment should be based on patient age and the presence or absence of posterior femoral neck comminution. Patients who exhibit severe spasticity and contracture should undergo primary prosthetic replacement whether the fracture is displaced or not. Because the classic contracture is a flexion-adduction deformity, prosthetic replacement should be combined with muscle and tendon releases to correct the contracture. Furthermore, an anterior approach is preferred to increase stability of the prosthesis and to avoid the potential for instability in flexion and adduction associated with the posterior approach.

Chronic Renal Failure

Patients with chronic renal failure develop renal osteodystrophy and are consequently at increased risk for fracture. Although the bone loss that occurs is primarily due to hyperparathyroidism, the concomitant osteomalacia is a result of both vitamin D deficiency and aluminum inhibition of osteoid calcification.[152] These patients are moreover subject to bone loss from age-related (involutional) osteoporosis.

Among the few authors who have studied this rather complex situation, Thornhill and Creasman reported on 43 patients (average age, 62 years) with chronic renal failure who had sustained 48 hip fractures, nearly 75% of them in the femoral neck region[153]; all the rest were intertrochanteric fractures except for one subtrochanteric fracture. The intertrochanteric fractures, treated with internal fixation, all united; 11 of the 36 femoral neck fractures (31%) were internally stabilized, and none united. As expected, the mortality rate was high in this patient population.

Chalmers and Irvine reported on a series of five elderly patients (average age, 76 years) with hyperparathyroidism who sustained a femoral neck fracture.[154] Two patients had underlying renal failure, and the remaining three had primary hyperparathyroidism due to parathyroid adenoma. All five patients were treated by internal fixation, but none of the fractures united. Based on this experience, the authors recommended primary prosthetic replacement.

Primary prosthetic replacement appears to be the treatment of choice for femoral neck fractures in patients with chronic renal failure. Because these patients are usually seated in low, semireclining chairs while undergoing dialysis, an anterior approach should be considered to decrease the risk of dislocation. Because heparinization is necessary for dialysis and is usually needed within 72 hours of surgery, hemostasis is of paramount importance.

Preexisting Osteoarthritis or Rheumatoid Arthritis

Femoral neck fractures in patients with preexisting rheumatoid arthritis or osteoarthritis are relatively uncommon.[33] In one retrospective review, radiographic evidence of ipsilateral osteoarthritis was found in 2% of patients with femoral neck fractures compared to 26% of patients with intertrochanteric fractures.[155] Similarly, approximately 3% to 8% of all femoral neck fractures have been reported to occur in patients with rheumatoid arthritis.[156,157]

Several studies have evaluated the results of internal fixation after femoral neck fracture in patients with rheumatoid arthritis; all reported high failure rates.[157–160] One study compared the results of internal fixation after femoral neck fracture in patients with rheumatoid arthritis ($n = 25$) to a nonrheumatoid control group ($n = 94$) utilizing the same treatment protocol.[157] In patients with rheumatoid arthritis, 1 of 5 (20%) nondisplaced femoral neck fractures developed late segmental collapse, whereas after displaced fracture, 19 of 20 (95%) developed loss of fixation, nonunion or late segmental collapse. Fourteen of these 20 patients (70%) required revision to total hip arthroplasty.

Primary total hip replacement is recommended for displaced femoral neck fractures in patients with symptomatic rheumatoid arthritis or osteoarthritis. Although some authors have reported successful results after hemiarthroplasty in patients who have osteoarthritis and have sustained a femoral neck fracture, the same is not true for fractures in patients with rheumatoid arthritis.[110,111,161–163] Total hip arthroplasty is thus generally preferred for displaced femoral neck fractures in all such patients.

Pathologic Fractures

The proximal femur is involved in over 50% of pathologic long bone fractures.[164] Reports in the literature vary as to the proportion of metastases to the femoral neck, intertrochanteric, and subtrochanteric regions; on average, the distribution seems to be equally divided.

Operative treatment is indicated for almost all pathologic femoral neck fractures.[165] This treatment approach maximizes patient function, alleviates pain, facilitates nursing care, decreases the duration and cost of hospitalization, and maximizes patient morale. Surgical contraindications, which are few, include (1) a patient whose medical condition is inadequate to tolerate the anesthesia and surgical procedure; (2) mental obtundation or alteration of consciousness

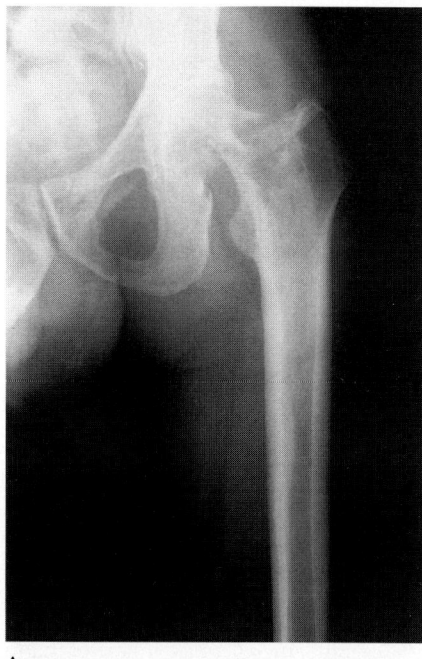 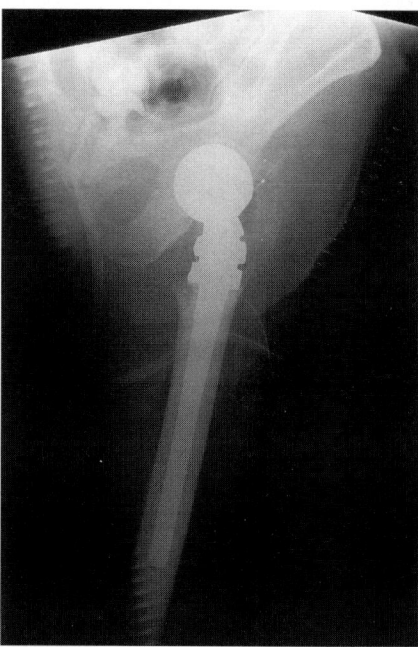

Figure 5.90. Pathologic femoral neck fracture (**A**) treated with prosthetic replacement (**B**).

that precludes the need for local measures to alleviate pain; and (3) markedly limited life expectancy (i.e., less than 1 month).[165]

Pathologic fractures of the femoral neck should be managed by prosthetic replacement (Figure 5.90). The temptation to attempt internal fixation, even of nondisplaced fractures, should be resisted.[165] These fractures have very high rates of nonunion associated with residual pain. The incidence of osteonecrosis is high, and advancement of the metastatic process may cause implant loosening and fixation failure despite the use of adjunctive methylmethacrylate.[165]

Surgical options include a unipolar or bipolar femoral endoprosthesis, proximal femoral replacement, and total hip arthroplasty, depending on the extent of metastatic involvement.[165] It is essential to obtain preoperative radiographs of the entire femur to identify other, more distal metastatic lesions. In most cases, a long-stemmed femoral component should be considered to reinforce the remaining femur. Although this adds to the expense of the component, it decreases the risk of periprosthetic fracture.[165]

Rehabilitation

Patients who have undergone surgery after femoral neck fracture—whether internal fixation, hemiarthroplasty, or total hip arthroplasty—are mobilized out of bed on postoperative day 1 and started on ambulation training. All such patients should be allowed to bear weight as tolerated. It is often difficult for elderly patients with decreased upper-extremity strength (and occasionally associated upper-extremity fractures) to comply with a non–weight-bearing or a partial weight-bearing protocol. Furthermore, in attempting to maintain partial weight bearing, considerable force is generated across the hip by the lower-extremity musculature.[166]

There is little biomechanical justification for restricted weight bearing after femoral neck fracture, since activities such as moving around in bed and use of a bedpan themselves generate forces across the hip approaching those resulting from unsupported ambulation.[166] Even foot and ankle range-of-motion exercises performed in bed produce substantial loads on the femoral head secondary to muscle contraction.[166]

Finally, it has been demonstrated in several studies that unrestricted weight bearing does not result in increased complication rates after femoral neck fracture stabilization. Cobb and Gibson reported on a series of 71 femoral neck fractures (43 nondisplaced, 28 displaced) stabilized with multiple cancellous screws.[10] Elderly patients were restricted to partial weight bearing, and younger patients with displaced femoral neck fractures remained non–weight bearing for 12 weeks. Sixty-five patients were available for follow-up at an average of 47 months. Four patients (6.2%), all with a displaced femoral neck fracture, developed loss of fixation or nonunion. The authors reported that they believed that weight-bearing status had no effect on loss of fixation.

Soreide et al. reported on a series of 50 patients who had a displaced femoral neck fracture stabilized with multiple screws and allowed immediate unrestricted weight bearing.[167] At 1-year follow-up, 10 fractures (20%) had loss of fixation, 8 of them requiring revision surgery. The authors attributed the high failure rate to poor screw positioning, not weight-bearing status.

In a prospective series performed at the Hospital for Joint Diseases to determine the effect of immediate unrestricted weight bearing on outcome after hip fracture, 95 patients with an internally stabilized femoral neck fracture were followed up for a minimum of 1 year.[168] Sixty-nine patients had a nondisplaced and 26 a displaced femoral neck fracture; 56 fractures were stabilized with multiple cancellous screws and 39 with multiple Knowles pins. Five fractures (5.3%) required revision surgery secondary to either loss of fixation (2 fractures) or nonunion (3 fractures); three of five patients requiring revision surgery had a nondisplaced and two a displaced femoral neck fracture. Among 74 of these patients who were followed up for a minimum of 2 years, four patients with femoral neck fractures (5.4%) developed symptomatic osteonecrosis requiring additional surgery; two of four patients had a nondisplaced and the other two a displaced femoral neck fracture. These results are comparable to other series in which patients had restricted weight bearing after femoral neck fracture fixation.

Ipsilateral Femoral Neck and Shaft Fractures

Fractures of the ipsilateral femoral neck and shaft are a rare and challenging combination of injuries (Figure 5.91). As of 1993, approximately 250 cases had been reported in the literature, with series ranging from to 2 to 46 patients.[169] The reported incidence of ipsilateral femoral neck and shaft fractures is increasing, due to several possible factors, including an increase in high-velocity trauma, better surveillance of this injury pattern, and advances in the field of emergency medicine, which has extended the survival of polytrauma patients.

Since the first report of this injury pattern by Delaney and Street in 1953,[170] the late diagnosis of an unrecognized femoral neck fracture associated with ipsilateral femoral shaft fracture has been problematic. Multiple series have reported an incidence of 19% to 31% missed femoral neck fracture in the face of an obvious femoral shaft fracture.[171,172] Furthermore, the literature is brimming with

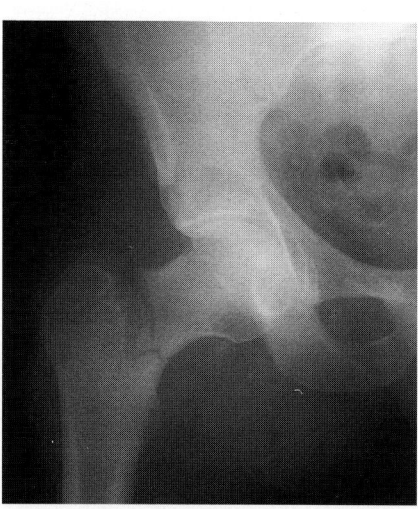 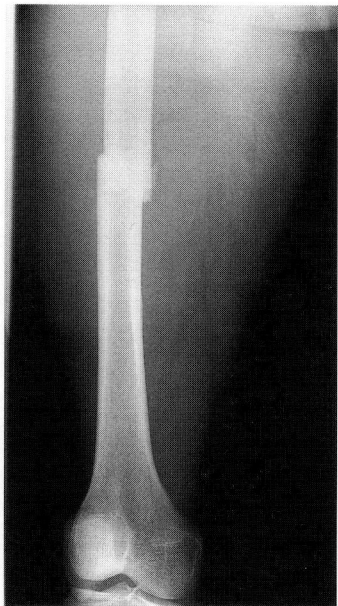

Figure 5.91. Ipsilateral femoral neck (**A**) and shaft fracture (**B**) in a 30-year-old man.

treatment approaches, including skeletal traction, spica cast immobilization, fixed-angle devices, sliding hip screws, cephalomedullary nails, and screws in combination with a retrograde-inserted intramedullary nail.[14,169–171,173–176] No single treatment protocol has achieved a consensus.

Incidence

Fracture of the ipsilateral femoral neck and shaft, although it can occur in anyone subjected to high-energy trauma, is primarily found in younger individuals, usually in their 20s or 30s.[171] The overall incidence of associated femoral neck and shaft fracture ranges between 2.5% and 6%, the majority of them resulting from a motor vehicle accident, a motorcycle accident, a fall from a height, or an industrial accident.[171,172]

Several authors have theorized that this injury typically arises from longitudinal compression of a flexed and abducted hip.[177] Most of the energy is dissipated by the femoral shaft fracture, which accounts for the high incidence of femoral shaft comminution; typically, the fracture occurs in the middle third of the femoral shaft. The femoral neck, because it is subjected to lower energy in this scenario, usually sustains a nondisplaced fracture, and the fracture line usually starts inferiorly, at the base of the femoral neck, and extends superiorly to the subcapital region (Figure 5.92).

Diagnosis

The evaluation of any severely traumatized patient should follow the principles of advanced trauma life support, with strict adherence to protocol. The deformity associated with femoral shaft fracture is usually obvious. Once this fracture has been confirmed radiographically, it is important to rule out an associated ipsilateral femoral neck fracture. If the pelvis film does not demonstrate a femoral neck fracture, an AP radiograph of the hip in internal rotation is recommended to exclude the diagnosis. Some have recommended bone scanning or tomograms for patients with persistent hip or groin pain following stabilization of a femoral shaft fracture in whom initial radiographs did not show a fracture.[178] Computed tomography (CT) has been recommended to identify occult hip fracture in polytraumatized patients, since most of these patients undergo routine abdominal and pelvic CT imaging during their initial trauma workup.[179]

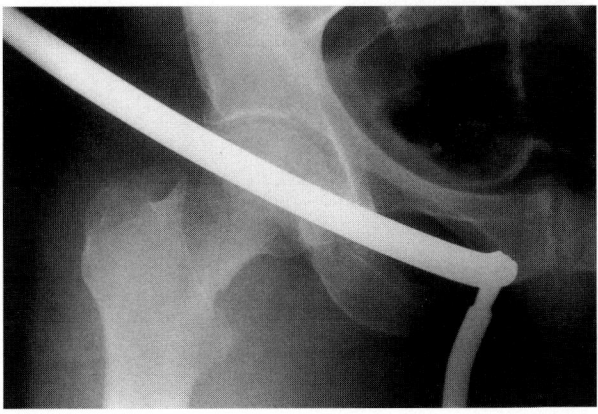

Figure 5.92. In an ipsilateral femoral neck and shaft fracture, the femoral neck fracture line usually starts inferiorly, at the base of the femoral neck, and extends superiorly to the subcapital region.

Treatment

Numerous options exist for the treatment of this complex injury pattern. The optimal timing of such surgery, however, is not controversial. Patients should have early femoral neck and long bone stabilization followed by rapid mobilization out of bed to minimize morbidity and mortality.[180]

Schatzker and Barrington recommended reduction and stabilization of the femoral shaft before stabilization of the femoral neck, reasoning that this would facilitate reduction of the femoral neck fracture.[181] Forty-two cases of ipsilateral femoral neck and shaft fractures were reported by Bennet et al., of which 19 (45%) had undergone antegrade nailing of the femoral shaft prior to treatment of the femoral neck fracture[169]; none developed osteonecrosis at 1-year follow-up.

Swiontkowski et al. recommended prompt reduction of the femoral neck and fixation with multiple cancellous lag screws, followed by extraarticular retrograde insertion of a locked intramedullary nail to stabilize the femoral shaft[176] (Figure 5.93). This method gave priority to the femoral neck in the hopes of avoiding the disastrous complication of osteonecrosis. Despite this attention, 2 of 12 (22%) patients developed osteonecrosis of the femoral head. Retrograde-inserted flexible nails can also be used to stabilize the femoral shaft fracture after fixation of the femoral neck. Flexible nail stabilization, however, is limited to stable femoral fracture patterns. Extraarticular retrograde femoral nailing has largely been replaced by retrograde locked femoral nailing through the intercondylar notch of the distal femur (Figure 5.94).

Another method of treating this combined injury is by use of a cephalomedullary nail (Figure 5.95). Wiss et al. reported on a series of 33 femoral neck and shaft fractures stabilized with either a cephalomedullary nail (14 patients) or a reversed first-generation interlocked nail to allow for locking

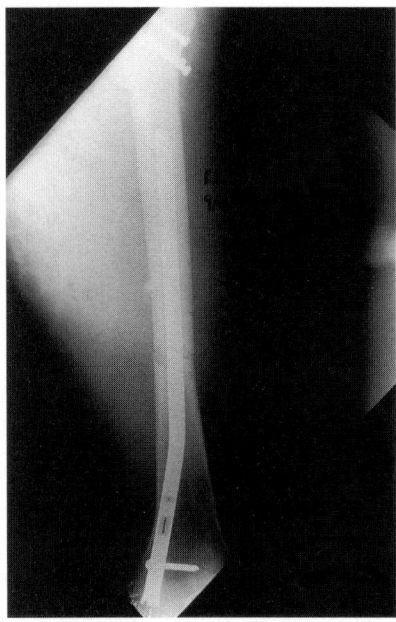

Figure 5.93. Ipsilateral femoral neck and shaft fracture stabilized with multiple cancellous lag screws for the femoral neck, followed by extraarticular retrograde insertion of a locked intramedullary nail to stabilize the femoral shaft.

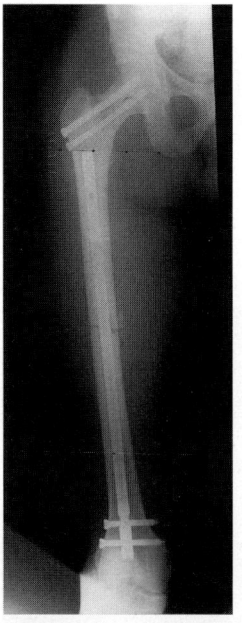

Figure 5.94. Ipsilateral femoral neck and shaft fracture stabilized with multiple cancellous lag screws for the femoral neck, followed by retrograde locked femoral nailing through the intercondylar notch of the distal femur.

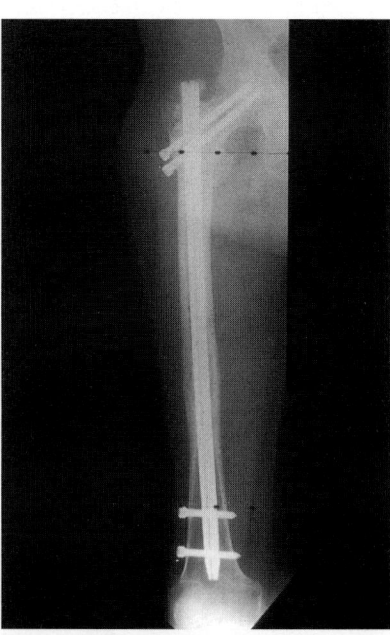

Figure 5.95. Ipsilateral femoral neck and shaft fracture stabilized with a cephalomedullary nail.

screw placement into the femoral head (19 patients).[182] Two patients (6%) developed a varus malunion of the femoral shaft and two patients (6%) developed osteonecrosis of the femoral head; both of the latter two patients had undergone open reduction and provisional stabilization of a displaced femoral neck fracture before intramedullary nailing.

Another technique that has been described involves antegrade intramedullary nailing of the femoral shaft fracture after reduction and provisional or definitive stabilization of the femoral neck with placement of cancellous lag screws around a locked intramedullary nail (Figure 5.96). Wu and Shih treated 22 of 42 (52%) ipsilateral neck and shaft fractures in this manner.[183] At 26-month follow-up, the authors reported a 100% union rate and 0% osteonecrosis. Chaturvedi and Sahu reported on a series of 17 such patients, of whom 13 of 17 (76%) had immediate stabilization of the femoral neck with multiple pins followed by antegrade nailing of the femoral shaft[184]; all fractures united by 6 months, with no cases of osteonecrosis.

If the femoral neck and shaft fractures are in close proximity, a sliding hip screw with a long sideplate may suffice; an antirotation screw should be placed into the femoral neck before insertion of the sliding hip screw. As the distance between the femoral neck and shaft fracture increases, this technique becomes less advisable.

Plate fixation of the femoral shaft with lag screw fixation of the femoral neck is yet another treatment option for this injury pattern (Figure 5.97). The advantages of this technique include reliable and familiar methods of fixation for each fracture. The disadvantages include increased blood loss and periosteal stripping of the femoral shaft with the potential need for bone grafting. Reimer et al. reported on a series of 10 ipsilateral femoral neck and shaft fractures, 9 of which had plate fixation of the femoral shaft.[171] The femoral neck

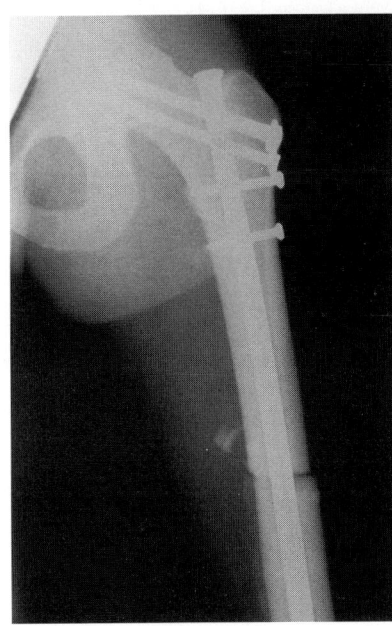

Figure 5.96. Ipsilateral femoral neck and shaft fracture stabilized by cancellous lag screws placed around an antegrade-inserted intramedullary nail.

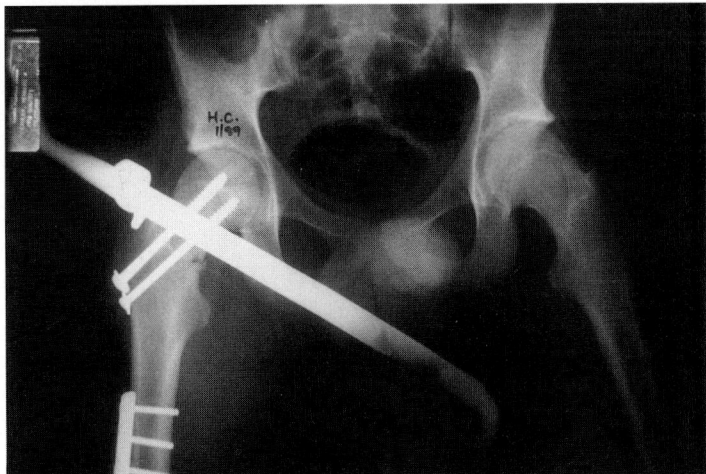

Figure 5.97. Ipsilateral femoral neck and shaft fracture stabilized by plate fixation of the femoral shaft with lag screw fixation of the femoral neck.

was subsequently stabilized using multiple cancellous lag screws. At an average follow-up of 21 months, there were no cases of osteonecrosis of the femoral head.

Complications

Complications following femoral neck fracture can be divided into three categories: (1) general complications relating to comorbidities, surgery, or anesthesia; (2) complications following the use of internal fixation devices; and (3) complications following the use of primary prosthetic replacement. Most complications specifically related to femoral neck fractures are discussed here; others are discussed in Chapter 6.

General Complications

The advanced age and medical fragility of many patients who sustain a femoral neck fracture increases their risk of experiencing a postoperative complication. Pneumonia, congestive heart failure, myocardial infarction, cardiac arrhythmia, electrolyte imbalance, urinary tract infection, decubitus ulcers, and thromboembolism are serious complications that occur with significant frequency. The incidence of clinically recognized thrombophlebitis in elderly hip fracture patients has been reported as 15–20%, while the incidence of radiographically documented thrombophlebitis has been reported as high as 50%.[185-189] Prophylactic anticoagulation using a variety of regimens, however, has been effective in decreasing the incidence of both thrombophlebitis and pulmonary embolism. Urinary tract infections and decubitus ulcers have been reported in 30% of patients with femoral neck fractures.[190,191] In one series, the presence of decubitus ulcers was associated with a 30% mortality rate.[192]

Many of these complications can be prevented by aggressive respiratory therapy, early surgical intervention followed by rapid mobilization, judicious management of fluid and electrolyte replacement, and meticulous nursing care. With conscientious care, the medical morbidity associated with femoral neck fracture can be decreased, as shown by the results of interdisciplinary care programs.[33,193] It is incumbent on the physician and nurses responsible for the care of these patients to anticipate problems that can occur and take steps to prevent them.

Complications Following Open Reduction and Internal Fixation

Infection

Superficial wound infection has been reported in up to 5% of cases after open reduction and internal fixation of femoral neck fractures.[57,81] Deep infection has also been reported in up to 5% of cases,[9,57,81,194] although one large series of 300 patients reported no deep infections.[68] Perioperative antibiotic prophylaxis has now become standard in the management of hip fracture patients and is responsible, in part, for the low rates of infection.

Wound hematoma may result in persistent wound drainage during the first several days after hip fracture surgery, particularly in obese, medically unstable, or nutritionally compromised patients. With the use of sterile pressure dressings and reduction in patient activities, such drainage often resolves uneventfully. In our institution, placement of elastic wraps in a spica arrangement (from the foot to the groin and across the abdomen) has been found to be effective in reducing wound drainage. Persistent serous or serosanguinous drainage is best treated aggressively. If it is copious, increasing, or does not resolve within 7 to 10 days, revision surgery should be considered to evacuate the hematoma and irrigate and débride the wound. Deep cultures should be taken and a Gram stain should be performed at surgery; we do not culture wound drainage at bedside, to avoid the risk of a positive skin contaminant culture. Appropriate antibiotics are initiated during surgery; after thorough débridement and irrigation, the wound is closed over suction drains. Antibiotics are discontinued if the final intraoperative culture results are negative. However, if bacterial organisms are recovered, the antibiotic coverage may need modification according to sensitivity tests and should be continued for several weeks.

Superficial wound infections should be treated with appropriate antibiotics, prompt débridement as needed, and open drainage, followed by secondary closure. If deep infection cannot be ruled out, it is much better to assume deeper tissue involvement and perform a formal irrigation and débridement. Deep infections may arise before or after fracture union, even several years after the initial surgery. Deep infections require surgical débridement and antibiotic coverage. If the fracture has not yet united and the fixation is stable, the implant should not be removed. If there is hip joint involvement or the implant is loose, however, removal of the internal fixation device and/or excisional arthroplasty is recommended.

Loss of Fixation

Fixation failure often becomes clinically apparent during the early postoperative period (Figure 5.98). The patient with unstable fixation generally complains of groin and/or buttock pain.[14] Radiographic studies may confirm displacement or angulation of the fracture, radiolucency around the implant, or backing out of the implant. Backout of the implant, however, can also occur with fracture settling as healing progresses and is facilitated by parallel insertion of multiple implants (Figure 5.99). Some degree of fracture settling is often associated with otherwise uneventful healing. Of the factors that predict fixation failure, patient age, preoperative fracture displacement, and the quality of fracture reduction have been found to be the most important.[33] Fixation failure early in the postoperative period is also related to comminution of the posterior femoral neck.

Because loss of fixation is probably related to failure of osteopenic bone around the implant, it may perhaps best be seen as a problem of patient selection.[14] Technical problems—such as fracture malreduction or the use of screws that are too short, have threads that do not completely cross the fracture line, or are widely divergent and prevent fracture settling—also play a role in fixation failure. Higher rates of nonunion and fixation failure have been reported with the use of a fixed-angle device or a sliding hip screw.

Early fixation failure (within 3 months after surgery) occurs in 12% to 24% of displaced femoral neck fractures.[8,37,195,196] Barnes reported a 14% early failure

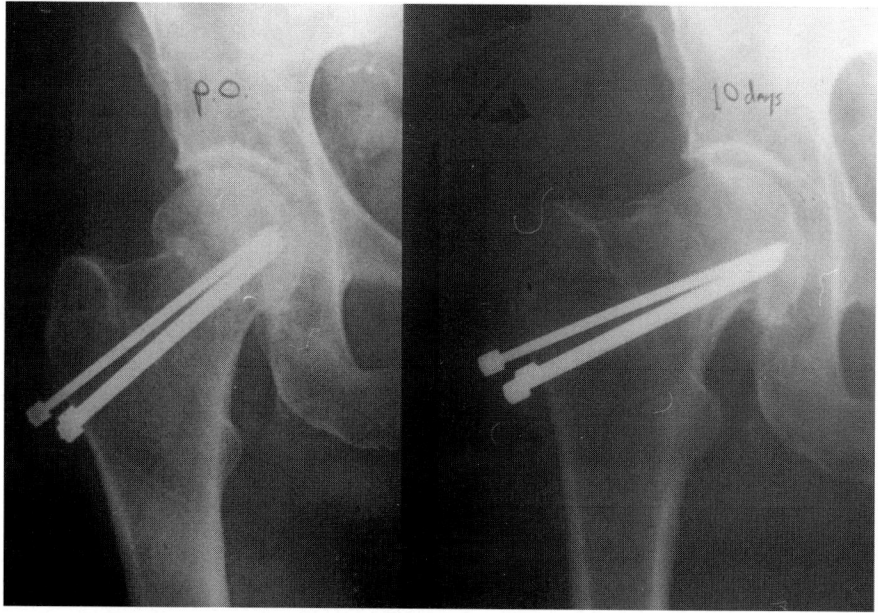

Figure 5.98. Loss of fixation 10 days after stabilization of a displaced femoral neck fracture using multiple pins. These pins were spaced too close together in the femoral head.

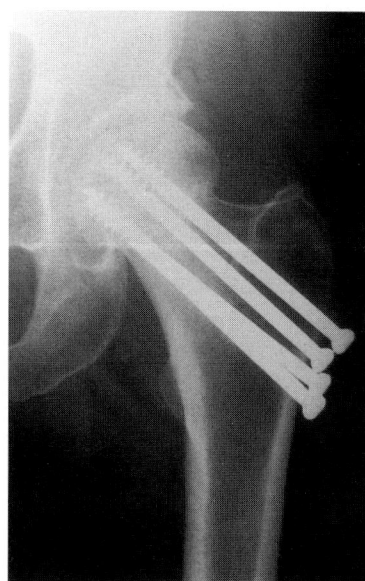

Figure 5.99. Backout of cancellous screws associated with uneventful fracture healing.

rate in a series of 1002 fractures using crossed screw fixation.[8] Brown reported a 24% failure rate at three months using a nail-plate device.[195] More recently, Stappaerts reported a 22% failure rate with use of Knowles pins or AO screws for stabilization of displaced femoral neck fractures.[196] He found that the most important factor associated with loss of fixation was patient age and an inaccurate fracture reduction. The presence of dementia, type of fracture (Garden type III or IV), surgical delay, and method of fixation (Knowles pins versus AO screws) were not significantly related to fixation failure. Other studies have shown the importance of nondisplaced versus displaced fracture type on the incidence of early fixation failure.[8,33] The importance of an anatomic reduction has been well documented in the literature and its importance is generally agreed upon.[8,195]

One report found that early loss of fixation occurred twice as frequently when the surgery was delayed for more than 7 days after injury.[37] Scheck and others have emphasized the importance of posterior comminution of the neck as a cause of unstable fixation leading to fixation failure and nonunion.[98,197]

In the face of loss of reduction and fixation failure, the choice of procedure depends on patient age, functional demands, medical condition, and bone quality. When these factors are favorable in an active individual, the surgeon should proceed with revision open reduction and internal fixation. Valgus osteotomy may also be considered. When these factors involve an older patient with poor bone quality and lower functional demands, hemiarthroplasty or total hip arthroplasty is the procedure of choice.

Nonunion

Nonunion after femoral neck fractures can be defined as a lack of radiographic evidence of union 6 months after fracture[33] (Figure 5.100). The diagnosis of nonunion is initially suspected clinically when the patient complains of groin or buttock pain, pain on hip extension, or pain with weight bearing. These symptoms occur earlier and are more severe than those associated with

Complications

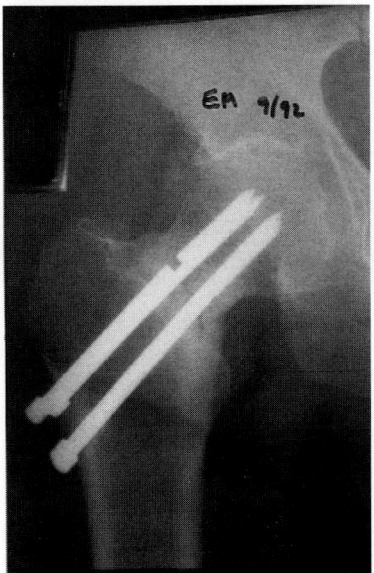

Figure 5.100. Femoral neck nonunion.

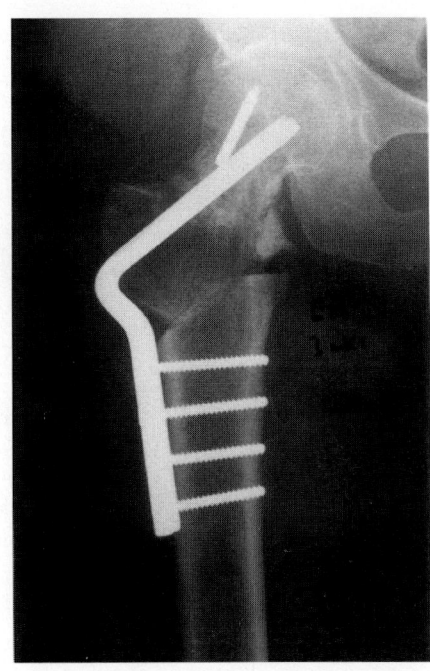

Figure 5.101. Femoral neck nonunion treated by a valgus osteotomy.

osteonecrosis. Radiographs may demonstrate a lucent zone at the fracture site; tomography may be necessary to confirm the diagnosis.

The incidence of nonunion is related to fracture displacement. In nondisplaced fractures (Garden types I and II), nonunion occurs in 0% to 5% of cases,[8,10,13,68] whereas in displaced fractures the reported incidence of nonunion ranges from 9% to 35%.[7,8–10,13,194,198,199] Nonunion is more common following an inadequate reduction.[8,200,201] The presence of posterior comminution is also associated with a higher rate of nonunion.[7,98]

The type of fixation also has an effect on the incidence of nonunion. The rate of nonunion with a nail-plate device is greater than with a sliding hip screw,[57] which in turn has a higher incidence of nonunion than multiple cancellous lag screws.[9,202]

As with fixation failure, the decision as to how to proceed is based on careful consideration of the patient's age, functioning, medical history, and bone quality. In the younger patient, if adequate bone remains in the femoral head, revision internal fixation with cancellous or muscle pedicle bone grafting is indicated. Many have used valgus osteotomy to convert the mechanical loading of the nonunion site from shear forces to compressive forces (Figure 5.101); in general, good results have been reported.[99,203,204] When the limb has shortened, valgus osteotomy is the procedure of choice because of the obligatory limb lengthening that results. The preferred treatment for symptomatic nonunion in the elderly patient is prosthetic replacement. Hemiarthroplasty or total hip replacement are acceptable options; the decision is based on the status of the acetabulum.

Osteonecrosis

The development of osteonecrosis following femoral neck fracture reflects the vulnerability of the femoral head vascularity to disruption (Figure 5.102). The

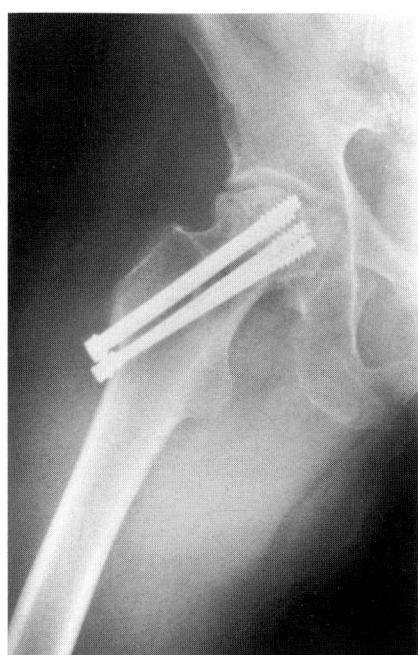

Figure 5.102. Osteonecrosis of the femoral head with segmental collapse following femoral neck fracture.

specific cause of the vascular insult remains controversial, but it probably involves disruption of the femoral head circulation at the time of fracture and/or compression of the vessels from increased intracapsular pressure that results from the hemarthrosis.[14,33] Some authors differentiate between osteonecrosis and late segmental collapse by characterizing the former as a microscopic process that may lead to the macroscopic problem of late segmental collapse[14]; segmental collapse causes loss of femoral head congruity, often resulting in secondary degenerative arthritis.[14] Unfortunately, this distinction is not universally accepted in the literature, making interpretation of the reported results somewhat difficult.[14]

The incidence of osteonecrosis following nondisplaced femoral neck fractures has been reported to be as high as 15%, but in general it ranges between 5% and 8%.[7,8,12,13,36,68,202] The incidence following displaced femoral neck fractures, in contrast, has been reported as being between 9% and 35%, with most series reporting between 20% and 35%.[7–9,11–13,68,202] Factors associated with increased incidence of osteonecrosis include inadequate fracture reduction, delay from injury to fracture reduction and fixation, and use of a sliding hip screw or nail plate device.[8,9,11,25,85] Garden linked the incidence of osteonecrosis directly to the adequacy of fracture reduction.[25] When his alignment index of reduction was acceptable, the incidence of osteonecrosis was 0%; mild deviations of postreduction alignment resulted in 6.6% incidence; moderate and severe alterations of the alignment index resulted in a 65% and 100% incidence of osteonecrosis, respectively. As previously indicated, a delay between injury and surgery is a risk factor for the development of osteonecrosis. Patients with normal bone stock have a higher risk of osteonecrosis, probably because greater energy is necessary to produce the hip fracture, resulting in greater soft tissue damage.

The majority of patients who develop osteonecrosis of the femoral head complain of groin, buttock, or proximal thigh pain. This pain, however, may not be functionally significant. It is generally true that the higher the functional demands on the hip, the more significant are the symptoms.[14] This is evidenced by the fact that the majority of patients younger than 50 years who develop posttraumatic femoral head osteonecrosis are sufficiently symptomatic to require a reconstructive procedure.[14] In contrast, only 33% of older patients with osteonecrosis have symptoms severe enough to warrant a second surgical procedure.[8,14]

The diagnosis of early osteonecrosis can be difficult. Tomography and CT scanning, because of their superior resolution, can show the changes of osteonecrosis (stippled areas of bone sclerosis, trabecular resorption, microfracture, and subchondral collapse) at an earlier stage than standard radiographs.[14] Bone scanning can also be used to diagnose early osteonecrosis. The bone scan may frequently be positive when standard radiographs are interpreted as negative. Magnetic resonance imaging has the potential for even earlier diagnosis of this condition, although ferrous metals (as in implants) and other materials distort magnetic resonance images.

Posttraumatic osteonecrosis is difficult to treat. Core decompression, even for treatment of nontraumatic osteonecrosis, has provided at best mixed results. Most authors doubt any favorable influence of core decompression on posttraumatic osteonecrosis, but adequate data remain unavailable.[14] In older patients with only mild to moderate symptoms and in whom radiographic findings may not correlate with function, observation is probably indicated. In those patients, arthroplasty is an excellent treatment option if symptoms increase. In younger patients, the acceptable options are limited. If the area of collapse involves less than 50% of the femoral head based on tomograms, CT, or standard radiographs obtained in various degrees of flexion and abduction, an osteotomy may provide acceptable improvement in function.[14] Hip arthrodesis is an option in the younger patient with high functional demands but is made more difficult by the presence of avascular bone.[14] Some authors have advocated bipolar prosthetic replacement in younger individuals, but long-term outcome studies are lacking.[14] Some authors have recommended total hip arthroplasty as the procedure of choice in younger patients, but studies have reported a high incidence of early component failure in younger patients.[14] The recent use of noncemented implants may offer a better option, but long-term data are not yet available. All factors considered, based on the lack of reliable reconstructive options in younger patients, every reasonable effort at prevention seems most appropriate.[14]

The preferred treatment for symptomatic osteonecrosis with collapse in the elderly is prosthetic replacement. Similar to nonunion after femoral neck fracture, hemiarthroplasty or total hip replacement are acceptable options; the choice depends on the status of the acetabular cartilage.

Complications Following Primary Prosthetic Replacement

Infection

The reported incidence of infection following primary prosthetic replacement after femoral neck fracture ranges between 2% and 20%.[104,109,114,205,206] Earlier studies are in general responsible for the higher rates, reflecting the fact that the population chosen for prosthetic replacement at the time was older and more debilitated than patients in more recent studies, in which generally lower rates (2% to 8%) have been reported.[81,201,207,208] The lower rates can be attributed not only to patient selection but also to the use of prophylactic perioperative antibiotics. Infections can be superficial or deep; they can occur early or late in the postoperative period. Early postoperative infections usually present with the classic signs of infection (e.g., erythema, swelling, pain, and drainage), whereas delayed infections are often difficult to diagnose because the symptoms are much more subtle. Deep infection may arise several years after surgery; symptoms can include hip pain, reduced hip range of motion, and elevated erythrocyte sedimentation rate and C-reactive protein. Elevated white blood cell count and fever are frequently absent unless acute sepsis develops. It is difficult to generalize regarding the incidence of superficial versus deep infection or early versus delayed infection, as many series do not categorize results in this way. It seems clear, however, that superficial infections are more common than deep infections and early infections more common than delayed ones. Furthermore, as indicated earlier, higher infection rates have been linked with a posterior approach, probably because of the proximity of the incision to the perineal region and the attendant potential for fecal contamination. Earlier concerns that the use of methylmethacrylate would increase the infection rate appear to have been unfounded.

Both superficial and deep wound infections should be treated aggressively. Superficial wound infections require appropriate antibiotics, prompt incision and débridement, followed by secondary closure. If deep infection cannot be

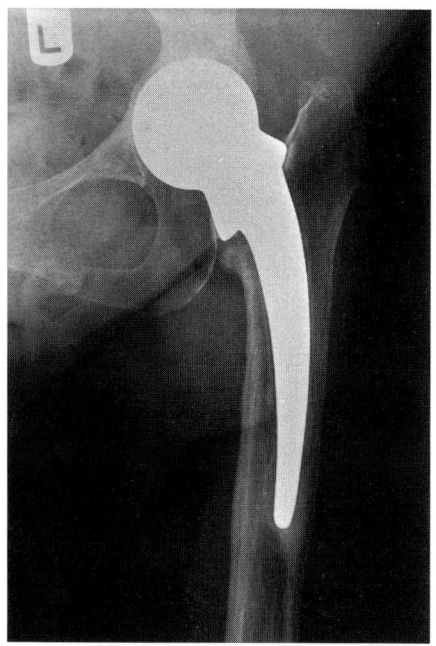

Figure 5.103. Acetabular erosion and protrusion associated with use of a cemented Thompson prosthesis.

ruled out, it is much better to assume deeper tissue involvement and to treat accordingly. Deep infections require meticulous surgical débridement and formal irrigation. Serious consideration should be given to implant removal, particularly if it is loose, followed by insertion of antibiotic-impregnated beads. Delayed prosthetic reimplantation can be considered after an appropriate delay if there have been no signs or symptoms of infection.

Dislocation

The reported incidence of dislocation following prosthetic replacement ranges between 0.3% and 10%.[110,114,119,209,210] The posterior approach is associated with a higher dislocation rate than the anterior approach.[114,208,211] Dislocation may occur less frequently with use of a bipolar prosthesis than after unipolar hemiarthroplasty.[119] Unfortunately, closed reduction of a bipolar prosthesis is more difficult to achieve.[33] Recurrent dislocation can be related to component malalignment or improper soft tissue tensioning. Revision surgery should be considered if the functional disability is significant.

Pain

Hip pain that develops after prosthetic replacement may have any of several causes, many of which are unrelated to the prosthesis.[33,212] The most important prosthesis-related causes of pain include acetabular erosion (groin pain) and prosthetic loosening (thigh pain). Acetabular erosion, which occurs as a result of contact between the prosthetic head and the acetabulum, may occur less frequently with use of a bipolar prosthesis than after implantation of a unipolar hemiarthroplasty[33] (Figure 5.103). Cement fixation of the femoral component is associated with a lower incidence of postoperative thigh pain, primarily because of the reduced risk of prosthetic loosening.[33] It is nevertheless important to remember that the incidence of revision surgery following prosthetic replacement in response to clinical symptoms is less than the radiographic incidence of significant acetabular erosion and prosthetic loosening.

Stress Fractures of the Femoral Neck

Fractures resulting from cyclic mechanical stresses can be classified as either fatigue or insufficiency fractures. A stress fracture that occurs in normal bone in a healthy young or middle-aged individual secondary to repetitive mechanical stress is defined as a *fatigue fracture,* one in which repetitive loading reduces the bone's failure strength. In the elderly, whose bone failure strength has already been lowered due to osteoporosis or another disease state, lower loads (such as those encountered in normal activities) or fewer loading cycles can result in osseous failure. This type of stress fracture is considered to be an *insufficiency fracture*. Recent work suggests that low levels of repetitive stress in normal bone can lead to increased bone remodeling, localized osteoporosis, and subsequent osseous weakening.

The incidence of femoral neck stress fractures is difficult to assess. Stoneham and Morgan reported a femoral neck stress fracture incidence of 0.3% in

1400 Royal Marine recruits whose age ranged from 16 to 27 years[213]; they noted that these fractures tended to occur near the end of basic training. In contrast, in a prospective study of 194 Israeli military recruits, Volpin et al. identified nine (4.7%) femoral neck stress fractures.[214]

Because many of the early series of femoral neck stress fractures studied male military recruits, the role of gender as a risk factor has been controversial. Lloyd-Smith et al., however, reported an equivalent distribution of exercise-induced femoral stress fractures in men and women.[215] A recent, large series by Zahger et al. reported a greater incidence of femoral neck stress fractures in Israeli female military recruits.[216] In the elderly, on the other hand, insufficiency fractures of the femoral neck are more common in women, probably reflecting their greater associated incidence of osteoporosis. Horiuchi et al. reported on a series of 42 patients who had sustained an insufficiency fracture of the femoral neck[217]; all were female.

Fatigue fractures, which occur predominantly in younger individuals, are most often the result of athletic activity. Competitive and recreational long-distance runners, ballet dancers, and military recruits are classic examples of those at increased risk for fatigue fractures. Fatigue fractures in these individuals can result from the initiation of a new athletic activity or an increase in the frequency or intensity of their current activity. Insufficiency fractures, which occur primarily in elderly females, occur most often secondary to normal activities of daily living. Conditions associated with an increased risk of insufficiency fractures include osteoporosis, osteomalacia, rheumatoid arthritis, diabetes, hyperparathyroidism, scurvy, and irradiation.[218,219]

Classification of Femoral Neck Stress Fractures

A system for classifying stress fractures of the femoral neck was first proposed by Devas in 1965.[220] He described two types, tension and compression, each with distinct radiographic and clinical characteristics. The tension (or transverse) type of femoral neck stress fracture is directed perpendicular to the line of force transmission in the femoral neck, originates at the superior surface of the femoral neck, and results from tension; this fracture pattern is at increased risk for displacement. The compression type of femoral neck stress fracture exhibits radiographic changes (evidence of internal callus formation) on the inferior femoral neck without apparent cortical disruption; Devas characterized this fracture pattern as mechanically stable.

Blickenstaff and Morris described three types of stress fracture of the femoral neck[221]:

- Type I: Fracture with periosteal reaction or callus formation along the inferior femoral neck without evidence of a fracture line.
- Type II: Visible nondisplaced fracture across the femoral neck.
- Type III: Completely displaced fracture.

More recently, Fullerton and Snowdy proposed three categories: tension, compression and displaced fractures[222] (Figure 5.104):

- *Tension stress fractures* occur on the superolateral aspect of the femoral neck and are at increased risk for fracture displacement. This type is similar to the tension fracture described by Devas.

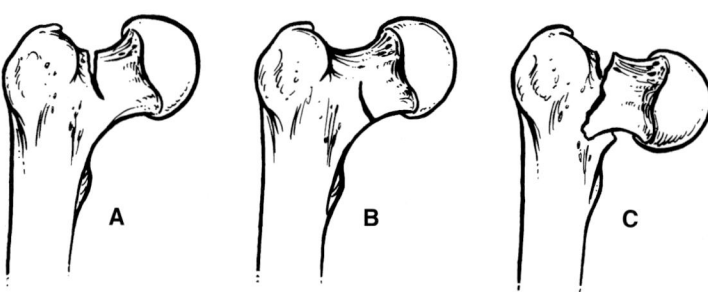

Figure 5.104. Fullerton and Snowdy classification of femoral neck stress fractures[222]: tension stress fractures occur on the superolateral aspect of the femoral neck and are at increased risk for fracture displacement (**A**); compression stress fractures occur on the inferomedial aspect of the femoral neck and have a lower risk for displacement (**B**); and displaced femoral neck fractures (**C**).

- *Compression stress fractures* are similar to the compression fracture described by Devas and the type I fracture described by Blickenstaff and Morris; they occur on the inferomedial aspect of the femoral neck and have a lower risk for displacement.
- *Displaced femoral neck fractures.*

Biomechanical Issues With Regard to Femoral Neck Stress Fractures

During walking or running, the loads on the femoral head can exceed three times body weight and are even higher if a weight, such as a backpack, is carried. These loads on the femoral head result from the torque caused by gravity acting on the center of mass of the body, which must be counteracted by contraction of the gluteus medius and gluteus minimus muscles. The total load on the femoral head is the sum of the forces producing these two torques.[223]

The force on the femoral head is transmitted through the femoral neck to the femoral shaft, creating stresses and strains in the femoral neck that act in both compression and bending.[223] Biomechanical analyses demonstrate that compressive forces on the femoral head are approximately three times greater than bending forces.[224] Strain-gauge studies have demonstrated that in normal single-leg stance, minimal tension or compressive strains occur in the superior aspect of the femoral neck and that increasing levels of compressive strain develop along the inferior aspect of the femoral neck.[224] Although the downward bending moment (force on femoral head × length of femoral neck) should induce tension stresses and strains in the superior aspect of the femoral neck, this is counteracted by contraction of the abductor muscles, producing a compensatory compressive strain on the superior aspect of the femoral neck. If the gluteus medius muscle is fatigued, this neutralizing effect is minimized, and unopposed strains develop along the superior aspect of the femoral neck.[224] The key to the biomechanics of the hip is therefore the gluteus medius muscle, which must be strong, reactive, and resistant to muscle fatigue.[223]

Bone is stronger in compression than in tension; unlike engineering materials, bone does not have a fatigue limit and in fact operates in normal activities of daily living close to its fatigue strength.[223] The fatigue process proceeds by the accumulation and consolidation of microcracks, which occur throughout the osseous structures (e.g., trabeculae, osteons, cement lines).[223] These structures have anisotropic (direction-dependent) mechanical properties that determine the initiation, orientation, and propagation of microfractures.[223] Cyclic testing in the laboratory of samples of bone at levels below its fracture strength allows identification of the microscopic features of damaged bone. The fatigue process is time dependent, as is the repair process; healing of these microfractures can occur given sufficient time without untoward loading.[223,224]

Tensile fatigue fractures, the result of cyclic loads, lead to osteon debonding and microfractures, which combine to form gross fatigue cracks. Fatigue cracks in effect decrease the area across which the force is applied, leading to higher stresses and rapid failure of the remaining osseous structure.[223] In compression, fatigue occurs under cyclic load with the production of shear microfractures (oriented at 45° to the applied force) that disrupt the osseous microcirculation. This results in local regions of bone necrosis, which are subsequently remodeled by osteoclastic response and creeping substitution.[223] The direction in which a fatigue crack propagates is dependent on the magnitude and direction of the applied load.

The level and distribution of stress and strain in the femoral neck are controlled by both gravitational and muscle forces. If gravitational forces are increased, as when one wears a knapsack, tensile stress in the femoral neck will increase correspondingly. If the abductor muscles fatigue and are unable to provide normal contraction, tensile stress in the femoral neck will also increase. Muscle fatigue from repetitive exercise can decrease the muscle's shock-absorbing capacity, resulting in higher peak stresses and strains in the femoral neck. Muscle fatigue also results in gait alterations that affect the position of the body's center of mass and alter the stress and strain patterns within the femoral neck.[223]

Clinical and Radiographic Presentation of Femoral Neck Stress Fractures

Stress fractures of the femoral neck can be difficult to diagnose. Clinically, the patient usually complains of a deep aching pain in the hip or groin that may radiate to the knee.[223] This pain may be associated with a particular activity and worsen with physical exertion. Patients usually deny specific trauma but may complain of hip pain that has been present for several days, weeks, or even months prior to presentation. On questioning, the patient may give a history of a recent change in the type, duration, or frequency of a physical activity. Older individuals must be questioned about their participation in low-impact activities. The patient may have difficulty walking; complaints of nighttime groin pain are common.[223] Physical examination may be unremarkable; the patient may be able walk without a limp. There is, however, usually tenderness in the inguinal area associated with pain at the extremes of hip motion.[223] Complaints of groin pain on heel percussion may or may not be present.

Evidence of radiographic abnormalities may be affected by both the location within the bone and the time from injury to examination. Radiographs may thus appear entirely normal at the time of initial presentation. In a prospective series of 250 U.S. Marine recruits presenting to sick call for stress-related complaints of the lower extremities, only 28% of stress fractures diagnosed by bone scan exhibited changes on standard radiographs.[225]

When radiographic changes consistent with femoral neck stress fracture are evident on standard radiographs, they usually appear as either an area of sclerosis or cortical deficiency on the superior or inferior aspect of the femoral neck[220-222] (Figure 5.105). Radiographs may show a fracture line beginning on

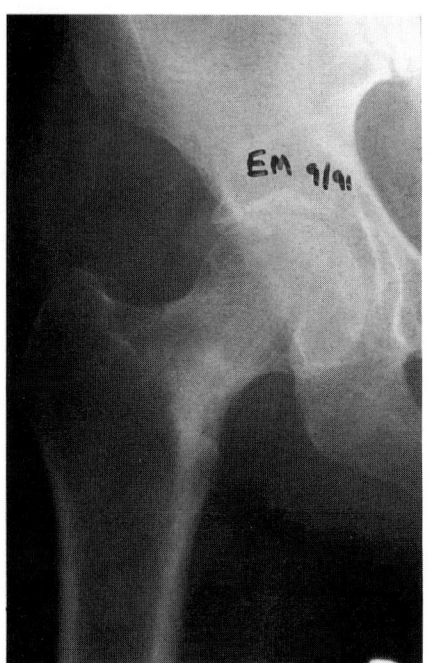

Figure 5.105. Stress fracture of the femoral neck.

the superior aspect of the femoral neck and oriented perpendicular to the axis of the femoral neck; these tension fractures must be distinguished from compression-type stress fractures, which are characterized by a small bony irregularity at the inferior aspect of the femoral neck. In the elderly, compression-type stress fractures are extremely uncommon; transverse (tension) fractures predominate. If the radiographs are negative and the patient's clinical history is suggestive of femoral neck stress fracture, a bone scan or magnetic resonance imaging study should be obtained.

Bone scintigraphy with technetium 99m medronate disodium is recognized as an early and reliable method for the detection of stress fractures.[225] Magnetic resonance imaging has been shown to be at least as accurate as bone scanning in the assessment of stress fractures of the femoral neck[226] and is preferred over bone scanning at our institution. Shin et al. prospectively evaluated 19 patients who had a suspected femoral neck stress fracture and negative radiographs with bone scans and magnetic resonance imaging.[226] The accuracy of bone scanning in identifying femoral neck stress fractures was 68%, as was its positive predictive value; magnetic resonance imaging was 100% sensitive, specific, and accurate.

Other methods for detection of stress fractures have recently been evaluated. In a study of female military recruits, quantitative ultrasound bone density screening was shown to be predictive for subsequent stress fracture.[227] Hisf et al. prospectively evaluated subjects using quantitative ultrasonography of the calcaneus with respect to velocity, speed of sound (SOS), and broadband ultrasonography.[227] The incidence of stress fractures in this population was 328 out of 3893 (8.4%); one-third of the recruits with an SOS value of 1498 m/s developed a stress fracture of the calcaneus during basic training.

Treatment of Femoral Neck Stress Fractures

Treatment of femoral neck stress fractures is type dependent. Tension fractures, because they are potentially unstable, require operative stabilization using multiple cancellous lag screws or a sliding hip screw.[220] Although the implant of choice for acute femoral neck fractures is a cancellous lag screw, the larger-diameter reamer required for insertion of the sliding hip screw may provide a greater stimulus for fracture healing. Fullerton and Snowdy allowed patients with a tension-type stress fracture of the femoral neck that was visible only on scintigraphy to be treated nonoperatively with frequent follow-up and protected weight bearing until they were pain free.[222] Our position, however, is that the risk of complications if fracture displacement occurs (osteonecrosis, malunion, and nonunion) in this potentially unstable fracture outweigh the benefits of nonoperative treatment. The region of the stress fracture can be curetted at surgery to induce a biological reaction and potentially increase the rate of fracture union.

Compression-type stress fractures of the femoral neck, on the other hand, are typically sufficiently stable to be treated nonoperatively. Treatment should consist of several days of rest followed by protected weight bearing. Frequent radiographs should be obtained to detect any changes in the fracture pattern or displacement; if evidence appears of fracture widening or displacement, fracture stabilization should be performed. A displaced femoral neck stress fracture in a young patient is an orthopaedic emergency and should be treated by open reduction and internal fixation. In the elderly, prosthetic replacement can also be considered.

Complications of Femoral Neck Stress Fractures

Complications of these fractures, most of which are associated with fracture displacement and/or a delay in diagnosis, include delayed union, nonunion, loss of fixation, refracture, and osteonecrosis of the femoral head.[219,228,229] Visuri et al. reported on a series of 12 displaced femoral neck stress fractures treated with open reduction and internal fixation[219]; 5 patients (42%) developed osteonecrosis, 1 patient (9%) developed a delayed union, and 1 patient (9%) developed a nonunion. Johansson et al. reported on a series of 23 patients who had sustained a femoral neck stress fracture with a mean delay in diagnosis of 14 weeks from the onset of symptoms (range, 3 to 104 weeks)[228]; 7 patients (30%) developed healing complications: osteonecrosis (3 patients), nonunion (1 patient), and refracture (3 patient). Five of the 7 patients (71%) had a displaced femoral neck stress fracture.

References

1. Pauwels F. *Biomechanics of the Normal and Diseased Hip*. New York: Springer-Verlag, 1976:83.
2. Pauwels F. De Schenkelhalsbruch, ein Mechanisches Problem: Grundlagen des Heilungsvorganges, Prognose und Kausale Therapie. Stuttgart: Ferdinand Enke Verlag, 1935.
3. DeLee JC. Fractures and dislocations of the hip. In: Rockwood CA, Green DP, Bucholz RW, Heckman JD, eds. *Rockwood and Green's Fractures in Adults*. Philadelphia: Lippincott-Raven, 1996:1659–1826.
4. Garden RS. Low-angle fixation in fractures of the femoral neck. *J Bone Joint Surg Br* 1961; 43:647–664.
5. Muller ME, Nazarian S, Koch P, Schatzker J. *Comprehensive Classification of Fractures of Long Bones*. Berlin: Springer-Verlag, 1990.
6. Frandsen PA, Andersen E, Madsen F, Skjodt T. Garden's classification of femoral neck fractures: an assessment of inter-observer variation. *J Bone Joint Surg Br* 1988; 70:588–590.
7. Banks HH. Factors influencing the result in fractures of the femoral neck. *J Bone Joint Surg Am* 1962; 44:931–964.
8. Barnes R, Brown JT, Garden RS, Nicoll EA. Subcapital fractures of the femur. A prospective review. *J Bone Joint Surg Br* 1976; 58:2–24.
9. Christie J, Howie C, Armoir P. Fixation of displaced femoral neck fractures: compression screw fixation versus double divergent pins. *J Bone Joint Surg Br* 1988; 70:199–201.
10. Cobb AG, Gibson PH. Screw fixation of subcapital fractures of the femur—a better method of treatment? *Injury* 1986; 17:259–264.
11. Linde F, Anderson E, Hvass I, et al. Avascular femoral head necrosis following fracture fixation. *Injury* 1986; 17:159–163.
12. Massie WK. Treatment of femoral neck fractures emphasizing long term follow-up observations on aseptic necrosis. *Clin Orthop* 1973; 92:16–62.
13. Stappaerts KH, Broos PL. Internal fixation of femoral neck fractures: a follow up study of 118 cases. *Acta Chir Belg* 1987; 87:247–251.
14. Swiontkowski MF. Intracapsular hip fractures. In: Browner BD, Levine AM, Jupiter JB, Trafton PG, eds. *Skeletal Trauma*, Vol 2. Philadelphia: WB Saunders, 1992:1751–1832.
15. Catto M. A histological study of avascular necrosis of the femoral head after transcervical fracture. *J Bone Joint Surg Br* 1965; 47:749–776.

16. Swiontkowski M, Tepic S, Ganz R, Perren SM. Laser Doppler flowmetry for measurement of femoral head blood flow. Experimental investigation and clinical application. *Helv Chir Acta* 1986; 53:55–59.
17. Swiontkowski MF, Tepic S, Rahn BA, Perren SM. The effect of femoral neck fracture on femoral head blood flow. *Orthop Trans* 1987; 11:344–345.
18. Vegter J, Klopper PJ. Effect of intracapsular hyperpressure on femoral head blood flow—laser Doppler flowmetry in dogs. *Acta Orthop Scand* 1991; 62:337–341.
19. Crawford EJP, Emery RJH, Hansell DM, et al. Capsular distention and intracapsular pressure in subcapital fractures of the femur. *J Bone Joint Surg Br* 1988; 70:195–198.
20. Grispigni C, Lazzerini A. Reduction and osteosynthesis of subcapital fractures of the femoral neck: possible repercussions on post-fracture hemarthrosis of the hip. *Italian Journal of Orthopaedic Traumatology* 1992; 18:539–542.
21. Harper WM, Barnes MR, Gregg PJ. Femoral head blood flow in femoral neck fractures: an analysis using intra-osseous pressure measurement. *J Bone Joint Surg Br* 1991; 73:73–75.
22. Holmberg S, Dalen N. Intracapsular pressure and caput circulation in nondisplaced femoral neck fractures. *Clin Orthop* 1987; 219:124–126.
23. Edholm P, Lindblom K, Maurseth K. Angulations in the fractures of the femoral neck with and without subsequent necrosis of the head. *Acta Radiol Scand* 1967; 6:329–336.
24. Garden RS. Stability and union in subcapital fractures of the femur. *J Bone Joint Surg Br* 1964; 46:630–647.
25. Garden RS. Malreduction and avascular necrosis in subcapital fractures of the femur. *J Bone Joint Surg Br* 1971; 53:183–197.
26. Smyth EHJ, Shah VM. The significance of good reduction and fixation in displaced subcapital fractures of the femur. *Injury* 1974; 5:197–209.
27. Claffey TJ. Avascular necrosis of the femoral head: an anatomical study. *J Bone Joint Surg Br* 1960; 42:802–809.
28. Brodetti A. The blood supply of the femoral neck and head in relation to the damaging effects of nails and screws. *J Bone Joint Surg Br* 1960; 42:794–801.
29. Stromqvist B, Hansson LI. Avascular necrosis associated with nailing of femoral neck fracture—two cases examined pre and postoperatively by tetracycline and radionuclide tracer techniques. *Acta Orthop Scand* 1983; 54:687–694.
30. Drake JK, Meyers MH. Intracapsular pressure and hemarthrosis following femoral neck fracture. *Clin Orthop* 1984; 182:172–176.
31. Melberg PE, Korner L, Lansinger O. Hip joint pressure after femoral neck fracture. *Acta Orthop Scand* 1986; 57:501–504.
32. Wingstrand H, Stomqvist B, Egund N, et al. Hemarthrosis in undisplaced cervical fractures: tamponade may cause reversible femoral head ischemia. *Acta Orthop Scand* 1986; 57:305–308.
33. Zuckerman JD. *Comprehensive Care of Orthopaedic Injuries in the Elderly*. Baltimore: Urban & Schwarzenberg, 1990.
34. Stromqvist B, Nilsson LT, Egund N, et al. Intracapsular pressure in undisplaced fractures of the femoral neck. *J Bone Joint Surg Br* 1988; 70:192–194.
35. Bentley G. Impacted fractures of the neck of the femur. *J Bone Joint Surg Br* 1968; 50:551–561.
36. Bentley G. Treatment of nondisplaced fractures of the femoral neck. *Clin Orthop* 1980; 152:93–101.
37. Holmberg S, Kalen R, Thorngren KG. Treatment and outcome of femoral neck fractures. An analysis of 2418 patients admitted from their own homes. *Clin Orthop* 1987; 218:42–51.
38. Peter R, Bedat B, Rossier J, Hoffmeyer P. Impacted Garden I fractures of the femoral neck (31-B1): operative vs. nonoperative treatment? Paper presented at the annual meeting of the Orthopaedic Trauma Association, Louisville, KY, 1997.
39. Smith-Petersen MN, Cave EF, Vangorder GW. Intracapsular fractures of the neck of the femur—treated by internal fixation. *Arch Surg* 1931; 23:715–759.
40. Johansson S. On the operative treatment of medial fractures of the femoral neck. *Acta Orthop Scand* 1932; 3:362–385.
41. Wescott HH. A method for the internal fixation of transcervical fractures of the femur. *J Bone Joint Surg* 1934; 16:372–378.
42. Henderson M. Internal fixation for recent fractures of the neck of the femur. *Ann Surg* 1938; 107:132–142.
43. Eyre-Brook AL, Pridie KH. Intracapsular fractures of the neck of the femur. Final results of 75 consecutive cases treated by the closed method of pinning. *Br J Surg* 1941; 23:115–138.

44. Thornton L. The treatment of trochanteric fracture of the femur: two new methods. *Piedmont Hospital Bulletin* 1937; 10:21–37.
45. Tronzo R. Hip nails for all occasions. *Orthop Clin North Am* 1974; 5:479–491.
46. Jewett EL. One piece angle nail for trochanteric fractures. *J Bone Joint Surg* 1941; 23:803–810.
47. Jewett E. Rigid internal fixation of intracapsular femoral neck fractures. *Am J Surg* 1956; 91:621–626.
48. Jewett E, Albee F, Stanford F. Treatment of all fractures of the upper end of the femur with the original one piece flange nail. *South Med J* 1953; 46:920–924.
49. Frangakis E. Intracapsular fractures of the neck of the femur—factors influencing nonunion and ischemic necrosis. *J Bone Joint Surg Br* 1966; 48:17–30.
50. Eaton G. Internal fixation in displaced intracapsular fracture of the femoral neck. *J Bone Joint Surg Am* 1956; 38:23–32.
51. Charnley J, Blockey N, Purser D. The treatment of displaced fractures of the neck of the femur by compression. A preliminary report. *J Bone Joint Surg Br* 1957; 39:45–65.
52. Hargaden E, Pearson J. Treatment of intracapsular fractures of the femoral neck with the Charnley compression screw. *J Bone Joint Surg Br* 1963; 45:305–311.
53. Pugh WL. A self-adjusting nail-plate for fractures about the hip joint. *J Bone Joint Surg Am* 1955; 37:1085–1093.
54. Jacobs B, Wade P, Match R. Intracapsular fractures of the femoral neck treated by the Pugh nail. *J Trauma* 1965; 5:751–760.
55. Fielding J. Pugh nail fixation of displaced femoral neck fractures. A long term follow-up. *Clin Orthop* 1975; 106:107–116.
56. Fielding JW, Wilson SA, Ratzan S. A continuing end result study of displaced intracapsular fractures of the neck of the femur treated with the Pugh nail. *J Bone Joint Surg Am* 1974; 56:1464–1472.
57. Svenningsen S, Benum P, Nesse O, Furset O. Internal fixation of femoral neck fractures: compression screw compared with nail-plate fixation. *Acta Orthop Scand* 1984; 55:423–429.
58. Nordkild P, Sonne-Holm S, Jensen J. Femoral neck fractures: sliding screw plate versus sliding nail plate—a randomized trial. *Injury* 1985; 17:449–454.
59. Moore AT. Fracture of the hip joint: treatment by extra-articular fixation with adjustable nails. *Surg Gynecol Obstet* 1937; 64:420–436.
60. Kimbrough E, Lunceford E, Kolibec A. 28 years experience with multiple Moore adjustable nail fixation of intracapsular fractures of the femur. *J Bone Joint Surg Am* 1965; 47:1282–1283.
61. Ackroyd C. Treatment of subcapital femoral fractures fixed with Moore's pins: a study of 34 cases followed for up to three years. *Injury* 1973; 5:100–108.
62. Modny M, Kaiser A. A special guide for insertion of multiple pins for fracture of the hip. *Clin Orthop* 1978; 137:144–147.
63. Green J, Gay F. High femoral neck fractures treated by multiple nail fixation. *Clin Orthop* 1958; 11:177–183.
64. Arnold WD, Lynden JP, Minkoff J. Treatment of intracapsular fractures of the femoral neck. With special reference to percutaneous Knowles pinning. *J Bone Joint Surg Am* 1974; 56:254–262.
65. McCutchen J, Carnesale P. Comparison of fixation in the treatment of femoral neck fractures. *Clin Orthop* 1982; 171:44–50.
66. Jarolem KL, Koval KJ, Zuckerman JD, Aharonoff G. A comparison of modified Knowles pins and cannulated cancellous screws for the treatment of nondisplaced or impacted femoral neck fractures. *Bull Hosp Jt Dis* 1993; 53:11–14.
67. Stromqvist B, Hansson L, Nilsson L, Thorngren K. Two-year follow-up of femoral neck fractures. Comparison of osteosynthesis methods. *Acta Orthop Scand* 1984; 55:521–525.
68. Stromqvist B, Hansson L, Nilsson L, Thorngren K. Hook pin fixation in femoral neck fractures: a two year follow-up study of 300 cases. *Clin Orthop* 1987; 218:58–62.
69. Deyerle WM. Impacted fixation over resilient multiple pins. *Clin Orthop* 1980; 152:102–122.
70. Metz C, Sellers T, Feagin J, et al. The displaced intracapsular fracture of the neck of the femur. Experience with the Deyerle method of fixation in sixty-three cases. *J Bone Joint Surg Am* 1970; 52:113–127.
71. Chapman MW, Stehr JH, Eberle CF, et al. Treatment of intracapsular hip fractures by the Deyerle method: a comparative review of one hundred and nineteen cases. *J Bone Joint Surg Am* 1975; 57:735–744.

72. Baker GI, Barrick EF. Deyerle treatment for femoral neck fractures. *J Bone Joint Surg Am* 1978; 60:269–271.
73. Madsen F, Linde F, Anderson E, et al. Fixation of displaced femoral fractures: a comparison between sliding screw plate and four cancellous bone screws. *Acta Orthop Scand* 1987; 58:212–216.
74. Husby T, Alho A, Ronningen H. Stability of femoral neck osteosynthesis: a comparison of fixation methods in cadavers. *Acta Orthop Scand* 1989; 60:299–302.
75. Husby T, Alho A, Hoiseth A, Fonstelien E. Strength of femoral neck fracture fixation. Comparison of six techniques in cadavers. *Acta Orthop Scand* 1987; 58:634–637.
76. Van Audekercke R, Martens M, Muiler JC, Stuyck J. Experimental study on the internal fixation of femoral neck fractures. *Clin Orthop* 1979; 141:203–212.
77. Mizrahi J, Harlon HS, Taylor JK, Solomon L. Investigation of load transfer and optimum pin configuration in the internal fixation by Muller screws of fractured femoral necks. *Med Biol Eng Comput* 1980; 18:319–325.
78. Swiontkowski MF, Harrington RM, Keller TS, Van Patten PK. Torsion and bending analysis of internal fixation techniques for femoral neck fractures: the role of implant design and bone density. *J Orthop Res* 1987; 5:433–444.
79. Kauffman JI, Simon JA, Kummer FJ, et al. Internal fixation of femoral neck fractures with posterior comminution: a biomechanical study. *J Orthop Trauma* 1999; 13(3):155–159.
80. Toolan BC, Koval KJ, Kummer FJ, et al. Effects of supine positioning and fracture post placement on the perineal countertraction force in awake volunteers. *J Orthop Trauma* 1995; 9:164–170.
81. Rodriguez J, Herrara A, Canales V, Serrano S. Epidemiologic factors, mortality and morbidity after femoral neck fractures in the elderly—a comparative study: internal fixation vs. hemiarthroplasty. *Acta Orthop Belg* 1987; 53:472–479.
82. Ewald FC, Christie MJ, Thomas WH. Total hip arthroplasty for failed hemiarthroplasty. Paper presented at the 52nd annual meeting of the American Academy of Orthopaedic Surgeons, Las Vegas, NV, January 28, 1985.
83. Graham J. Early or delayed weight-bearing after internal fixation of transcervical fracture of the femur. *J Bone Joint Surg Br* 1968; 50:562–569.
84. Kyle RF, Dahl M, Mattson P. Femoral fractures in young adults. Paper presented at the 51st annual meeting of the American Academy of Orthopaedic Surgeons, Atlanta, GA, 1984.
85. Manninger J, Kazar G, Fekete G, et al. Avoidance of avascular necrosis of the femoral head, following fractures of the femoral neck, by early reduction and internal fixation. *Injury* 1985; 16:437–448.
86. Kirschner PT, Simon MA. Current concepts review: radioisotopic evaluation of skeletal disease. *J Bone Joint Surg Am* 1981; 63:673–681.
87. Lucie RS, Fuller S, Burdickes DC, Johnson RM. Early prediction of avascular necrosis of the femoral head following femoral neck fracture. *Clin Orthop* 1981; 161:207–214.
88. Meyers MH, Telfer N, Moore TM. Determination of the vascularity of the femoral head with technetium 99m-sulfur-colloid: diagnostic and prognostic significance. *J Bone Joint Surg Am* 1977; 59:658–664.
89. Turner JH. Post-traumatic avascular necrosis of the femoral head predicted by preoperative technetium-99m antimony colloid scan. *J Bone Joint Surg Am* 1983; 65:786–797.
90. Stromqvist B. Femoral head vitality after intracapsular hip fracture; 490 cases studied by intravital tetracycline labeling and TC-MDP radionuclide imaging. *Acta Orthop Scand* 1983; 54:5–71.
91. Broeng L, Hansen LB, Sperling K, Kanstrup IL. Postoperative Tc-scintimetry in femoral neck fracture: a prospective study of 46 cases. *Acta Orthop Scand* 1994; 65:171–174.
92. Asnis SE, Gould ES, Bansal M, et al. Magnetic resonance imaging of the hip after displaced femoral neck fractures. *Clin Orthop* 1994; 298:191–198.
93. Speer KP, Spritzer CE, Harrelson JM, Nunley JA. Magnetic resonance imaging of the femoral head after acute intracapsular fracture of the femoral neck. *J Bone Joint Surg Am* 1990; 72:98–103.
94. Speer KP, Quarles LD, Harrelson JM, Nunley JA. Tetracycline labeling of the femoral head following acute intracapsular fracture of the femoral neck. *Clin Orthop* 1991; 267:224–227.

References

95. Garden RS. Reduction and fixation of the subcapital fractures of the femur. *Orthop Clin North Am* 1974; 5:683–712.
96. Green JT. Management of fresh fractures of the neck of the femur. *Instr Course Lect* 1960; 17:94–105.
97. Lowell JD. Results and complications of femoral neck fractures. *Clin Orthop* 1980; 152:162–172.
98. Scheck M. The significance of posterior comminution in femoral neck fractures. *Clin Orthop* 1980; 152:138–142.
99. Meyers MH. The role of posterior bone grafts (muscle-pedicle) in femoral neck fractures. *Clin Orthop* 1980; 152:143–146.
100. Smyth EH, Ellis JS, Manifold MC, Dewey PR. Triangle pinning for fracture of the femoral neck. *J Bone Joint Surg Br* 1964; 46:664–673.
101. Meyers MH, Harvey JPJ, Moore TM. Treatment of displaced subcapital and transcervical fractures of the femoral neck by muscle-pedicle bone grafts and internal fixation. *J Bone Joint Surg Am* 1973; 55:257–274.
102. Baksi D. Internal fixation of ununited femoral neck fractures combined with muscle-pedicle bone grafting. *J Bone Joint Surg Br* 1986; 68:239–245.
103. Baksi D. Treatment of osteonecrosis of the femoral head by drilling and muscle-pedicle bone grafting. *J Bone Joint Surg Br* 1991; 73:241–245.
104. Carnesale PG, Anderson LD. Primary prosthetic replacement for femoral neck fractures. *Arch Surg* 1975; 110:27–29.
105. Coates R. Proceedings: a retrospective survey of eighty-one patients with hemiarthroplasty for subcapital fracture of the femoral neck. *J Bone Joint Surg Br* 1975; 57:256.
106. Kofoed H, Kofod J. Moore prosthesis in the treatment of fresh femoral neck fractures. A critical review with special attention to secondary acetabular degeneration. *Injury* 1983; 14:531–540.
107. Salvati EA, Artz T, Aglietti P, Asnis SE. Endoprostheses in the treatment of femoral neck fractures. *Orthop Clin North Am* 1977; 5:757–777.
108. Soreide O, Lillestol J, Alho A, Hvidsten K. Acetabular protrusion following endoprosthetic hip surgery. A multifactorial study. *Acta Orthop Scand* 1980; 51:943–948.
109. Whittaker RP, Abeshaus MM, Scholl HW, Chung SML. Fifteen years' experience with metallic endoprosthetic replacement of the femoral head for femoral neck fractures. *J Trauma* 1972; 12:799–806.
110. D'Arcy J, Devas M. Treatment of fractures of the femoral neck by replacement with the Thompson prosthesis. *J Bone Joint Surg Br* 1976; 58:279–286.
111. Gingras MB, Clarke J, Evarts C. Prosthetic replacement in femoral neck fractures. *Clin Orthop* 1980; 152:147–157.
112. Higgins RW, Hughes JL. Preliminary results of eight-one hip replacements with the Bateman endoprosthesis. *Orthop Trans* 1983; 7:411–412.
113. Kwok DC, Cruess RL. A retrospective study of Moore and Thompson hemiarthroplasty. A review of 599 surgical cases and an analysis of the technical complications. *Clin Orthop* 1982; 169:179–185.
114. Chan RNW, Hoskinson J. Thompson prosthesis for fractured neck of the femur: a comparison of surgical approaches. *J Bone Joint Surg Br* 1975; 57:437–443.
115. Lu-Yao GL, Keller RB, Littenberg B, Wennberg JE. Outcomes after displaced fractures of the femoral neck: a meta-analysis of one hundred and six published reports. *J Bone Joint Surg Br* 1994; 76:15–25.
116. Hunter GA. Should we abandon primary prosthetic replacement for fresh displaced fractures of the neck of the femur? *Clin Orthop* 1980; 152:158–161.
117. Sikorski JM, Barrington R. Internal fixation versus hemiarthroplasty for the displaced subcapital fracture of the femur: a prospective randomized study. *J Bone Joint Surg Br* 1981; 63:357–361.
118. Holmberg S, Thorngren KG. Rehabilitation after femoral neck fracture. 3053 patients followed for 6 years. *Acta Orthop Scand* 1985; 36:305–308.
119. Bochner RM, Pellicci PM, Lyden JP. Bipolar hemiarthroplasty for fracture of the femoral neck: clinical review with special emphasis on prosthetic motion. *J Bone Joint Surg Am* 1988; 70:1001–1010.
120. Eiskjaer S, Gelineck J, Soballe K. Fractures of the femoral neck treated with cemented bipolar hemiarthroplasty. *Orthopedics* 1989; 12:1545–1550.
121. Franklin A, Gallannaugh SC. The bi-articular hip prosthesis for fractures of the femoral neck—a preliminary report. *Injury* 1983; 15:159–162.

122. Lausten GS, Vedel P, Nielsen PM. Fractures of the femoral neck treated with a bipolar endoprosthesis. *Clin Orthop* 1987; 218:63–67.
123. Phillips TW. The Bateman bipolar femoral head replacement. A fluoroscopic study of movement over a four-year period. *J Bone Joint Surg Br* 1987; 69:761–764.
124. Yamagata M, Chao EY, Illstrup DM, et al. Fixed-head and bipolar hip endoprosthesis. *J Arthroplasty* 1987; 2:327–341.
125. Wathne RA, Koval KJ, Aharonoff GB, et al. Modular unipolar versus bipolar prosthesis: a prospective evaluation of functional outcome after femoral neck fracture. *J Orthop Trauma* 1995; 9:298–302.
126. Beckenbaugh RD, Tressler HA, Johnson EW. Results after hemiarthroplasty of the hip using a cemented femoral prosthesis: a review of 109 cases with an average follow-up of 36 months. *Mayo Clin Proc* 1977; 52:349–353.
127. Soreide O, Lerner AP, Thunold J. Primary prosthetic replacement in acute femoral neck fracture. *Injury* 1975; 6:286–293.
128. Welch RB, Taylor LW, Wynne GF, White AH. Results with the cemented hemiarthroplasty for displaced fractures of the femoral neck. Paper presented at the Fifth Open Scientific Meeting of the Hip Society, St. Louis, MO, 1977.
129. Wrighton LD, Woodyard JE. Prosthetic replacement for subcapital fractures of the femur: a comparative study. *Injury* 1971; 2:287–293.
130. Follacci FM, Charnley J. A comparison of the results of femoral head prosthesis with and without cement. *Clin Orthop* 1969; 62:156–161.
131. Coates RL, Armour P. Treatment of subcapital femoral fractures by primary total hip replacement. *Injury* 1979; 11:132–135.
132. Pun WK, Ip FK, So YC, Chow SP. Treatment of displaced subcapital femoral fractures by primary total hip replacement. *J R Coll Surg Edinb* 1987; 32:293–297.
133. Sim FH, Stauffer RN. Management of hip fractures by total hip arthroplasty. *Clin Orthop* 1980; 152:191–197.
134. Sim FH, Stauffer RN. Total hip arthroplasty in acute femoral neck fractures. *Instr Course Lect* 1980:9–16.
135. Sim FH, Sigmond ER. Acute fractures of the femoral neck, managed by total hip replacement. *Orthopedics* 1986; 9:35–38.
136. Taine WH, Armour PC. Primary total hip replacement for displaced subcapital fractures of the femur. *J Bone Joint Surg Br* 1985; 67:214–217.
137. Delamarter R, Moreland JR. Treatment of acute femoral neck fractures with total hip arthroplasty. *Clin Orthop* 1987; 218:68–74.
138. Greenbough CG, Jones JR. Primary total hip replacements for displaced subcapital fracture of the femur. *J Bone Joint Surg Br* 1988; 70:639–643.
139. Coughlin L, Templeton J. Hip fractures in patients with Parkinson's disease. *Clin Orthop* 1980; 148:192–195.
140. Eventor I, Moreno M, Geller E, et al. Hip fractures in patients with Parkinson's syndrome. *J Trauma* 1983; 23:98–101.
141. Rothermel JE, Garcia A. Treatment of hip fractures in patients with Parkinson's syndrome on levodopa therapy. *J Bone Joint Surg Am* 1972; 54:1251–1254.
142. Staeheli JW, Frassica FJ, Sim FH. Prosthetic replacement of the femoral head for fracture of the femoral neck in patients who have Parkinson's disease. *J Bone Joint Surg Am* 1988; 70:565–568.
143. Barry HC. Fractures of the femur in Paget's disease of bone in Australia. *J Bone Joint Surg Am* 1967; 49:1359–1370.
144. Dove J. Complete fractures of the femur in Paget's disease of bone. *J Bone Joint Surg Br* 1980; 62:12–17.
145. Grundy M. Fractures of the femur in Paget's disease of bone. *J Bone Joint Surg Br* 1970; 52:252–263.
146. Lake M. Studies of Paget's disease (osteitis deformans). *J Bone Joint Surg Br* 1951; 32:323–335.
147. Nicholas JA, Killoran P. Fracture of the femur in patients with Paget's disease. *J Bone Joint Surg Am* 1965; 47:450–461.
148. Milgram JW. Orthopaedic management of Paget's disease of bone. *Clin Orthop* 1977; 127:63–69.
149. Stauffer RN, Sim FH. Total hip arthroplasty in Paget's disease of the hip. *J Bone Joint Surg Am* 1976; 58:476–478.
150. Soto-Hall R. Treatment of transcervical fractures complicated by certain common neurological conditions. *Instr Course Lect* 1960; 17:117–120.
151. McClure J, Goldsborough S. Fractures neck of femur and contra-lateral intracerebral lesions. *J Clin Pathol* 1986; 39:920–922.

152. Malluche HH, Smith AJ, Abreo K, Faugere MC. The use of deferoxamine in the management of aluminum accumulation in bone in patients with renal failure. *N Engl J Med* 1984; 311:140–144.
153. Thornhill TS, Creasman C. Hip Fractures in patients with renal failure. Paper presented at the 52nd annual meeting of the American Academy of Orthopaedic Surgeons, Las Vegas, NV, January 24, 1985.
154. Chalmers J, Irvine GB. Fractures of the femoral neck in elderly patients with hyperparathyroidism. *Clin Orthop* 1988; 229:125–130.
155. Colhoun EN, Johnson V, Fairclough JA. Bone scanning for hip fractures in patients with osteoarthritis: brief report. *J Bone Joint Surg Br* 1988; 70:848.
156. Julkunen H. Medical aspects in the treatment of femoral neck fractures with rheumatoid arthritis. *Scand J Rheumatol* 1974; 3:13–16.
157. Stromqvist B, Kelly I, Lidgren L. Treatment of hip fractures in rheumatoid arthritis. *Clin Orthop* 1988; 28:75–78.
158. Bogoch ER, Ovellette G, Hastings DE. Failure of internal fixation of femoral neck fractures in rheumatoid arthritis patients. Paper presented at the 56th annual meeting of the American Academy of Orthopaedic Surgeons, Las Vegas, NV, February 1989.
159. Stephen IBM. Subcapital fractures of the femur in rheumatoid arthritis. *Injury* 1979–1980; 11:233–241.
160. Vahvanen V. Femoral neck fracture of the rheumatoid hip joint. *Acta Rheumatol Scand* 1971; 17:125–136.
161. Hagglund G, Nordstrom B, Lidgren L. Total hip replacement after nailing failure in femoral neck fractures. *Arch Orthop Trauma Surg* 1984; 103:125–127.
162. Jensen JS, Holstein P. A long term follow-up of Moore arthroplasty in femoral neck fractures. *Acta Orthop Scand* 1975; 46:764–774.
163. Johnsson R, Bendjellou H, Ekelund L, et al. Comparison between hemiarthroplasty and total hip replacement following failure of nailed femoral neck fractures focused on dislocations. *Arch Orthop Trauma Surg* 1984; 102:187–190.
164. Harrington K. *Orthopaedic Management of Metastatic Bone Disease*. St. Louis: CV Mosby, 1988.
165. Walling A, Bahner R. Pathological fractures. In: Koval K, Zuckerman J, eds. *Fractures in the Elderly*. Philadelphia: Lippincott-Raven, 1998:247–259.
166. Nordin M, Frankel VH. Biomechanics of the hip. In: Nordin M, Frankel VH, eds. *Basic Biomechanics of the Musculoskeletal System*. Malvern, PA: Lea & Febiger, 1989:135–151.
167. Soreide O, Molster A, Raugstad TS. Immediate weight bearing after internal fixation of femoral fractures using Von Bahr screws. *J Bone Joint Surg Br* 1977; 48:659–664.
168. Koval K, Friend K, Aharonoff G, Zuckerman J. Weightbearing after hip fracture: a prospective series of 596 geriatric hip fracture patients. *J Orthop Trauma* 1996; 10:526–30.
169. Bennet F, Zinar D, Kilgus D. Ipsilateral hip and femoral shaft fractures. *Clin Orthop* 1993; 296:168–177.
170. Delaney W, Street D. Fracture of the femoral shaft with fracture of neck of same femur. *J Int Coll Surg* 1953; 19:303–312.
171. Riemer B, Butterfield S, Ray R, Daffner R. Clandestine femoral neck fractures with ipsilateral diaphyseal fractures. *J Orthop Trauma* 1993; 7:443–449.
172. Swiontkowski MF. Ipsilateral femoral shaft and hip fractures. *Orthop Clin North Am* 1987; 18:73–84.
173. Bose WJ, Corces A, Anderson LD. A preliminary experience with the Russell-Taylor reconstruction nail for complex femoral fractures. *J Trauma* 1992; 32:71–76.
174. Casey MJ, Chapman MW. Ipsilateral concomitant fractures of the hip and femoral shaft. *J Bone Joint Surg Am* 1979; 61:503–509.
175. Kang S, McAndrew MP, Johnson KD. The reconstruction locked nail for complex fractures of the proximal femur. *J Orthop Trauma* 1995; 9:453–463.
176. Swiontkowski MF, Hansen ST Jr, Kellam J. Ipsilateral fractures of the femoral neck and shaft. A treatment protocol. *J Bone Joint Surg Am* 1984; 66:260–268.
177. Swiontkowski MF, Winquist RA, Hansen ST Jr. Fractures of the femoral neck in patients between the ages of twelve and forty-nine years. *J Bone Joint Surg Am* 1984; 66:837–846.
178. Zettas J, Zettas P. Ipsilateral fractures of the femoral neck and shaft. *Clin Orthop* 1981; 160:63–73.
179. Hughes S, Voit G, Kates S. The role of computerized tomography in the diagnosis of an occult femoral neck fracture associated with an ipsilateral femoral shaft fracture: a case report. *J Trauma* 1991; 31:296–298.

180. Wolinsky P, Johnson K. Ipsilateral femoral neck and shaft fractures. *Clin Orthop* 1995; 318:81–90.
181. Schatzker J, Barrington T. Fractures of the femoral neck associated with fractures of the same femoral shaft. *Can J Surg* 1968; 11:297–305.
182. Wiss DA, Sima W, Brien WW. Ipsilateral fractures of the femoral neck and shaft. *J Orthop Trauma* 1992; 6:159–166.
183. Wu C, Shih C. Ipsilateral femoral neck and shaft fractures. *Acta Orthop Scand* 1991; 62:346–351.
184. Chaturvedi S, Sahu S. Ipsilateral concomitant fractures of the femoral neck and shaft. *Injury* 1993; 24:243–246.
185. Culver D, Crawford JS, Gardiner JH, Wiley AM. Venous thrombosis after fracture of the upper end of the femur: A study of incidence and site. *J Bone Joint Surg Br* 1970; 52:61–69.
186. Hamilton HW, Crawford JS, Gardiner JH, Wiley AM. Venous thrombosis in patients with fractures of the upper end of the femur: a phlebographic study of the effect of prophylactic anticoagulation. *J Bone Joint Surg Br* 1970; 52:268–289.
187. Moskovitz PA, Ellenberg SS, Feffer HL, et al. Low-dose heparin for prevention of venous thromboembolism in total hip arthroplasty and surgical repair of hip fractures. *J Bone Joint Surg Am* 1978; 60:1065–1070.
188. Pini M, Spadini E, Carluccio L, et al. Dextran/aspirin versus heparin/dihydroergotamine in preventing thrombosis after hip fractures. *J Bone Joint Surg Br* 1985; 67:305–309.
189. Rorbach-Madsen M, Jakobsen BW, Pederson J, Sorenson B. Dihydroergotamine and the thromboprophylactic effect of dextran 70 in emergency hip surgery. *Br J Surg* 1988; 75:364–365.
190. Jensen TT, Junker Y. Pressure sores common after hip operations. *Acta Orthop Scand* 1987; 58:209–211.
191. Mullen JO. Relationship of admission mental status, hospital confusion, and mortality in hip fractures: a prospective study. Paper presented at the 52nd annual meeting of the American Academy of Orthopaedic Surgeons, Las Vegas, NV, January 24, 1985.
192. Kyle RF. Trauma: Hip Fracture. *Orthopaedic Knowledge Update II*. Rosemont, IL: American Academy of Orthopaedic Surgeons, 1987:357–368.
193. Zuckerman JD, Sakales SK, Fabian DR, Frankel VH. Hip fractures in geriatric patients. Results of an interdisciplinary hospital care program. *Clin Orthop* 1992; 274:213–225.
194. Skinner PW, Powles D. Compression screw fixation for displaced subcapital fracture of the femur: success or failure. *J Bone Joint Surg Br* 1986; 68:78–82.
195. Brown TIS, Court-Brown C. Failure of sliding nail-plate fixation in subcapital fractures of the femoral neck. *J Bone Joint Surg Br* 1979; 61:342–346.
196. Stappaerts KH. Early fixation failure in displaced femoral neck fractures. *Arch Orthop Trauma Surg* 1985; 104:314–318.
197. Banks HH. Nonunion in fractures of the femoral neck. *Orthop Clin North Am* 1974; 5:865–885.
198. Calandruccio RA, Anderson WE. Post-fracture avascular necrosis of the femoral head: correlation of experimental and clinical studies. *Clin Orthop* 1980; 152:49–84.
199. Soreide O, Molster A, Raugstad TS. Internal fixation versus primary prosthetic replacement in acute femoral neck fractures: a prospective, randomized clinical study. *Br J Surg* 1979; 66:56–60.
200. Arnold WD. The effect of early weight-bearing on the stability of femoral neck fractures treated with Knowles pins. *J Bone Joint Surg Am* 1984; 66:847–852.
201. Cassebaum WH, Nugent G. The predictability of bony union in displaced intracapsular fractures of the hip. *J Trauma* 1963; 3:421–424.
202. Scott WA, Allum RL, Wright K. Implant induced trabecular damage in cadaveric femoral necks. *Acta Orthop Scand* 1985; 56:145–146.
203. Meyer S, Weiland AJ, Willenegger H. The treatment of infected non-union of fractures of long bones: study of sixty-four cases with a five to twenty-one year follow-up. *J Bone Joint Surg Am* 1975; 57:836–842.
204. Meyers MH, Harvery JP, Moore TM. Delayed treatment of subcapital and transcervical fractures of the neck of the femur with internal fixation and a muscle-pedicle bone graft. *Orthop Clin North Am* 1974; 5:743–756.
205. Anderson LD, Hamsa WR, Waring TL. Femoral-head prosthesis; a review of three hundred and fifty-six operations and their results. *J Bone Joint Surg Am* 1964; 46:1049–1065.

References

206. Hinchey JJ, Day PL. Primary prosthetic replacement in fresh femoral-neck fractures. *J Bone Joint Surg Am* 1964; 46:223–240.
207. Bray TJ, Smith-Hoefer E, Hooper A, Timmerman L. The displaced femoral neck fracture: internal fixation versus bipolar endoprosthesis. Results of a prospective, randomized comparison. *Clin Orthop* 1988; 230:127–140.
208. Wood MR. Femoral head replacement following fracture: an analysis of the surgical approach. *Injury* 1979–1980; 11:317–320.
209. Johnston CE, Ripley LP, Bray CB. Primary endoprosthetic replacement for acute femoral neck fractures. *Clin Orthop* 1982; 167:123–130.
210. Lunt HR. The role of prosthetic replacement of the head of the femur as primary treatment for subcapital fractures. *Injury* 1971; 3:107–110.
211. Hunter GA. A comparison of the use of internal fixation and prosthetic replacement for fresh fractures of the femur. *Br J Surg* 1969; 56:229–232.
212. Schon L, Zuckerman JD. Hip pain in the elderly: evaluation and diagnosis. *Geriatrics* 1988; 43:48–62.
213. Stoneham MD, Morgan NV. Stress fractures of the hip in Royal Marine recruits under training: a retrospective analysis. *Br J Sports Med* 1989; 25:145–148.
214. Volpin G, Hoerer D, Groisman G, et al. Stress fractures of the femoral neck following strenuous activity. *J Orthop Trauma* 1990; 4:394–398.
215. Lloyd-Smith R, Clement DB, McKenzie DC, Taunton JE. A survey of overuse and traumatic hip and pelvic injuries in athletes. *Physician Sportsmedicine* 1985; 13:131–141.
216. Zahger D, Abramovitz A, Zelikovsky L, et al. Stress fractures in female soldiers: an epidemiologic investigation of an outbreak. *Mil Med* 1988; 153:448–450.
217. Horiuchi T, Igarashi M, Karube S, et al. Spontaneous fractures of the hip in the elderly. *Orthopedics* 1988; 11:1277–1280.
218. Daffner RH, Pavlov H. Stress fractures: current concepts. *AJR Am J Roentgenol* 1992; 159:245–252.
219. Visuri T, Vara S, Meurman KOM. Displaced stress fractures of the femoral neck in young male adults: a report of twelve operative cases. *J Trauma* 1988; 28:1562–1569.
220. Devas MB. Stress fractures of the femoral neck. *J Bone Joint Surg Br* 1965; 47:728–737.
221. Blickenstaff LD, Morris JM. Fatigue fracture of the femoral neck. *J Bone Joint Surg Am* 1966; 48:103–104.
222. Fullerton LR, Snowdy HA. Femoral neck stress fractures. *Am J Sports Med* 1988; 16:365–377.
223. Egol K, Koval K, Kummer F, Frankel V. Stress fractures of the femoral neck. *Clin Orthop* 1998; 348:72–78.
224. Nordin M, Frankel VH. *Biomechanics of Bone. Basic Biomechanics of the Musculoskeletal System*. Malvern, PA: Lea & Febiger, 1989:3–29, 135–151, 149–177.
225. Greaney RB, Gerber FH, Laughlin RL, et al. Distribution and natural history of stress fractures in U.S. Marine recruits. *Radiology* 1983; 146:339–346.
226. Shin AY, Morin WD, Gorman JD, et al. The superiority of magnetic resonance imaging in differentiating the cause of hip pain in endurance athletes. *Am J Sports Med* 1996; 24:168–176.
227. Hisf L, White M, Laurin MJ. Quantitative ultrasound predicts stress fracture risk during basic military training in female soldiers. *Transactions of the Orthopaedic Research Society* 1997; 186:31.
228. Johansson C, Ekenman I, Tornkvist H, Eriksson E. Stress fractures of the femoral neck in athletes. *Am J Sports Med* 1990; 18:524–528.
229. Mendez A, Eyster RL. Displaced nonunion stress fracture of the femoral neck treated with internal fixation and bone graft. *Am J Sports Med* 1992; 20:230–233.
230. Muller ME, Nazarian S, Koch P, Schatzker J. *The Comprehensive Classifications of Fractures of Long Bones*. Berlin: Springer-Verlag, 1990.

Chapter 6
Intertrochanteric Fractures

Because they are located distal to the anatomic limits of the hip joint capsule, fractures in the region between the greater and lesser trochanters are characterized as *extracapsular fractures* (Figure 6.1). The cancellous bone in this intertrochanteric region is well vascularized. Therefore, one rarely encounters the problems of nonunion and osteonecrosis that can complicate intracapsular fractures.

Classification

For many years, the standard system for classifying intertrochanteric hip fractures was the one devised by Boyd and Griffin[1] (Figure 6.2). They described four fracture types based on the fracture pattern and the amount of comminution: nondisplaced intertrochanteric fractures (type I), comminuted intertrochanteric fractures (type II), intertrochanteric fractures with subtrochanteric extension (type III), and oblique fractures of the proximal femur (reverse obliquity) (type IV).

An important step toward understanding intertrochanteric hip fractures was taken by Evans in 1949 with the introduction of his classification system based on the stability of the fracture pattern and the potential to convert an unstable fracture pattern to a stable reduction[2] (Figure 6.3). Evans observed that the key to a stable reduction was restoration of posteromedial cortical continuity. He accordingly divided intertrochanteric hip fractures into two types differentiated by the status of this anatomic area. In stable fracture patterns, the posteromedial cortex remains intact or has minimal comminution, making it possible to obtain a stable reduction. Unstable fracture patterns, on the other hand, are characterized by greater comminution of the posteromedial cortex; although they are inherently unstable, these fractures can be converted to a stable reduction if medial cortical opposition is obtained. Evans further observed that the reverse obliquity pattern is inherently unstable because of the tendency for medial displacement of the femoral shaft. The adoption of this system was important not only because it emphasized the important distinction between stable and unstable fracture patterns, but also because it helped define the characteristics of a stable reduction.

Evans's system was refined by Jensen and Michaelsen in 1975[3] and later, in 1979, by Kyle.[4] In Jensen and Michaelsen's classification, decreasing stability is linked to the number of associated lesser and greater trochanteric fracture segments (Figure 6.4). Type IA (nondisplaced) and type IB (displaced) fractures

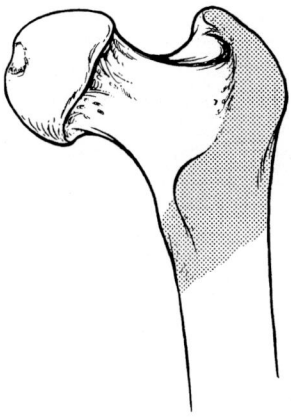

Figure 6.1. Intertrochanteric fractures occur in the region between the greater and lesser trochanters.

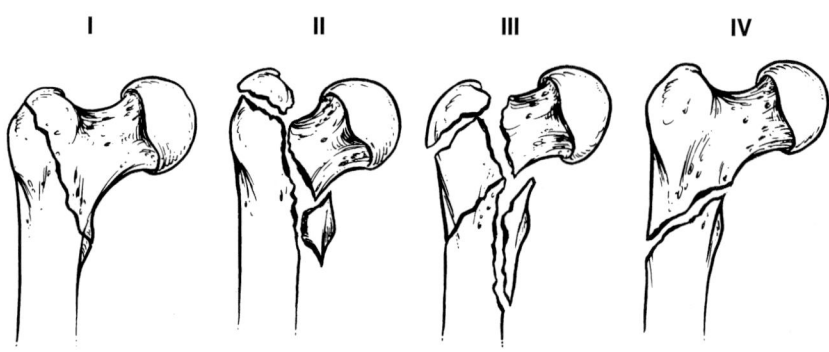

Figure 6.2. The Boyd and Griffin classification system for intertrochanteric fractures[1]: type I, nondisplaced; type II, comminuted; type III, intertrochanteric fractures with subtrochanteric extension; and type IV, oblique fractures of the proximal femur (reverse obliquity).

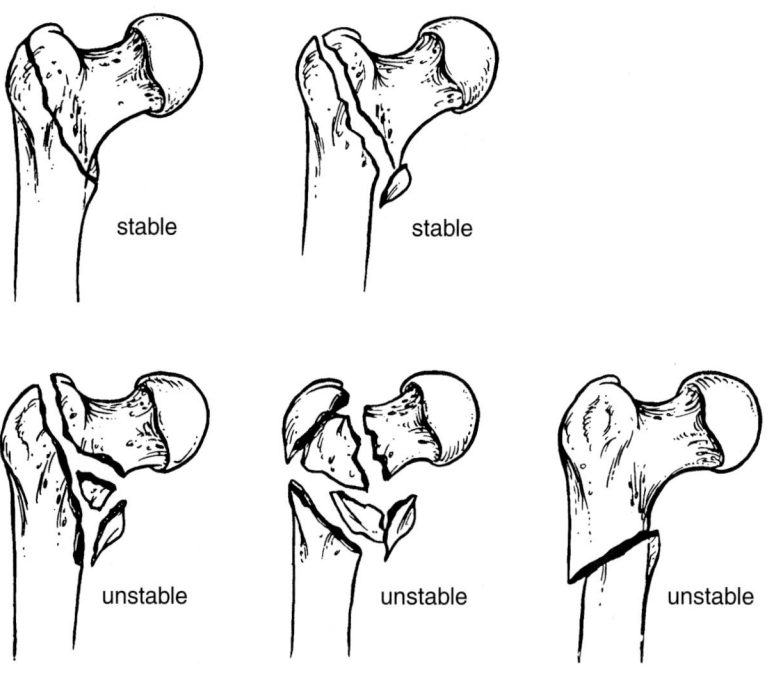

Figure 6.3. The Evans classification system for intertrochanteric fractures, based on the stability of the fracture pattern and the potential to convert an unstable fracture pattern to a stable reduction.[2] In stable fracture patterns the posteromedial cortex remains intact or has minimal comminution, making it possible to obtain a stable reduction. Unstable fracture patterns, on the other hand, are characterized by greater comminution of the posteromedial cortex; although they are inherently unstable, these fractures can be converted to a stable reduction if medial cortical opposition is obtained. Evans further observed that the reverse obliquity pattern is inherently unstable because of the tendency for medial displacement of the femoral shaft.

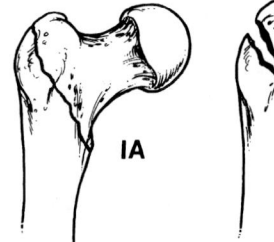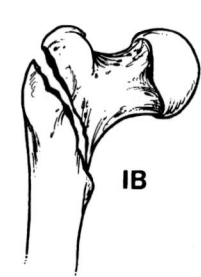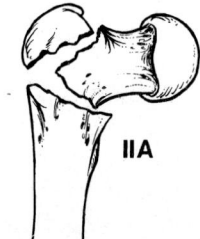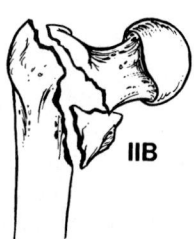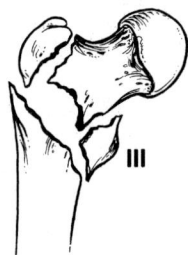

Figure 6.4. The Jensen and Michaelsen classification system for intertrochanteric fractures[3]: type IA (nondisplaced) and type IB (displaced) fractures are simple, stable two-part fractures. Type IIA fractures are three-part fractures with a separate greater trochanteric fragment. Type IIB fractures are three-part fractures involving the lesser trochanter. Type III fractures are four-part fractures involving both greater and lesser trochanteric fragments.

are simple, stable, two-part fractures. Type IIA fractures are three-part fractures with a separate greater trochanteric fragment; these fractures are more difficult to reduce but are stable if medial cortical apposition is obtained. Type IIB fractures are three-part fractures involving the lesser trochanter; these fractures are inherently unstable but can be converted to a stable reduction if the medial cortical buttress is reestablished. Type III fractures are four-part fractures involving both greater and lesser trochanteric fragments; these fractures are also inherently unstable.

In Kyle's four-type classification[4] (Figure 6.5), based on Evans's system, type I fractures are two-part fractures that are nondisplaced and stable; type II fractures (stable) are displaced into varus with a small lesser trochanteric fragment but with an essentially intact posteromedial cortex; type III fractures (four-part, unstable) are displaced into varus with posteromedial cortical comminution and a greater trochanteric fragment; and type IV fractures (unstable) are similar to type III fractures but have fracture extension into the subtrochanteric region.

In the AO/ASIF group's uniform alphanumeric fracture classification that incorporates prognosis and suggests treatment for every element of the human skeleton, intertrochanteric hip fractures make up type 31A[5] (Figure 6.6). These fractures are divided into three groups, and each group is further divided into subgroups based on the obliquity of the fracture line and the degree of comminution. Group 1 fractures are simple (two-part) fractures, with the typical oblique fracture line extending from the greater trochanter to the medial cortex; the lateral cortex of the greater trochanter remains intact. Group 2 fractures are comminuted with a posteromedial fragment; the lateral cortex of the greater trochanter, however, remains intact. Fractures in this group are generally unstable, depending on the size of the medial fragment. Group 3 fractures are those in which the fracture line extends across both the medial and lateral cortices; this group includes the reverse obliquity pattern.

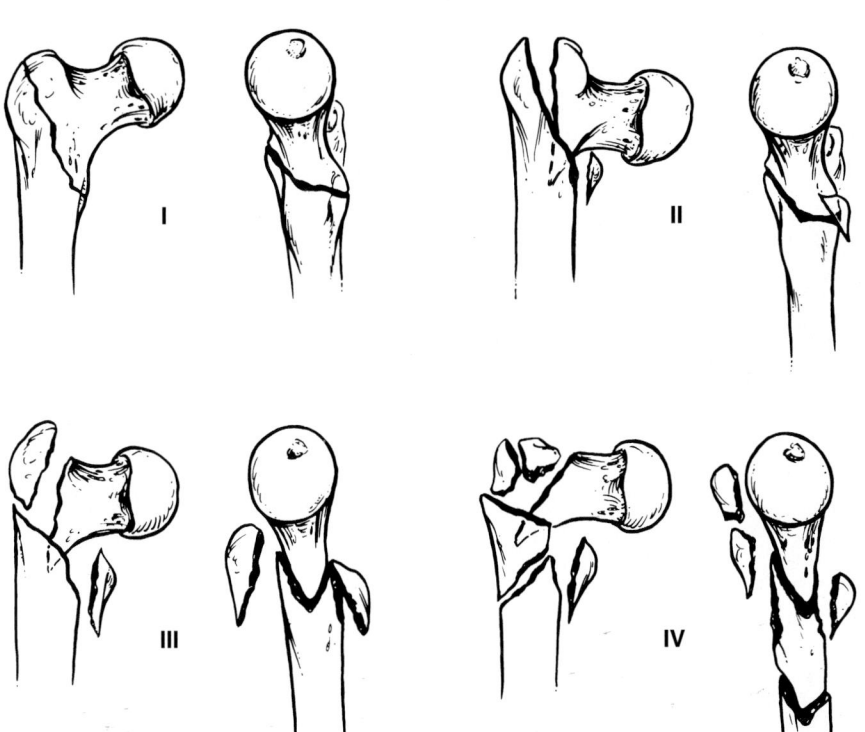

Figure 6.5. The Kyle classification system for intertrochanteric fractures[4]: type I fractures are two-part fractures that are nondisplaced and stable; type II fractures (stable) are displaced into varus with a small lesser trochanteric fragment, but with an essentially intact posteromedial cortex; type III fractures (four-part, unstable) are displaced into varus with posteromedial cortical comminution and a greater trochanteric fracture; and type IV fractures (unstable) are similar to type III fractures but have fracture extension into the subtrochanteric region.

Figure 6.6. The AO/ASIF alphanumeric fracture classification for intertrochanteric fractures. Intertrochanteric hip fractures comprise type 31A.[5] These fractures are divided into three groups, and each group is further divided into subgroups based on obliquity of the fracture line and degree of comminution. Group 1 fractures are simple (two-part) fractures, with the typical oblique fracture line extending from the greater trochanter to the medial cortex; the lateral cortex of the greater trochanter remains intact. Group 2 fractures are comminuted with a posteromedial fragment; the lateral cortex of the greater trochanter, however, remains intact. Group 3 fractures are those in which the fracture line extends across both the medial and lateral cortices; this group includes the reverse obliquity pattern.

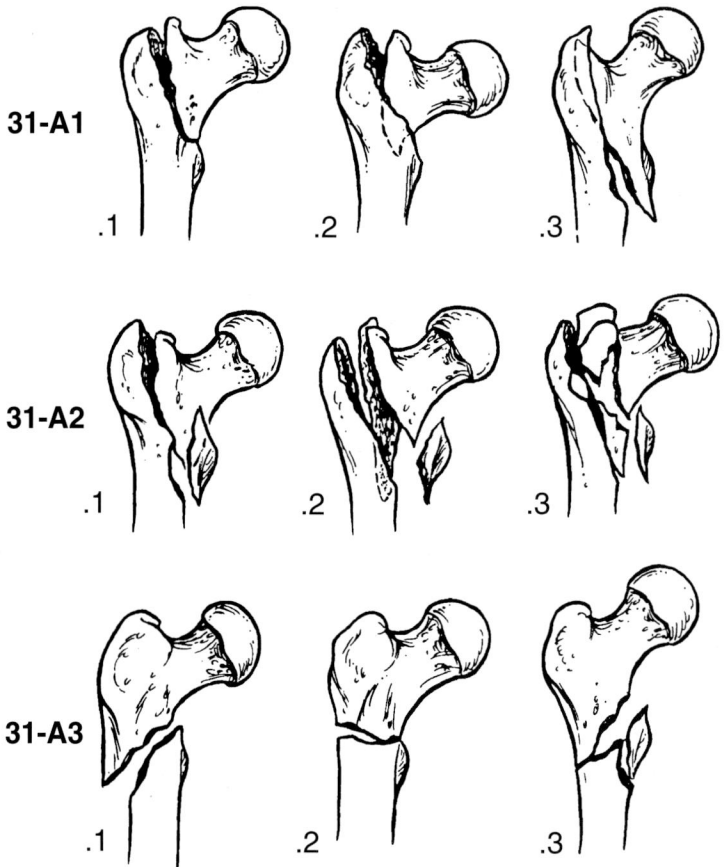

Studies have documented poor reproducibility of the different intertrochanteric fracture classification systems.[6] Therefore, we prefer simply to classify intertrochanteric fractures as either stable or unstable, depending on the status of the posteromedial cortex (Figure 6.7). Unstable fracture patterns include those with comminution of the posteromedial cortex, subtrochanteric extension, or a reverse obliquity pattern.

Figure 6.7. Stable intertrochanteric fracture with an intact posteromedial cortex (**A**). Unstable intertrochanteric fracture characterized by comminution of the posteromedial cortex (**B**).

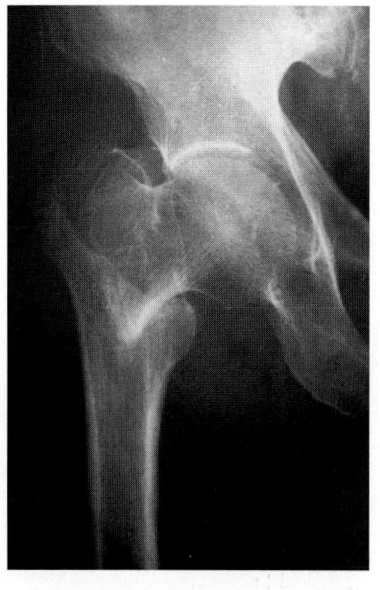
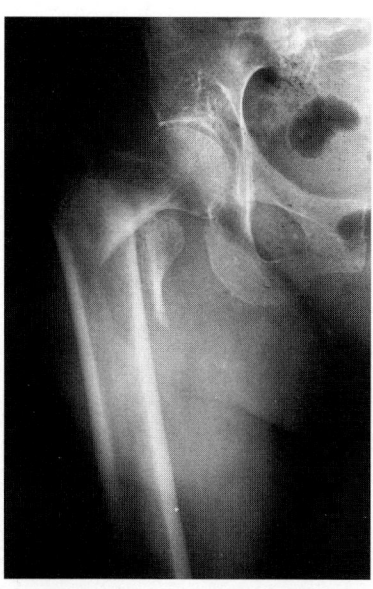

Treatment

Nonoperative Treatment

Before the introduction of suitable fixation devices, treatment for intertrochanteric fractures was nonoperative, consisting of prolonged bed rest in traction until fracture healing occurred (usually in 10 to 12 weeks), followed by a lengthy program of ambulation training (Figure 6.8). In elderly patients, this approach was associated with high complication rates[7]; typical problems included decubitus ulcers, urinary tract infection, joint contractures, pneumonia, and thromboembolic complications, resulting in a high mortality rate. In addition, fracture healing was generally accompanied by varus deformity and shortening because of the inability of traction to effectively counteract the deforming muscular forces.[7]

Over the past 30 years, the techniques of operative fixation have changed dramatically, and the problems associated with early fixation devices have largely been overcome. Operative management, consisting of fracture reduction and stabilization, has thus become the treatment of choice for intertrochanteric fractures; operative management allows early patient mobilization, minimizing many of the complications that would result from prolonged bed rest. There nevertheless remain situations when surgery cannot be performed and treatment must be nonoperative. One example of such a situation is an elderly person whose medical condition carries an excessively high risk of mortality from anesthesia and surgery (e.g., one who has sustained a recent myocardial infarction). Furthermore, nonambulatory patients who have minimal discomfort after fracture should be treated nonoperatively and permitted early bed-to-chair mobilization.

Historically, nonoperative management protocols took one of two different approaches. In the first approach, directed at early mobilization within the limits of the patient's discomfort, the patient was out of bed and in a chair within a few days of the injury. Ambulation was delayed, but the early bed-to-chair mobilization helped prevent many of the complications of prolonged recumbency. This approach does not attempt to treat the fracture specifically and accepts the deformity that invariably ensues (Figure 6.9).

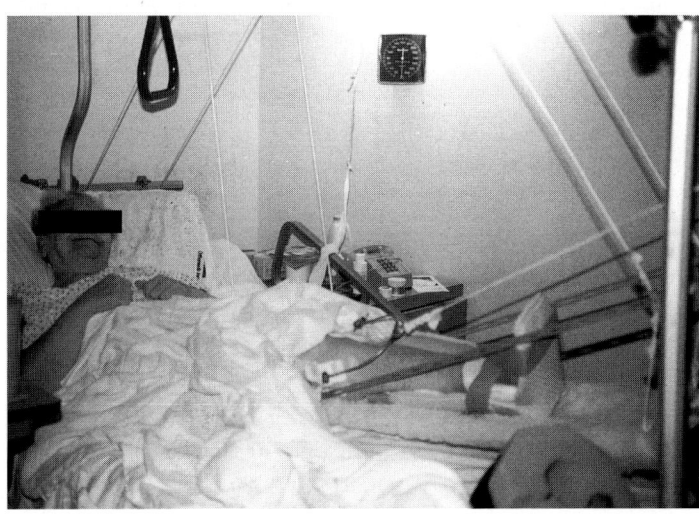

Figure 6.8. Elderly hip fracture patient in skeletal traction.

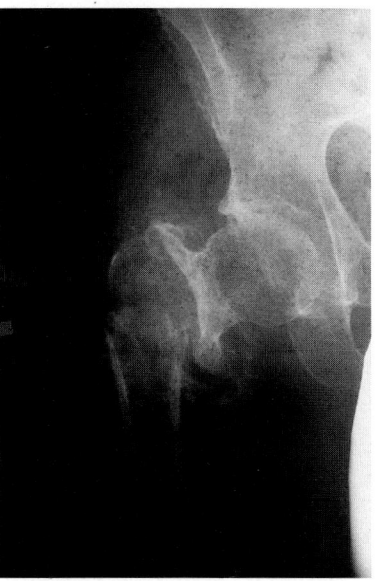

Figure 6.9. Displaced intertrochanteric fracture treated nonoperatively that united with deformity.

In contrast, the second approach attempted to establish and maintain a reasonable reduction via skeletal traction until fracture union occurred. As outlined previously, traction using this technique was prolonged, and an acceptable position was difficult to achieve and maintain. Nursing care was also exceedingly difficult. In addition, this approach was subject to all the complications noted previously.

When nonoperative management is required in the elderly, we prefer the first approach directed at early mobilization and acceptance of deformity. We believe that avoiding the complications inherent in prolonged bed rest is more important than attempting the often unsuccessful task of maintaining a reduction in traction. In a review of approximately 400 intertrochanteric fractures treated at the Hospital for Joint Diseases between 1985 and 1994, only four fractures have been treated nonoperatively. Two patients, each of whom had recently sustained a pulmonary embolism, required ongoing anticoagulation therapy that could not be discontinued. The patients both underwent late reconstructive surgery when anticoagulation could be safely discontinued. The other two patients were nonambulators with severe medical problems as well as Alzheimer's dementia; within a few days after fracture, both of these patients had minimal pain, were mobilized from bed to chair, and returned to their prefracture living environment.

Operative Treatment

Operative management, which allows early rehabilitation and offers the patient the best chance for functional recovery, is the treatment of choice for virtually all intertrochanteric fractures.

Evolution of Surgical Techniques

Although it is unnecessary to review every one of the multitude of implants that have been used to stabilize intertrochanteric fractures, it is important to understand the principles behind their evolution. The first implants to be used with success were fixed-angle nail-plate devices (e.g., Jewett nail, Holt nail) consisting of a triflanged nail fixed to a plate at an angle between 130° and 150° (Figure 6.10). Although these devices provided stabilization of the femoral head and neck fragment to the femoral shaft, they did not allow fracture impaction. If significant impaction of the fracture site occurred, the implant would either penetrate into the hip joint or cut out through the superior portion of the femoral head and neck. If, on the other hand, no impaction occurred, lack of bone contact would result in either plate breakage or separation of the plate and screws from the femoral shaft (Figure 6.11). These complications occurred much more frequently when these devices were used to treat unstable fractures.

The experience with fixed-angle nail-plate devices indicated the need for a device that allowed controlled fracture impaction. This gave rise to sliding nail-plate devices (e.g., Massie nail, Ken-Pugh nail), which consisted of a nail that provided proximal fragment fixation and a sideplate that allowed the nail to "telescope" within a barrel (Figure 6.12). Impaction provided bone-on-bone contact, which promoted fracture union; implant sliding also decreased the moment arm and stresses on the implant, thereby lowering the risk of implant failure. In a retrospective study, Kyle et al. reported a lower incidence of nail breakage and fewer cases of nail penetration with a Massie sliding nail than with a fixed-angle Jewett nail for the treatment of unstable intertrochanteric fractures. In a subsequent prospective series, they reported fixation failure rates of 1.5% when the Massie nail was used in stable intertrochanteric fractures, 6.8% in unstable intertrochanteric fractures, and 13.2% in combined intertrochanteric–subtrochanteric fractures.[4]

The sliding nail-plate devices gave rise to sliding hip screw devices (Figure 6.13). The nail portion was replaced by a blunt-ended screw with a large outside thread diameter. Theoretically, this was to result in improved proximal fragment fixation and decrease the risk of screw cutout by eliminating the

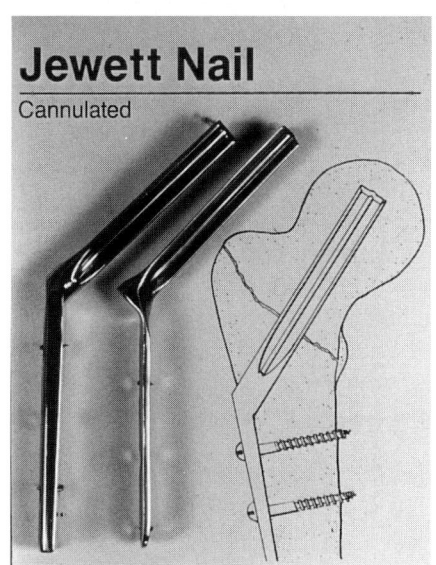

Figure 6.10. Photograph and drawing of a Jewett nail (courtesy of R. A. Calandruccio, The Campbell Clinic Foundation, Memphis TN).

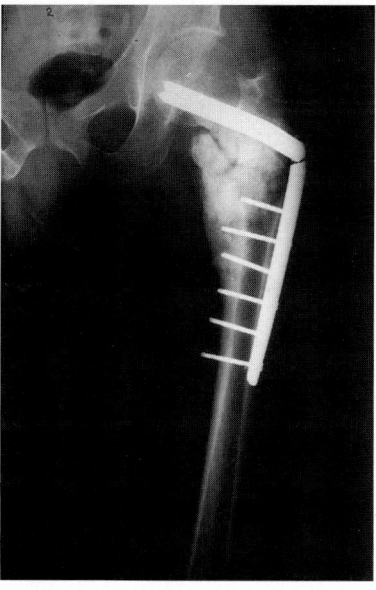

Figure 6.11. Intertrochanteric nonunion with a broken Jewett nail.

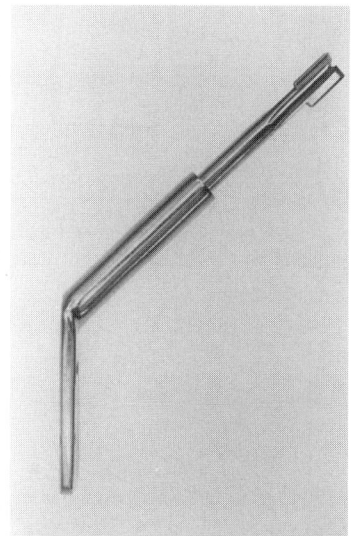

Figure 6.12. Photograph of a Massie nail.

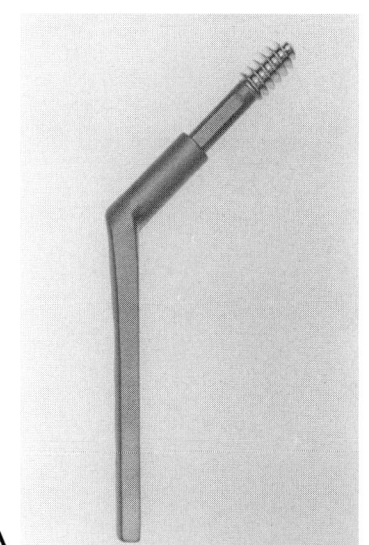 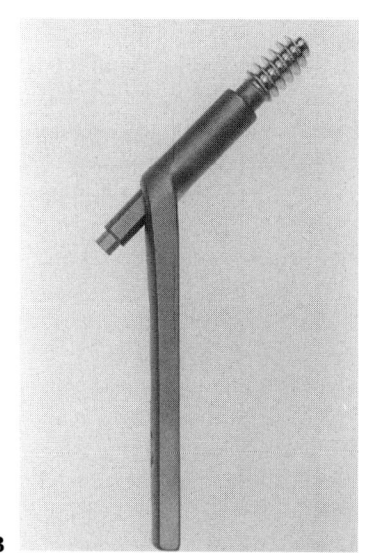 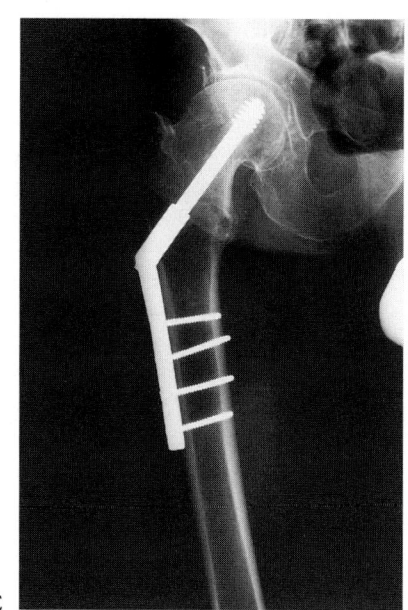

Figure 6.13. Photographs of a sliding hip screw (**A**), demonstrating sliding of the lag screw within the plate barrel (**B**). AP radiograph of a healed intertrochanteric fracture stabilized with a sliding hip screw (**C**).

sharp edges found on triflanged nails. Numerous series have reported excellent results with sliding hip screws for intertrochanteric fracture fixation,[7–9] and currently this device is the most widely used implant for this application.

Heyse-Moore et al. retrospectively compared the results of 107 intertrochanteric fractures stabilized with a sliding hip screw to 103 fractures treated with a Jewett nail.[10] In patients with comparable fractures, those treated with the sliding hip screw had shorter hospitalization stays and a lower incidence of fixation failure. Bannister et al., in a prospective randomized study of 155 intertrochanteric fractures stabilized using similar devices, found that fractures stabilized with a sliding hip screw had a significantly lower risk of mechanical failure and a lower incidence of revision surgery.[11] Jacobs et al. reported on a series of 173 intertrochanteric fractures treated with internal fixation, 72 with a Jewett nail and 101 with a sliding hip screw.[12] Treatment failure—defined as either loss of fixation, symptomatic joint penetration, osteonecrosis, malunion, or nonunion—occurred in 25% of fractures stabilized with a Jewett nail and in 6% of fractures stabilized using a sliding hip screw.

One early modification to the sliding hip screw maximized fracture impaction by allowing the proximal lag screw to telescope within the plate barrel and the plate to slide axially along the femoral shaft. To accomplish this bidirectional sliding, the plate was modified by replacing the round screw holes with slotted screw holes (Egger's plate). More recently, a two-component plate device was introduced (Medoff plate, Medpac, Culver City, CA) in which a central vertical channel constrains an internal sliding component (Figure 6.14). Both devices have been used successfully for the treatment of stable and unstable intertrochanteric fractures.

In a nonrandomized study, Medoff and Maes compared the use of a Medoff plate (25 patients) to the use of a sliding hip screw (61 patients) for fixation of unstable intertrochanteric fractures.[13] In patients who received a standard sliding hip screw, the technical failure rate was 12%, whereas no fracture that was stabilized with the Medoff plate had loss of fixation. Furthermore, a larger proportion of patients who received the Medoff plate were able to ambulate 50 feet independently by the time of hospital discharge.

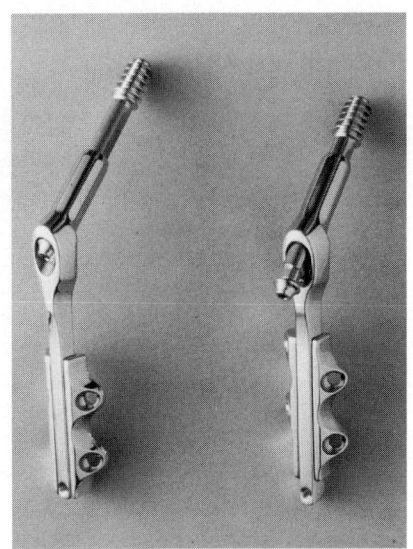 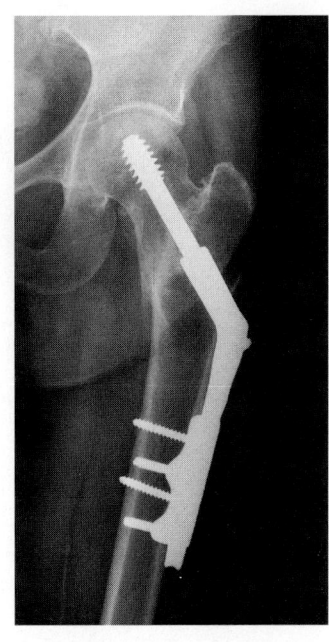

Figure 6.14. The Medoff plate, which allows sliding of the lag screw within the plate barrel as well as axial plate sliding along the femoral shaft (**A**). AP radiograph of a healed intertrochanteric fracture stabilized with a Medoff plate (**B**).

Watson et al. compared the Medoff plate to a standard sliding hip screw in a prospective randomized series of 160 stable and unstable intertrochanteric fractures[14]; follow-up averaged 9.5 months (range, 6 to 26 months). Ninety-one fractures were treated using the standard sliding hip screw and 69 with the Medoff sliding plate. Although stable fracture patterns united without complication in both treatment groups, there was a significantly higher failure rate with use of the sliding hip screw for unstable fractures (14% versus 3%). No differences were observed between the two devices in terms of length of hospitalization, return to prefracture ambulatory status, postoperative living status, or need for postoperative analgesic medication. For all fracture types, however, use of the Medoff plate was associated with significantly greater blood loss and operating time.

The Alta expandable dome plunger (Howmedica, Rutherford, NJ) is a modified sliding hip screw designed to improve fixation of the proximal fragment by facilitating cement intrusion into the femoral head (Figure 6.15). Cement is kept away from the plate barrel so that the device's sliding potential is maintained. The device is inserted in a fashion similar to that used for the sliding hip screw except that the dome unit is manually pushed into the prereamed femoral neck and head; proximal fixation is achieved as the plunger is then advanced, expanding the dome in the cancellous bone of the femoral head and extruding the contained cement. Although this device was demonstrated to be superior to a standard sliding hip screw system in the laboratory,[15] improved efficacy has not been shown in clinical trials.

Intramedullary devices have also been used to stabilize intertrochanteric fractures. Such implants are subjected to smaller bending moments than plate-and-screw devices because they are positioned closer to the mechanical axis of the femur (Figure 6.16). The most experience has been gained with the use of flexible intramedullary nails (Ender nails) (Figure 6.17). For stabilization of intertrochanteric fractures, these devices are inserted under image intensification in a retrograde manner through portals in the distal femur. From there they are passed up into the proximal femur, without the need for

Figure 6.15. Photograph of the Alta dome plunger and lag screw, both of which telescope within a plate barrel (**A**). Radiograph of the dome plunger with cement intrusion into the femoral head (**B**).

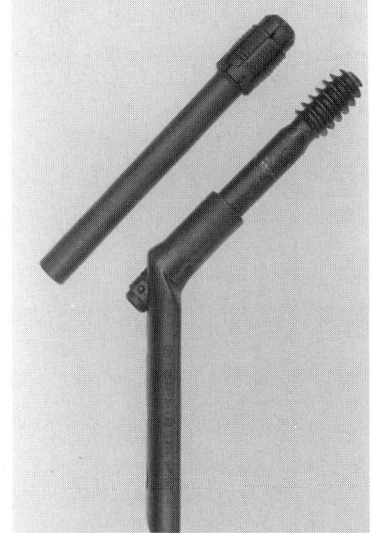
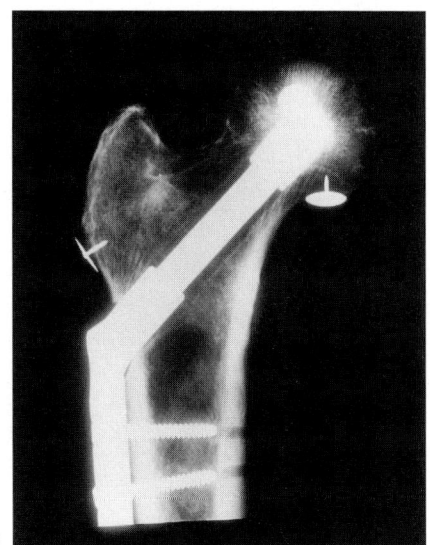

Figure 6.16. Intramedullary nails (**B**, **C**) are subjected to smaller bending moments than plate-and-screw devices (**A**) because they are positioned closer to the mechanical axis of the femur.

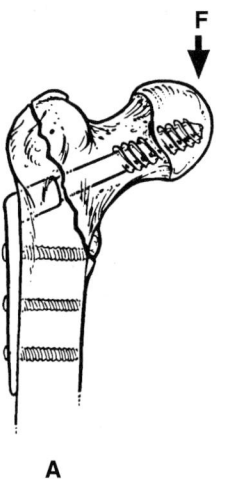
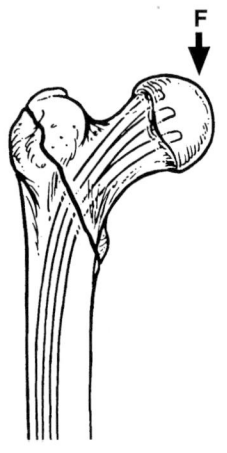
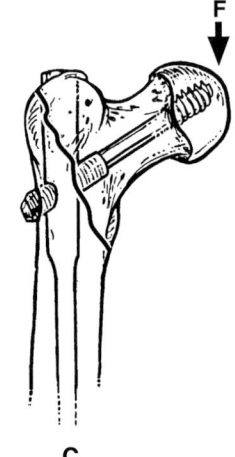

Figure 6.17. Photograph and drawing of Ender nails (**A**) (courtesy of R. A. Calandruccio, The Campbell Clinic Foundation, Memphis TN). Radiograph of a healed intertrochanteric fracture stabilized with retrograde-inserted Ender nails (**B**).

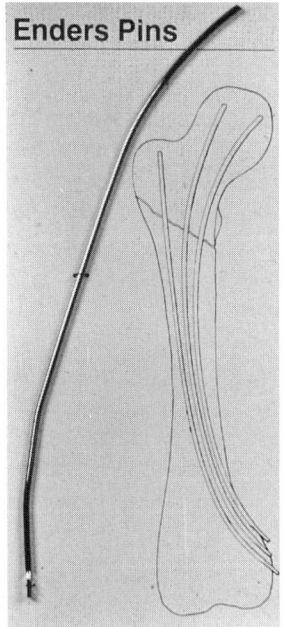
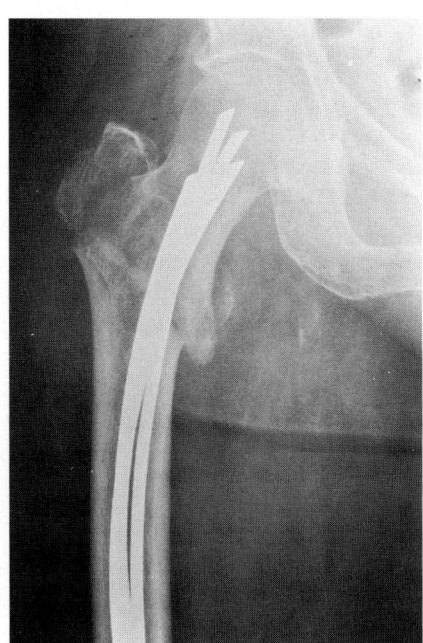

direct fracture exposure. Although the advantages of this procedure were supposed to include reductions in blood loss, anesthetic use, operating time, and mortality rate, in actuality their use has been associated with a significant incidence of complications, including rotational deformity, supracondylar femur fracture, proximal migration of the nails through the femoral head, and backout of the nails with resultant knee pain and stiffness[16–21] (Figure 6.18). Levy et al., studying a series of 200 hip fractures stabilized using Ender nails, reported that 50% of patients exhibited distal pin migration, 76% experienced knee pain, and 36% developed a significant external rotation deformity.[22]

Sernbo et al. compared use of Ender nails to use of a sliding hip screw for the treatment of unstable intertrochanteric hip fractures in a prospective randomized trial.[23] There were more than 100 patients in each treatment group; minimum follow-up was 6 months. There were more secondary operations for patients whose fractures were stabilized using Ender nails, and more of these patients experienced loss of fixation. Rao et al. reported similar findings in a retrospective analysis of 77 cases of stable and unstable intertrochanteric fractures[24]; fractures stabilized using Ender nails had more complications than those stabilized with a sliding hip screw. Waddell, however, reported excellent results with the use of Ender nails in a large series of patients who had sustained a pertrochanteric fracture[25]; he concluded, contrary to the experience of other investigators, that Ender nails are the implants of choice for unstable intertrochanteric fractures. These widely divergent conclusions about the same device underline the importance of surgeon experience.

Intramedullary sliding hip screw devices have recently been developed for stabilization of pertrochanteric fractures (e.g., Gamma nail [Howmedica, Rutherford, NJ], Intramedullary Hip Screw [IMHS] [Smith+Nephew, Memphis, TN]). These devices couple a sliding hip screw with a locked intramedullary nail (Figure 6.19). This design offers several potential advantages: (1) an intramedullary fixation device, because of its location, has the theoretical advantage of providing more efficient load transfer than does a sliding hip screw; (2) the shorter lever arm of the intramedullary device can be expected to decrease tensile strain on the implant, thereby decreasing the risk of implant failure; (3) because the intramedullary fixation device incorporates a sliding hip screw, the advantage of controlled fracture impaction is maintained; and (4) insertion of an intramedullary hip screw theoretically requires shorter operative

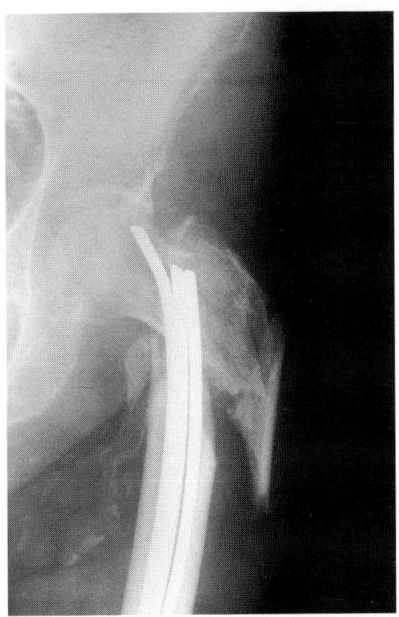
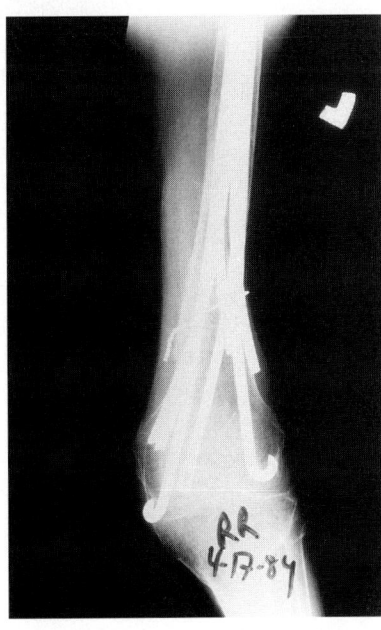

Figure 6.18. Complications associated with use of Ender nails for stabilization of intertrochanteric fractures include: loss of fixation (**A**) and knee pain secondary to backout of the implant (**B**).

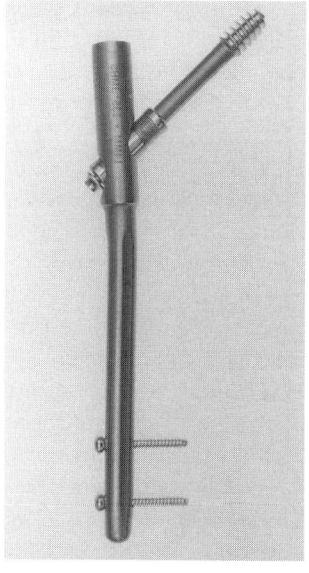
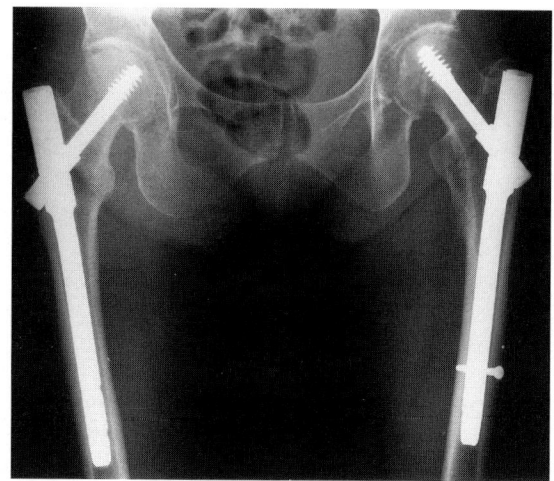

Figure 6.19. Photograph of the Smith+Nephew's Intramedullary Hip Screw (**A**). Use of the intramedullary hip screw device to stabilize bilateral intertrochanteric fractures (**B**).

A   B

time and less soft tissue dissection than insertion of a sliding hip screw, potentially resulting in decreased overall morbidity.

Most studies comparing an intramedullary hip screw to a sliding hip screw have found no significant differences with respect to operating time, duration of hospital stay, infection rate, wound complications, implant failure, screw cutout, or screw sliding.[26,27] Patients treated with an intramedullary hip screw, however, are at increased risk for femoral shaft fracture at the nail tip and the insertion sites of the distal locking screws[28–30] (Figure 6.20).

Butt et al. reported on a prospective, randomized controlled trial that compared results in 95 consecutive patients who sustained a pertrochanteric fracture of the femur and were treated using a sliding hip screw ($n = 48$) or a

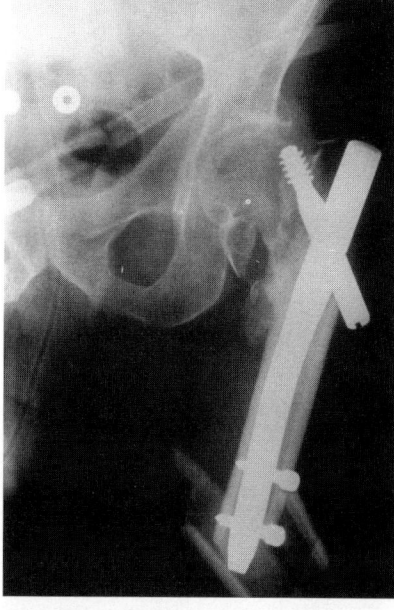

Figure 6.20. Radiograph demonstrating femoral shaft fracture that occurred at the tip of an intramedullary hip screw as well as lag screw cutout of the femoral head.

Gamma nail ($n = 47$).[31] Whereas clinical and radiological outcomes were similar, the Gamma nail was associated with a higher incidence of complications—in particular, femur fracture distal to the implant.

Aune et al. reported on a series of 378 intertrochanteric and subtrochanteric hip fractures prospectively randomized to treatment with either a Gamma nail (177 fractures) or a sliding hip screw (201 fractures).[32] At an average follow-up of 17 months, 15 patients needed revision surgery: 13 in the Gamma nail group and 2 in the sliding hip screw group. Ten patients, all stabilized with a Gamma nail, sustained a femoral shaft fracture, either along the nail or at its distal tip. Lag screw cutout or femoral head penetration occurred in 5 patients, 3 in the Gamma nail group and 2 in the sliding hip screw group.

Leung et al. reported on a prospective series of 186 peritrochanteric fractures stabilized with either a Gamma nail or a sliding hip screw.[27] Gamma nails were inserted in a significantly shorter operative time using a smaller incision and were associated with a smaller estimated blood loss. There was, however, no significant differences between the two groups with regard to 6-month mortality rate, postoperative mobility, or hip function at follow-up. A higher number of intraoperative complications occurred in fractures stabilized with a Gamma nail.

Baumgaertner et al. reported on a series of 131 patients (135 fractures) who sustained an intertrochanteric fracture and were randomly assigned to treatment with either a sliding hip screw or an intramedullary hip screw (IMHS).[33] In patients with unstable intertrochanteric fractures, the intramedullary device was associated with significantly less surgical time and blood loss; however, use of the intramedullary hip screw in patients who had a stable fracture pattern required significantly greater fluoroscopy time. Intraoperative complications occurred exclusively in the intramedullary hip screw group. At latest follow-up, there was no difference in the percentage of functional recovery between the two fixation groups.

Hardy et al. performed a prospective, randomized study comparing use of a sliding hip screw to use of an intramedullary hip screw (IMHS) for stabilization of 100 intertrochanteric fractures in patients age 60 years or older.[34] The operative time was significantly greater with use of the intramedullary device; however, estimated intraoperative blood loss was significantly lower. There was one intraoperative femur fracture and two greater trochanter fractures associated with use of the intramedullary hip screw, but no late postoperative fractures. One fracture stabilized with a sliding hip screw had loss of fixation. The in-hospital and 6-month mortality rates were similar between the two treatment groups. Patients whose fractures were stabilized using the intramedullary hip screw had significantly better mobility at 1- and 3-month follow-up. This difference was no longer seen at 6 and 12 months, although patients who received the intramedullary device had significantly better walking ability outside the home at all time periods. The intramedullary hip screw was associated with significantly less screw sliding and limb shortening than the sliding hip screw, particularly when used to stabilize unstable fracture patterns. Based on the results of this study, the authors concluded that routine use of the intramedullary hip screw cannot be recommended for stabilization of intertrochanteric hip fractures.

A biomechanical laboratory evaluation of the Gamma nail performed at the Hospital for Joint Diseases in a stable and unstable intertrochanteric fracture model demonstrated that this device transmits decreasing load to the calcar femorale with decreasing fracture stability.[35] Virtually no osseous strain was identified in four-part fractures with the posteromedial fragment removed. The insertion of distal locking screws did not change the pattern of proximal femoral strain. These results were attributed to the inherent stiffness of the implant.

Implant Choice

Based on the available literature, we believe that a sliding hip screw is the implant of choice for most intertrochanteric hip fractures. Use of the Alta bolt may be appropriate in patients with severe osteopenia of the femoral head; one might also consider methylmethracylate augmentation in these patients. Use of the Medoff plate or an intramedullary hip screw (e.g., Gamma nail, IMHS) may be indicated in patients who have intertrochanteric fractures with subtrochanteric extension (including the reverse-obliquity fracture). Use of Ender nails should be reserved for patients who have proximal soft tissue compromise so that the benefits of this distally inserted implant outweigh the risks.

Reduction Techniques

Before devices became available that allowed postoperative fracture impaction, one had to achieve fracture stability at surgery to minimize the risk of healing complications. In the absence of a stable medial buttress, the incidence of implant failure and hip joint penetration was unacceptably high. Methods subsequently developed to achieve stable medial cortical opposition included medial-displacement osteotomy (Dimon-Hughston osteotomy), valgus osteotomy (Sarmiento osteotomy), and lateral-displacement osteotomy (Wayne County osteotomy).[7]

A medial-displacement osteotomy alters the pathologic anatomy of the unstable fracture such that it is converted to a stable, albeit nonanatomic, position[36,37] (Figure 6.21). The surgical technique involves (1) transverse osteotomy of the proximal femoral shaft at the level of the lesser trochanter; (2) osteotomy (if necessary) and proximal displacement of the greater trochanter and the attached abductor muscles; (3) medial displacement of the femoral

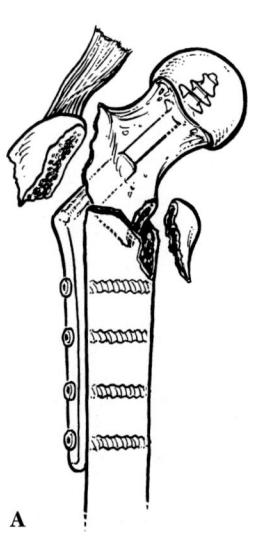 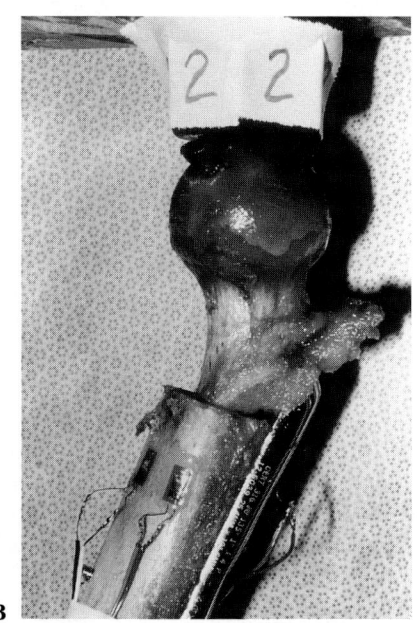

Figure 6.21. Drawing (**A**) and cadaveric example (**B**) of a medial displacement osteotomy stabilized with a sliding hip screw.

Treatment

shaft; and (4) impaction of the proximal fragment into the medullary canal of the femoral shaft. If the proximal fragment is firmly impacted into the femoral shaft, a stable construct will result. Dimon and Hughston reported improved results with Jewett nail fixation of unstable intertrochanteric fractures using this osteotomy technique.[36] However, to the extent that the proximal fragment is impacted into the femoral shaft, limb shortening will occur. This can be at least partially counteracted by a valgus positioning of the proximal fragment—which may, however, adversely affect the function and appearance of the knee. In addition, the level of functioning and proximal migration of the greater trochanteric fragment significantly compromises abductor function, increasing the stress on the implant and impairing the patient's ability to regain his or her ambulatory ability.

Sarmiento recommended a valgus osteotomy for unstable intertrochanteric fractures to provide a medial cortical buttress[38,39] (Figure 6.22). This technique involves (1) an oblique osteotomy of the proximal femoral shaft, extending from the base of the greater trochanter to a medial position, 1 cm distal to the apex of the fracture; (2) implant placement into the proximal fragment, 90° to the fracture surface; and (3) reduction and impaction of the osteotomy surfaces. Several possible pitfalls are associated with this technique: (1) creation of an excessively valgus osteotomy, which increases the force required by the abductor muscles to stabilize the pelvis in single-stance phase and results in increased joint reaction forces; (2) excessive limb shortening; and (3) an external rotation deformity. Although Sarmiento reported success using this technique, his results have rarely been reproduced.

A Wayne County or lateral-displacement osteotomy involves lateral displacement of the femoral shaft to create medial cortical overlap[40] (Figure 6.23). This technique is applicable to relatively unstable fractures with a small posteromedial fragment. It has not been used widely.

Since the advent of sliding hip screw devices, there has been renewed interest in anatomic alignment. Anatomic alignment differs from anatomic fracture reduction in that the goal is simply to align the head and neck fragment with the shaft rather than to reduce and stabilize all fracture fragments.[7] A sliding hip screw is used to control fracture impaction.

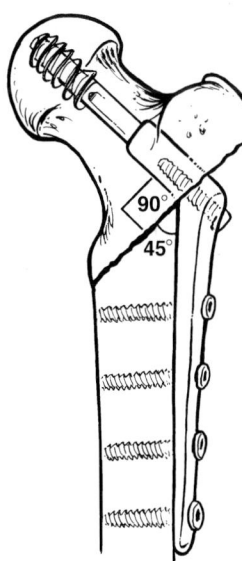

Figure 6.22. Drawing of a valgus osteotomy stabilized with a sliding hip screw.

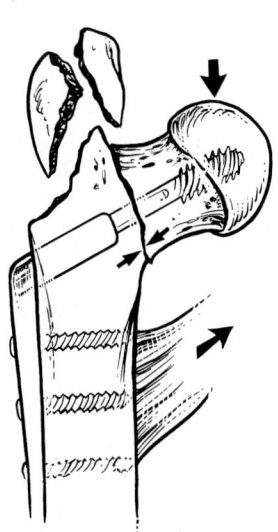

Figure 6.23. Drawing of a lateral displacement osteotomy stabilized with a sliding hip screw.

The need for proximal femoral osteotomy (medial displacement osteotomy, valgus osteotomy) to stabilize unstable intertrochanteric fractures has been largely eliminated since the development of sliding hip screw and nail systems. In a laboratory study performed at the Hospital for Joint Diseases, we determined that, in terms of load transmission and plate strain, a formal medial displacement osteotomy is inferior to anatomic reduction—with or without fixation of the posteromedial fragment.[41] Because a sliding hip screw allows controlled fracture collapse, anatomically aligned unstable fractures stabilized with a properly inserted sliding hip screw usually impact spontaneously to a stable, medially displaced position (Figure 6.24).

Hopkins et al. reported on a retrospective series of 55 unstable intertrochanteric fractures treated with an anatomic-alignment or a medial-displacement osteotomy and stabilized using a sliding hip screw.[42] Eighty-nine percent of fractures that were anatomically aligned subsequently collapsed into a medially displaced position; 97% of these same fractures united without a complication. The authors reported that the only advantage of formal medial-displacement osteotomy was a slightly lower rate of trochanteric bursitis resulting from less fracture impaction and screw sliding.

Gargan et al. performed a prospective randomized study of 100 consecutive unstable intertrochanteric fractures stabilized with a sliding hip screw to compare anatomic alignment with two types of osteotomy (medial displacement and valgus).[43] The patient groups were similar in terms of age, gender, mental test score, and fracture configuration. Patients in the osteotomy groups experienced a higher rate of fixation failure and had increased operative time. The authors concluded that there was no benefit to either type of osteotomy and recommended that unstable intertrochanteric fractures be treated by anatomic alignment and stabilization with a sliding hip screw.

In a similar study, Desjardins et al. compared anatomic alignment to medial-displacement osteotomy in unstable intertrochanteric fractures stabilized using a sliding hip screw.[44] One hundred twenty-seven consecutive patients were randomized and prospectively followed up. At an average follow-up of 11

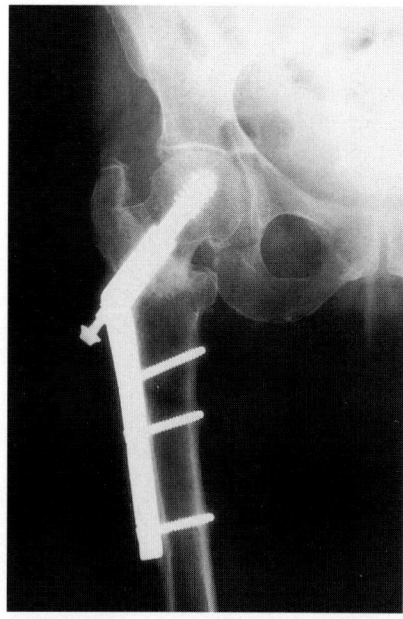

Figure 6.24. Radiograph of an anatomically aligned intertrochanteric fracture stabilized with a sliding hip screw that impacted into a medially displaced position.

Treatment

months, no difference was found in walking ability or incidence of fixation failure between the two groups of patients. However, operative time and estimated blood loss were significantly higher in patients who underwent medial-displacement osteotomy.

Sliding Hip Screw

The sliding hip screw is currently the most commonly used implant for stabilization of intertrochanteric fractures. It is a two-piece device consisting of a large-diameter cannulated lag screw that articulates within a sideplate and barrel (Figure 6.25). Sliding hip screws are available with plate angles from 125° to 155°; the 135° and 150° devices are the most popular (Figure 6.26). Much has been written about the advantages and disadvantages of the various plate

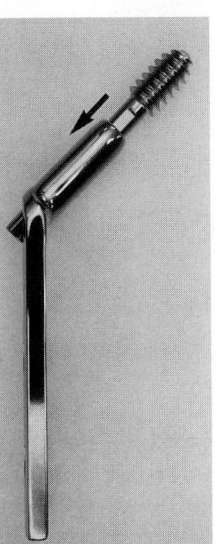

Figure 6.25. Photograph of a sliding hip screw.

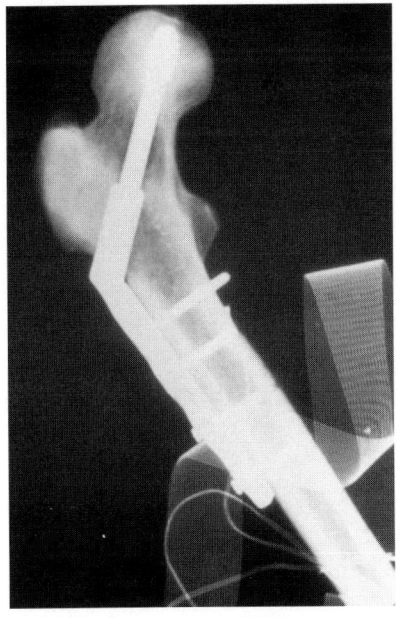
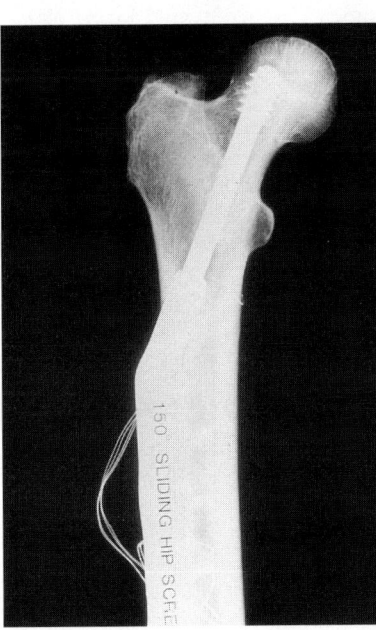

Figure 6.26. Anatomic specimens stabilized with a 135° (**A**) and 150° (**B**) sliding hip screw. Note the distal entry site required for insertion of the 150° implant as well as the superior position of the lag screw within the femoral head.

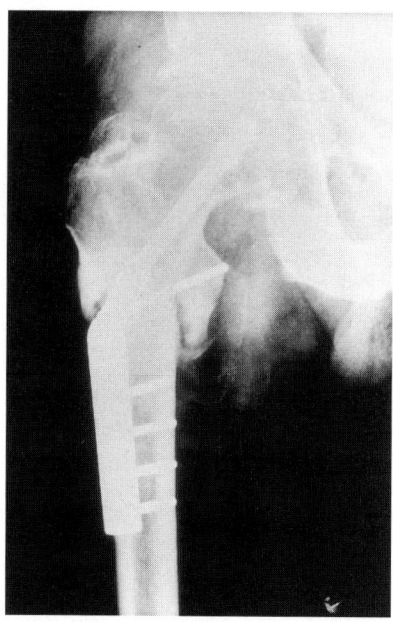

Figure 6.27. Stress fracture of the proximal femur at the 150° plate insertion site.

angles.[45–47] Proponents of the 150° implant cite the following advantages: (1) the higher angle more closely approximates the weight-bearing axis of the proximal femur, thereby reducing the varus moment arm and decreasing the stress on the implant; and (2) the higher angle facilitates lag screw sliding, thereby improving fracture impaction. Proponents of the 135° device cite the problems inherent in the use of the 150° device—specifically, (1) the higher angle makes it difficult to insert the nail in the desired central portion of the head; and (2) the higher plate angle requires a more distal entry point in the femoral shaft, through diaphyseal cortical bone rather than metaphyseal cancellous bone, and results in a significant potential stress riser effect[7] (Figure 6.27).

Biomechanical studies performed at the Hospital for Joint Diseases evaluated the strain distribution in the proximal femur for sliding hip screw plate angles ranging from 130° to 150°.[48] An unstable intertrochanteric fracture pattern was produced in cadaveric femurs and stabilized with an anatomic reduction. Optimal strain distribution (highest compressive strain in the area of the medial cortex and lowest tensile strain on the sideplate) was identified with 135° and 140° devices. The 150° device demonstrated better lag screw sliding, but in five of six of these specimens, the lag screw cut out through the superior portion of the femoral head. Furthermore, several clinical series have either failed to demonstrate the superiority of the 150° devices or failed to find any difference between them and the 135° devices.[45,46] Our preference, based on our laboratory and clinical experience, is to use the 135° plate for virtually all intertrochanteric fractures.

Operative Technique for Insertion of a Sliding Hip Screw

The patient is positioned supine on a fracture table with both lower extremities resting in padded foot holders (Figure 6.28). A padded perineal post is placed in the ipsilateral groin, with care taken that there is no impingement of the labia or scrotum (Figure 6.29). Furthermore, in female patients it is impor-

Treatment

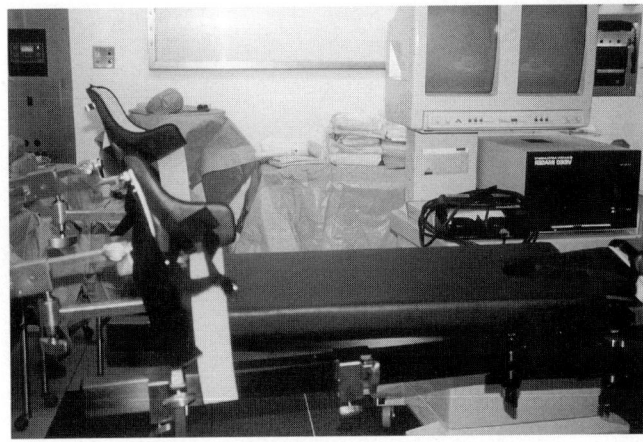

A

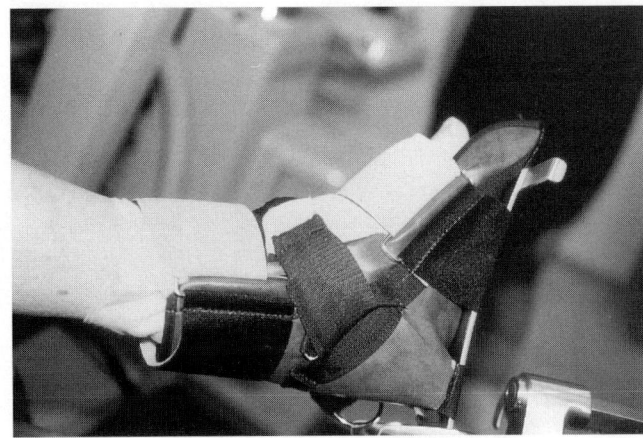

B

Figure 6.28. For intertrochanteric fracture reduction and sliding hip screw insertion, the patient is positioned supine on a fracture table (**A**) with both lower extremities resting in padded foot holders (**B**).

tant to verify that the mucosa of the labia is not everted against the perineal post. (In one young woman, this labial positioning was not recognized, and the patient developed a slough of her entire labia majora.)

Once the patient is properly positioned, the fracture is reduced. Intertrochanteric hip fractures can be reduced using gentle longitudinal traction with the leg externally rotated followed by internal rotation (Figure 6.30). The uninvolved leg is then flexed, abducted, and externally rotated to allow positioning of the image intensifier for a lateral view (Figure 6.31). Alternatively, the contralateral extremity can be abducted with the hip and knee extended (Figure 6.32); this maneuver, however, places greater post pressure on the perineum.[49]

The surgeon must assess the fracture reduction before preparing and draping the operative site and must be certain that unobstructed biplanar radiographic visualization of the entire proximal femur, including the hip joint, is obtainable (Figure 6.33). Inadequate visualization of the entire proximal femur can result in inappropriate lag screw length or positioning (Figure 6.34). The surgeon must be prepared to deal with residual varus angulation, posterior

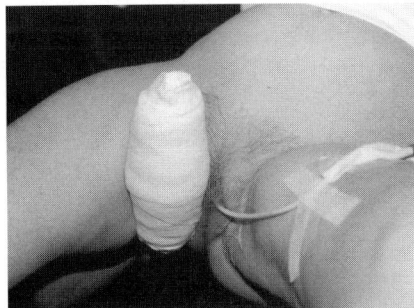

Figure 6.29. A padded perineal post is placed in the ipsilateral groin, with care taken that there is no impingement of the labia or scrotum. In female patients, it is important to verify that the mucosa of the labia is not everted against the perineal post.

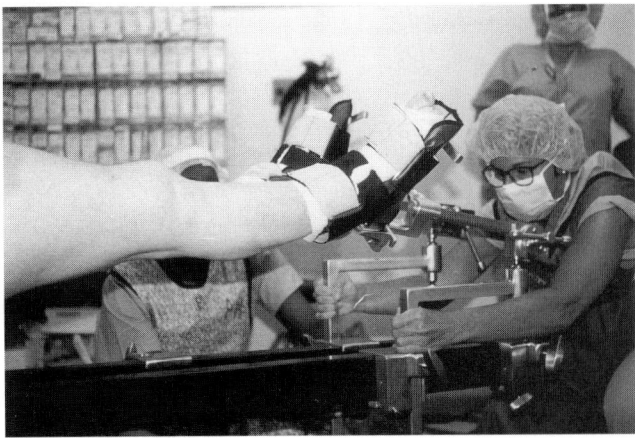

Figure 6.30. An intertrochanteric fracture can be reduced using longitudinal traction with the leg externally rotated, followed by internal rotation.

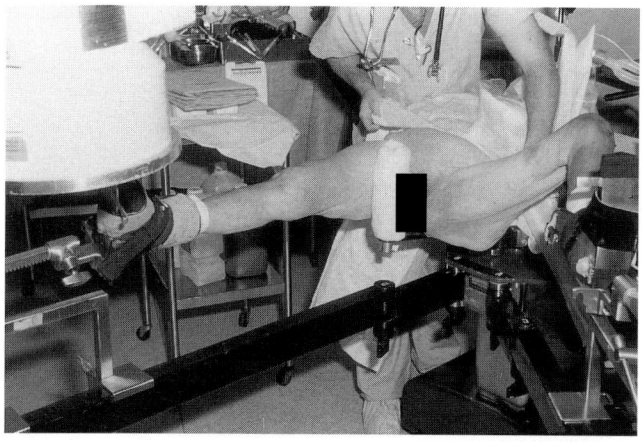

Figure 6.31. Flexion, abduction, and external rotation of the contralateral lower extremity to allow positioning of the image intensifier for a cross-table lateral view.

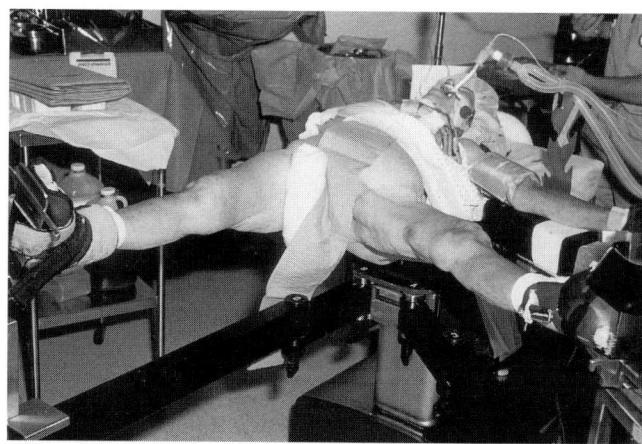

Figure 6.32. Alternative positioning of the contralateral extremity in abduction with the hip and knee extended; this maneuver, however, places greater post pressure on the perineum.[49]

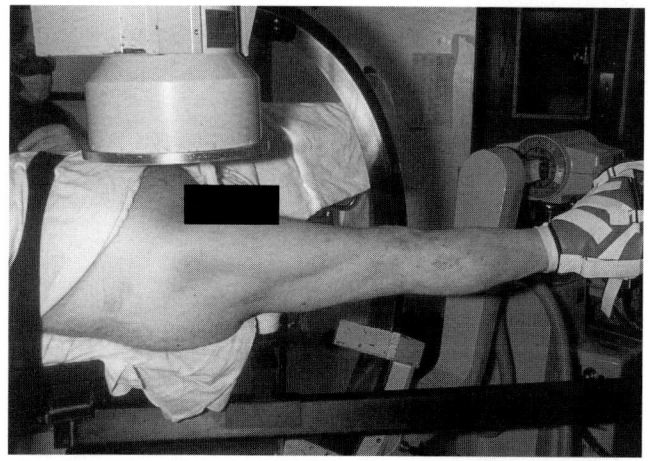

A

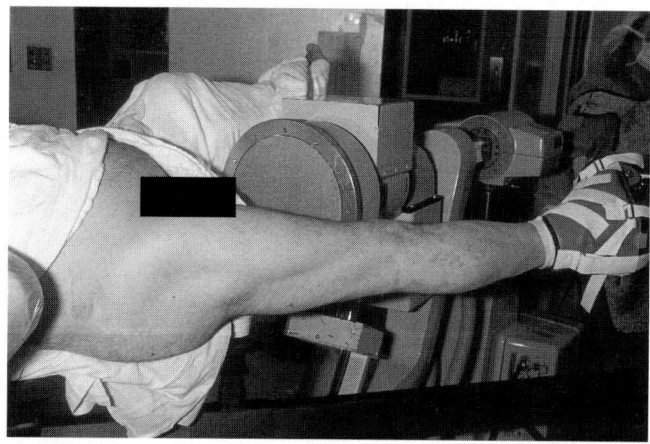

B

Figure 6.33. AP (**A**) and lateral (**B**) positioning of the image intensifier to obtain unobstructed visualization of the proximal femur (**C, D**).

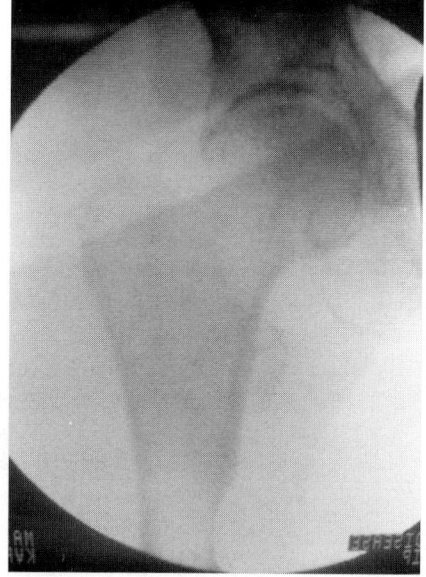

C

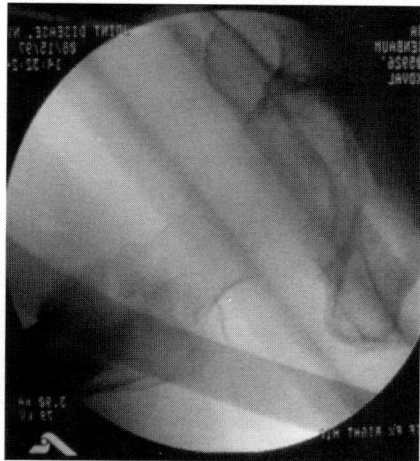

D

Treatment

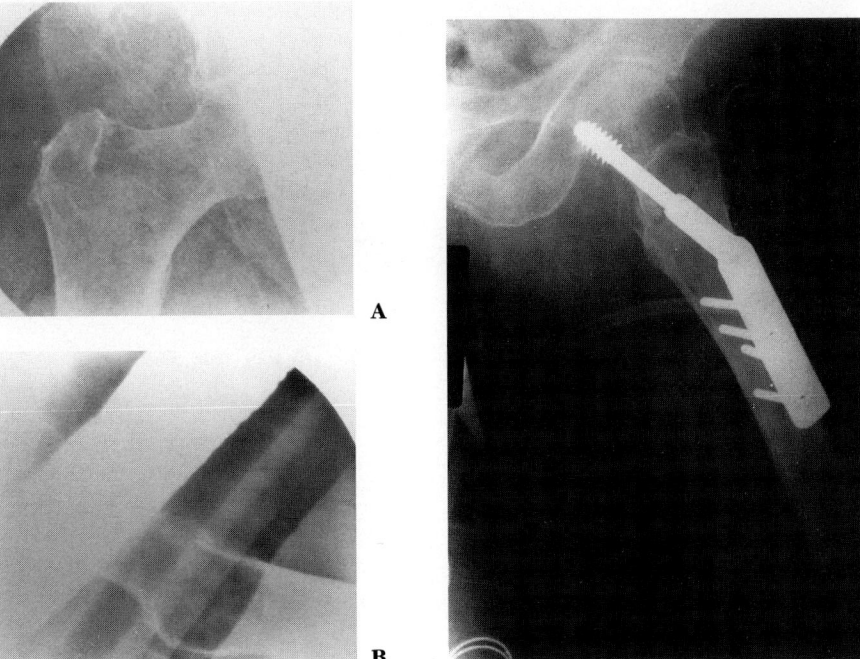

Figure 6.34. Inadequate visualization of the proximal femur (**A, B**) resulted in posterior femoral head penetration by the lag screw (**C**).

sag, or malrotation. Fracture reduction with varus angulation or posterior sag will result in difficulty centering the lag screw in the femoral neck and head (Figure 6.35). Varus angulation can usually be corrected by placing additional traction on the lower extremity to disengage the fracture fragments, followed by a second fracture reduction. Occasionally, one may have to abduct the lower extremity to correct a varus malreduction. If residual varus remains, one should check the position of the fracture fragments on the lateral radiographic view, as posterior sag may prevent adequate fracture reduction. In this situation, traction should be released and the fracture manipulated to disengage

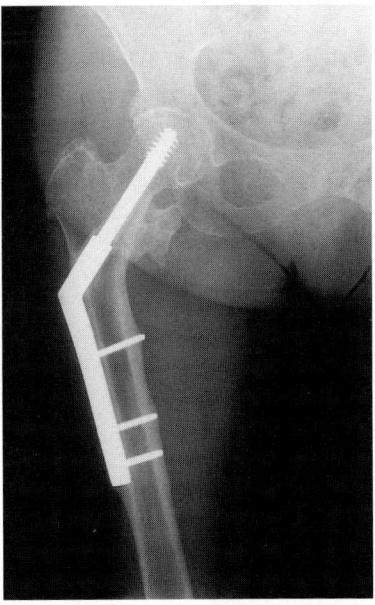

Figure 6.35. Varus fracture reduction resulted in lag screw placement in the inferior femoral neck and superior femoral head.

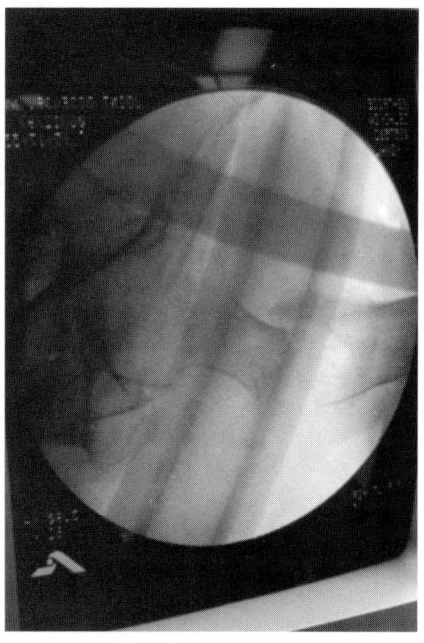 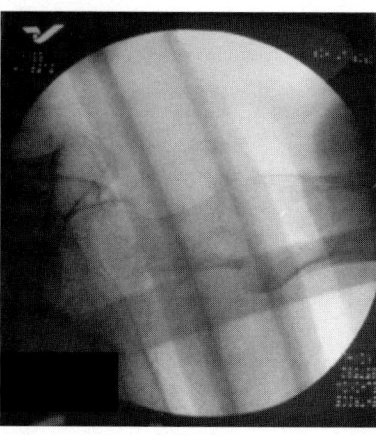 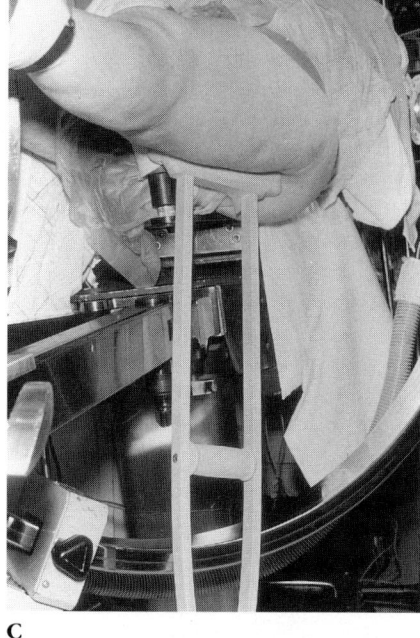

A B C

Figure 6.36. Posterior sag (**A**) can be corrected (**B**) with use of a crutch placed under the proximal thigh (**C**).

the fragments. Posterior sag requires manual correction using a crutch, a bone hook, or a periosteal elevator (Figure 6.36). If unrecognized, posterior sag results in positioning the guide pin in the anterior femoral neck and posterior femoral head. Finally, we rotate the lower extremity under fluoroscopic control to determine whether the fracture fragments move as a single unit. In patients in whom the femoral shaft moves independently from the proximal fragment, excessive internal rotation of the leg is avoided. Instead, the lower extremity is placed in neutral or slight external rotation. Once the fracture is reduced, the patient is prepared and draped; for this purpose we prefer an isolation screen (Figure 6.37).

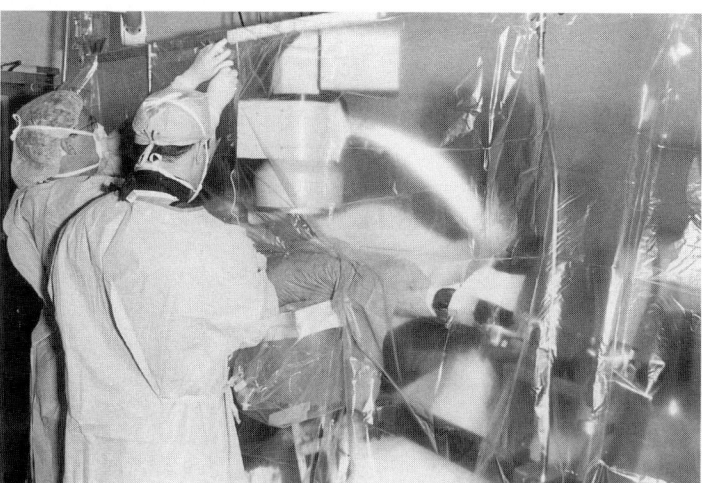

Figure 6.37. Use of an isolation screen.

Stable Fractures

A straight 8- to 10-cm lateral incision is made, starting at the base of the greater trochanter and extending distally (Figure 6.38). The incision is deepened through the subcutaneous tissue, and the iliotibial band is incised in line with its fibers, with care taken to remain posterior to the tensor fasciae latae muscle (Figure 6.39). This exposes the vastus lateralis muscle and its covering fascia (Figure 6.40). Rather than using a muscle-splitting approach through the vastus lateralis muscle, we prefer to incise the fascia of the vastus lateralis and reflect the muscle from the intermuscular septum (Figure 6.41). One should take care to identify and ligate the perforators from the profunda femoris artery (Figure 6.42); otherwise, if cut, they may retract posteriorly through the intermuscular septum, making them difficult to control. The lateral aspect of the proximal femur is cleared of soft tissue using a periosteal elevator, and the vastus lateralis muscle is retracted anteriorly with a Hohmann retractor (Figure 6.43).

Using image intensification, a starting point is identified on the lateral cortex of the proximal femur (Figure 6.44). This is usually at the level of the lesser trochanter, centered between the anterior and posterior cortical margins. A drill hole is made and a guide pin inserted into the femoral neck and head under image intensification using the 135° guide (Figure 6.45). One can place a guide pin anterior to the femoral neck to estimate femoral neck anteversion, although we find this unnecessary. The position of the guide pin is adjusted until it lies in the center of the femoral head and neck on both the AP and lateral planes (Figure 6.46). Peripheral placement in any direction is avoided,

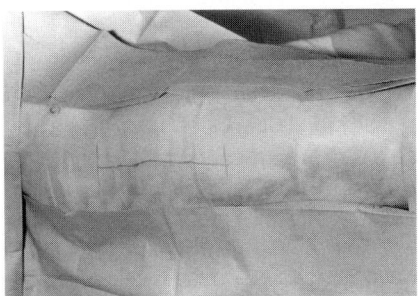

Figure 6.38. A straight 8- to 10-cm lateral incision is made, starting at the base of the greater trochanter.

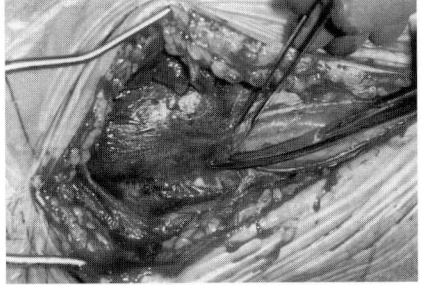

Figure 6.39. The iliotibial band is incised in line with its fibers, with care taken to remain posterior to the tensor fasciae latae muscle.

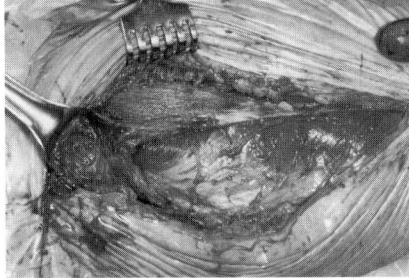

Figure 6.40. Exposure of the vastus lateralis muscle.

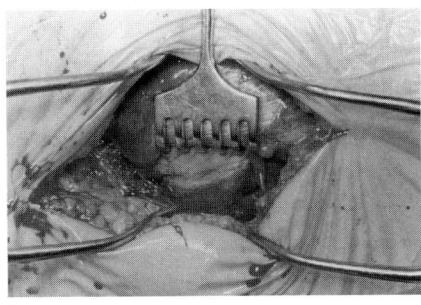

A

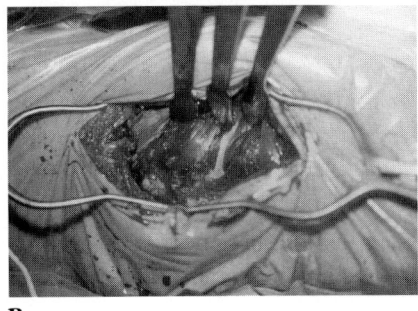

B

Figure 6.41. Anterior retraction of the vastus lateralis muscle (**A**), and exposure of a perforating branch of the profunda femoris artery (**B**).

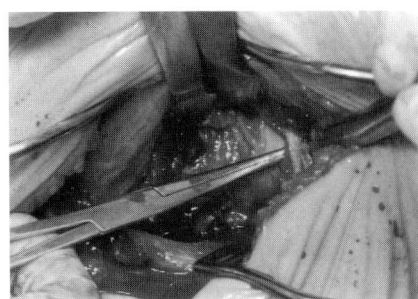

Figure 6.42. Ligation of a perforator from the profunda femoris artery.

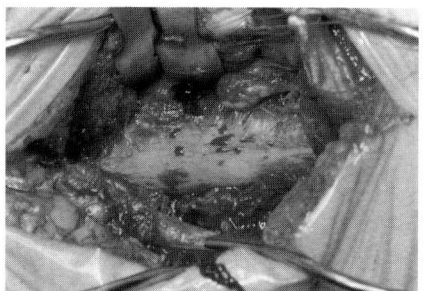

Figure 6.43. Exposure of the lateral aspect of the proximal femur.

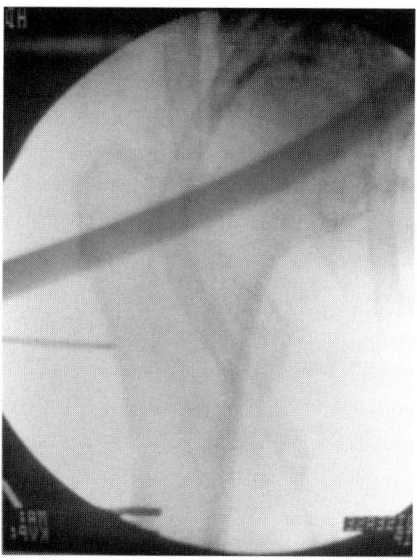

Figure 6.44. Identification of the starting point on the lateral cortex of the proximal femur at the level of the lesser trochanter.

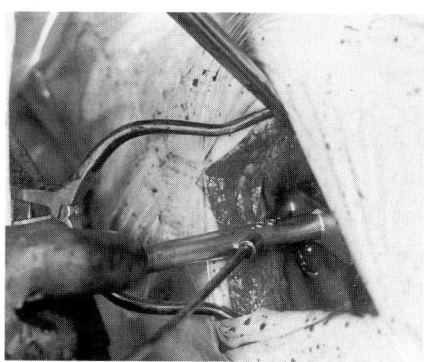

Figure 6.45. Use of the 135° guide to insert a guide pin into the femoral neck and head.

because only with the pin directed centrally in both views can the screw be safely advanced to within 5 to 10 mm of the joint line without risking joint penetration. Central and deep placement allows screw purchase in the best bone available as well as allowing maximal collapse of the screw before its threads engage the plate barrel. If the guide pin cannot be positioned appropriately in the femoral head and neck, the fracture reduction and plate angle should be reassessed, particularly for residual varus and posterior sag. Occasionally, a 130° or 140° plate is needed to optimize lag screw position.

Baumgaertner et al. devised the concept of tip–apex distance (TAD) to determine lag screw position within the femoral head.[50] This measurement,

Figure 6.46. The position of the guide pin is adjusted until it lies in the center of the femoral head and neck on both the AP (**A**) and lateral (**B**) planes.

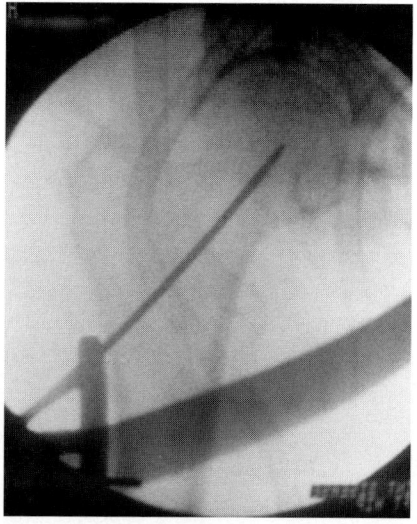

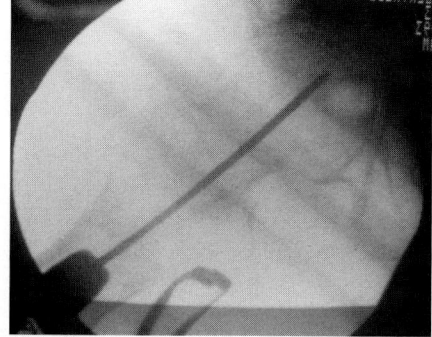

expressed in millimeters, is the sum of the distances from the tip of the lag screw to the apex of the femoral head on both the AP and lateral radiographic views (after controlling for radiographic magnification) (Figure 6.47). Peripheral malpositioning of the lag screw is not differentiated from shallow lag screw positioning; only the actual distance from the tip of the lag screw to the apex of the femoral head is considered.

Baumgaertner et al. demonstrated the utility of utilizing the TAD in a series of 198 intertrochanteric fractures[50]; 16 fractures (8%) had loss of fixation secondary to lag screw cutout of the femoral head. Regardless of patient age, fracture stability, quality of fracture reduction, or type or angle of implant used, no lag screw cutout occurred when the TAD was 27 mm or less. Conversely, the rate of lag screw cutout increased to 60% when the TAD was greater than 45 mm. Using multivariate logistic regression statistical techniques, Baumgaertner et al. demonstrated that screw position as measured by the TAD was the strongest (though not the only) independent predictor of lag screw cutout. (Unstable fractures and increasing patient age were also predictive of lag screw cutout.) It was therefore recommended that if guide pin location yields a TAD greater than 25 mm, the surgeon should reassess the fracture reduction and reposition the guide pin.

A subsequent study by Baumgaertner and Solberg assessed the impact of the TAD on the management of intertrochanteric fractures in a single hospital setting.[51] These authors compared 198 fractures treated before the application of the TAD method to 118 fractures treated after its adoption by a group of surgeons. The TAD significantly decreased from a mean of 25 mm in the early group to 20 mm in the study group. Concurrently, the proportion of mechanical failures by lag screw cutout decreased from 8% to 0%.

When the guide pin is confirmed to be in the desired position, it is advanced to the level of the subchondral bone and the length of the lag screw is determined (Figure 6.48). In stable intertrochanteric fractures, significant fracture impaction is not anticipated, and therefore a screw length is chosen that maximizes screw-barrel engagement, allows for about 5 mm of impaction, and lies within 1 cm of the subchondral bone. For example, if the guide pin measures 100 mm to the subchondral bone, a 90-mm lag screw might be selected; once fully seated 5 mm from the subchondral bone, the lag screw would be inset 5 mm into the plate barrel.

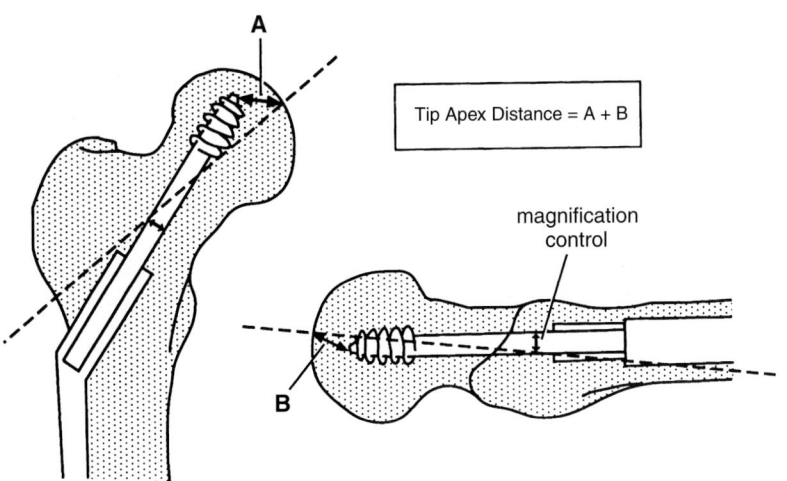

Figure 6.47. The tip-apex distance (TAD) is the sum of the distances from the tip of the lag screw to the apex of the femoral head on both the AP and lateral radiographic views (after controlling for radiographic magnification). From Baumgaertner et al.[50]

Figure 6.48. Use of the cannulated depth gauge to determine the length of the lag screw.

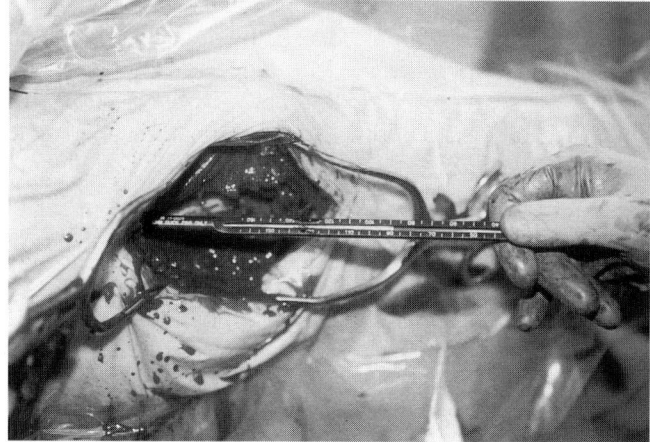

Reaming of the femoral neck and head over the guide pin is performed under image intensification to the desired final position of the lag screw (Figure 6.49). The position of the guide pin during reaming must be monitored to detect possible binding of the guide pin within the reamer, which might result in advancement of the guide pin and penetration of the femoral head (Figure 6.50). The position of the guide pin may be lost during reamer removal; one can replace the guide pin either by using a guide pin repositioner available in many sliding hip screw sets (Figure 6.51) or by inserting a free lag screw backwards into the reaming channel. We believe that the reamed tract should be tapped, even in elderly patients, to prevent femoral head rotation during lag screw insertion. The lag screw is then inserted to within 1 cm of the subchondral bone (Figure 6.52).

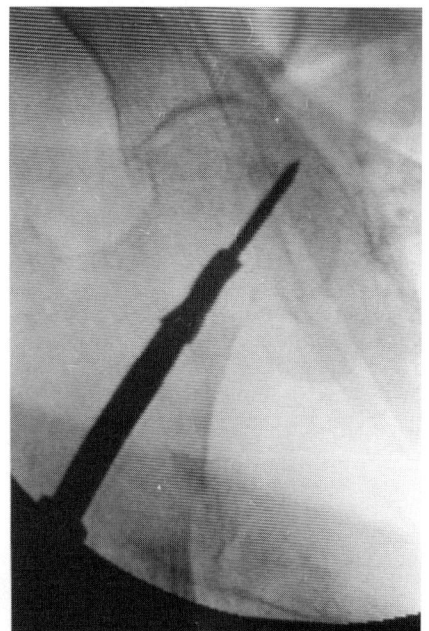

Figure 6.49. Reaming of the femoral neck and head over the guide pin is performed under image intensification to the desired final position of the lag screw.

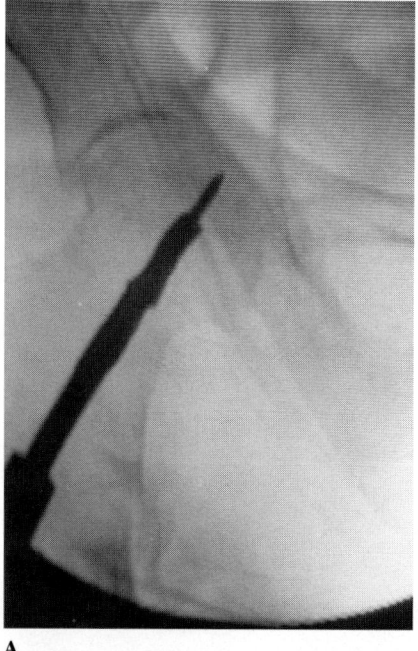

A

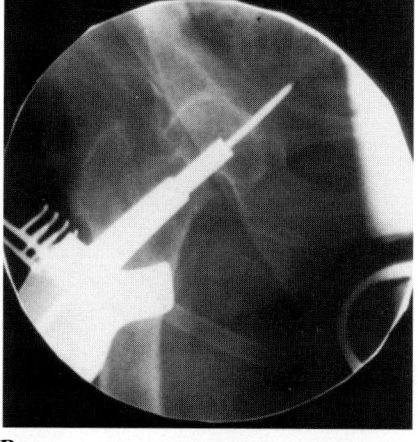

B

Figure 6.50. The position of the guide pin during reaming must be monitored (**A**) to detect possible binding of the guide pin within the reamer, which might result in guide pin advancement and femoral head penetration (**B**).

Treatment

Figure 6.51. Use of a guide pin repositioner (**A, B**) to replace the guide pin that was lost during reamer removal.

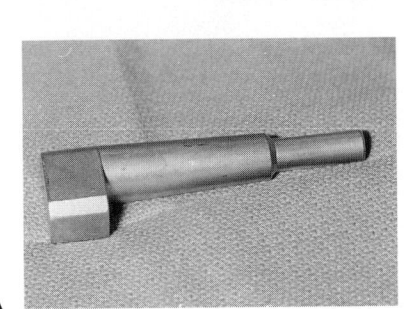
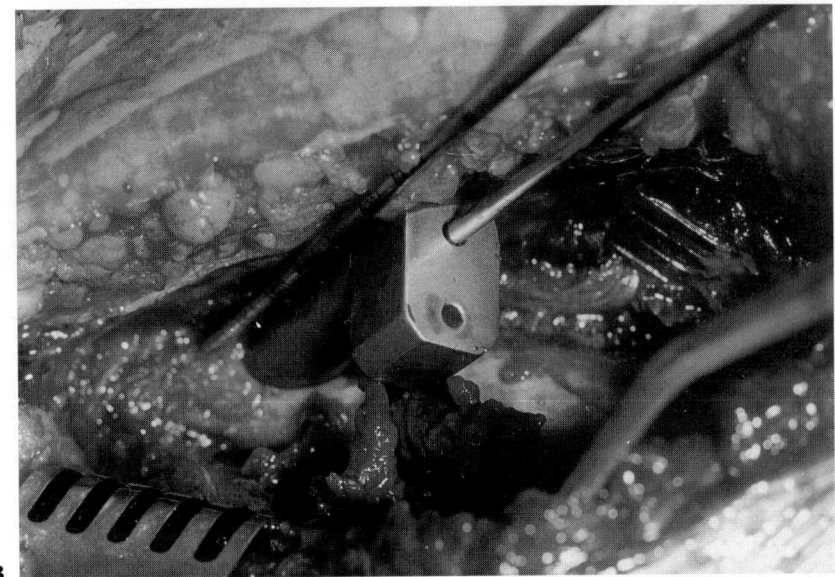

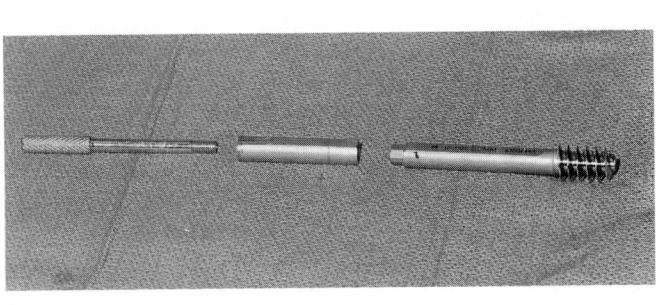
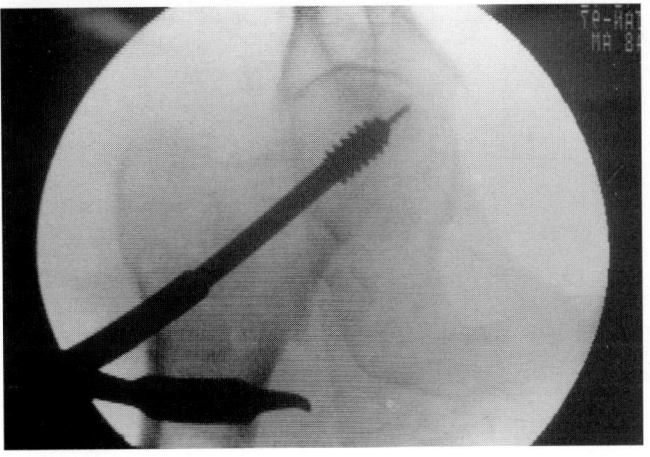

Figure 6.52. Assembly (**A**) and insertion (**B**) of the lag screw.

When the proper position of the lag screw within the femoral head is confirmed, a three- or four-hole 135° sideplate is placed over the screw (Figure 6.53). We routinely use a three-hole plate for fixation of both stable and unstable intertrochanteric fractures and have not encountered mechanical failure secondary to loss of plate fixation from the lateral femur. Biomechanical studies have demonstrated no added benefit of a fourth holding screw for sideplate stabilization in stable and unstable intertrochanteric fracture models.[52,53]

We prefer to use a "keyed" sliding hip screw system (Figure 6.54). In a keyed system, the lag screw is captured within the plate barrel such that the screw can slide along the barrel but cannot rotate. This mechanism theoretically maximizes the rotational stability of the femoral head and neck compared to a nonkeyed system in which the lag screw can rotate within the plate barrel. Use of a keyed sliding hip screw system, however, requires that the lag screw be oriented so that the plate can be properly positioned along the femoral shaft.

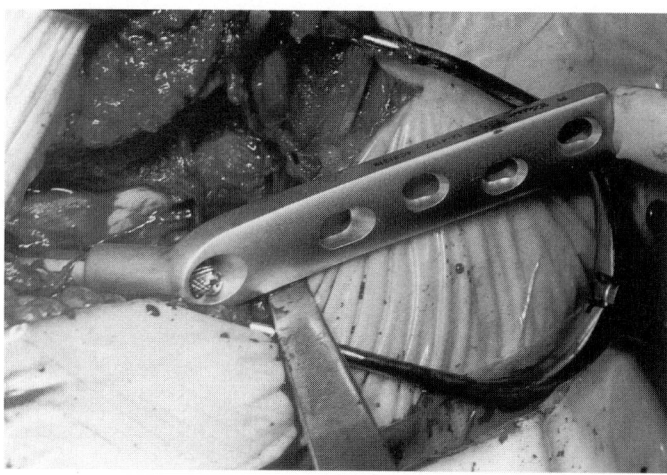

Figure 6.53. Insertion of the sideplate over the lag screw.

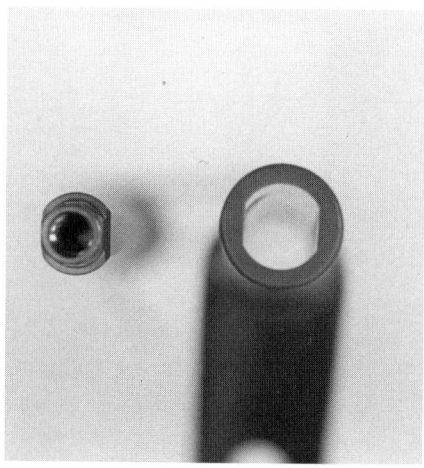

Figure 6.54. In a keyed lag screw system, the lag screw is captured within the plate barrel such that the screw can slide along the barrel but cannot rotate.

A standard (long-barrel) plate is used for most intertrochanteric fractures (Figure 6.55). The longer barrel maximizes the amount of screw-barrel engagement and minimizes the likelihood of the lag screw "jamming" within the plate barrel. However, a short-barrel plate is used if a lag screw shorter than 85 mm has been inserted. This helps to prevent postoperative impaction that exceeds the sliding capacity of the device. If screw sliding brings the screw threads into contact with the plate barrel, additional impaction will not be possible and the device becomes the biomechanical equivalent of a rigid nail plate.

The minimum amount of available screw-barrel slide necessary to reduce the risk of fixation failure with use of a sliding hip screw has been estimated to be 10 mm. Gundle et al. reported on a prospective series of 100 consecutive patients who had sustained an unstable intertrochanteric fracture that was stabilized using a sliding hip screw.[54] In fractures stabilized with less than 10 mm of available slide, the risk of fixation failure was more than three times greater than in fractures with at least 10 mm of available slide. Based on the

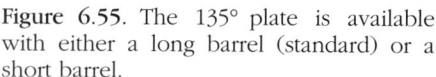

Figure 6.55. The 135° plate is available with either a long barrel (standard) or a short barrel.

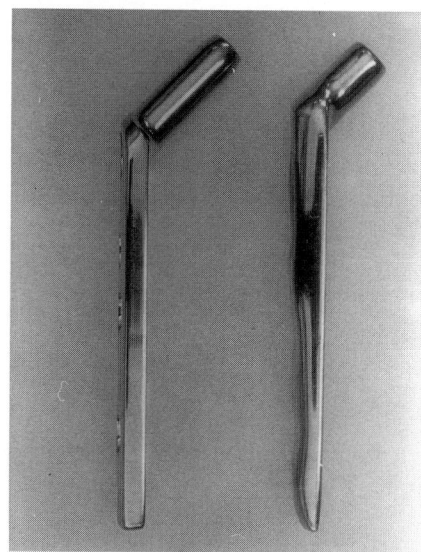

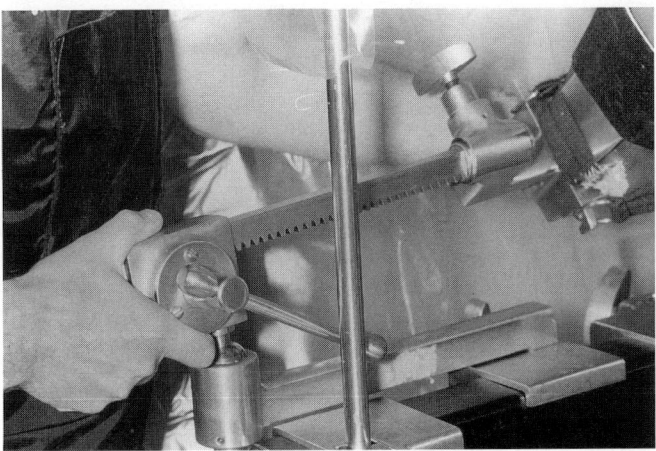

Figure 6.56. With the plate loosely clamped to the femur, the fracture is impacted by releasing the traction on the extremity and gently displacing the femoral shaft toward the proximal fragment.

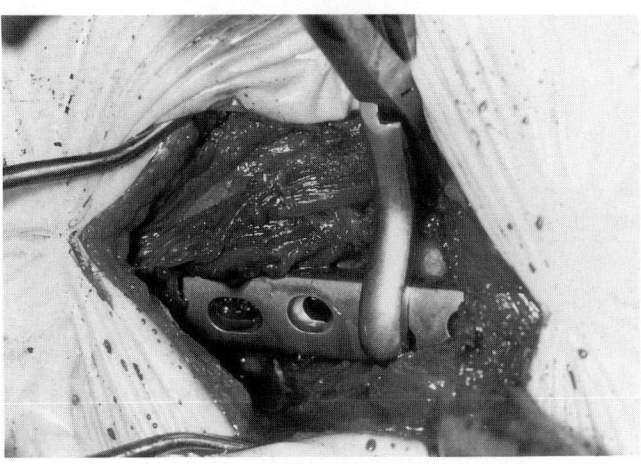

Figure 6.57. The plate clamp is tightened and the fracture position reassessed.

specifications for the particular lag screw and sideplate used in this study (DHS, Synthes, Paoli, PA), Gundle advocated use of a short-barrel sideplate when using lag screws of 85 mm or less.

The plate is loosely clamped to the femoral shaft and the fracture is impacted by releasing the traction on the extremity and gently displacing the femoral shaft toward the proximal fragment (Figure 6.56). The plate clamp is then tightened (Figure 6.57) and the fracture position is reassessed. This impaction maneuver enhances fracture stability and helps prevent fracture distraction that might result in excessive postoperative screw-barrel slide. The plate-holding screws are then inserted (Figure 6.58). The need for a compression screw is determined by direct visualization of the lag screw within the plate barrel (Figure 6.59); a compression screw is inserted if there is risk of postoperative screw-barrel disengagement. The compression screw is not used to achieve fracture impaction. A compression screw is not used routinely because (1) it is an added expense and (2) the compression screw often loosens (even during uneventful fracture healing) and can become a source of lateral thigh pain (Figure 6.60). The wound is closed in layers over suction drains (Figure 6.61).

Unstable Fractures

The most frequently encountered unstable intertrochanteric fractures are characterized by loss of the posteromedial buttress[7] (Figure 6.62). Another type of unstable intertrochanteric fracture is the reverse obliquity pattern, which begins just proximal to the lesser trochanter and extends laterally and distally with an oblique orientation (Figure 6.63).

The general treatment approach for fractures with posteromedial comminution is similar to that described for stable fracture patterns in the preceding section: anatomic fracture alignment followed by internal fixation using a sliding hip screw. In older patients, the posteromedial fragment is usually ignored. In younger patients, an attempt should be made to stabilize large posteromedial fragments in a nearly anatomic position to prevent excessive screw-barrel slide, which would result in limb shortening (Figure 6.64).

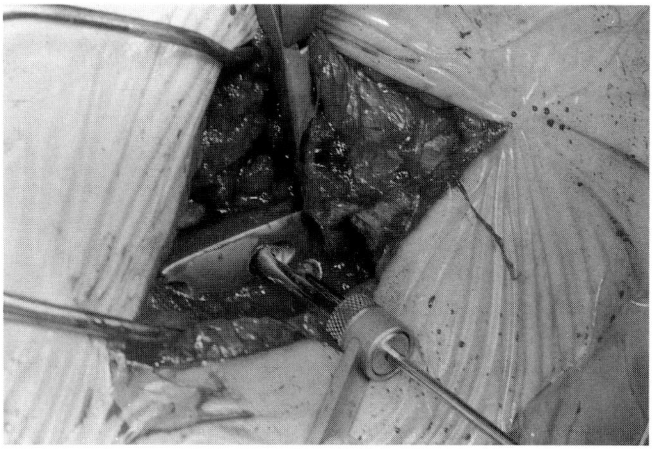

Figure 6.58. Placement of the plate-holding screws (**A–C**).

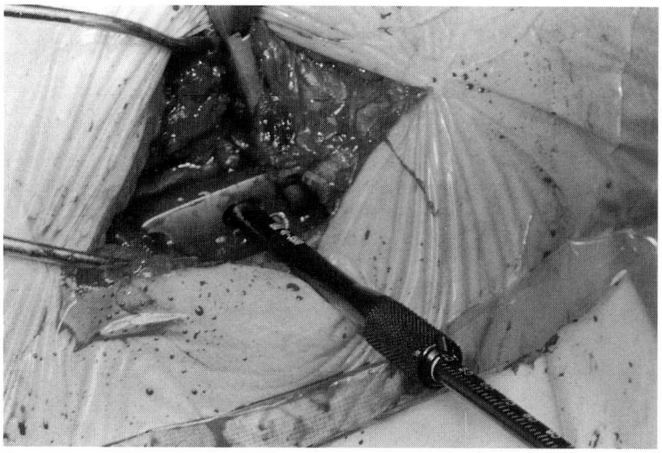

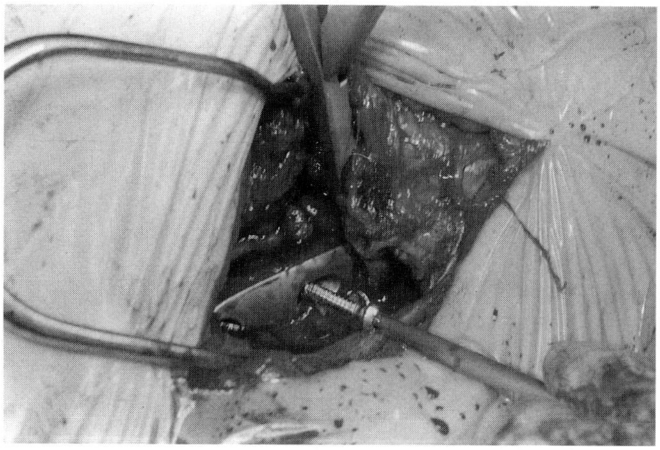

Figure 6.59. Direct visualization of the lag screw within the plate barrel (**A**) indicates that there is no need for use of a compression screw (**B**).

Furthermore, axial loading studies of unstable fractures have confirmed that reduction and fixation of the posteromedial fragment becomes progressively more important with increasing fragment size.[55] According to a study by Apel and colleagues, anatomic reduction of a large posteromedial fragment increased load resistance by 57% compared with identical fractures with the

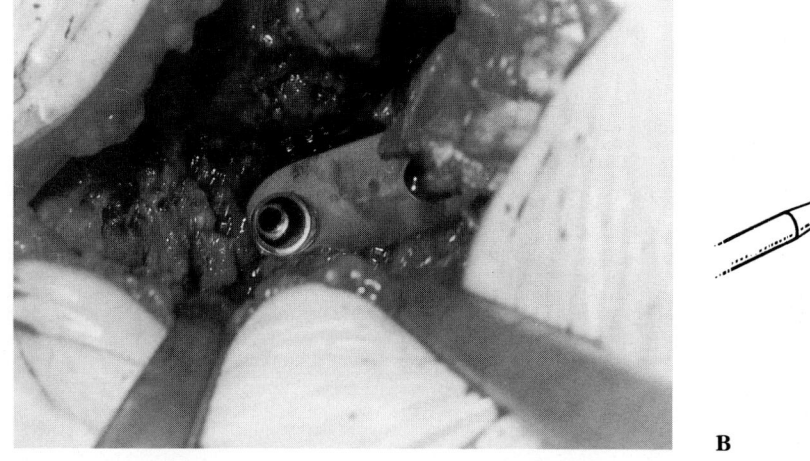
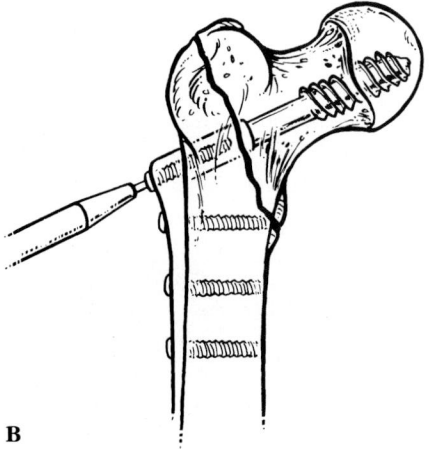

Treatment

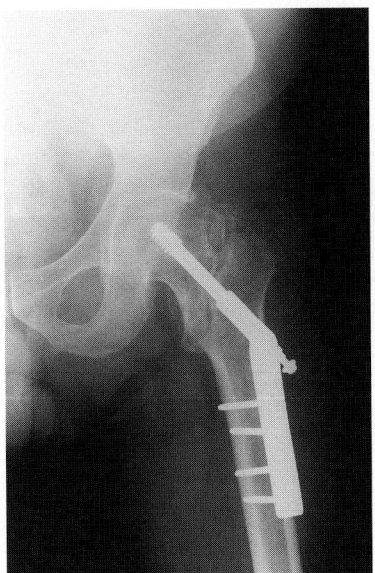

Figure 6.60. Radiograph demonstrating loosening and prominence of the compression screw.

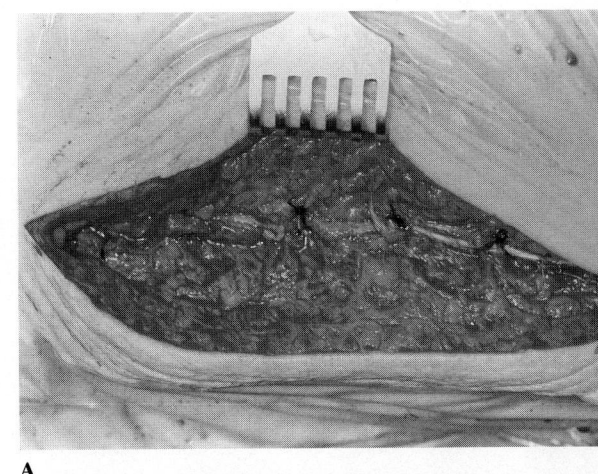

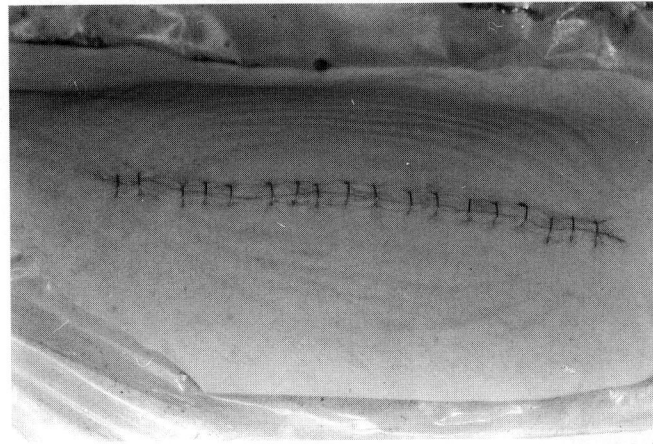

Figure 6.61. Wound closure (**A, B**).

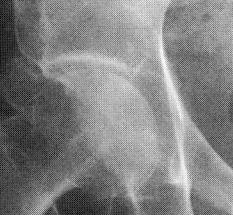

Figure 6.62. Unstable intertrochanteric fracture characterized by loss of the posteromedial buttress.

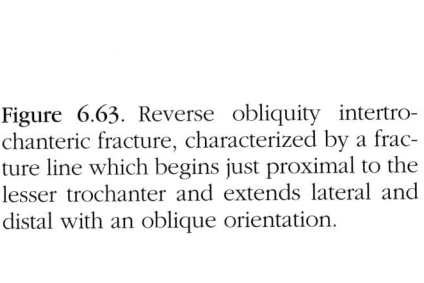

Figure 6.63. Reverse obliquity intertrochanteric fracture, characterized by a fracture line which begins just proximal to the lesser trochanter and extends lateral and distal with an oblique orientation.

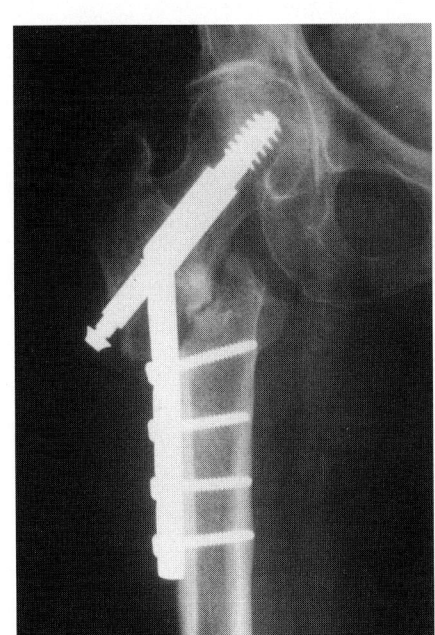

Figure 6.64. Fixation of the posteromedial fragment using a lag screw helped to prevent excessive screw-barrel slide.

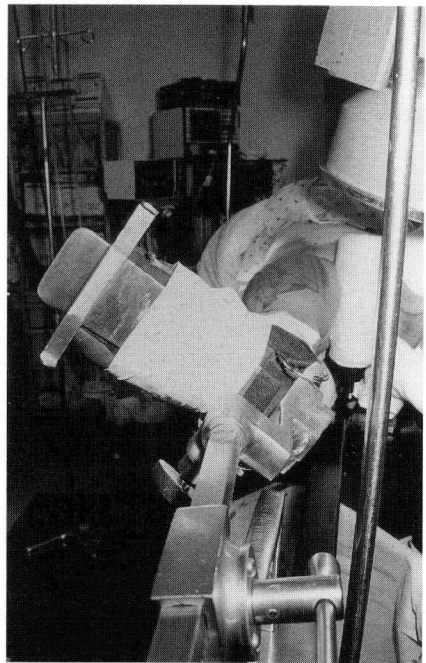

Figure 6.65. To mobilize and reduce the posteromedial fragment, there should be no traction on the lower extremity; the extremity is externally rotated to expose the posteromedial area of the femoral shaft.

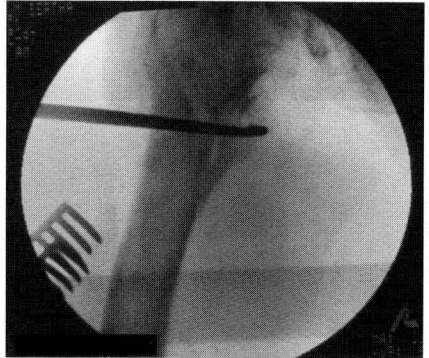

Figure 6.66. Reduction of the posteromedial fragment using a bone hook.

fragment excluded.[55] Fixation of a small posteromedial fragment increased stability by only 17%.

Reduction and stabilization of the posteromedial fragment can be performed either before or after lag screw and sideplate application. We prefer the former, as this method facilitates anatomic fracture reduction of the posteromedial fragment. If the main fracture fragments are reduced and stabilized primarily, it may be impossible to reduce the posteromedial fragment anatomically.

To mobilize and reduce the posteromedial fragment, there should be no traction on the lower extremity; since the iliopsoas is attached to the lesser trochanter, traction results in proximal migration of the posteromedial fragment. The extremity is externally rotated to better expose the posteromedial area of the femoral shaft (Figure 6.65). The posteromedial fragment can be reduced using a bone hook (Figure 6.66) and can be provisionally stabilized using a Verbrugge or standard reduction clamp. Definitive fracture fixation involves use of either one or more cerclage wires or one or more lag screws directed from anterolateral to posteromedial (Figure 6.67). These screws cannot be inserted through the proximal hole of the plate. Proper angulation cannot be achieved because of the limitations of the screw hole and its position distal to the involved area. Once the posteromedial fragment is stabilized, traction is placed on the lower extremity and the head and neck fragment reduced. The sliding hip screw is then inserted as previously described (Figure 6.68).

We have developed an auxiliary buttress plate to facilitate fixation of the posteromedial fragment after application of the sliding hip screw (Figure 6.69). This plate is attached to the proximal screw hole of any standard sliding hip screw sideplate. It has two superior extensions, each providing two additional screw holes (anterior and posterior), permitting insertion of 3.5- or 4.0-mm screws for fixation of the posteromedial fragment. These extensions are malleable for adjustment and their holes can accommodate up to 30° angulation of the supplemental fixation screws.

After insertion of the sliding screw, the buttress plate is attached to the sliding hip screw sideplate with a screw placed through the buttress plate and the most proximal screw hole in the sideplate. The posteromedial fragment is reduced and provisionally stabilized with either a cerclage wire or a bone

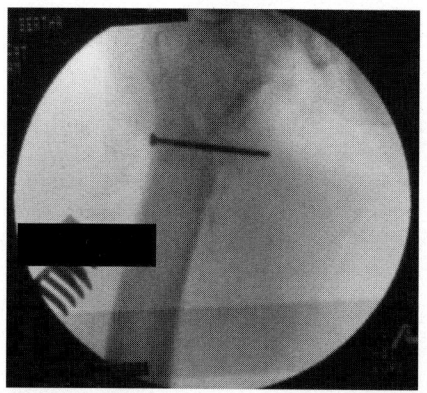 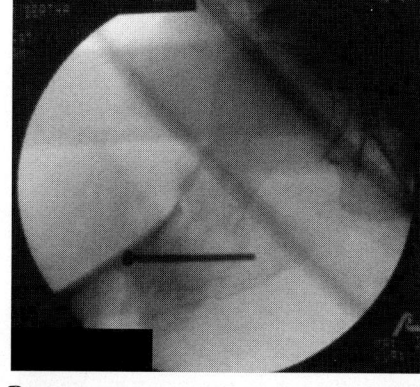

A **B**

Figure 6.67. Use of a lag screw directed from anterolateral to posteromedial to stabilize the posteromedial fragment (**A, B**); alternatively, one or more cerclage wires can be used for fixation of the posteromedial fragment.

Treatment

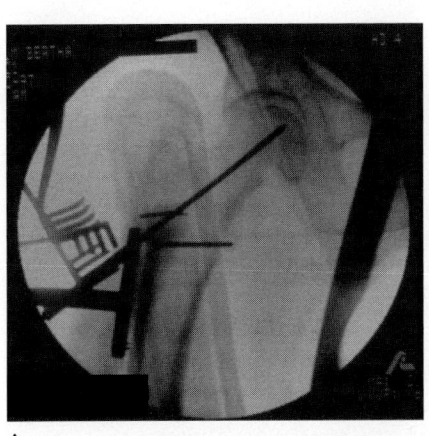
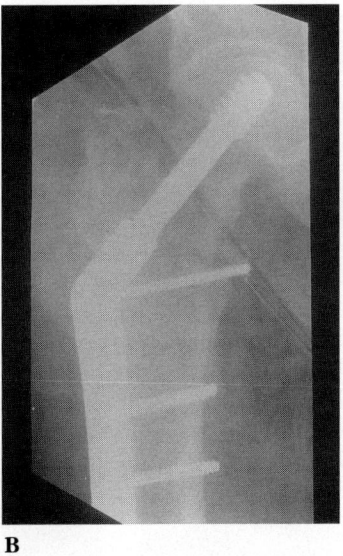
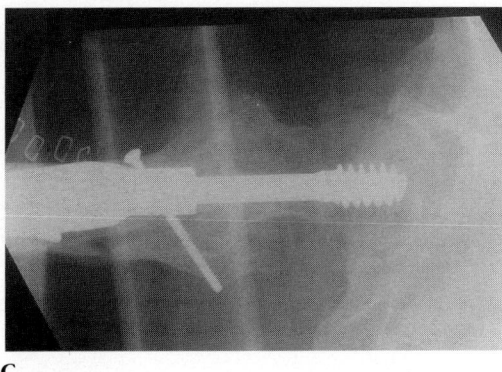

A B C

Figure 6.68. Once the posteromedial fragment is stabilized, traction is placed on the lower extremity, and the head and neck fragment reduced. The sliding hip screw is inserted using standard technique (**A–C**).

clamp. One or two lag screws are then inserted through the anterior holes in the plate extension to definitively stabilize the posteromedial fragment (Figure 6.70).

This buttress plate has been used on 12 patients. All patients were able to have the medial fragment reduced and stabilized using the buttress plate, typically with two lag screws. In the 8 patients available for follow-up, all fractures united without loss of reduction of the posteromedial fragment.

Medoff Plate

The Medoff plate utilizes a lag screw (from the standard sliding hip screw set) to allow compression along the axis of the femoral neck. In place of the standard femoral sideplate, however, it utilizes a coupled pair of sliding components that enable the fracture to impact parallel to the longitudinal axis of the femur (Figure 6.71). A locking set screw may be used to prevent independent sliding of the lag screw within the plate barrel; if the locking set screw is applied, the plate can only slide axially on the femoral shaft (uniaxial dynamization) (Figure 6.72). If, however, the surgeon applies the implant without placement of the locking set screw, sliding may occur along both the femoral neck and the femoral shaft (biaxial dynamization). For most intertrochanteric fractures, biaxial dynamization is suggested.[56]

The design of the sliding plate requires consideration of certain factors before application. If the fracture line is distal to the entry hole of the lag screw (as in a pure subtrochanteric fracture), no modification of the lateral femoral cortex is required. If, however, the fracture is proximal, through, or just distal to the lag screw entry site (as in a typical intertrochanteric fracture), it is necessary to distally enlarge the lag screw entry site by approximately 2.5 cm to prevent the sideplate barrel from impinging on the lateral cortex of the distal fragment and obstructing dynamic axial compression[13,56–59] (Figure 6.73).

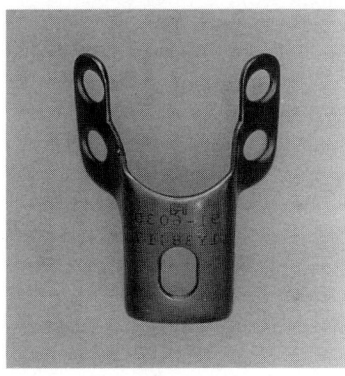

Figure 6.69. The buttress plate developed by the authors to facilitate stabilization of the posteromedial fragment after application of the sliding hip screw.

Figure 6.70. AP (**A**) and lateral (**B**) radiographs demonstrating use of the buttress plate for stabilization of an unstable intertrochanteric fracture.

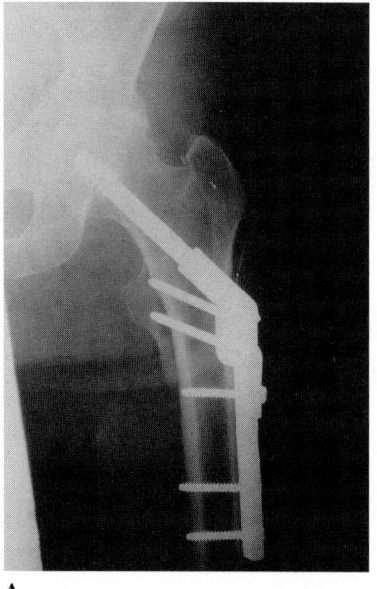
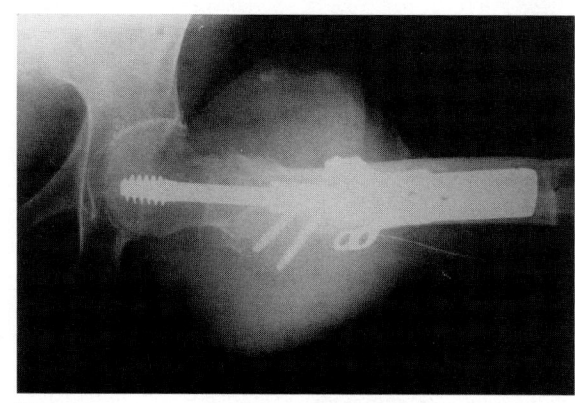

Figure 6.71. The six-hole and four-hole Medoff plates (**A**). AP radiograph demonstrating use of the Medoff plate to stabilize an unstable intertrochanteric fracture (**B**).

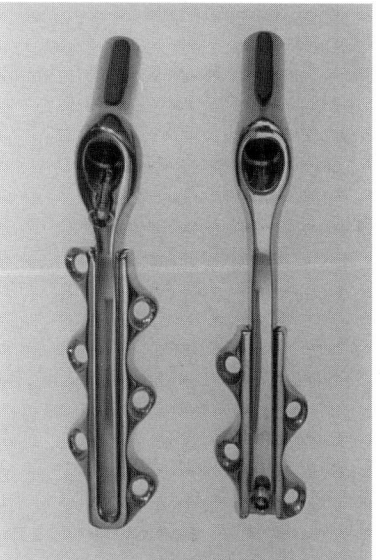
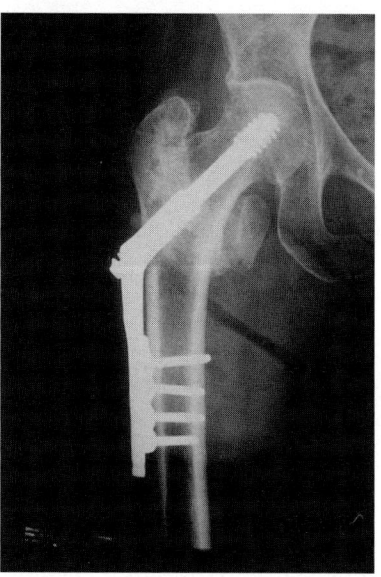

Figure 6.72. A locking set screw may be used to prevent independent sliding of the lag screw within the plate barrel (**A**); if the locking set screw is applied, the plate can only slide axially on the femoral shaft (uniaxial dynamization) (**B**). However, if the surgeon applies the implant without placement of the locking set screw, sliding may occur along both the femoral neck and the femoral shaft (biaxial dynamization) (**C**).

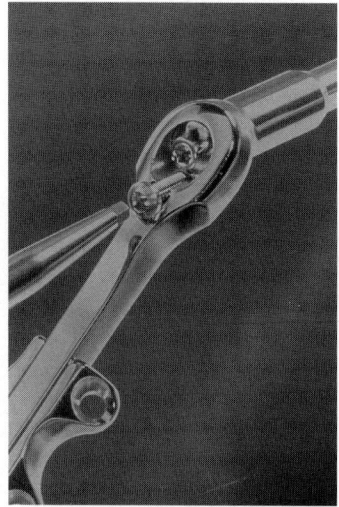
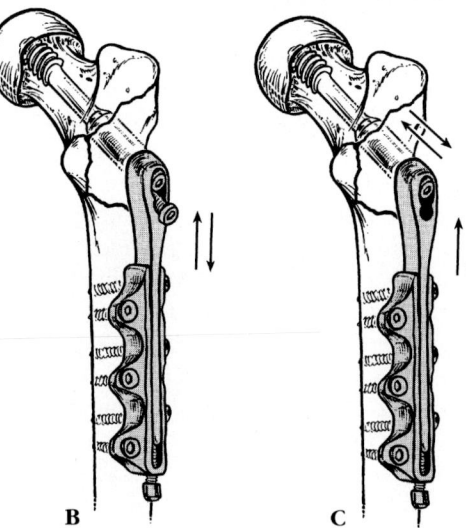

Treatment

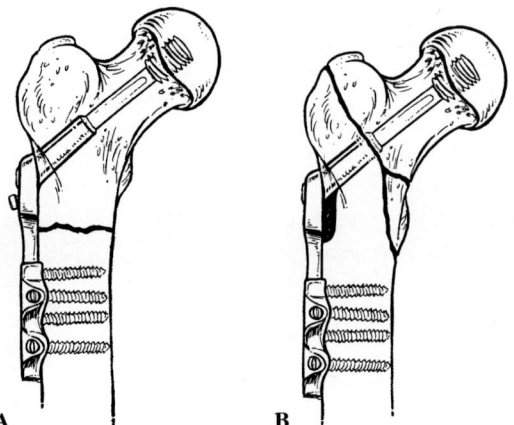

Figure 6.73. If the fracture line is distal to the entry hole of the lag screw (i.e., pure subtrochanteric fracture), no modification of the lateral cortex is required (**A**). If, however, the fracture line extends into the intertrochanteric region, it is necessary to enlarge the distal aspect of the lag screw entry hole by approximately 2.5 cm to prevent the sideplate barrel from impinging on the lateral cortex of the distal fragment and obstructing dynamic axial slide (**B**).

Operative Technique for Insertion of the Medoff Plate

Insertion of the Medoff plate is similar to that of a standard sliding hip screw. After fracture reduction, a standard lag screw guide pin is inserted into the center of the femoral head and neck (Figure 6.74). The Medoff plate is currently available with only a 135° angle, so the proper angle guide should be used for guide pin insertion. The length of the lag screw is determined and the proximal femur is reamed and tapped (Figure 6.75). If the site of entry for the reamer in the lateral cortex enters the distal fragment, as is usual with intertrochanteric fractures, the barrel of the sideplate will contact the lateral cortex of the distal fragment and prevent axial sliding. In this circumstance, the entry hole should be slotted to allow the sideplate to slide axially. The hole can be slotted by placing a second unicortical guide pin through the lateral cortex approximately 1 cm distal to the distal extent of the reamed hole (Figure 6.76). The reamer is then collapsed to its lowest limit, and a second hole is reamed more distally in the lateral cortex (Figure 6.77). A rongeur or burr is used to smooth out the connection between the holes into a slot (Figure 6.78). Alternatively, the slot may be made entirely with a rongeur or burr, by removing bone from the lateral cortex distal to the initial reamed hole. Because this distal extension (slot) must be wide enough to allow unimpeded axial plate

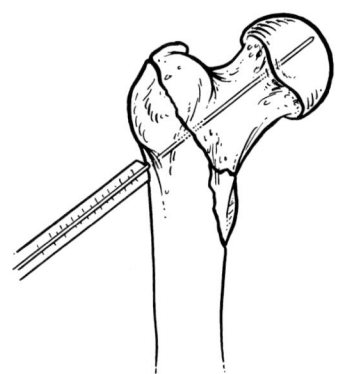

Figure 6.74. After insertion of the lag screw guide pin into the center of the femoral head and neck, the length of the lag screw is measured.

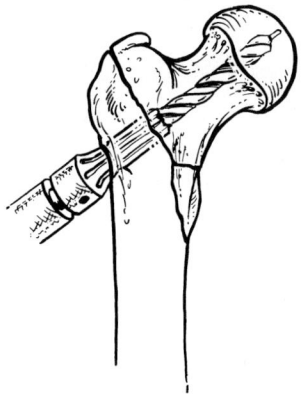

Figure 6.75. Reaming of the proximal femur over the guide pin.

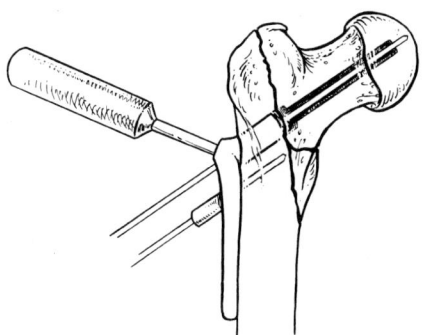

Figure 6.76. Creation of the slotted hole by placing a second unicortical guide pin through the lateral cortex approximately 1 cm distal to the distal extend of the reamed hole.

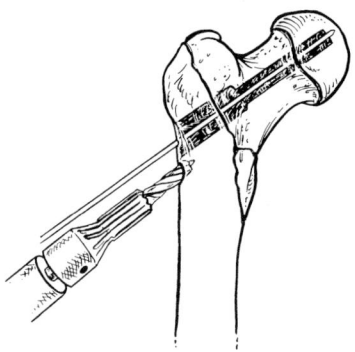

Figure 6.77. The reamer is collapsed to its lowest limit, and a second hole is reamed more distally in the lateral cortex.

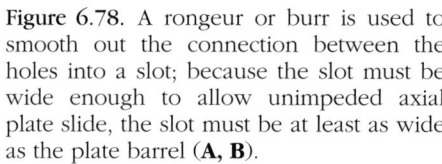

Figure 6.78. A rongeur or burr is used to smooth out the connection between the holes into a slot; because the slot must be wide enough to allow unimpeded axial plate slide, the slot must be at least as wide as the plate barrel (**A, B**).

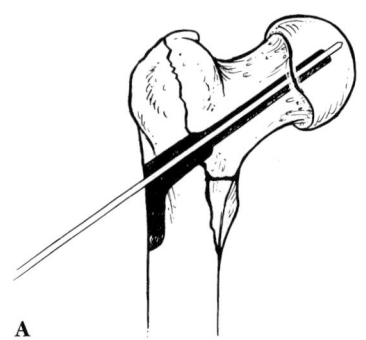

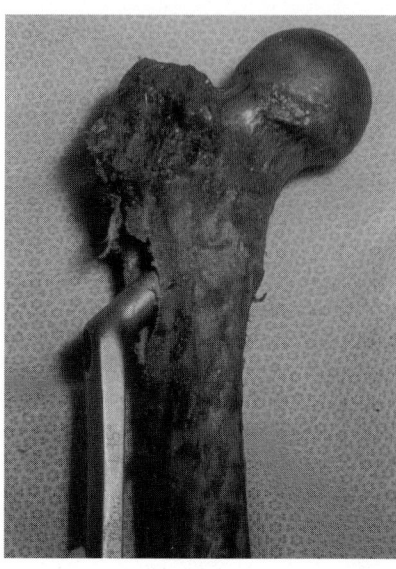

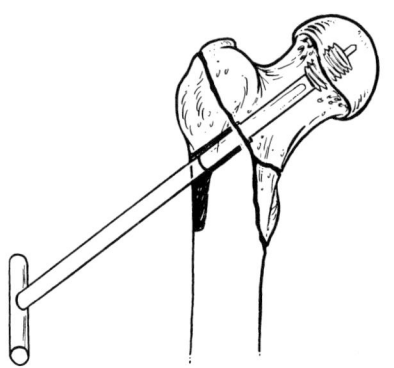

Figure 6.79. Insertion of the lag screw.

slide, the slot must be at least as wide as the plate barrel. The lag screw is then inserted (Figure 6.79). The Medoff sideplate is adjusted so that 1.5 to 2.0 cm of plate slide is available; it is then inserted over the lag screw (Figure 6.80). Sideplates are available in two lengths, having four and six holes; the four-hole plate is used for intertrochanteric fractures and the six-hole plate is used for subtrochanteric fractures. The plate is curved slightly to fit around the femoral shaft. The screw holes are designed to direct the anterior and posterior plate-holding screws to converge at a 30° angle (Figure 6.81). Because of this arrangement, securing the plate to the femoral shaft is facilitated by first inserting the anterior screws and then internally rotating the lower extremity and inserting the posterior screws (Figure 6.82). One should not attempt to angle the holding screws greater than 15° to 30° from the horizontal; otherwise, the screws will not fully seat within the plate. The fracture is manually

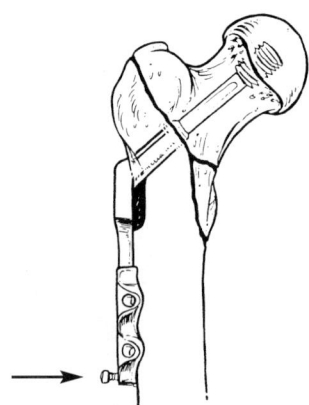

Figure 6.80. The Medoff sideplate is adjusted so that 1.5 to 2.0 cm of plate slide is available; it is then inserted over the lag screw. Note the screw that can be used to hold the two plate components together during insertion (arrow); this screw is removed after placement of the plate-holding screws.

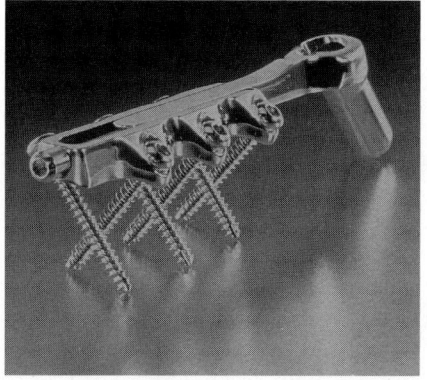

Figure 6.81. The screw holes are designed to direct the anterior and posterior plate-holding screws to converge at a 30° angle.

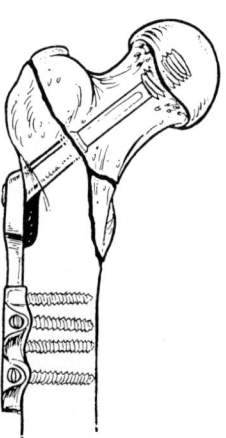

Figure 6.82. Insertion of the plate-holding screws.

impacted after releasing traction from the fracture table. Although it is possible to insert a set screw to prevent screw-barrel slide along the femoral neck and permit only axial slide along the femoral shaft (unixial slide) (Figure 6.83), this configuration is not recommended for most intertrochanteric fractures.[56]

Intramedullary Hip Screw

An intramedullary hip screw is a sliding hip screw coupled to a locked intramedullary nail. Two such devices are currently available: the Gamma nail (Howmedica, Rutherford, NJ) and the Intramedullary Hip Screw (IMHS) (Smith+Nephew, Memphis, TN). Both devices offer the theoretical mechanical advantage of decreasing implant bending strain by moving the shaft fixation from the lateral cortex to the intramedullary canal, thereby decreasing the lever arm on the implant. Both devices also offer the biological advantage of a potentially closed technique with periosteal disruption limited to that caused by the fracture itself. Each features a slight proximal valgus bend to allow device insertion through the tip of the greater trochanter. Both devices are short intramedullary nails without a sagittal bow, so they can be used on either the left or the right side. Finally, both nails have bowed left and right "long-stem" versions, although distal interlocking using these nails requires a freehand technique.

The Gamma nail has a 12-mm lag screw with a grooved shank that articulates with an intramedullary nail. A set screw prevents rotation of the lag screw but allows it to back out through the nail, similar to the design of the Zickel nail. The Gamma nail is available in several angles and widths; the distal interlocking screws are 6 mm in diameter. The Smith+Nephew IMHS uses a 12.7-mm lag screw from the sliding hip screw set, which articulates with a keyed "sleeve" of similar proportion to the barrel of a sliding hip screw sideplate; this sleeve is placed through the intramedullary nail and is locked to the nail with a set screw (Figure 6.84). The screw can slide but cannot rotate within the sleeve; a compression screw is available to facilitate fracture impaction and prevent implant disassembly. The 4.5-mm distal interlocking screws are the same as those used with the sliding hip screw system to stabilize the sideplate.

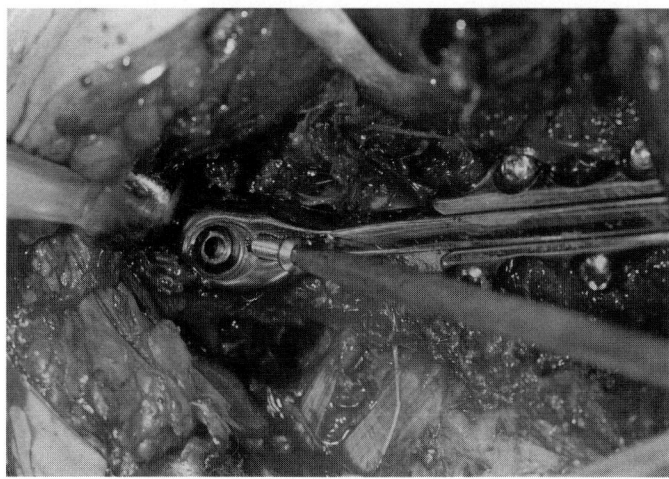

Figure 6.83. Use of a set screw to prevent screw-barrel slide along the femoral neck and permit only axial slide along the femoral shaft (unixial slide).

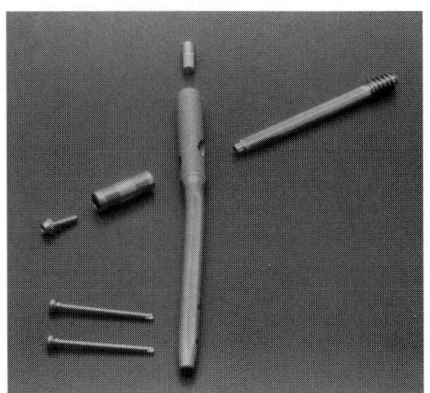
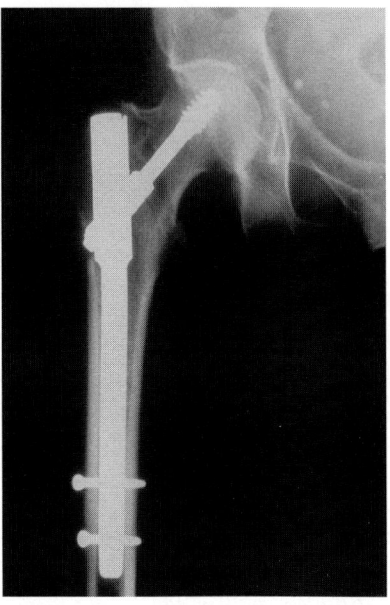

Figure 6.84. Photograph of the Smith+Nephew Intramedullary Hip Screw (**A**). Radiograph demonstrating use of the Intramedullary Hip Screw to stabilize an intertrochanteric fracture (**B**).

Operative Technique for Insertion of the Short-Stem Intramedullary Hip Screw

The surgical technique for insertion of the Gamma nail is similar to that for the Smith+Nephew IMHS; only the latter is presented here.

Preoperative radiographs and templates are used to evaluate the appropriateness of an intramedullary device and to estimate nail diameter, lag screw angle, and lag screw length. If there is a severe bow to the affected femur or associated deformity, use of an intramedullary device may be contraindicated. The IMHS is manufactured in three diameters (12, 14, and 16 mm) and two angles (130° and 135°). In general, we have found it best to use the 12-mm 135° angle intramedullary hip screw. Breakage of the 12-mm nail is unlikely; little is gained in placing large-diameter nails, which are stiffer, making insertion and later removal more difficult. As previously noted with regard to the sliding hip screw, higher-angle devices have superior screw sliding characteristics.

The patient is positioned supine on a fracture table, with both lower extremities resting in padded foot holders. The fracture is reduced as described with use of a sliding hip screw, and the leg is placed in neutral position or slight adduction to facilitate nail insertion through the greater trochanter; the contralateral leg is positioned to allow an unimpeded lateral radiograph. Fracture reduction is then assessed, with particular attention given to residual varus angulation, posterior sag, and malrotation. As described with use of a sliding hip screw, varus angulation can usually be corrected by placing additional traction on the lower extremity. Since it is extremely difficult to insert an intramedullary nail with the hip abducted, abduction of the lower extremity is not used to correct a varus malreduction. Although it is possible to insert the intramedullary nail component of the device with the fracture unreduced and the leg adducted, followed by fracture reduction and lag screw insertion with the leg abducted, this can be technically difficult to perform. Therefore, if a varus reduction cannot be corrected without placement of the leg in abduction, we prefer either to perform an open reduction with direct fracture expo-

Treatment

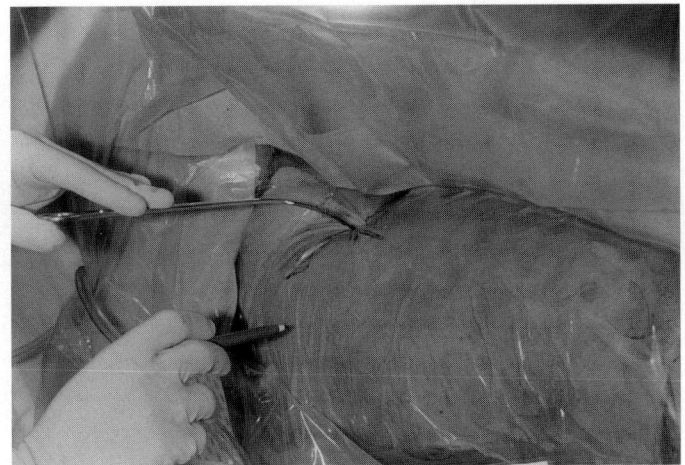 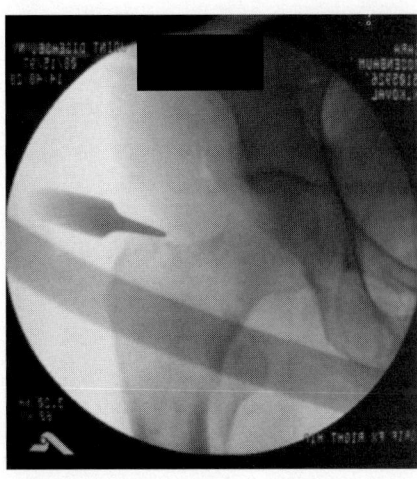

Figure 6.85. After fracture reduction, a straight lateral incision is made from the tip of the greater trochanter, extending proximally for 4 to 6 cm (**A**). One can use the image intensifier to help identify the tip of the greater trochanter (**B**).

sure or to use a sliding hip screw for fracture stabilization. Posterior sag can be corrected with use of a crutch, a bone hook, or a periosteal elevator.

Once the fracture is reduced, the extremity is prepared and draped from the pelvis to the distal thigh. A straight lateral incision is made from the tip of the greater trochanter extending proximally for 4 to 6 cm (Figure 6.85); the gluteus maximus muscle is dissected in line with its fibers. If an open reduction is required, one can extend the incision distally, incising the iliotibial band in line with the skin incision. In this case, the vastus lateralis muscle is reflected anteriorly to expose the proximal femoral shaft as described previously.

The entry point for the IMHS is at the tip of the greater trochanter, halfway between its anterior and posterior extent. One can use a curved awl to open the medullary canal, carefully assessing the awl's position using biplanar image intensification (Figure 6.86). Alternatively, one can use a guidewire and a special cannulated one-step graduated reamer to enter and prepare the proximal femur (Figure 6.87). In younger individuals, particularly those with subtrochanteric fractures, it may be necessary to ream the femoral isthmus to accommodate the intramedullary nail; a ball-tipped guidewire can be placed down the femoral shaft and a flexible cannulated reamer used to enlarge the proximal shaft to the appropriate diameter. In elderly patients who have larger-diameter medullary canals, this step is usually not necessary. The appropriate intramedullary nail is then assembled with its corresponding intramedullary angle guide attachment. There are two intramedullary angle guide attachments, corresponding to the 130° and 135° nails. It is imperative that the appropriate angle guide be matched to the device chosen, otherwise it will be impossible to insert the lag screw. One should verify that the angle guide targets the proximal and distal holes in the nail using the drill sleeves and guide pin before inserting the device (Figure 6.88). The nail is inserted by hand through the greater trochanter into the proximal femur (Figure 6.89). In most cases, the device can be inserted without use of a guidewire. One should avoid use of excessive force, which may produce comminution of the proximal femoral shaft. It is also important that one use frequent fluoroscopic evaluation to follow the progress of the nail as it is inserted.

The nail is positioned to allow lag screw placement into the center of the femoral neck and head. The drill sleeves are inserted into the angle attachment and pushed to the lateral femoral cortex (Figure 6.90). It is important that the sleeves rest against bone and not the vastus lateralis muscle. The

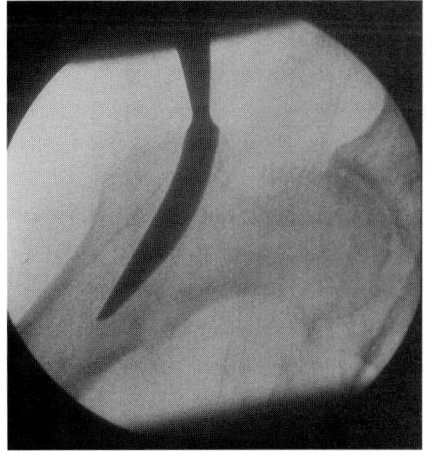

Figure 6.86. Use of a curved awl to open the medullary canal; the entry point for the intramedullary hip screw is at the tip of the greater trochanter, halfway between its anterior and posterior extent.

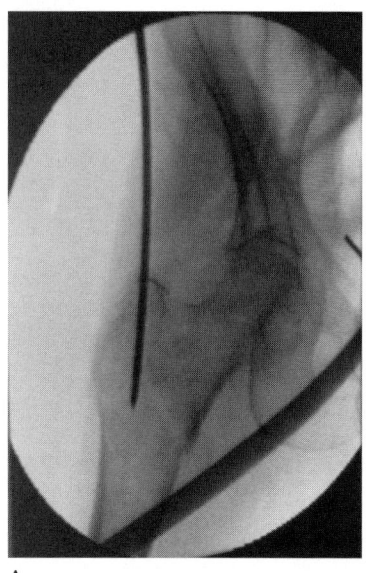 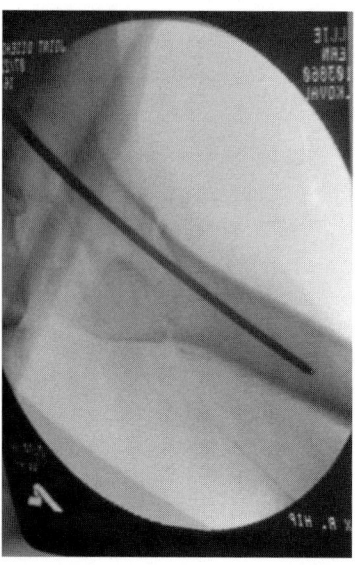 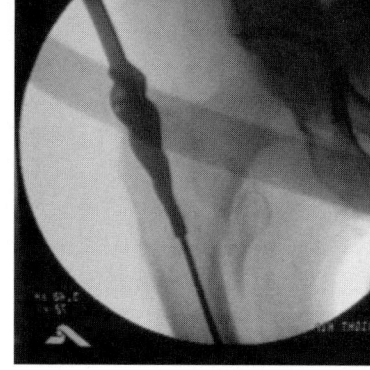

Figure 6.87. Use of a guidewire (**A, B**) and a special cannulated one-step graduated reamer (**C**) to enter and prepare the proximal femur.

threaded guide pin is inserted through the sleeves into the femoral neck and head using image intensification and advanced until it is 5 to 10 mm from the hip joint (Figure 6.91). As with the sliding hip screw, the guide pin should lie in the center of the femoral head and neck on both AP and lateral radiographic views. If the guide pin is not correctly positioned, it should be removed and the nail height and rotation adjusted. The length of the lag screw is determined using a direct-reading depth gauge (Figure 6.92).

A cannulated reamer is advanced over the guide pin to the appropriate depth (Figure 6.93); periodic assessment of the guide pin position is necessary during reaming to detect guide pin advancement. Guide pin advancement can

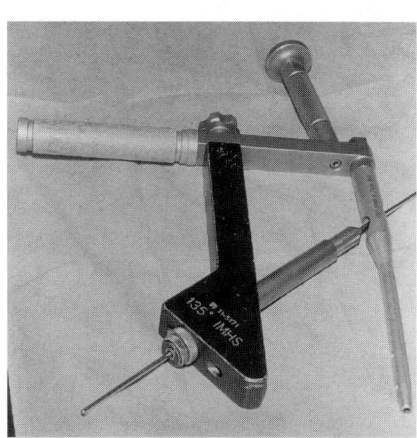 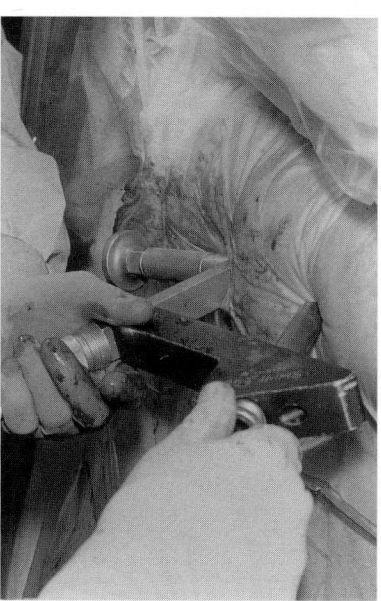 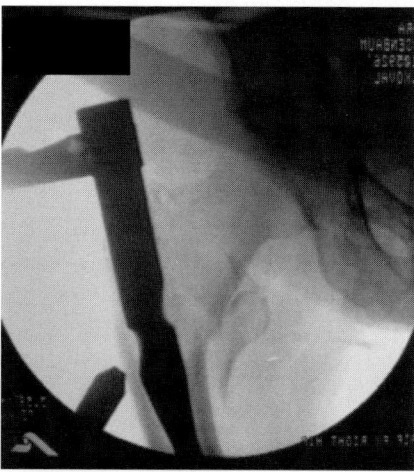

Figure 6.88. Verification that the angle guide targets the proximal and distal holes in the nail using the drill sleeves and guide pin before insertion of the device.

Figure 6.89. Insertion of the nail by hand through the greater trochanter into the proximal femur.

Figure 6.90. Positioning of the nail to allow lag screw placement into the center of the femoral neck and head. The drill sleeves are inserted into the angle guide and pushed to the lateral femoral cortex. It is important that the sleeves rest against bone and not the vastus lateralis muscle.

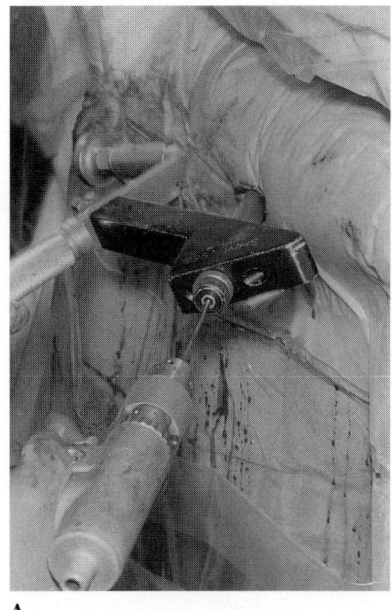 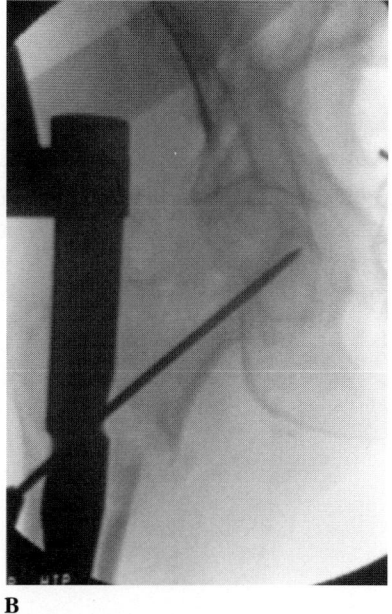 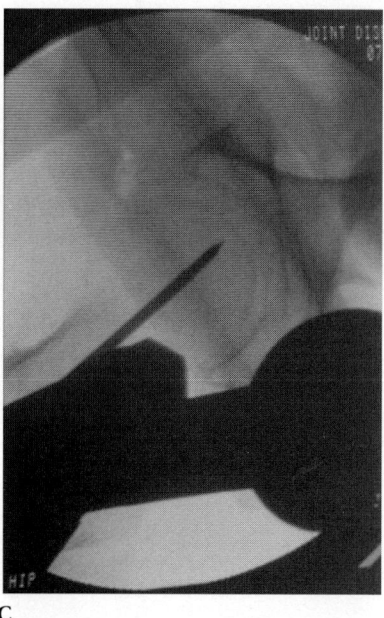

A B C

lead to intraarticular or intrapelvic penetration, resulting in a potentially life-threatening situation. The larger-diameter cannulated sleeve reamer is next used and advanced until the stop makes contact with the drill sleeve (Figure 6.94); this step enables insertion of the large-diameter sleeve, which centers the lag screw in the intramedullary nail. The femoral neck and head are then tapped to the desired lag screw position to avoid rotation of the femoral neck and head during screw insertion.

The lag screw and screw-centering sleeve are attached to the lag screw insertion wrench, and the screw is advanced into the femoral head under

Figure 6.91. Insertion of the threaded guide pin through the drill sleeves (**A**) into the femoral neck and head (**B, C**). Similar to the sliding hip screw, the guide pin should lie in the center of the femoral head and neck on both AP and lateral radiographic views.

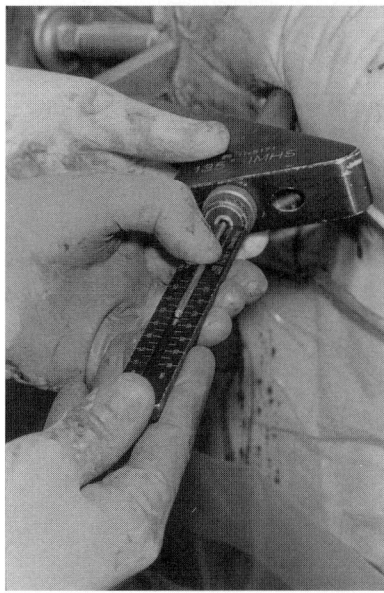 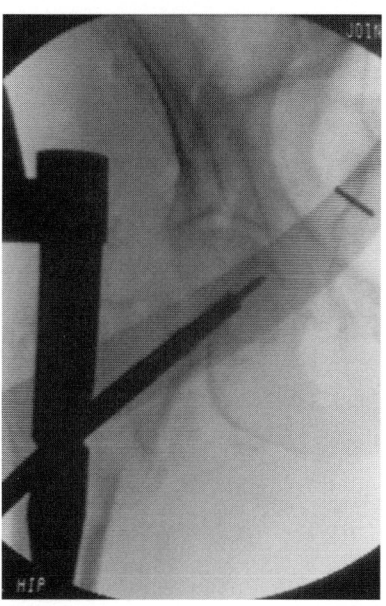 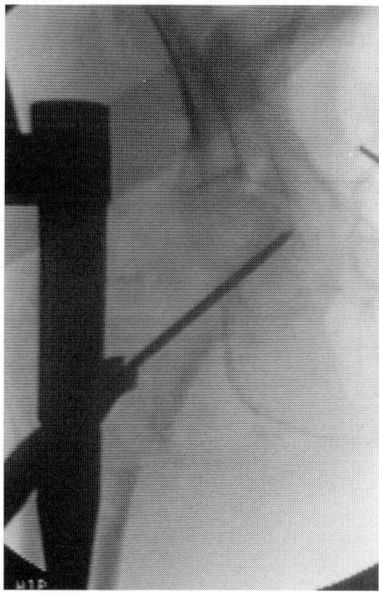

Figure 6.92. The length of the lag screw is determined using a direct-reading depth gauge.

Figure 6.93. Reaming of the proximal femur over the guide pin.

Figure 6.94. Use of the larger-diameter cannulated sleeve reamer; this reamer is advanced until the stop makes contact with the drill sleeve.

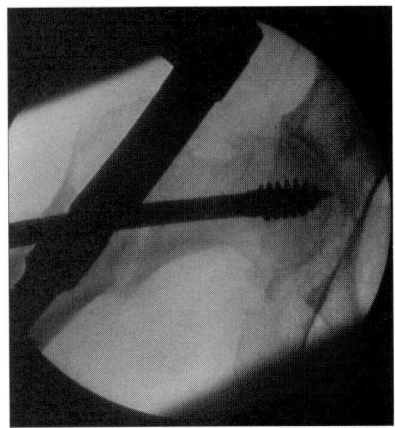

Figure 6.95. Placement of the lag screw.

radiographic control until it lies within 1 cm of the subchondral bone (Figure 6.95). The insertion wrench handle is removed and a cannulated impactor is used to push the centering sleeve into the nail using image intensification (Figure 6.96). One should verify that the centering sleeve is correctly positioned within the nail (Figure 6.97). The nail driver attachment is removed and the set screw is inserted into the top of the nail and tightened using a torque wrench until there is an audible snap (Figure 6.98). This set screw keys the centering sleeve and lag screw within the nail; after set screw insertion, the lag screw will no longer be able to rotate but will be able to slide. Although it is rarely indicated, a compression screw can be inserted.

Distal targeting, when necessary, is performed using the angle guide and drill sleeves (Figure 6.99). Although biomechanical and clinical studies have

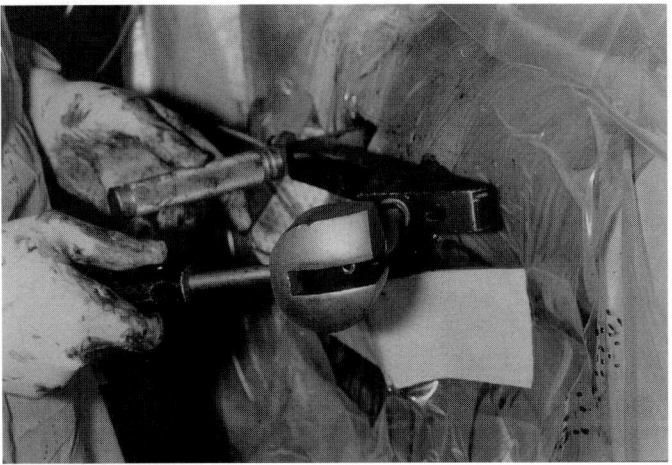

Figure 6.96. Use of the cannulated impactor to push the centering sleeve into the nail.

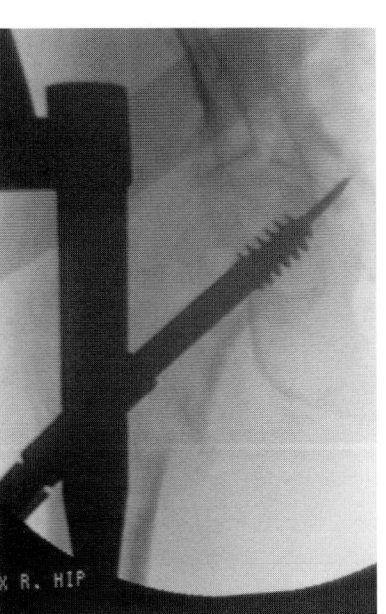

Figure 6.97. Verification that the centering sleeve is correctly positioned within the nail.

Figure 6.98. Insertion of the set screw (**A**) through the top of the nail (**B**). This set screw keys the centering sleeve and lag screw within the nail; after set screw insertion, the lag screw will no longer be able to rotate but will be able to slide.

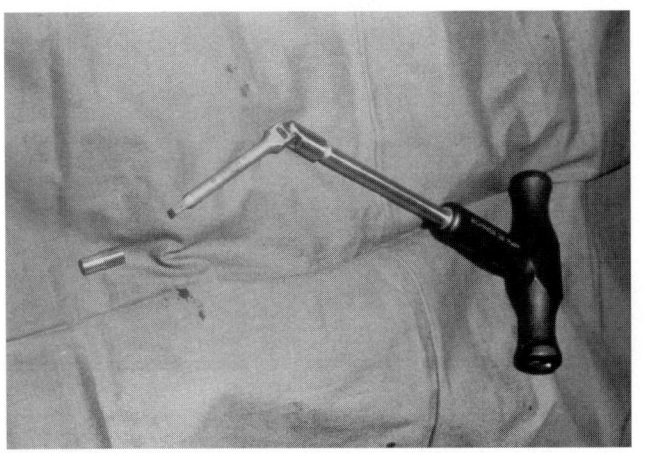

A
B

Treatment

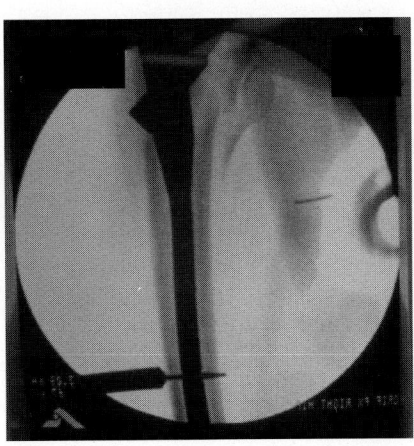
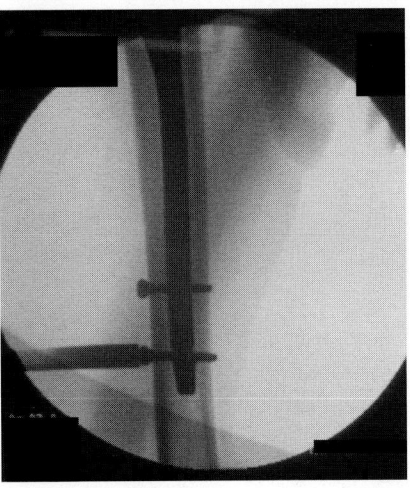

Figure 6.99. Distal targeting is performed using the angle guide and drill sleeves (**A, B**).

questioned the need for routine interlocking of stable and even of unstable fractures, we distally lock unstable intertrochanteric fractures. One must radiographically verify that the distal screws have passed through the nail. The angle guide is removed and the incision is closed in layers over suction drains (Figure 6.100).

Basicervical Fractures

Basicervical hip fractures are located just proximal to or at the intertrochanteric line. Although it is generally acknowledged that basicervical fractures are extracapsular, this may not always be true.[60] Basicervical fractures are thus at greater risk for osteonecrosis than the more distal intertrochanteric fractures. Since basicervical fractures are located adjacent to the femoral neck region, some authors have advocated the use of multiple cancellous screws for fracture stabilization.[61-63] The fracture pattern seen with a basicervical fracture, however, is more lateral than either the subcapital or transcervical fracture,

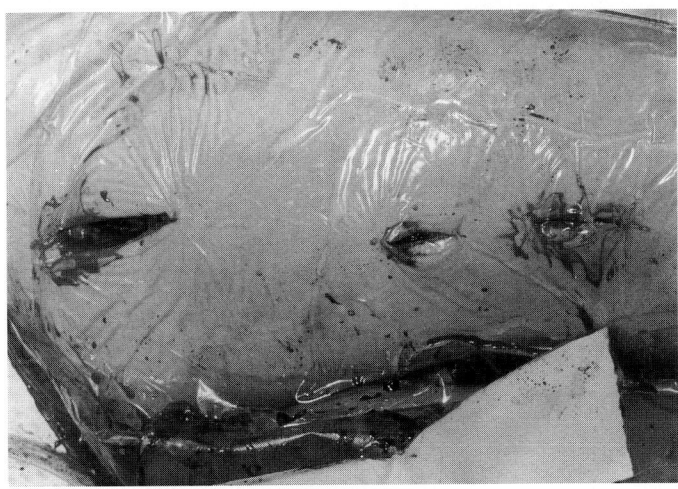

Figure 6.100. The angle guide is removed and the incision is closed in layers.

thereby creating an increased varus moment at the fracture site. This, in turn, may result in toggling of multiple cancellous screws at their insertion points through the lateral cortex. The sideplate of the sliding hip screw prevents screw toggling, theoretically reducing the risk of varus displacement. In addition, a sliding screw-plate device permits controlled fracture impaction.

We performed a biomechanical cadaver study to compare the stability and ultimate strength of three standard fixation techniques in a basicervical hip fracture model[64]: (1) three parallel 6.5-mm cannulated cancellous screws; (2) a 135° sliding hip screw with a four-hole sideplate; and (3) a 135° sliding hip screw with a four-hole sideplate and an additional 6.5-mm cannulated cancellous screw placed proximal and parallel to the sliding screw. The multiple cancellous screw group had a significantly lower ultimate axial load to failure than either sliding hip screw group. Based on these results, we believe that the implant of choice for basicervical fracture fixation is a sliding hip screw.

When using a sliding hip screw for treatment of basicervical fractures, however, one must make a few modifications to the surgical technique from the technique used for more distal intertrochanteric fractures. Because insertion of the lag screw into the femoral head and neck may cause the proximal fragment to rotate, two guide pins are inserted, one in an inferior position and the second more superior. The sliding hip screw is placed over the inferior guide pin, while the proximal guide pin (or cannulated cancellous screw) helps to prevent rotation of the femoral head and neck segment (Figure 6.101).

Intertrochanteric Fractures With Subtrochanteric Extension

Sliding hip screws were initially not recommended for fractures extending into the subtrochanteric region, but improvements in material properties and design have broadened the indications for these devices. Mullaji et al., reporting on a series of 42 peritrochanteric and subtrochanteric fractures so treated, found that at an average follow-up of 11 months, 91% had united satisfactorily.[65]

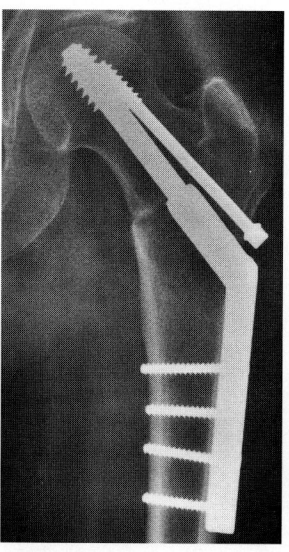
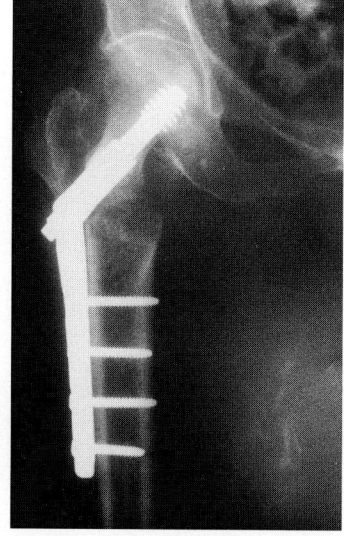

Figure 6.101. Use of a sliding hip screw and antirotation pin to stabilize a basicervical fracture (**A**). Malrotation deformity that resulted from failure to prevent rotation of the proximal fragment during lag screw insertion (**B**).

Treatment

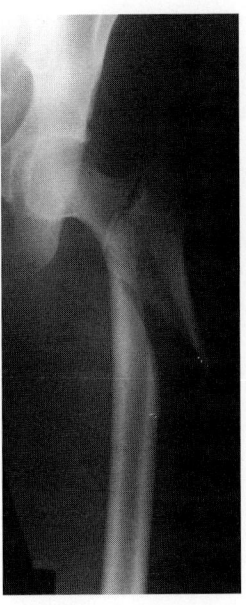 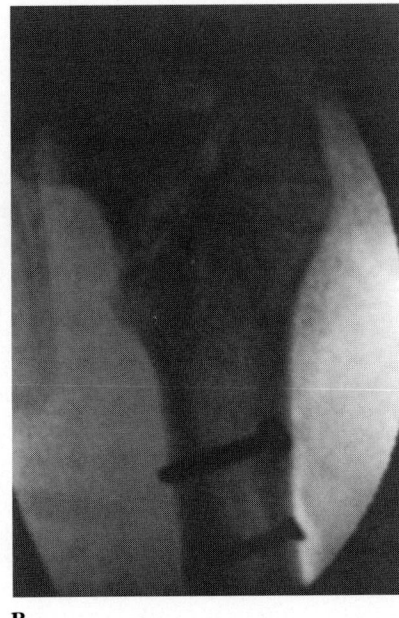 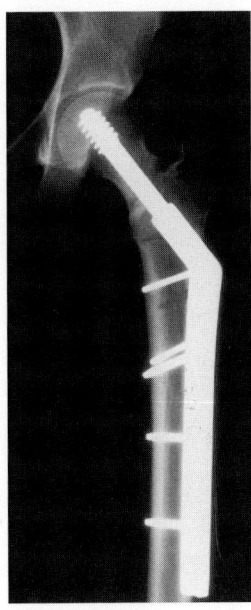

A B C

Figure 6.102. Use of a sliding hip screw to stabilize an intertrochanteric fracture with subtrochanteric extension (**A**). The subtrochanteric component is reduced and stabilized using lag screws or cerclage wire (**B**), followed by reduction and stabilization of the intertrochanteric fracture component (**C**).

When treating an intertrochanteric fracture with subtrochanteric extension using a sliding hip screw, one should reduce and provisionally stabilize the subtrochanteric component, using lag screws or cerclage wire, before inserting the sliding hip screw (Figure 6.102). This can be accomplished on the fracture table by releasing the traction and manipulating the extremity as needed. Once the subtrochanteric component has been reduced and stabilized, traction is reapplied and the position of the femoral head and neck component is checked on both AP and lateral views. Placement of the sliding hip screw then proceeds as described previously. Whenever possible, screws passed through the plate should be placed as lag screws to stabilize the subtrochanteric fracture component. The distal extension of the fracture necessitates a longer plate to obtain adequate shaft fixation than with a pure intertrochanteric fractures.

Intertrochanteric fractures with subtrochanteric extension can also be stabilized using an intramedullary nail, a 95° fixed-angle plate, or a Medoff plate. Reverse obliquity intertrochanteric fractures, which are considered subtrochanteric fractures, are best stabilized with these same devices. The relevant surgical techniques are described in Chapter 7.

Fractures With Comminution and Displacement of the Greater Trochanter

Because of the importance of the greater trochanter as the site of insertion for the abductor muscles, fractures that result in comminution or displacement of the greater trochanter require special attention. If the greater trochanter is displaced, a tension-banding technique is used to reattach it and preserve or restore abductor function. A cerclage wire is placed under the abductor tendon and passed around the plate barrel (Figure 6.103). With the plate stabilized to the femoral shaft, the cerclage wire is tightened to provide secure reattachment.

Figure 6.103. Use of a cerclage wire placed under the abductor tendons and passed around the plate barrel to stabilize a displaced greater trochanter fragment associated with an intertrochanteric fracture.

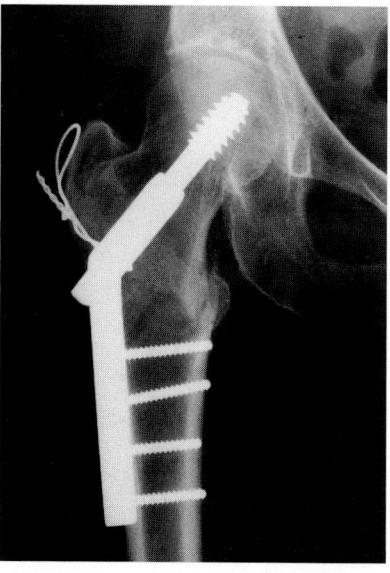

Prosthetic Replacement

Primary prosthetic replacement, while an important treatment option for displaced femoral neck fractures, has had limited use in the management of acute intertrochanteric fractures. The anatomic location of femoral neck fractures makes prosthetic replacement a reasonable option because the distal portion of the femoral neck remains intact, providing excellent prosthetic support; in addition, the greater trochanter–abductor mechanism remains undisturbed. Neither condition applies when endoprosthetic replacement is used for comminuted intertrochanteric fractures. The prosthesis selected must replace the calcar, with provisions for greater trochanteric reattachment to restore abductor function (Figure 6.104). In general, this requires a more extensive surgical procedure than does internal fixation and entails greater blood loss, longer

Figure 6.104. Use of a calcar replacement prosthesis for treatment of a comminuted intertrochanteric fracture.

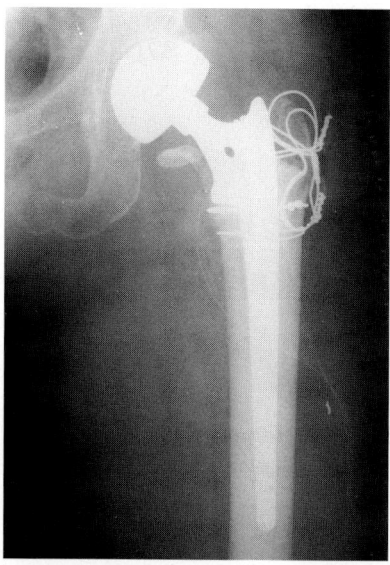

surgical and anesthetic time, and the potential for more frequent complications, not to mention greater cost of the implant. On the other hand, in certain situations, prosthetic replacement may expedite patient mobilization and ambulation and thereby maximize the patient's functional recovery. Utilizing this technique, some studies have reported reduced lengths of hospital stay—to some extent justifying the greater cost of the prosthesis as compared with internal fixation devices.[66,67]

Several authors have reported satisfactory results using either a unipolar or a bipolar prosthetic design for intertrochanteric hip fractures.[67–69] In a series reported by Stern and Goldstein, of 29 intertrochanteric fractures stabilized using a Leinbach (unipolar) proximal femoral replacement, 86% of patients were ambulatory within 1 week of surgery.[69] Stern and Angerman reported on a series of 105 unstable intertrochanteric fractures treated with a Leinbach prosthesis[67]; 94% of patients regained their prefracture ambulatory status. Green et al. reported on a series of 20 elderly patients who had sustained an unstable intertrochanteric fracture and underwent cemented bipolar prosthetic replacement.[66] At an average follow-up of 13.2 months, 12 of 16 (75%) surviving patients were ambulatory; they reported no dislocations or infections, although 25% of patients had residual thigh or groin pain.

Stappaerts et al. reported on a series of 90 patients, 70 years of age or older, who sustained an unstable pertrochanteric fracture[70]; patients were randomized to either open reduction and internal fixation using a sliding hip screw or cemented hemiarthroplasty and followed for three months after surgery. No difference between the two treatment groups was found with respect to surgical time, wound complications, or short-term mortality; however, patients treated with prosthetic replacement had higher transfusion requirements. Severe fracture collapse or loss of fixation occurred in 26% of patients treated with the sliding hip screw, two of whom required additional surgery. One patient treated with prosthetic replacement required revision surgery for recurrent dislocations.

Haentjens et al. reported on a series of 100 patients, 75 years of age or older, who were treated with either a cemented bipolar arthroplasty (91 patients) or total hip arthroplasty (9 patients) for an unstable intertrochanteric or subtrochanteric fracture.[71] Good to excellent results were noted in 78% of patients; however, 45% of total hip arthroplasty patients sustained a hip dislocation, compared with 3% in the bipolar group. Hip dislocation was associated with an increased incidence of pressure sores and pulmonary complications. Other complications included loss of greater trochanter fixation in four cases, one fracture distal to the femoral component, and one femoral nonunion.

In a separate study, Haentjens et al. reported a prospective series comparing 37 consecutive patients over 75 years of age who were managed by either bipolar arthroplasty or internal fixation.[72] The authors concluded that the arthroplasty group had an easier and faster rehabilitation, with a lower incidence of pressure sores, pulmonary infection, and atelectasis, which they attributed to earlier return to full weight bearing. A 5% dislocation rate was noted in the arthroplasty group.

The indications for primary prosthetic replacement remain ill-defined. Most authors cite as the primary indication elderly, debilitated patients with a comminuted, unstable intertrochanteric fracture in severely osteoporotic bone—an assessment that is difficult to quantitate at best. Many patients with pertrochanteric fractures that fit this description have been successfully treated by internal fixation. However, some elderly patients who sustain a comminuted unstable intertrochanteric fracture experience loss of reduction or fixation and require revision surgery. This population of patients would benefit the most from primary prosthetic replacement. However, it is virtually impossible to identify these patients before surgery.

At the Hospital for Joint Diseases, our only indications for primary prosthetic replacement (either hemiarthroplasty or total hip replacement) after intertrochanteric fracture are (1) symptomatic ipsilateral degenerative hip disease (total hip replacement) and (2) attempted open reduction and internal fixation that cannot be performed because of extensive comminution and poor bone quality; in this situation, it would be necessary to abort the planned internal fixation and proceed with prosthetic replacement (hemiarthroplasty). The rate of revision surgery after open reduction and internal fixation of unstable intertrochanteric fractures, despite immediate unrestricted weight bearing, is low (less than 5%). Primary prosthetic replacement is a much more extensive and invasive procedure than open reduction and internal fixation, with the potential for increased morbidity and complications, including prosthetic dislocation. Furthermore, the cost of the prosthesis is high; comparative studies would need to demonstrate significantly improved patient outcomes to justify the added expense of the implant over a sliding hip screw.

Composite Fixation

The use of adjunctive methylmethacrylate ("bone cement") has been advocated in patients with severe osteopenia who have sustained a comminuted, unstable intertrochanteric fracture; the technique was introduced by Harrington as a means of enhancing internal fixation[73] (Figure 6.105). Muhr et al. emphasized that the purpose of the cement is to maintain stability of the fracture–implant construct until osseous union occurs[74]; these authors, who treated 231 intertrochanteric fractures with cement augmentation, believed that the cement provided the stability necessary for immediate weight bearing after surgery. Bartucci et al. compared unstable intertrochanteric fractures treated with and without cement augmentation[75]; fractures treated with cement augmentation had significantly fewer fixation failures than those with-

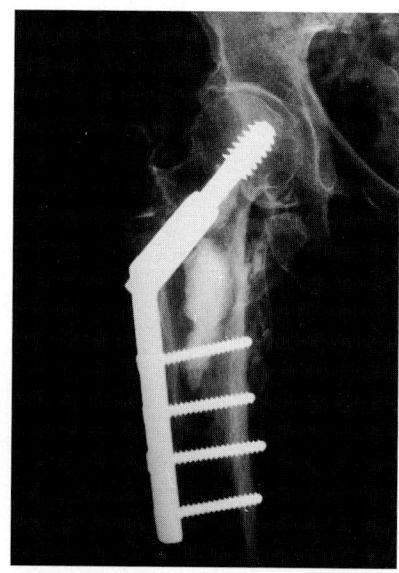

Figure 6.105. Use of adjunctive methylmethacrylate to augment fixation of an unstable intertrochanteric fracture stabilized with a sliding hip screw.

out. Hip function scores, however, were significantly lower in the cement augmentation group—for reasons that could not be explained.

Cheng et al. reported on a series of 38 unstable intertrochanteric fractures whose treatment included cement augmentation[76]; 76% had a good or excellent result at an average follow-up of 3.7 years (range, 2 to 5 years). Late complications occurred in six patients (16%) and included nonunion, screw protrusion, partial destruction of the femoral head, subcapital fracture of the femoral neck, and osteonecrosis of the femoral head. All complications occurred a year or more after surgery and were attributed to inappropriate placement and/or excessive amount of cement resulting in inadequate new bone formation.

Methylmethacrylate can be used to enhance lag screw fixation within the femoral head or fixation of the plate-holding screws, depending on the area of compromised fixation. When employing this technique, it is essential to obtain good fracture impaction at surgery. In addition, introduction of the cement must be well controlled so as to avoid cement intrusion into the fracture site, which could interfere with healing, as well as extravasation into the surrounding soft tissues.

The technique for methylmethacrylate enhancement of the lag screw and plate-holding screws is similar and involves inserting and then removing the screw, injecting liquid methylmethacrylate by syringe into the empty screw hole, and reinserting the screw. Precooling the cement monomer gives the surgeon more time for the procedure. It is interesting to note that if the screw is turned as the methylmethacrylate sets, its holding power is diminished; similarly, if the methylmethacrylate hardens and the screw tract is then drilled and tapped, its holding power is also diminished. Therefore, the screw should be fully placed in the cement while it is still soft and tightened after the cement has set.

SRS (Norian Corporation, Cupertino, CA), an injectable, fast-setting paste, is in clinical trials for the augmentation of unstable intertrochanteric fractures.[77] The paste cures in vivo to form an osteoconductive carbonated apatite with chemical and physical characteristics similar to the mineral phase of bone. SRS has higher compressive strength (55 MPa) and lower tensile and shear strength than cancellous bone.[77] It can be used as a space-filling grout to facilitate the geometric reconstruction and healing of bone with defects and/or fractures. The osteoconductive nature of SRS allows it to be integrated into the bone-healing process. Over time, it is remodeled and incorporated into the newly formed bone tissue.[77] Use of SRS may enhance fracture stability and fill residual defects commonly associated with unstable intertrochanteric fracture without adverse effects on fracture healing.

Pathologic Fractures

The proximal femur is involved in more than 50% of pathologic long-bone fractures.[78] The distribution of metastases to the femoral neck and to the intertrochanteric and subtrochanteric regions appears to be equal.

Operative treatment is indicated for most pathologic intertrochanteric fractures.[79] This treatment approach maximizes patient functioning, alleviates pain, facilitates nursing care, decreases the duration and cost of hospitalization, and improves morale. Surgical contraindications are few and include (1) a patient whose medical condition is inadequate to tolerate the anesthesia and surgical procedure; (2) mental obtundation or alteration of consciousness that precludes the need for local measures to alleviate pain; and (3) markedly limited life expectancy (e.g., less than 1 month).

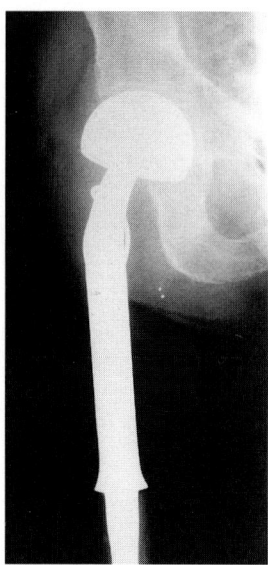

Figure 6.106. Pathologic intertrochanteric fracture treated by proximal femoral replacement.

There are three basic operative approaches to pathologic intertrochanteric fractures[79]: (1) composite fixation, consisting of a sliding hip screw supplemented with methylmethacrylate to fill the voids left by removal of macroscopic tumor; (2) locked intramedullary nailing; and (3) proximal femoral replacement (Figure 6.106). Composite fixation with a sliding hip screw has been described by Walling.[79] The technique utilizes a standard lateral approach to the proximal femur and guide pin placement for positioning the lag screw. A generous cortical window is then made around the guide pin to enable removal of gross tumor and structurally inadequate bone. After reaming and tapping for the lag screw, the appropriate screw-sideplate combination is selected and a trial reduction is performed. The sideplate should extend well below the area of tumor involvement, into normal bone. The entire assembly is then removed, leaving only the guide pin; the methylmethacrylate is prepared and inserted into the defect created by removal of bone and tumor. It is important to insert the cement distally into the femoral canal and to use the cement to reconstitute any cortex that was removed. The cement should fill the femoral neck and trochanteric area and extend distally into the shaft. The lag screw and sideplate are then inserted and the guide pin is removed. After the cement has set, the plate-holding screws are inserted. This composite provides a strong construct and has the advantage of not disturbing the natural attachment of the hip abductors.

Cephalomedullary interlocked nails (e.g., reconstruction nail [Smith +Nephew, Memphis, TN]) can be used to treat pathologic pertrochanteric fractures, but their use should be limited to lesions that are small, have reasonable medial cortical integrity, and have shown radiosensitivity or are at least expected to be radiosensitive.[79] One concern with the use of these devices is that further progression of the tumor might lead to osseous instability (and pain) more quickly than with either composite fixation or prosthetic replacement.[79]

Proximal femoral replacement can be used for lesions that are too extensive for composite fixation.[79] The main disadvantage of proximal femoral replacement is the mandatory reattachment of the hip abductors. However, proximal femoral replacement with a long-stem component has the advantage of providing prophylactic fixation of more distal femoral shaft lesions.

Polytrauma Patients

Young adults with hip fractures are often the victims of high-energy trauma resulting from a motor vehicle accident or a fall from a height. Polytrauma patients should undergo immediate stabilization of all long-bone fractures. Several studies have stressed the advantage of early fixation of long-bone fractures, which should include fixation of pertrochanteric fractures to facilitate patient mobilization.[80,81]

Ipsilateral intertrochanteric–femoral shaft fractures occur less frequently than do concomitant femoral neck–shaft fractures.[82,83] The choice of fixation for ipsilateral intertrochanteric–femoral shaft fractures depends on the two fracture patterns as well as the surgeon's expertise. If the hip and shaft fractures are in close proximity, a sliding hip screw with a long sideplate may suffice; this is by far the simplest and most effective means of stabilizing the two adjacent fractures.[83] As the distance between the intertrochanteric fracture and shaft fracture increases, fixation techniques become more complicated. An attractive treatment option is to stabilize the intertrochanteric fracture with a sliding hip screw and the femoral shaft fracture with an interlocked retrograde nail. If the femoral shaft fracture is transverse and not comminuted, retrograde-inserted Ender nails can be used for femoral shaft fixation in conjunction with a sliding hip screw. Use of a cephalomedullary nail, with screws anchored in the femoral head and neck, is possible but has had poorer reported results for stabilization of ipsilateral intertrochanteric–femoral shaft fractures than for ipsilateral femoral neck–shaft fractures (Figure 6.107). Finally, one can consider using a compression plate for fixation of a femoral shaft fracture that is located significantly distal to an intertrochanteric fracture.

Ipsilateral intertrochanteric–supracondylar distal femur fractures can be treated as two separate fractures. The intertrochanteric fracture can be stabilized using a sliding hip screw and the distal femur fracture can be stabilized with either a 95° fixed-angle plate or a retrograde-inserted interlocked nail.

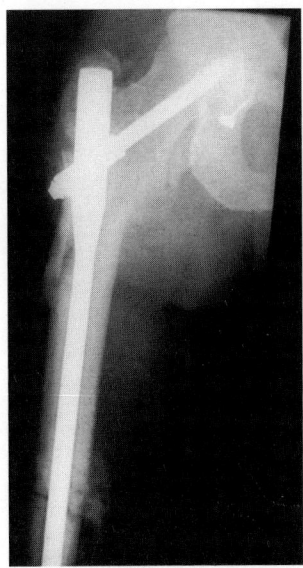

Figure 6.107. Ipsilateral intertrochanteric–femoral shaft fracture stabilized with a cephalomedullary nail.

Rehabilitation

Patients are mobilized out of bed and ambulation training is initiated on postoperative day 1. We believe that all patients who have sustained a femoral neck or intertrochanteric fracture and who have been surgically treated with either internal fixation or prosthetic replacement should be allowed to bear weight as tolerated. It is often difficult for elderly patients with decreased upper-extremity strength—and especially those with associated upper-extremity fractures—to comply with even a partial weight-bearing protocol. Furthermore, in attempting to maintain partial weight bearing, considerable force is generated across the hip by the lower-extremity musculature.[84]

There is little biomechanical justification for restricted weight bearing after intertrochanteric or femoral neck fracture, since activities such as moving around in bed and use of a bedpan generate forces across the hip approaching those resulting from unsupported ambulation.[84] Even foot and ankle range-of-motion exercises performed in bed produce substantial loads on the femoral head secondary to muscle contraction.[84]

Several studies have demonstrated that unrestricted weight bearing does not increase complication rates following fixation of intertrochanteric fractures.[85,86] Ecker et al. reported on a series of 62 intertrochanteric fractures stabilized with a sliding hip screw.[85] Twenty-two patients were allowed early weight bearing, 33 patients remained non–weight-bearing for at least 6 weeks, and ambulation was not attempted in 7 patients. Patient follow-up averaged 15 months. Three fractures (4.8%) required revision surgery secondary to nonunion; all three occurred in unstable fractures. There was no effect of weight bearing on the need for revision surgery.

A prospective series was performed at the Hospital for Joint Diseases to determine the effect of immediate unrestricted weight bearing on outcome after hip fracture surgery.[86] Two hundred eight patients who sustained an intertrochanteric fracture were followed up for a minimum of 1 year, 138 patients with a stable and 70 with an unstable fracture pattern. Six intertrochanteric fractures (2.9%) required revision surgery; five of these six revisions could be attributed to poor surgical technique. Three patients who required revision surgery had a stable intertrochanteric fracture and three had an unstable intertrochanteric fracture for a revision surgery rate of 2.2% for stable and 4.3% for unstable intertrochanteric fractures.

Complications

Complications following intertrochanteric fracture can be divided into medical and surgical complications. Many elderly patients are at increased risk for developing both types of complications because of preexisting medical comorbidities. The rates of urinary tract infection, decubitus ulcers, cardiopulmonary problems, and deep venous thrombosis are similar to those described for femoral neck fractures. The mortality rate after intertrochanteric fracture does not differ significantly from that associated with femoral neck fracture.[7,87]

Loss of Fixation

The most common mode of fixation failure with either a sliding hip screw or an intramedullary hip screw is varus collapse of the proximal fragment with cutout of the lag screw from the femoral head[83] (Figure 6.108). The incidence of fixation failure is reported to be as high as 20% in unstable fracture patterns[83]; rarely is it reported to be less than 4%.[83] Lag screw cutout from the femoral head generally occurs within 3 months of surgery and is usually due to one of the following[7]: (1) eccentric placement of the lag screw within the femoral head; (2) improper reaming that creates a second channel; (3) inability to obtain a stable reduction; (4) excessive fracture collapse such that the sliding capacity of the device is exceeded; (5) inadequate screw-barrel engagement, which prevents sliding; or (6) severe osteopenia, which precludes secure fixation. Retrospective reviews of cases with loss of fixation often indicate technical problems that may have been contributory. Achieving a stable reduction with proper insertion of the sliding hip screw remains the best way of preventing postoperative loss of fixation. Rarely, fixation failure results from loss of fixation of the plate-holding screws (Figure 6.109); however, we have not experienced this complication in over 400 intertrochanteric fractures treated and followed at our hospital.

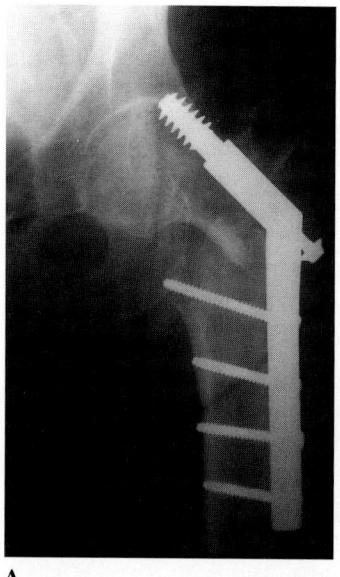
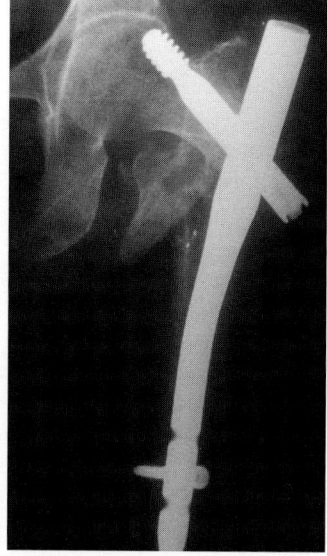

Figure 6.108. Loss of fixation with cutout from the femoral head secondary to superior lag screw placement associated with use of a sliding hip screw (**A**) and an intramedullary hip screw (**B**).

A **B**

Complications

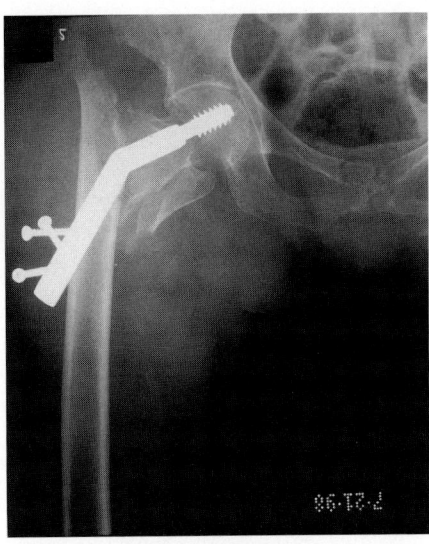

Figure 6.109. Fixation failure secondary to pullout of the plate-holding screws.

When fixation failure occurs, management choices include (1) acceptance of the deformity; (2) revision open reduction and internal fixation, which may require injection of methylmethacrylate; and (3) conversion to prosthetic replacement. Acceptance of the deformity should be considered in marginal ambulators who are a poor surgical risk. Revision open reduction and internal fixation is indicated in younger patients, whereas conversion to prosthetic replacement (unipolar, bipolar, or total hip replacement) is preferred in elderly patients with osteopenic bone.

Nonunion

Nonunion after surgical treatment of intertrochanteric fracture is rare, occurring in less than 2% of patients[1,4,88–90]; this low figure is largely due to the fact that the fracture occurs through well-vascularized cancellous bone. The incidence of nonunion is highest in unstable fracture patterns; Mariani and Rand reported on 20 nonunions, 19 of which (95%) occurred in fractures with loss of posteromedial support.[91] Most intertrochanteric nonunions follow unsuccessful operative stabilization, with subsequent varus collapse and screw cutout through the femoral head. Another possible cause of intertrochanteric nonunion is an osseous gap secondary to inadequate fracture impaction. This can occur as a result of "jamming" of the lag screw within the plate barrel or mismatch of the lag screw and plate barrel length leading to loss of available screw-barrel slide. Both of these problems can be avoided with proper attention to the details of device insertion.

A diagnosis of intertrochanteric nonunion should be suspected in a patient with persistent hip pain and radiographs revealing a persistent radiolucency at the fracture site 4 to 7 months after fracture fixation[83] (Figure 6.110). Progressive loss of alignment strongly suggests nonunion, although union may occur after an initial change in alignment, particularly if fragment contact is improved.[83] Abundant callus formation may be present, making the diagnosis of nonunion difficult to confirm. Tomographic evaluation may help to confirm the diagnosis; otherwise the diagnosis may not be possible until the time of surgical exploration. As with any nonunion, the possibility of an occult infection

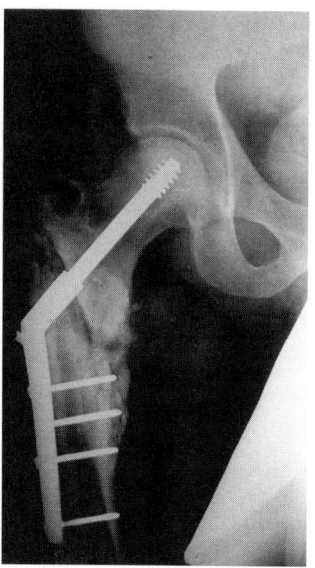

Figure 6.110. Intertrochanteric nonunion with persistent radiolucency at the fracture 9 months after surgery.

must be considered and excluded. In some cases, with good bone stock, a second internal fixation combined with a valgus osteotomy and bone grafting can be considered. However, in most elderly individuals, conversion to a calcar replacement prosthesis is preferred.

Malrotation Deformity

Malrotation deformity usually results from internal rotation of the distal fragment at the time of internal fixation. In unstable fracture patterns, the proximal and distal fragments may move independently; in such cases, the distal fragment should be placed in either neutral position or slight external rotation during fixation of the plate to the shaft. When malrotation is severe and interferes with ambulation, revision surgery with plate removal and rotational osteotomy of the femoral shaft should be considered.

Wound Drainage and Infection

Wound hematoma may result in persistent drainage for several days after hip fracture surgery, particularly in obese, medically unstable, or nutritionally compromised patients. With reduction in patient activities and sterile pressure dressings, such drainage often resolves uneventfully. We have found that placement of elastic wraps in a spica arrangement (from the foot to the groin and across the abdomen) is an effective method to reduce wound drainage after hip fracture.

We do not culture wound drainage at the bedside. The results of such cultures are typically unreliable and misleading. If persistent wound drainage necessitates that cultures be obtained, a strict protocol should be followed. The skin edges should be prepared with povidone-iodine and a sterile cotton swab should be interposed between the skin edges corresponding to the area of drainage. The swab should be inserted into the deeper tissues until resistance is met. We have found this to be a more reliable method of obtaining cultures.

Persistent wound drainage is best treated aggressively. If it is copious or if it increases, changes in appearance, or does not resolve within 7 to 10 days, revision surgery should be considered for irrigation, débridement, and evacuation of hematoma. Gram stain and deep cultures should be obtained. Appropriate antibiotics are initiated during surgery; after thorough débridement and irrigation, the wound is closed over suction drains. Antibiotics are discontinued if the final intraoperative culture results are negative. If bacterial organisms are recovered, however, the antibiotic coverage may need modification (based on the results of sensitivity testing) and should be continued for several weeks.

The incidence of postoperative wound infection after hip fracture surgery ranges between 0.15% and 15%.[83] The lowest figures have been obtained in studies that used perioperative prophylactic antibiotics.[83,92] In a double-blind, prospective study, Burnett demonstrated the value of prophylactic antibiotics in reducing the incidence of wound infection after hip fracture.[93] The value of perioperative antibiotics in hip fracture surgery is now generally accepted.

Postoperative wound infections can be classified as either superficial or deep. Risk factors for wound infection include urinary tract infection, decubitus ulcer, prolonged surgical time, patient disorientation that interferes with proper wound care, and proximity of the incision to the perineum. Superficial wound infections occur early in the postoperative period and are characterized by wound swelling, erythema, and discharge with or without persistent fever. Superficial wound infections should be treated with appropriate antibiotics, prompt débridement as needed, and open drainage followed by secondary closure. If deep infection cannot be ruled out, it is much better to assume deeper tissue involvement and perform a formal irrigation and débridement.

Deep infections may arise before or after fracture union, even several years after surgery. It can be difficult to diagnose late deep infection; patient symptoms may include unexplained hip pain, decreased range of hip motion, and an increased erythrocyte sedimentation rate and C-reactive protein. An increased white blood cell count or fever is frequently absent unless acute sepsis develops. Deep infections require surgical débridement and antibiotic coverage. If the fracture has not yet united and the fixation is stable, the implant should not be removed. In this situation, an extensive débridement with retention of the internal fixation device can be attempted. However, if the infection persists or recurs, removal of hardware and/or resection arthroplasty will be necessary. If there is hip joint involvement or the implant is loose, however, removal of the internal fixation device and/or excisional arthroplasty is recommended.

Decubitus Ulcers

Sacral and heel decubitus ulcers are common complications in patients who have sustained a hip fracture. Agarwal et al. reported an incidence of 20% in patients with fracture of the proximal femur.[94] The mortality rate in patients who have developed a decubitus ulcer has been reported to be as high as 27%.[95] Pressure caused by the weight of the involved part can create tissue necrosis if maintained for as little as 2 hours. Prevention—avoidance of such pressure—is particularly important when skin sensation or protective mobility is impaired. A team approach to avoidance of skin decubitus ulcers is imperative. Frequent turning of the patient is a time-honored protective measure, but is difficult and painful preoperatively for patients who have sustained a fracture of the proximal femur. Special beds, flotation mattresses, early fracture fixation, and constant vigilance by physicians, nurses, and therapists are all helpful in decreasing the incidence and severity of pressure sores after hip fracture.

Other Complications

Osteonecrosis of the femoral head is rare following intertrochanteric fracture[4,96-99] (Figure 6.111). No association has been established between location of the implant within the femoral head and the development of osteonecrosis, although one should avoid the posterior superior aspect of the femoral head because of the vicinity of the lateral epiphyseal artery system.

Various case reports have documented unusual complications relating to separation of the lag screw and sideplate (Figure 6.112) and migration of the lag screw into the pelvis.[100-103] Lag screw–sideplate separation can be prevented by using a compression screw if one feels there is inadequate screw-barrel engagement. Most cases of migration of the lag screw into the pelvis occur in unstable fractures and are associated with improper reaming and violation of the hip joint or the presence of inadequate screw-barrel engagement.

Laceration of the superficial femoral artery by a displaced lesser trochanter fragment has been reported,[104] as has binding of the guide pin within the reamer, resulting in advancement of the guide pin and subsequent intraarticular or intrapelvic penetration[7] (Figure 6.113).

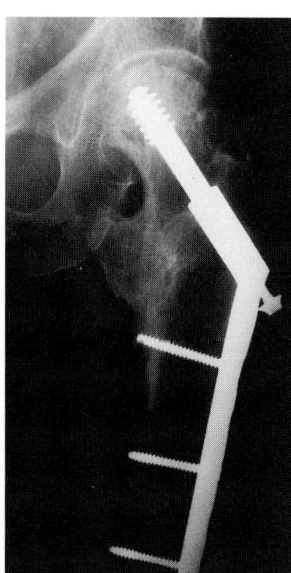

Figure 6.111. Osteonecrosis of the femoral head following intertrochanteric fracture.

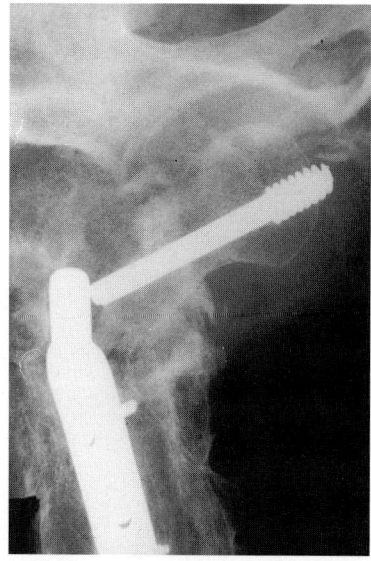

Figure 6.112. Disengagement of the lag screw and sideplate.

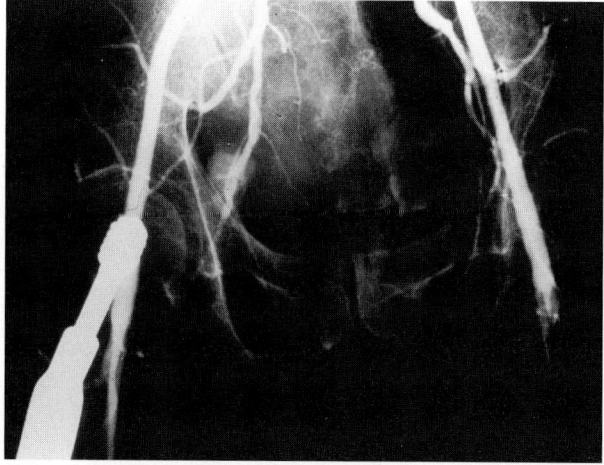

Figure 6.113. Arteriogram depicting injury to the obturator artery secondary to guide pin advancement into the pelvis by the reamer.

Greater Trochanteric Fractures

Isolated greater trochanteric fractures are rare and are typically encountered in older patients following a direct blow to the area.[105] Patients usually report a fall and complain of pain about the lateral aspect of the hip and buttock, which may increase with range of hip motion and weight bearing.[7] Ecchymosis about the lateral aspect of the hip may be noted but is uncommon. Radiographic evaluation includes an AP view of the pelvis (for comparison with the opposite hip) and an AP and a cross-table lateral view of the involved hip. Displaced fractures are easily recognized (Figure 6.114). The greater trochanter is usually displaced superiorly and posteriorly; Milch maintained that the primary deforming force arises from the external rotators and not the abductor muscles.[106] Nondisplaced greater trochanteric fractures, however, may be difficult to recognize on standard radiographs.[7] If a fracture is suspected, a bone scan, computed tomographic scan, or magnetic resonance image may be indicated. It is important to carefully evaluate the radiographs to avoid overlooking an associated nondisplaced intertrochanteric fracture.

Treatment of greater trochanteric fractures is usually nonoperative. Since only a portion of the greater trochanter is usually involved, abductor muscle function is largely preserved; even fractures displaced more than 1 cm can be expected to heal by osseous or fibrous union with restoration of abductor function.[106] Treatment should be symptomatic, with use of nonnarcotic analgesics.[7] Ambulation should be encouraged with initial use of assistive devices to decrease the displacing forces on the fragment. Gradual return to preinjury ambulatory function can be anticipated in the majority of cases. Operative management can be considered in younger active patients who have a widely displaced greater trochanter. Tension band wiring of the displaced fragment and the attached abductor muscles is the preferred technique (Figure 6.115).

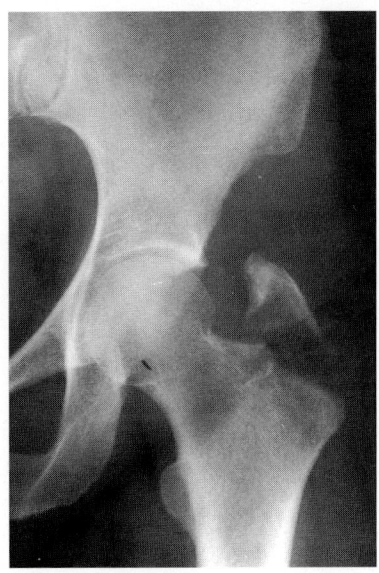

Figure 6.114. Displaced greater trochanteric fracture.

Lesser Trochanteric Fractures

Isolated lesser trochanteric fractures are most common in adolescence, secondary to forceful contracture of the iliopsoas muscle, resulting in avulsion of the lesser trochanteric apophysis.[107] In the elderly, lesser trochanteric fractures were once believed to result from the loss of resistance to iliopsoas muscle contraction secondary to osteoporosis.[108] More recently, however, isolated lesser trochanteric fractures have been recognized as pathognomic for pathologic lesions of the proximal femur.[7,109-111] Therefore, it is essential to evaluate the possibility of pathologic fracture in all elderly patients who present with an isolated lesser trochanteric fracture. If a pathologic process is identified, treatment will be based on the nature of the lesion and the extent of involvement. If there is no evidence of a pathologic lesion, treatment should be symptomatic, directed at regaining range of hip motion and ambulatory function.[7] Similar to fractures of the greater trochanter, it is important to carefully evaluate the radiographs to avoid overlooking an associated nondisplaced intertrochanteric fracture.

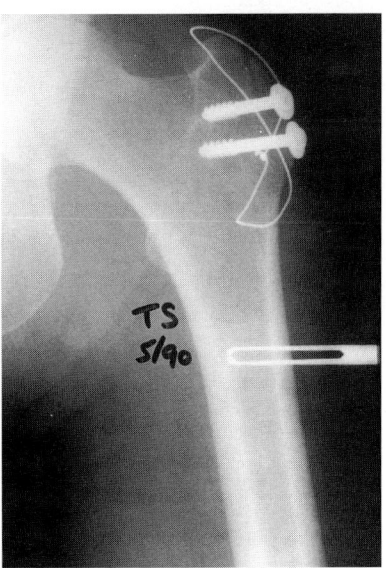

Figure 6.115. Tension band wiring of the greater trochanter.

References

1. Boyd HB, Griffin LL. Classifications and treatment of trochanteric fractures. *Arch Surg* 1949; 58:853–866.
2. Evans E. The treatment of trochanteric fractures of the femur. *J Bone Joint Surg Br* 1949; 31:190–203.
3. Jensen JS, Michaelsen M. Trochanteric femoral fractures treated with McLaughlin osteosynthesis. *Acta Orthop Scand* 1975; 46:795–803.
4. Kyle RF, Gustilo RB, Premer RF. Analysis of six hundred and twenty-two intertrochanteric hip fractures. *J Bone Joint Surg Am* 1979; 61:216–21.
5. Muller ME, Nazarian S, Koch P, Schatzker J. *The Comprehensive Classifications of Fractures of Long Bones*. Berlin: Springer-Verlag, 1990.
6. Gehrchen PM, Nielsen JO, Olesen B. Poor reproducibility of Evan's classification of the trochanteric fracture. *Acta Orthop Scand* 1993; 64:71–72.
7. Zuckerman JD. *Comprehensive Care of Orthopaedic Injuries in the Elderly*. Baltimore: Urban & Schwarzenberg, 1990.
8. Kyle RF, Cabanela ME, Russell TA, et al. Fractures of the proximal part of the femur. *Instr Course Lect* 1995; 44:227–253.
9. Zuckerman J. Current concepts: hip fracture. *N Engl J Med* 1996; 334:1519–1525.
10. Heyse-Moore GH, MacEachern AG, Evans DCJ. Treatment of intertrochanteric fractures of the femur. *J Bone Joint Surg Br* 1983; 65:262–267.
11. Bannister G, Gibson A, Ackroyd C, Newman J. The fixation and prognosis of trochanteric fractures: a randomized prospective controlled trial. *Clin Orthop* 1990; 254:242–246.
12. Jacobs R, Armstrong H, Whitaker J, Pazell J. Treatment of intertrochanteric hip fractures with a compression hip screw and a nail plate. *J Trauma* 1976; 16:599–603.
13. Medoff RJ, Maes K. A new device for the fixation of unstable pertrochanteric fractures of the hip. *J Bone Joint Surg Am* 1991; 73:1192–1199.
14. Watson J, Moed B, Cramer K, Karges D. Comparison of the compression screw with the Medoff sliding plate for intertrochanteric fractures. *Clin Orthop* 1998; 348:79–86.
15. Choueka J, Koval KJ, Kummer FJ, et al. Biomechanical comparison of the sliding hip screw and the dome plunger. Effects of material and fixation design. *J Bone Joint Surg Br* 1995; 77:277–283.
16. Chapman MW, Bowman WE, Csongradi JJ, et al. The use of Enders pins in extracapsular fractures of the hip. *J Bone Joint Surg Am* 1981; 63:14–28.
17. Cobelli N, Sadler A. Ender rod versus compression screw fixation of hip fractures. *Clin Orthop* 1985; 201:123–129.
18. Elabadien BSZ, Olerud S, Karlstrom G. Ender nailing of peritrochanteric fractures. Results at follow-up evaluation after one year. *Clin Orthop* 1984; 191:53–63.
19. Harper MC, Walsh T. Ender nailing for pertrochanteric fractures of the femur: an analysis of indications, factors related to mechanical failure, and postoperative results. *J Bone Joint Surg Am* 1985; 67:79–88.
20. Iwegbu CG, Patel RJ. Difficulties and complications of the Ender method of treatment of trochanteric fractures of the femur. *Injury* 1981; 13:116–124.
21. Jensen JS, Sonne-Holm S, Tondevold E. Unstable trochanteric fractures: a comparative analysis of four methods of internal fixation. *Acta Orthop Scand* 1980:949–962.
22. Levy RN, Siegel M, Sedlin ED, Siffert R. Complications of Ender-pin fixation in basicervical, intertrochanteric and subtrochanteric fractures of the hip. *J Bone Joint Surg Am* 1983; 65:66–69.
23. Sernbo I, Johnell O, Gentz G, Nilsson J. Unstable intertrochanteric fractures of the hip: treatment with Ender pins compared with compression hip Screws. *J Bone Joint Surg Am* 1988; 70:1297–1303.
24. Rao JP, Banzon MT, Weiss AB, Rayhack J. Treatment of unstable intertrochanteric fractures with anatomic reduction and compression hip screw fixation. *Clin Orthop* 1983; 175:65–71.
25. Waddell J, Czitrom A, Simmons EH. Ender nailing in fractures of the proximal femur. *J Trauma* 1987:911–916.
26. Halder SC. The Gamma nail for peritrochanteric fractures. *J Bone Joint Surg Br* 1992; 74:340–344.
27. Leung KS, So WS, Shen WY, Hui PW. Gamma nails and dynamic hip screws for pertrochanteric fractures. A randomized prospective study in elderly patients. *J Bone Joint Surg Br* 1992; 74:345–351.
28. Boriani S, Bettelli G, Zmerly H, et al. Results of the multicentric Italian experience on the Gamma nail: a report on 648 cases. *Orthopedics* 1991; 14:1307–1314.

References

29. Bridle SH, Patel AD, Bircher M, Calvert P. Fixation of intertrochanteric fractures of the femur: a randomized prospective comparison of the gamma nail and the dynamic hip screw. *J Bone Joint Surg Br* 1991; 73:330–334.
30. Radford PJ, Needoff M, Webb JK. A prospective randomized comparison of the dynamic hip screw and the gamma locking nail. *J Bone Joint Surg Br* 1993; 75:789–793.
31. Butt M, Krikler S, Naffe S, Ali M. Comparison of dynamic hip screw and gamma nail: a prospective, randomized, controlled trial. *Injury* 1995; 26:615–618.
32. Aune AK, Ekeland A, Odegaard B, et al. Gamma nail vs compression screw for trochanteric femoral fractures: 15 reoperations in a prospective, randomized study of 378 patients. *Acta Orthop Scand* 1994; 65:127–130.
33. Baumgaertner M, Curtin S, Lindskog D. Intramedullary versus extramedullary fixation for the treatment of intertrochanteric hip fractures. *Clin Orthop* 1998; 348:87–94.
34. Hardy D, Descamps P, Krallis P, et al. Use of an intramedullary hip-screw compared with a compression hip-screw with a plate for intertrochanteric femoral fractures. A prospective, randomized study of one hundred patients. *J Bone Joint Surg Am* 1998; 80:618–630.
35. Rosenblum SF, Zuckerman JD, Kummer FJ, Tam BS. A biomechanical evaluation of the Gamma nail. *J Bone Joint Surg Br* 1992; 74:352–357.
36. Dimon JH, Hughston JC. Unstable intertrochanteric fractures of the hip. *J Bone Joint Surg Am* 1967; 49:440–450.
37. Dimon JH. The unstable intertrochanteric fracture. *Clin Orthop* 1973; 92:100–107.
38. Sarmiento A. Intertrochanteric fractures of the femur: 150-degree-angle nail-plate fixation and early rehabilitation. A preliminary report of 100 cases. *J Bone Joint Surg Am* 1963; 45:706–722.
39. Sarmiento A, Williams EM. The unstable intertrochanteric fracture: treatment with a valgus osteotomy and I-beam nail-plate. *J Bone Joint Surg Am* 1970; 52:1309–1318.
40. Kaufer H, Matthews LS, Sonstegard D. Stable fixation of intertrochanteric fractures: a biomechanical evaluation. *J Bone Joint Surg Am* 1974; 56:899–907.
41. Chang WS, Zuckerman JD, Kummer FJ, Frankel VH. Biomechanical evaluation of anatomic reduction versus medial displacement osteotomy in unstable intertrochanteric fractures. *Clin Orthop* 1987; 225:141–146.
42. Hopkins CT, Nugent JT, Dimon JH. Medial displacement osteotomy for unstable intertrochanteric fractures. Twenty years later. *Clin Orthop* 1989; 245:169–172.
43. Gargan MF, Gundle R, Simpson AH. How effective are osteotomies for unstable intertrochanteric fractures? *J Bone Joint Surg Br* 1994; 76:789–792.
44. Desjardins AL, Roy A, Paiement G, et al. Unstable intertrochanteric fracture of the femur: a prospective randomized study comparing anatomical reduction and medical displacement osteotomy. *J Bone Joint Surg Br* 1993; 75:445–447.
45. Mulholland RC, Gunn DR. Sliding screw plate fixation of intertrochanteric femoral fractures. *J Trauma* 1972; 12:581–591.
46. Wolfgang GL, Bryant MH, O'Neil JP. Treatment of intertrochanteric fracture of the femur using sliding screw plate fixation. *Clin Orthop* 1982; 163:148–158.
47. Kyle RF, Wright TM, Burstein AH. Biomechanical analysis of the sliding characteristics of compression hip screws. *J Bone Joint Surg Am* 1980; 62:1308–1314.
48. Meislin RJ, Zuckerman JD, Kummer FJ, Frankel VH. A biomechanical analysis of the sliding hip screw: the question of plate angle. *J Orthop Trauma* 1990; 4:130–136.
49. Toolan BC, Koval KJ, Kummer FJ, et al. Effects of supine positioning and fracture post placement on the perineal countertraction force in awake volunteers. *J Orthop Trauma* 1995; 9:164–170.
50. Baumgaertner MR, Curtin SL, Lindskog DM, Keggi J. The value of the tip-apex distance in predicting failure of fixation of peritrochanteric fractures of the hip. *J Bone Joint Surg Am* 1995; 77:1058–1064.
51. Baumgaertner M, Solberg B. Awareness of the tip-apex distance reduces failure of fixation of trochanteric fractures of the hip. *J Bone Joint Surg Br* 1997; 79:969–971.
52. Reich S, Jaffe W, Kummer F. Biomechanical determination of the optimal number of fixation screws for the sliding hip screw. *Bull Hosp Jt Dis* 1993; 53:43–44.
53. Yian E, Banerji I, Mathews L. Optimal side plate fixation for unstable intertrochanteric hip fractures. *J Orthop Trauma* 1997; 11:254–259.
54. Gundle R, Gargan MF, Simpson AHRW. How to minimize failures of fixation of unstable intertrochanteric fractures. *Injury* 1995; 26:611–614.
55. Apel DM, Patwardhan A, Pinzur MS, Dobozi WR. Axial loading studies of unstable intertrochanteric fractures of the femur. *Clin Orthop* 1989; 246:156.

56. Olsson O, Ceder L, Lunsjo K, Hauggaard A. Biaxial dynamization in unstable intertrochanteric fractures. Good experience with a simplified Medoff sliding plate in 94 patients. *Acta Orthop Scand* 1997; 68:327–331.
57. Ceder L, Lunsjo L, Olson O, et al. Different ways to treat subtrochanteric fractures with the Medoff sliding plate. *Clin Orthop* 1998; 348:101–106.
58. Lunsjo K, Ceder L, Stigsson L, Hauggaard A. One-way compression along the femoral shaft with the Medoff sliding plate: the first European experience of 104 intertrochanteric fractures with a 1 year follow-up. *Acta Orthop Scand* 1995; 66:343–346.
59. Lunsjo K, Ceder L, Stiggson L, Hauggaard A. Two-way compression along the shaft and the neck of the femur with the Medoff sliding plate. *J Bone Joint Surg Br* 1996; 78:387–390.
60. Swiontkowski MF. Intracapsular hip fractures. In: Browner BD, Levine AM, Jupiter JB, Trafton PG, eds. *Skeletal Trauma,* Vol 2. Philadelphia: WB Saunders, 1992:1751–1832.
61. Madsen F, Linde F, Anderson E, et al. Fixation of displaced femoral fractures: a comparison between sliding screw plate and four cancellous bone screws. *Acta Orthop Scand* 1987; 58:212–216.
62. Skinner PW, Powles D. Compression screw fixation for displaced subcapital fracture of the femur: success or failure. *J Bone Joint Surg Br* 1986; 68:78–82.
63. Swiontkowski MF, Harrington RM, Keller TS, Van Patten PK. Torsion and bending analysis of internal fixation techniques for femoral neck fractures: the role of implant design and bone density. *J Orthop Res* 1987; 5:433–444.
64. Blair B, Koval KJ, Kummer F, Zuckerman JD. Basicervical fractures of the proximal femur. A biomechanical study of 3 internal fixation techniques. *Clin Orthop* 1994; 306:256–263.
65. Mullaji AB, Thomas TL. Low-energy subtrochanteric fractures in elderly patients: results of fixation with the sliding screw plate. *J Trauma* 1993; 34:56–61.
66. Green S, Moore T, Proano F. Bipolar prosthetic replacement of unstable intertrochanteric hip fractions in the elderly. *Clin Orthop* 1986; 224:169–177.
67. Stern MB, Angerman A. Comminuted intertrochanteric fractures treated with a Leinback prosthesis. *Clin Orthop* 1987; 218:75–80.
68. Rosenfeld RT, Schwartz DR, Alter AH. Prosthetic replacement for trochanteric fractures of the femur. *J Bone Joint Surg Am* 1973; 55:420.
69. Stern MB, Goldstein TB. The use of the Leinback prosthesis in intertrochanteric fracture of the hip. *Clin Orthop* 1977; 128:325–331.
70. Stappaerts KH, Deldycke J, Broos PLO, et al. Treatment of unstable peritrochanteric fractures in elderly patients with a compression hip screw or with the Vandeputte (VDP) endoprosthesis: a prospective randomized study. *J Orthop Trauma* 1995; 9:292–297.
71. Haentjens P, Casteleyn P, Opdecam P. Primary bipolar arthroplasty or total hip replacement for the treatment of unstable intertrochanteric and subtrochanteric fractures in elderly patients. *Acta Orthop Belg* 1994; 60:124–128.
72. Haentjens P, Casteleyn PP, De Boeck H, et al. Treatment of unstable intertrochanteric and subtrochanteric fractures in elderly patients: primary bipolar arthroplasty compared with internal fixation. *J Bone Joint Surg Am* 1989; 71:1214–1255.
73. Harrington KD. The use of methylmethacrylate as an adjunct in the internal fixation of unstable comminuted intertrochanteric fractures in osteoporotic patients. *J Bone Joint Surg Am* 1975; 57:744–750.
74. Muhr C, Tscherne H, Thomas R. Comminuted trochanteric femoral fractures in geriatric patients: the result of 231 cases treated with internal fixation and acrylic cement. *Clin Orthop* 1979; 138:41–44.
75. Bartucci EJ, Gonzalez MH, Cooperman DR, et al. The effect of adjunctive methylmethacrylate on failures of fixation and function in patients with intertrochanteric fractures and osteoporosis. *J Bone Joint Surg Am* 1985; 67:1094–1107.
76. Cheng CL, Chow SP, Pun WK, Leong JC. Long-term results and complications of cement augmentation in the treatment of unstable trochanteric fractures. *Injury* 1989; 20:134–138.
77. Goodman SB, Bauer TW, Carter D, et al. Norian SRS cement augmentation in hip fracture treatment. Laboratory and initial clinical results. *Clin Orthop* 1998; 348:42–50.
78. Harrington K. Orthopaedic *Management of Metastatic Bone Disease.* St. Louis: CV Mosby, 1988.

References

79. Walling A, Bahner R. Pathological fractures. In: Koval K, Zuckerman J, eds. *Fractures in the Elderly*. Philadelphia: Lippincott-Raven, 1998:247–259.
80. Bone L, Bucholz R. The management of fractures in the patient with multiple trauma. *J Bone Joint Surg Am* 1986; 68:945–949.
81. Johnson KD, Cadambi A, Seibert GB. Incidence of adult respiratory distress syndrome in patients with multiple musculoskeletal injuries: effect of early operative stabilization of fractures. *J Trauma* 1985; 25:375–384.
82. Swiontkowski MF. Ipsilateral femoral shaft and hip fractures. *Orthop Clin North Am* 1987; 18:73–84.
83. Baumgaertner MR, Chrostowski JH, Levy RN. Intertrochanteric hip fractures. In: Browner BD, Levine AM, Jupiter JB, Trafton PG, eds. *Skeletal Trauma*, Vol 2. Philadelphia: WB Saunders, 1992:1833–1881.
84. Nordin M, Frankel VH. Biomechanics of the hip. In: Nordin M, Frankel VH, eds. *Basic Biomechanics of the Musculoskeletal System*. Malvern, PA: Lea & Febiger, 1989:135–151.
85. Ecker ML, Joyce JJI, Kohl EJ. The treatment of trochanteric hip fractures using a compression screw. *J Bone Joint Surg Am* 1975; 57:23–27.
86. Koval K, Friend K, Aharonoff G, Zuckerman J. Weightbearing after hip fracture: a prospective series of 596 geriatric hip fracture patients. *J Orthop Trauma* 1996; 10:526–530.
87. Aharonoff GB, Koval KJ, Skovron ML, Zuckerman JD. Hip fractures in the elderly: predictors of one year mortality. *J Orthop Trauma* 1997; 11:162–165.
88. Altner PC. Reasons for failure in treatment of intertrochanteric fractures. *Orthop Rev* 1982; 11:117.
89. Boyd HB, Lipiniski SW. Nonunion of trochanteric and subtrochanteric fractures. *Surg Gynecol Obstet* 1957; 104:463–470.
90. Hunter GA. The results of operative treatment of trochanteric fractures of the femur. *Injury* 1975; 6:202–205.
91. Mariani EM, Rand JA. Nonunion of intertrochanteric fractures of the femur following open reduction and internal fixation: results of second attempt to gain union. *Clin Orthop* 1987; 218:81–89.
92. Bodoky A, Neff U, Heberer M, Harder F. Antibiotic prophylaxis with two doses of cephalosporin in patients managed with internal fixation for a fracture of the hip. *J Bone Joint Surg Am* 1993; 75:61–65.
93. Burnett JW, Gustilo RB, Williams DN, Kind A. Prophylactic antibiotics in hip fractures. A double-blind, prospective study. *J Bone Joint Surg Am* 1980; 62:457–462.
94. Agarwal N, Reyes JD, Westerman DA, Cayten C. Factors influencing DRG 201 (hip fracture) reimbursement. *J Trauma* 1986; 26:426–431.
95. Versluysen M. Pressure sores in elderly patients: the epidemiology related to hip operations. *J Bone Joint Surg Br* 1985; 67:10–13.
96. Claffey TJ. Avascular necrosis of the femoral head: an anatomical study. *J Bone Joint Surg Br* 1960; 42:802–809.
97. Cleveland M, Bosworth DM, Thompson FR, et al. A ten year analysis of intertrochanteric fractures of the femur. *J Bone Joint Surg Am* 1959; 41:1399–1408.
98. Mann RJ. Avascular necrosis of the femoral head following intertrochanteric fractures. *Clin Orthop* 1973; 92:108–115.
99. Taylor GM, Newfield AJ, Nickel VL. Complications and failures in the operative treatment of intertrochanteric fractures of the femur. *J Bone Joint Surg Am* 1955; 37:306–316.
100. Brodell JD, Leve AR. Disengagement and intrapelvic protrusion of the screw from a sliding screw plate device, a case report. *J Bone Joint Surg Am* 1983; 65:697–701.
101. Joseph KN. Acetabular penetration of sliding screw. A case of trochanteric hip fracture. *Acta Orthop Scand* 1986; 57:245–246.
102. Lichtblau S. A pitfall in the insertion of a sliding screw. *Bull Hosp Jt Dis* 1986:60–62.
103. Manoli A. Malassembly of the sliding screw-plate device. *J Trauma* 1986; 26:916–922.
104. Soballe K. Laceration of the superficial femoral artery by an intertrochanteric fracture fragment. *J Bone Joint Surg Am* 1987; 69:781–783.
105. Merlino AF, Nixon JE. Isolated fractures of the greater trochanter. *Int Surg* 1969; 52:117–124.
106. Milch H. Avulsion fracture of the great trochanter. *Arch Surg* 1939; 38:334–350.
107. Poston H. Traction fracture of the lesser trochanter of the femur. *Br J Surg* 1921–1922; 9:256–258.

108. Kewenter Y. A case of isolated fracture of the lesser trochanter. *Acta Orthop Scand* 1931; 2:160–165.
109. Bertin KC, Horstman J, Coleman SS. Isolated fracture of the lesser trochanter in adults: an initial manifestation of metastatic malignant disease. *J Bone Joint Surg Am* 1984; 66:770–773.
110. Gradwohl JR, Mailliard JA. Cough induced avulsion of the lesser trochanter. *Nebr Med J* 1987; 72:280–281.
111. Phillips C, Pope T, Jones J, et al. Nontraumatic avulsion of the lesser trochanter: a pathognomonic sign of metastatic disease. *Skeletal Radiol* 1988; 17:106–110.

Chapter Seven
Subtrochanteric Fractures

Subtrochanteric fractures—those between the lesser trochanter and the isthmus (narrowest portion) of the femoral shaft (Figure 7.1) —account for approximately 5% to 34% of all hip fractures.[1] Boyd and Griffin, in a review of 300 hip fractures, classified 26.7% as subtrochanteric.[2] Michelson et al. reported that 14% of hip fractures in patients over age 50 years were located in the subtrochanteric region.[3] At the Hospital for Joint Diseases, subtrochanteric fractures account for approximately 5% of hip fractures in patients over 65 years of age. A review of retrospective studies reveals that the incidence of these fractures exhibits a bimodal age distribution, with high-energy injuries occurring more frequently in younger individuals and low-energy injures occurring more frequently in the elderly.[4-7]

The subtrochanteric region is the site of very high mechanical stresses; the medial and posteromedial cortices are subject to high compressive forces, whereas the lateral cortex experiences high tensile forces. According to Koch's analysis of mechanical stresses on the femur during weight bearing, compression stresses in a 200-lb man can exceed 1200 lb/in^2 in the medial subtrochanteric area 1 to 3 in distal to the level of the lesser trochanter[8] (Figure 7.2); lateral tensile stresses are approximately 20% less. Koch's analysis, however, did not take into account the additional effects of muscle forces. Frankel and Burstein, studying the effects of stresses on proximal femoral fixation devices in patients during bed rest, demonstrated that significant forces are placed on the hip and proximal femur during hip flexion and extension, even while the patient is recumbent.[9] This asymmetric high-stress-loading pattern is an important consideration in the selection of an internal fixation device and in understanding the causes of fixation failure and healing disturbances. Furthermore, the cortical bone in the subtrochanteric region is less vascular than the cancellous bone in the intertrochanteric region; therefore, the risk of healing complications is greater with subtrochanteric fractures than with intertrochanteric fractures.

Because there are several sites of muscle attachment in the proximal femur, certain characteristic deformity patterns arise after subtrochanteric fracture (Figure 7.3). The proximal fragment may be flexed, abducted, and externally rotated secondary to the forces exerted by the iliopsoas muscle, the gluteus medius and minimus muscles, and the short external rotators. The gluteus medius and minimus muscles abduct the proximal fragment through their attachment onto the greater trochanter. The iliopsoas muscle flexes and externally rotates the proximal fragment if the lesser trochanter is attached. The short external rotators externally rotate the proximal fragment. The adductors and hamstrings cause shortening and adduction of the distal fragment.

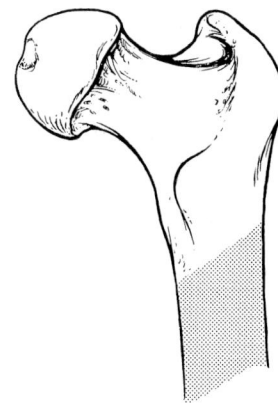

Figure 7.1. The subtrochanteric region can be defined as the area between the lesser trochanter and the isthmus (narrowest portion) of the femoral shaft.

Figure 7.2. The subtrochanteric region is the site of very high mechanical stresses; the medial and posteromedial cortex are subject to high compressive forces, while the lateral cortex experiences high tensile forces. According to Koch's analysis of mechanical stresses on the femur during weight bearing, compression stresses in a 200-lb man can exceed 1200 lb/in^2 in the medial subtrochanteric area 1 to 3 in distal to the level of the lesser trochanter.[8]

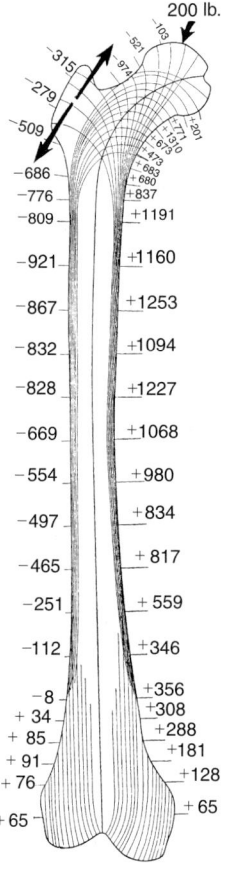

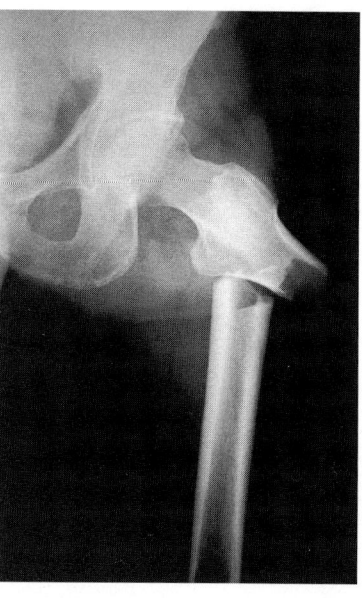

Figure 7.3. AP radiograph of a subtrochanteric fracture demonstrating the typical deformity of the proximal fragment: flexion, abduction, and external rotation.

Mechanism of Injury

The majority of subtrochanteric fractures result from complex loading patterns. Nevertheless, there are specific loading patterns that produce characteristic fractures:

1. In pure bending, the convex side of the femur is loaded in tension and the concave side in compression; in this scenario, the side subjected to tension fails, resulting in a transverse fracture.
2. When bending is associated with axial compression, bending produces a transverse fracture line on the convex side of the bone; axial compression converts the transverse fracture to an oblique fracture pattern on the concave side of the loaded bone, frequently producing a butterfly fragment.
3. Pure torsion results in a spiral fracture with the fracture line oriented approximately 45° to the axis of torque application.

Low-energy trauma usually results in a minimally comminuted oblique or spiral fracture, frequently in osteopenic bone with a wide medullary canal and thin cortices. Fractures from high-energy trauma are often comminuted, posing the risk for significant damage to the soft tissues (even in closed injuries) as well as devascularization of the fracture fragments. In the United States, gunshot wounds are a common source of high-energy subtrochanteric trauma—accounting for approximately 10% of subtrochanteric fractures at the Campbell Clinic.[10] Excluding penetrating trauma, the majority of subtrochanteric fractures are caused either by direct lateral forces to the proximal thigh (e.g., side impact in a motor vehicle accident or a fall from a height) or by axial loading.

The mechanism of injury varies with the age of the patient. As noted earlier, in younger individuals, these fractures are more commonly the result of high-energy trauma—motor vehicle accident, vehicle–pedestrian accident, fall from a height, or penetrating injury—whereas in elderly persons they are more commonly secondary to low-energy trauma (e.g., simple fall).[10] Berman et al., in a review of subtrochanteric fractures at a level I trauma center, reported a mean age of 40.6 years among those who sustained these fractures as a result of high-energy trauma and 76.2 years among those who sustained low-energy trauma.[4]

The subtrochanteric region of the femur is also frequently the site of pathologic fracture arising from neoplastic disease; these account for 17% to 35% of reported subtrochanteric fractures.[11,12]

Associated Injuries

In patients who sustain subtrochanteric fractures from low-energy trauma, significant associated injuries are unusual. Although contusions and abrasions are the most common, cranial and vertebral injuries must also be considered.[10] When subtrochanteric fracture is the result of high-energy trauma, total system examination is required, as with all polytrauma patients. Bergman et al. noted that 16 of 31 (52%) patients who sustained a high-energy subtrochanteric fracture had other injuries to the long bones, pelvis, spine, or abdominal organs.[11] Waddell's retrospective review of eight hospitals over a 6-year period found associated injuries of the cranium, thorax, and/or abdomen that required surgical treatment in 27 of 130 patients (21%) who sustained a subtrochanteric fracture.[7] Jekic and Jekic, reporting on a series of 63 subtrochanteric fractures (53 of which resulted from a high-energy injury), noted that 38 patients (60%) had sustained polytrauma, defined as a multiply injured person with a life-threatening injury of at least one of the following body parts: head, neck, thorax, abdomen, spine, extremities with neurovascular compromise, or pelvic girdle.[13] Russell and Taylor reported a high incidence of ipsilateral patellar and tibial fractures associated with high-energy subtrochanteric fractures[10]; they noted that these associated injuries can compromise knee flexion and ankle motion, which, together with possible compromise of hip function, may severely limit the patient's functional ability.

In high-energy injuries, one should perform the standard ABCs of trauma care followed by a secondary survey to look for injuries involving any organ system. The four extremities should be examined for any swelling, crepitus, or abnormal motion; the extremities' sensorimotor function and neurovascular status should be documented. Long-bone injuries must be identified and immobilized to minimize the risk of fat embolization. Early stabilization of long-bone and pelvic fractures facilitates patient mobilization and helps to optimize respiratory function, the main source of morbidity and mortality in the polytrauma patient.[14,15]

Classification

Several classification systems have been proposed for subtrochanteric fractures; it is important to recognize that an intact (or at least reconstructible) posteromedial cortical buttress—because of asymmetric proximal femoral loading—is the key to stabilization. If posteromedial cortical continuity can be reestablished, internal fixation devices will act as a tension band, and compression forces will be transmitted along the medial cortex. If, however, fracture configuration (especially steep obliquity) or comminution prevents reestablishment of posteromedial continuity, the consequent bending stresses on the internal fixation device greatly increase the risk of implant failure.

Among the first systems of subtrochanteric fracture classification to become widely accepted was that proposed by Fielding and Magliato, whose typology was organized in terms of fracture location in relation to the lesser trochanter.[16] (Figure 7.4) According to their system, type I fractures are at the level of the lesser trochanter, type II fractures are distal to but still within 1 in of the lower border of the lesser trochanter, and type III fractures are 1 to 2 in from the lower border. Although this classification did not take into account fracture comminution, it was useful to the extent that it alerted the surgeon to type III (distinctly distal) fractures, which had a poorer result with the available internal fixation devices.

Waddell's classification shifted the emphasis to the degree of medial comminution[7] (Figure 7.5). In his system, type 1 is a transverse or short oblique fracture without medial comminution; type 2 is a long oblique or spiral fracture with minimal medial comminution; and type 3 is any fracture that exhibits marked medial comminution. Waddell reported that the outcome of fracture treatment was dependent on the quality of reduction and the ability to restore the medial buttress. Fixation of type 3 fractures using the implants then available held the highest risk for healing complications.

Seinsheimer's classification, still currently in use, is based on the fracture's location, pattern, amount of displacement, and degree of comminution, as follows[17] (Figure 7.6):

- Type I: Fractures with less than 2 mm displacement
- Type II: Displaced two-part fractures with:
    IIA: Transverse fracture pattern

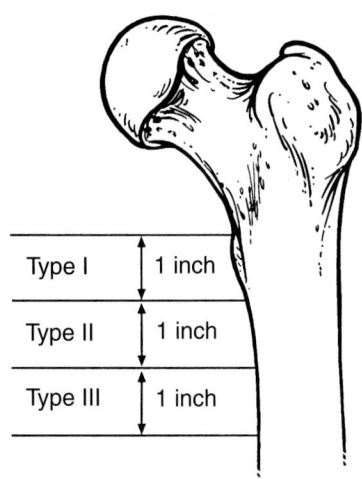

Figure 7.4. The Fielding and Magliato classification system for subtrochanteric fractures[16]: type I fractures are at the level of the lesser trochanter, type II fractures are distal to but still within 1 in of the lower border of the lesser trochanter, and type III fractures are 1 to 2 in from the lower border of the lesser trochanter.

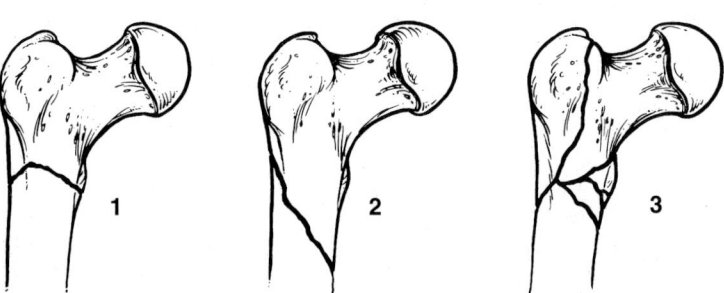

Figure 7.5. The Waddell classification for subtrochanteric fractures[7]: type 1 is a transverse or short oblique fracture without medial comminution; type 2 is a long oblique or spiral fracture with minimal medial comminution; and type 3 is a fracture with marked medial comminution.

Classification

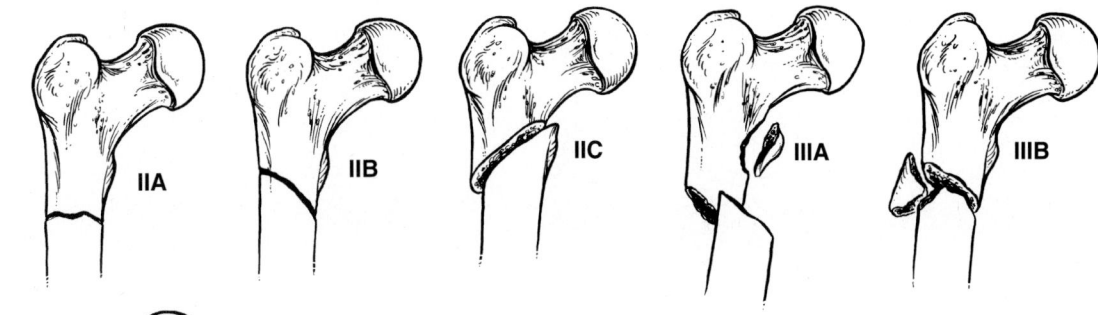
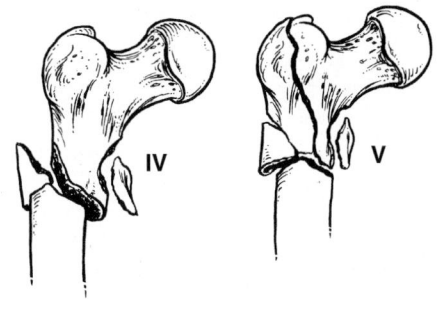

Figure 7.6. The Seinsheimer classification for subtrochanteric fractures[17]: type I is a fracture with less than 2 mm displacement. Type IIA is a displaced two-part fracture with a transverse fracture pattern. Type IIB is a displaced two-part fracture with an oblique fracture pattern, with the lesser trochanter attached to the proximal fragment. Type IIC is a displaced two-part fracture with an oblique fracture pattern, with the lesser trochanter attached to the distal fragment. Type IIIA is a displaced three-part fracture in which the lesser trochanter is a separate fragment. Type IIIB is a displaced three-part fracture in which the lesser trochanter is attached to either the proximal or distal fragment. Type IV is a displaced four-part fracture. Type V is a subtrochanteric fracture with fracture extension into the greater trochanter.

    IIB: Oblique fracture pattern, with the lesser trochanter attached to the proximal fragment
    IIC: Oblique fracture pattern, with the lesser trochanter attached to the distal fragment
- Type III: Displaced three-part fractures where:
    IIIA: Lesser trochanter is a separate fragment
    IIIB: Lesser trochanter is attached to either the proximal or the distal fragment
- Type IV: Displaced four-part fractures
- Type V: Fractures with extension through the greater trochanter

The usefulness of this classification is that it identifies fractures with loss of medial stability (types IIIA and IV) that are at increased risk for healing complications.

The comprehensive classification of long-bone fractures described by the AO/ASIF group ranges from 32A1 to 32C3 (where 32 is the femoral diaphysis)[18] (Figure 7.7). This classification is based on fracture pattern and degree of comminution; it does not take into account the degree of fracture displacement.

- 32A: Two-part fractures
  A1: Spiral
  A2: Oblique
  A3: Transverse
- 32B: Fractures with a butterfly fragment and:
  B1: A spiral wedge,
  B2: A bending wedge
  B3: A comminuted wedge
- 32C: Complex, comminuted fractures
  C1: Comminuted spiral
  C2: Segmental
  C3: Irregular pattern

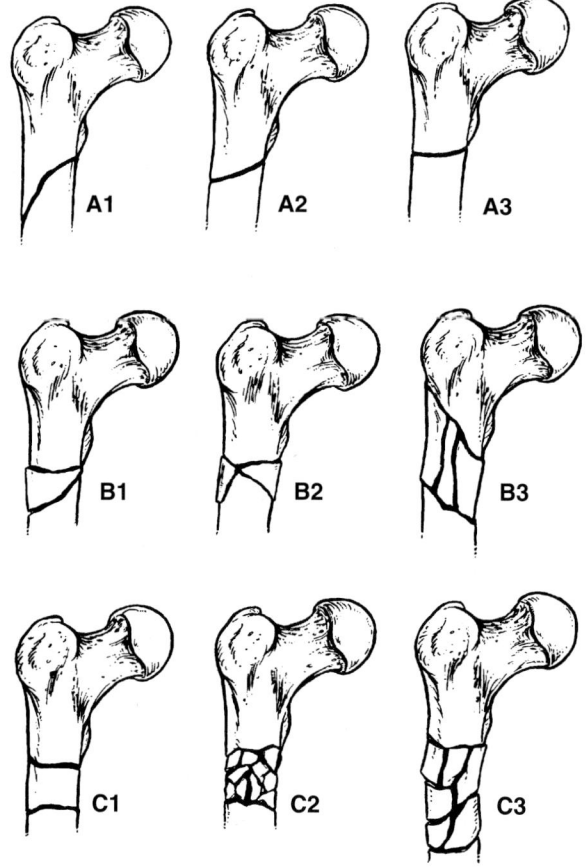

Figure 7.7. The AO/ASIF classification for subtrochanteric fractures.[18]
32A—Two-part fractures: A1, spiral; A2, oblique; and A3, transverse.
32B—Fractures with a butterfly fragment and: B1, a spiral wedge; B2, a bending wedge; and B3, a comminuted wedge.
32C—Complex, comminuted fractures. C1—Comminuted spiral. C2—Segmental. C3—Irregular pattern.

The AO/ASIF classification contains further subdivisions. It is important to note that in this classification system, subtrochanteric fractures with intertrochanteric extension are considered trochanteric fractures. For a variety of reasons, the AO classification system is useful primarily for research purposes.

The Russell-Taylor classification of subtrochanteric fractures was created in response to the development of first- and second-generation interlocked nails[10] (Figure 7.8). Because it can be used as a guide to treatment—for example, in helping the surgeon to select the appropriate device for fracture stabilization—it is the system we prefer to use. In the Russell-Taylor classification, subtrochanteric fractures are divided into stable and unstable types:

- Type 1: Fractures with an intact piriformis fossa in which:
  1A: The lesser trochanter is attached to the proximal fragment (This fracture type is amenable to standard antegrade nailing using a first-generation interlocked nail.)
  1B: The lesser trochanter is detached from the proximal fragment (This fracture type is amenable to intramedullary nailing but will require a second-generation interlocked nail—e.g., reconstruction nail—in which the nail has screw fixation into the femoral head and neck.)
- Type 2: Fractures that extend into the piriformis fossa and that:
  2A: Have a stable medial construct (posteromedial cortex)
  2B: Have comminution of the piriformis fossa and lesser trochanter, associated with varying degrees of femoral shaft comminution.

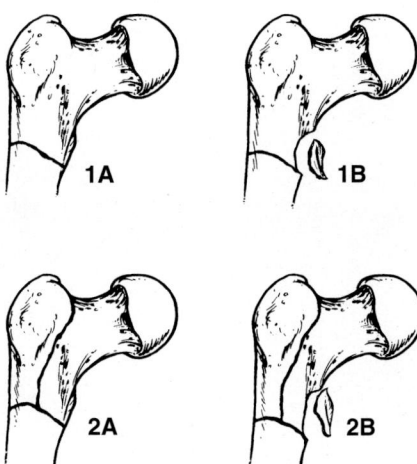

Figure 7.8. The Russell-Taylor classification for subtrochanteric fractures[10]: type 1 are subtrochanteric fractures with an intact piriformis fossa. In type 1A, the lesser trochanter is attached to the proximal fragment, whereas in type 1B, the lesser trochanter is detached from the proximal fragment. Type 2 are subtrochanteric fractures that extend into the piriformis fossa. Type 2A have a stable medial construct (posteromedial cortex), while type 2B have comminution of the piriformis fossa and lesser trochanter, associated with varying degrees of femoral shaft comminution.

Russell-Taylor type 2 fractures are difficult to stabilize with an intramedullary device and are perhaps better treated with a sliding hip screw or a 95° fixed-angle device using indirect reduction techniques.

Treatment

Nonoperative Treatment

Although nonoperative management of subtrochanteric fractures is rarely considered, it is important to discuss the basic principles of this approach. Nonoperative management generally consists of skeletal traction followed by placement of a spica cast or cast brace. Because of the deforming forces on the proximal femur, skeletal traction usually involves placement of the limb in a 90/90 position (Figure 7.9). Skeletal traction is usually applied through a distal femoral pin to avoid pulling across the knee, although tibial traction has also been used successfully. The limb is suspended with both the hip and knee flexed to 90°. The leg and foot are placed in a well-padded short leg cast, with the ankle in a neutral or dorsiflexed position to avoid an equinus contracture. For the average adult, initial traction is 30 to 40 lb (13.6 to 18.2 kg). Appropriate adjustments of the traction apparatus are made, with radiographic monitoring, until a satisfactory reduction is obtained in both AP and lateral views: less than 5° of varus or valgus angulation and more than 25% fracture fragment apposition on both views. Shortening by more than 1 cm is avoided. As it is difficult to obtain adequate radiographic views of the proximal femur with the extremity suspended in a 90/90 position, physician-directed radiographs may be necessary. It is also important to assess proper limb rotation to avoid a rotational deformity.

After approximately 3 to 4 weeks, as the patient's symptoms subside, the leg is gradually lowered into a less flexed position, with abduction as necessary to prevent varus angulation. When clinical consolidation has been obtained—as indicated by restoration of mechanical continuity (e.g., rotation of the distal thigh producing rotation of the greater trochanter) and callus formation evident

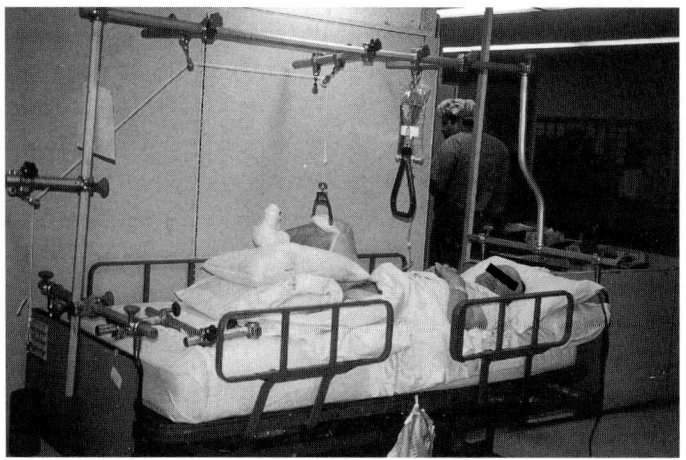

Figure 7.9. Use of skeletal traction with the limb placed in a 90/90 position to stabilize a subtrochanteric fracture.

on radiographs—the patient may be placed in a cast brace with a pelvic band and a proximal quadrilateral mold. At this point, the patient is allowed out of bed and ambulation is initiated with touch-down weight bearing on the injured extremity. Radiographs should be taken weekly; if signs of lost reduction appear, manipulation and recasting or traction should be instituted as necessary.

Nonoperative treatment is poorly tolerated, particularly in the elderly and multiply injured because of the need for prolonged bed rest and the potential for skin problems associated with use of a spica cast. In general, reported results of nonoperative management indicate increased rates of morbidity and mortality as well as nonunion, delayed union, and malunion compared to open treatment.[6,7] Waddell retrospectively reviewed traction treatment of nondisplaced and displaced fractures in patients who were medically unsuitable for surgical treatment.[7] Although the patients with nondisplaced fractures did well with nonoperative treatment, only 4 of 11 patients (36%) who had a displaced subtrochanteric fracture had a satisfactory result with traction. Velasco and Comfort reported that 11 of 22 (50%) adults who had a subtrochanteric fracture treated with skeletal traction had an unsatisfactory result with significant shortening or angular deformity.[6]

Another drawback to nonoperative treatment of subtrochanteric fractures is that it usually requires a much longer hospital stay than does operative treatment, making it financially undesirable given the reimbursement methods in effect for most American health care institutions.

For all these reasons, we believe that nonoperative management should be reserved for high-risk patients for whom surgery is not a reasonable option. It must nevertheless be kept in mind that these same patients are usually poor candidates for prolonged traction treatment as well. Such cases represent a true dilemma. Some proximal subtrochanteric fractures or intertrochanteric–subtrochanteric fractures in nonambulators may be amenable to nonoperative management consisting of early bed-to-chair mobilization if the pain level permits. More distal subtrochanteric fractures, however, particularly those with a spiral pattern, cannot be treated in this manner because of the risk of conversion to an open fracture. Thus, we favor operative management whenever possible and reserve nonoperative management for carefully selected patients who are clearly not surgical candidates.

Operative Treatment

Operative management of subtrochanteric fractures is the treatment of choice to achieve the goals of early rehabilitation and optimal functional recovery. If surgery is anticipated within 24 hours of admission, one can place a pillow under the knee of the injured extremity or apply 5 lb of Buck's skin traction. When a longer delay is anticipated, a distal femoral or proximal tibial pin should be inserted to maintain reasonable fracture alignment and length and prevent additional soft tissue injury from displaced fracture fragments. The distal femoral pin should be inserted from medial to lateral to avoid injury to the femoral artery; the proximal tibial pin is inserted from lateral to medial to avoid injury to the common peroneal nerve. If the fracture is to be stabilized with an interlocked nail, the distal femoral pin is placed anterior in the femoral condyle to avoid the intended path of the femoral nail. Furthermore, with use of an interlocked nail, one should ascertain that the fracture has been brought out to length before surgery; this is best determined on a cross-table lateral radiograph. Establishment of limb length decreases the amount of traction required at surgery to effect fracture reduction and may minimize the risk of fracture table–induced pudendal nerve palsy.

Evolution of Surgical Techniques

From the 1940s to the 1960s, the most commonly utilized device for subtrochanteric fracture stabilization was the Jewett nail, consisting of a triflanged nail fixed to a plate at angles ranging from 130° to 150° (Figure 7.10). Although it provided adequate fixation of the proximal fragment and stabilization to the femoral shaft, the Jewett nail did not make allowances for postoperative fracture impaction. If significant impaction of the fracture site occurred, it resulted in penetration of the nail into the hip joint or "cutting out" of the nail through the superior portion of the femoral head. If fracture impaction did not occur, loading on the device secondary to lack of bone contact resulted in either breakage of the device at the nail–plate junction (Figure 7.11) or separation of the plate and screws from the femoral shaft. Although some authors reported satisfactory experiences with use of the Jewett nail for treatment of subtrochanteric fractures, in general, the overall results were disappointing.[16,19,20]

Hanson and Tullos, reporting on nonpathologic subtrochanteric fractures stabilized using a Jewett nail, found that 42 of 48 (88%) united successfully after a single operative procedure[19]; six patients (12%) developed a nonunion and required further surgery. Fielding et al. reviewed 46 subtrochanteric fractures stabilized with a Jewett nail and reported a 26% rate of nonunion.[16] The latter authors' failure rate is representative of other authors' experiences. Teitge in 1976 recommended avoiding use of a Jewett nail for stabilization of subtrochanteric fractures.[20]

The AO/ASIF 95° fixed-angle condylar blade plate gained popularity in the 1970s. The 95° design allows two or more cortical screws to be inserted through the plate into the calcar region, providing additional fixation of the proximal fracture fragment (Figure 7.12). An additional benefit of this device is that it can be inserted into a small proximal fragment before fracture reduction; when correctly used, the device restores femoral alignment and provides stable fixation. Placement of the 95° condylar blade plate, however, is a technically demanding procedure requiring exact three-plane insertion. Incorrect

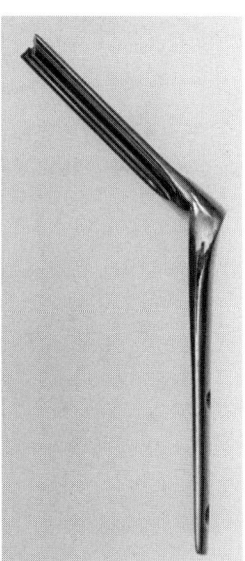
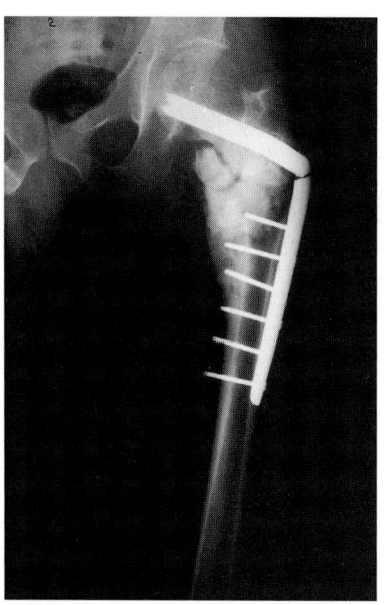
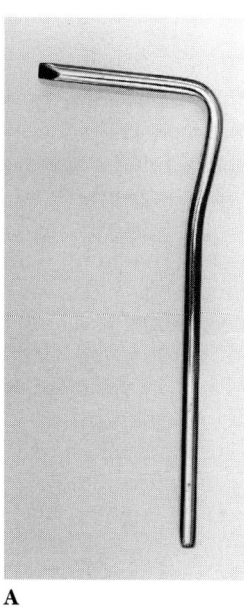
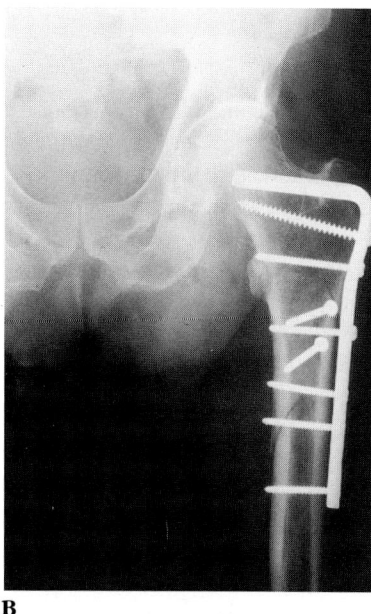

Figure 7.10. Photograph of a Jewett nail.

Figure 7.11. A subtrochanteric nonunion with failure of the Jewett nail at the nail-plate junction.

Figure 7.12. Photograph of a 95° fixed-angle condylar blade plate (**A**). AP radiograph demonstrating use of the blade plate to stabilize a subtrochanteric fracture (**B**).

use of either this device or the 95° dynamic condylar screw can lead to angular malalignment.

Initially, the highest success rates with use of a condylar blade plate were reported in subtrochanteric fractures with a transverse fracture pattern.[21] Whatley et al. reported on a series of 23 such fractures, 21 of which were available for follow-up; 17 fractures (74%) united primarily within 6 months, 2 were delayed unions that united by 12 months, and 2 were nonunions that experienced device failure requiring revision surgery and bone grafting before healing.[21] These authors concluded that the 95° fixed-angle blade plate provided adequate stabilization and fixation with a high union rate in subtrochanteric fractures.

Asher et al. reported on the use of the 95° condylar blade plate for stabilization of 11 acute subtrochanteric fractures, of which 10 were available for follow-up.[22] Of the 10 fractures, 7 (70%) united without complication; the other 3 experienced loss of fixation: 2 united in varus, and in 1 device, fixation failure occurred with resultant nonunion. The poor results were attributed to technical errors, including improper implant placement into the femoral head and neck fragment, blade protrusion posteriorly, and failure to obtain medial contact of the fracture fragments.

Of the 40 consecutive subtrochanteric fractures studied by Van Meeteren et al., all stabilized using a 95° blade plate, 36 (90%) united (despite deep postoperative wound infection in three cases)[23]; three patients died prior to fracture union secondary to multiple injuries, and one patient developed a delayed union that ultimately resulted in fatigue failure of the plate.

Kinast et al. studied a series of 47 subtrochanteric femur fractures stabilized with a 95° condylar blade plate to determine the effect of two surgical techniques.[24] One group of 24 patients (group I) had been treated using an older technique involving extensive visualization of the fracture lines, anatomic reduction of all fracture fragments, internal fixation with the 95° blade plate, and optional autologous bone grafting. The other group, consisting of 23 patients (group II), were treated using a newer, indirect reduction technique that abandoned visualization of the fracture lines and bone grafting and instead attempted to gain overall fracture alignment and stability without achieving anatomic fracture reduction. The average time to osseous union for the fractures that healed primarily was 5.4 months in group I and 4.2 months in group II. Delayed union or nonunion was found in 16.6% of patients in group I and in 0% of those in group II; the infection rate was 20.8% in group I and 0% in group II. The functional end result was similar in both groups. The authors concluded that use of an indirect reduction technique that preserves the vascularity of the medial fragments and osseous compression were the two most important prerequisites for a successful outcome using a 95° condylar blade plate.

The 95° dynamic condylar screw is a two-piece device with the same basic design as the 95° condylar blade plate but with the blade replaced by a large-diameter cannulated lag screw that is inserted over a guide pin after its channel is reamed and tapped (Figure 7.13). The device is technically easier to insert than the blade plate: varus/valgus malalignment of the guide pin is easily corrected, and flexion/extension can be adjusted by rotation of the lag screw. Moreover, the 95° dynamic condylar screw may provide better purchase in osteopenic bone than does the condylar blade plate. It does not, however, provide as much control of the proximal fragment as does the 95° blade plate, and it requires insertion of an additional screw through the plate into the proximal fragment for rotational stability.

Several authors have reported good results using the 95° dynamic condylar screw for subtrochanteric fracture stabilization.[25] Sanders and Regazzoni reported on a consecutive series of subtrochanteric fractures in which 22 patients were available for follow-up at an average of 23.8 months.[25] Fractures were classified according to the radiographic criteria of Seinsheimer and results were reported using a hip function rating system. The union rate was 77% (17 of 22), with functional results rated as good or excellent in 68% (15 of

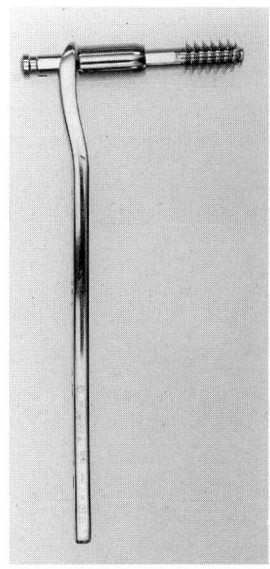
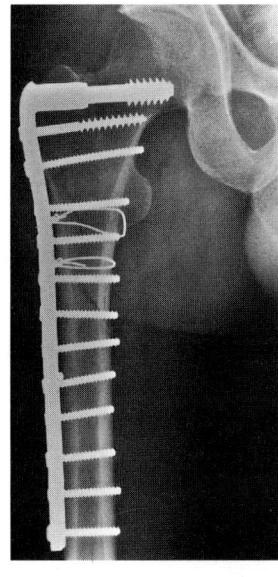

Figure 7.13. Photograph of a 95° dynamic condylar screw (**A**). AP radiograph demonstrating use of the 95° dynamic condylar screw to stabilize a subtrochanteric fracture (**B**).

22). All five technical failures were associated with extensive bone comminution; of these, four were not bone grafted.

Pai reported on 16 subtrochanteric fractures with greater trochanteric fracture extension stabilized using the 95° dynamic condylar screw.[26] All patients were treated using the principles of indirect reduction to achieve overall fracture alignment rather than anatomic reduction, without bone grafting, followed by delayed weight bearing. The overall union rate was 93.7% (15 of 16).

Nungu et al. reported on a series of 15 subtrochanteric fractures stabilized using the 95° dynamic condylar screw.[27] Patient age averaged 70 years (range, 20 to 95 years); patients were followed up for 18 to 30 months. Three patients (20%) developed healing disturbances, two of whom had insufficient medial cortical bone support. The fixation device failed in two cases and loosened in one.

The popularity of the sliding hip screw in the early 1970s led to use of this device for stabilization of subtrochanteric fractures (Figure 7.14). The sliding mechanism allows impaction of fracture surfaces as well as medial displacement of the femoral shaft relative to the proximal fragment, which serves to reduce the bending moment on the implant and thus decrease the possibility of varus displacement or device failure. For impaction to occur, however, the sliding mechanism must cross the fracture site and the plate must not be fixed to the proximal fragment, a situation that can be obtained only in proximal subtrochanteric fractures—specifically, those with both subtrochanteric and intertrochanteric involvement. In practice, the sliding hip screw is often used to stabilize a variety of subtrochanteric fracture patterns, reflecting, at least in part, surgeons' desire to use a familiar device. When the sliding hip screw is used to reduce more distal fractures or comminuted fractures, it is essential to reconstruct the posteromedial cortical buttress to minimize the risk of varus displacement and device failure.

Excellent results have been reported with use of the sliding hip screw to treat subtrochanteric fractures.[4,28–30] Wile et al., reporting on a series of 25 subtrochanteric fractures stabilized using a high-angle sliding hip screw, found no mechanical failures, delayed unions, or nonunions; malunion occurred in two cases, at least one of which was the result of technical error at the time of fracture reduction.[28] Osseous union occurred at a mean time of 3.6 months. Similar results were reported by Berman et al., who found no instance of device

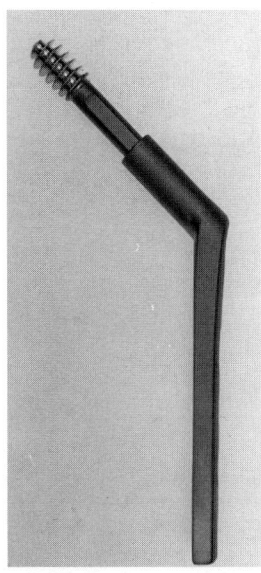 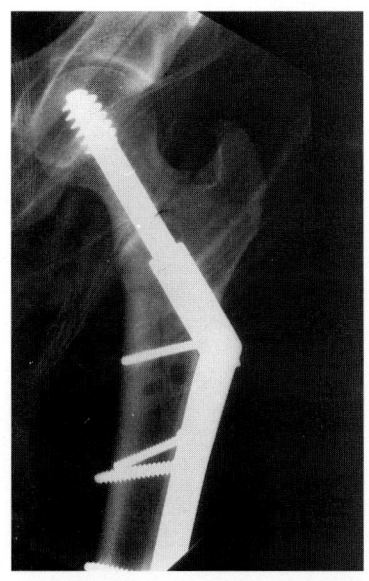

Figure 7.14. Photograph of a sliding hip screw (**A**). AP radiograph demonstrating use of a sliding hip screw to stabilize an intertrochanteric–subtrochanteric fracture (**B**).

Treatment

failure in a series of 38 subtrochanteric fractures stabilized using a sliding hip screw and bone graft.[4] Ruff and Lubbers reported fracture union in 43 of a series of 45 subtrochanteric fractures (95%) treated with a sliding screw-plate device.[29] Fractures were stabilized in a valgus position (mean angle: 140°), with primary medial displacement of the femoral shaft in 25 patients. Radiographic analysis of the degree of postoperative impaction of the fragments correlated with fracture pattern: fractures with medial cortical comminution were at the greatest risk for fracture-related complications.

Mullaji and Thomas reported the results of low-energy subtrochanteric fractures in 31 elderly patients 70 years of age or older whose fractures were stabilized using a sliding hip screw.[30] Interfragmentary lag screws were placed whenever possible. Of the 22 surviving patients at 6-month follow-up, 20 (91%) had successful union. Parker et al. reported on a prospective series of 103 consecutive patients who sustained a subtrochanteric fracture. Among the 74 fractures stabilized with a sliding hip screw, there were only 6 failures of fixation (8%).

A modification of the sliding hip screw, the Medoff sliding plate (Wright Medical, Arlington, TN) was designed to allow compression along both the axis of the femoral neck and the longitudinal axis of the femoral shaft (Figure 7.15). Although it uses a large-diameter lag screw, similar to a sliding hip screw, to allow compression along the axis of the femoral neck, instead of the usual sideplate of the sliding hip screw it employs a sliding component to enable the fracture to impact parallel to the longitudinal axis of the femur. A distal compression screw allows intraoperative longitudinal compression along the femoral shaft. A locking set screw may be used to prevent independent sliding of the lag screw (Figure 7.16); if the locking set screw is engaged to prevent sliding of the lag screw within the barrel, the plate can only slide axially on

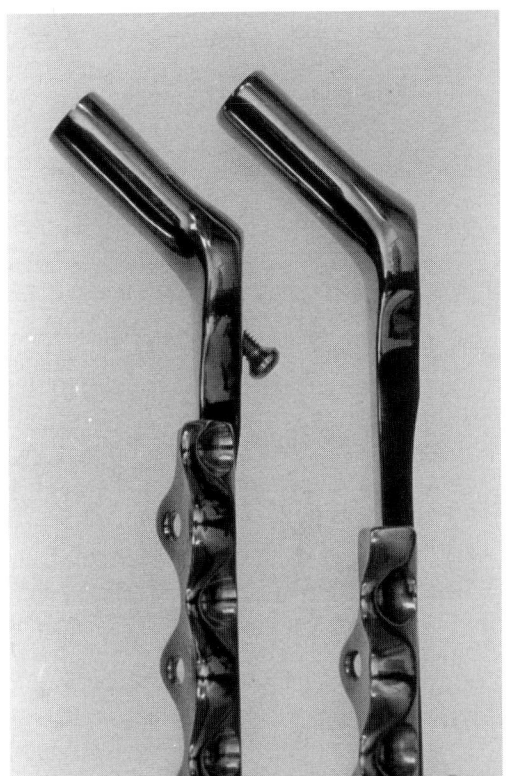
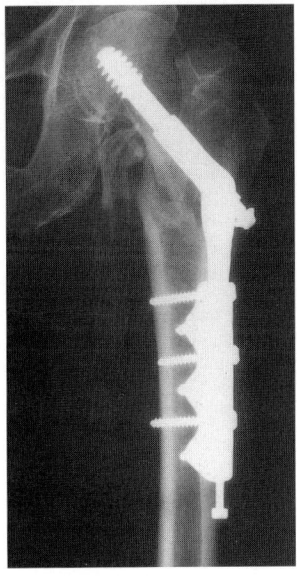

Figure 7.15. Photograph of the Medoff sliding plate (**A**). AP radiograph demonstrating use of the Medoff sliding plate to stabilize a subtrochanteric fracture (**B**).

Figure 7.16. A locking set screw may be used to prevent independent sliding of the lag screw; if the locking set screw is engaged to prevent sliding of the lag screw within the barrel, the plate can only slide axially on the femoral shaft (uniaxial dynamization). If, however, the surgeon implants the device without the locking set screw in place, sliding may occur along the femoral neck and the femoral shaft (biaxial dynamization).

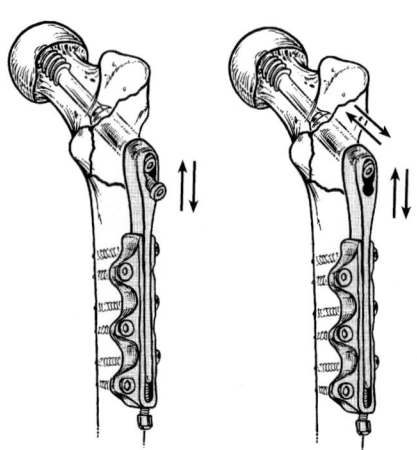

the femoral shaft (uniaxial dynamization). If, however, the surgeon implants the device without the locking set screw in place, sliding may occur along the femoral neck and the femoral shaft (biaxial dynamization). This device has some of the features of an intramedullary nail when used for subtrochanteric fracture fixation; it can act as an extramedullary dynamically locked device. It may be most useful for subtrochanteric fracture fixation by surgeons unfamiliar or uncomfortable with closed intramedullary nailing techniques.

Although good results have been reported with use of the Medoff plate for stabilization of intertrochanteric fractures, there are few reports regarding the use of this device in subtrochanteric fractures. Ceder et al. reported the results of 32 consecutive subtrochanteric fractures stabilized using the Medoff sliding plate and followed up prospectively for 1 year.[31] Two patients died during the first postoperative year; of the remaining 30, 29 (97%) of the fractures united. Two types of plate dynamization schema were used: uniaxial (in 17 patients) and biaxial (in 15 patients). With uniaxial dynamization, plate sliding averaged 12 mm along the femoral shaft without medialization of the femoral shaft. With biaxial dynamization along both the femoral shaft and the neck, plate sliding averaged 11 mm and screw-barrel sliding averaged 9 mm; medialization of the femoral shaft ranged from 0 to 35% of the femoral shaft diameter. Three fractures treated with uniaxial dynamization exhibited migration of the lag screw within the femoral head; all three fractures united without further screw migration after secondary or staged biaxial plate dynamization was performed. Based on these results, the authors concluded that uniaxial dynamization was preferred in pure subtrochanteric fractures, with staged biaxial dynamization reserved for combined intertrochanteric and subtrochanteric fractures, or if the early postoperative radiographs demonstrate complete plate sliding.

For most subtrochanteric femur fractures, the implant of choice is an intramedullary nail. Biomechanically, these devices offer several advantages over plate and screw fixation:

1. Because the intramedullary canal is closer to the central axis of the femur than the usual plate position on the external surface of the bone, intramedullary nails are subjected to smaller bending loads than plates and are thus less vulnerable to fatigue failure (Figure 7.17);
2. Intramedullary nails act as load-sharing devices in fractures that have cortical contact of the major fragments. If the nail is not locked at both the proximal and distal ends, it will act as a gliding splint and allow continued compression as the fracture is loaded;

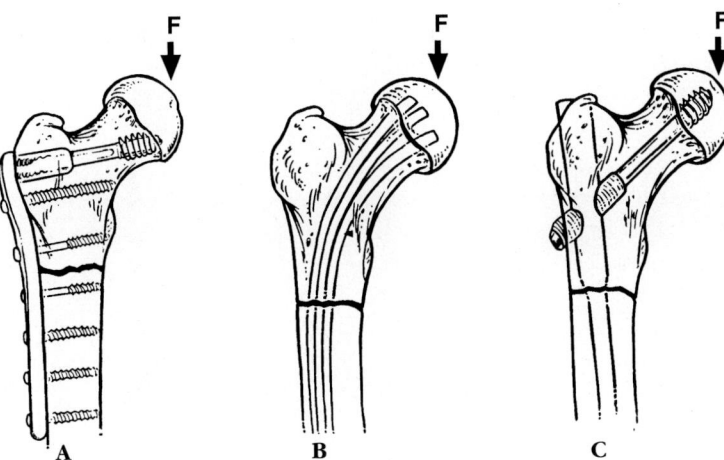

Figure 7.17. Because the intramedullary canal is closer to the central axis of the femur than the usual plate position on the external surface of the bone, intramedullary nails (**B,C**) are subjected to smaller bending loads than plates (**A**) and are thus less vulnerable to fatigue failure.

3. Stress shielding with resultant cortical osteopenia, commonly seen with plates and screws, is avoided with intramedullary devices; and
4. Refracture after implant removal is rare with the use of intramedullary devices, secondary to the lack of cortical osteopenia and the minimum number of stress risers created in the cortical bone.

Intramedullary devices also offer significant biological advantages over other fixation methods. Although insertion can be technically demanding, intramedullary implants do not usually require the extensile exposures required for plate application. With use of image intensification, these devices can be implanted in a "closed" manner, without exposing the fracture site. These "closed" techniques result in low infection and high union rates, with a minimum of soft tissue scarring. One review of the literature reported an infection rate for closed intramedullary femoral nailing of femoral shaft fractures of 0.4%, with a nonunion rate of 1.0%.[32] Early range of motion of the extremity is allowable, even desirable, and in stable fractures, weight bearing is permitted—another advantage conferred by the biomechanical properties of these devices.

Intramedullary nails can be categorized as either centromedullary, condylocephalic, or cephalomedullary.[10] Centromedullary nails are contained within the medullary canal and are usually inserted from the piriformis fossa; if the centromedullary nail is of the interlocked variety, the locking screws are inserted into the metaphyseal–diaphyseal region proximally and distally. Condylocephalic nails (e.g., Ender nails) are inserted from the femoral condyle and extend into the femoral head and neck. Cephalomedullary nails are interlocked centromedullary nails with screw/blade devices that can be inserted cephalad into the femoral head and neck; examples are the Zickel nail and the Russell-Taylor reconstruction nail.

Intramedullary devices became popular for the treatment of subtrochanteric fractures in part because of the problems encountered with the use of fixed-angle nail plates. The Zickel nail, introduced in the early 1970s, is pre-bent to accommodate the anterior bow of the femur (Figure 7.18). The trochanteric section is wide, but it tapers distally to accommodate the midshaft area in sizes ranging from 11 to 15 mm. Fixation of the proximal fragment is supplemented by a modified triflanged nail that is passed through the proximal portion of the nail into the femoral neck. Initially implanted in an open procedure with exposure of the fracture site, the Zickel nail can be implanted using a closed technique. Despite reports of successful use of the Zickel nail for stabilization

Figure 7.18. Photograph and drawing of the Zickel nail (**A**) (courtesy of R. A. Calandruccio, The Campbell Clinic Foundation, Memphis, TN). Radiograph demonstrating use of a Zickel nail to stabilize a subtrochanteric fracture (**B**).

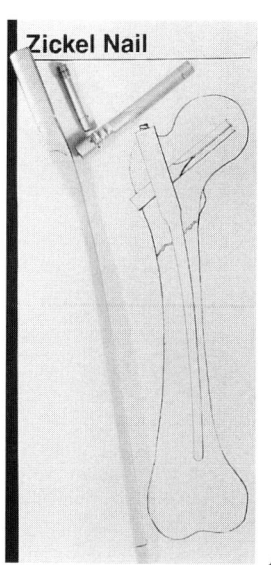 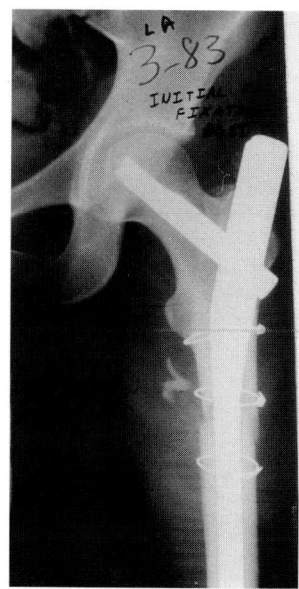

of pathologic subtrochanteric fractures, one must keep in mind that it has no distal locking capability and may require supplemental fracture fixation such as cerclage wiring for axial and torsional stability.

Among the several reports of satisfactory results using Zickel nails to stabilize subtrochanteric fractures is the one by Bergman et al., who studied a series of 131 such fractures with patients divided into four clinical groups[11]: (1) elderly patients with fracture secondary to minor trauma; (2) patients with fracture due to high-energy trauma; (3) patients with a pathologic fracture; and (4) patients with a fracture that previously had been treated unsuccessfully with internal fixation. Overall satisfactory results were obtained in 90% of cases, with a nonunion rate of 5%. Iatrogenic proximal femoral shaft fracture, however, has been reported to occur during removal of Zickel nails.[11,33] This appears to be a result of the excessive stress on the proximal femur due to the anterior and valgus angulation of the nail. The development of first- and second-generation interlocked nails have supplanted the Zickel nail for stabilization of subtrochanteric fractures.

Ender nails have been used extensively for subtrochanteric fracture stabilization, with varying results (Figure 7.19). These flexible nails are usually inserted retrograde into the femoral canal in a stacked fashion to provide fracture stability. As with the Zickel nail, use of flexible Ender nails may require supplemental fracture fixation such as cerclage wire for axial and torsional stability. The theoretical advantages of Ender nails include limited surgical exposure, lower blood loss, and decreased operative time compared with plate-and-screw fixation. These advantages are somewhat blunted, however, if comminution or an inability to obtain a closed reduction make it necessary to expose the fracture site.

High complication rates have been reported with use of Ender nails for stabilization of subtrochanteric fractures. The most common complications include nail migration, loss of fixation, malrotation deformity, and knee pain[34–38] (Figure 7.20). Early revision surgery rates ranging from 10% to 32% have been reported.[34–38] Furthermore, use of Ender nails has been associated with restricted knee motion and knee pain secondary to nail backout (Figure 7.21) and iatrogenic distal femur fracture secondary to the stress riser effect of the medial and/or lateral portals required for nail insertion. Consequently, use of

Treatment

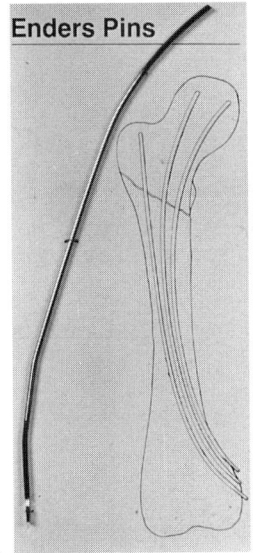
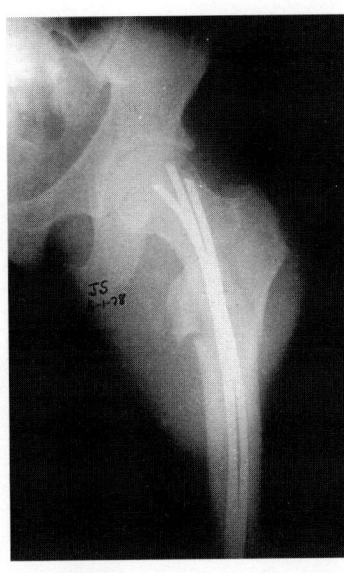

Figure 7.19. Photograph and drawing of Ender nails (**A**) (courtesy of R. A. Calandruccio, The Campbell Clinic Foundation, Memphis, TN). Radiograph of a subtrochanteric fracture stabilized with retrograde-inserted Ender nails (**B**).

Ender nails for subtrochanteric femur stabilization is generally indicated only in (1) debilitated elderly patients who are such poor operative candidates that they can tolerate only minimal operative intervention; or (2) patients with severe soft tissue injury around the proximal thigh in whom distal retrograde implant insertion is desirable. The advent of interlocked nails designed specifically for retrograde insertion however, may result in abandonment of Ender nails for even the limited indications cited above.

Virtually any subtrochanteric fracture, regardless of fracture pattern or degree of comminution, can be stabilized using an interlocked nail. The favorable mechanical characteristics of interlocking nails have eliminated the requirement of surgically reconstituting the medial femoral cortex. Conventional

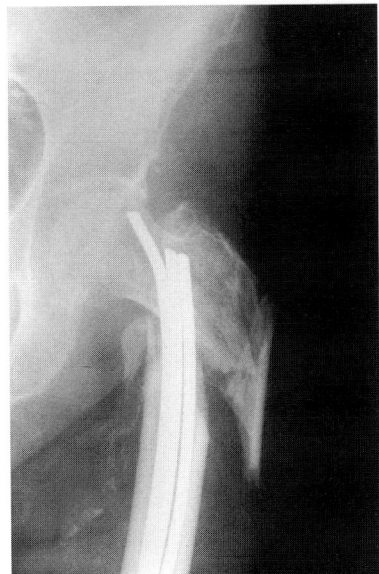

Figure 7.20. Loss of fixation in a subtrochanteric fracture stabilized with multiple Ender nails.

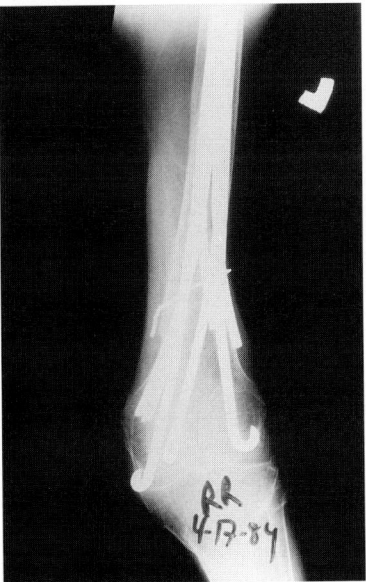

Figure 7.21. Backout of the Ender nails at the knee.

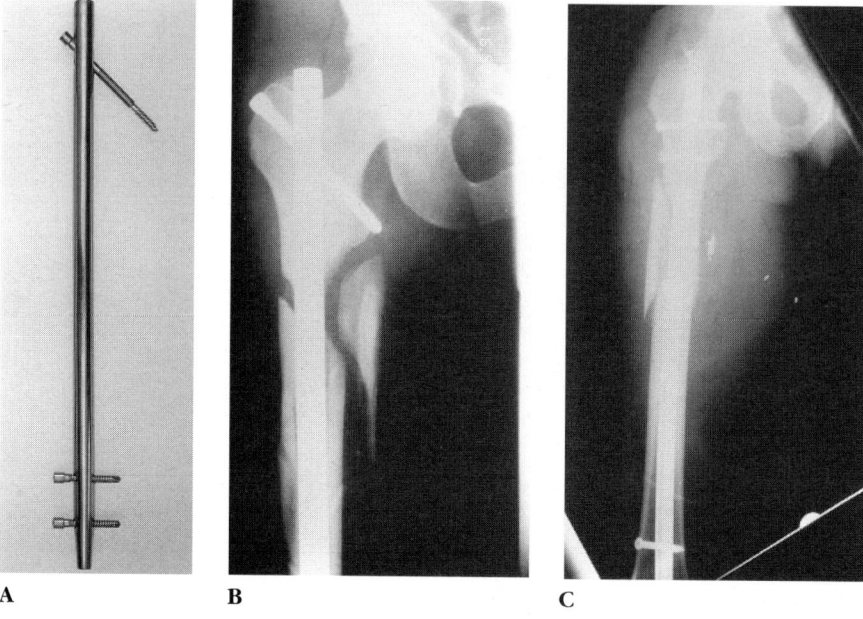

Figure 7.22. Photograph of a centromedullary (first-generation) interlocked nail (**A**). Radiograph of a centromedullary nail with an oblique proximal locking bolt (**B**) and one with transverse proximal locking bolts (**C**).

(first-generation) interlocked nails are inserted through the piriformis fossa, and their transverse or oblique proximal locking bolts are directed into the subtrochanteric region (Figure 7.22). Consequently, they require that the lesser trochanter be attached to the proximal fragment for adequate fracture stabilization. Cephalomedullary (second-generation) interlocked nails (e.g., reconstruction nail [Smith+Nephew, Memphis, TN]) provide fixation of the femoral head and neck and can be used to stabilize proximal fractures that lack an intact posteromedial support (Figure 7.23).

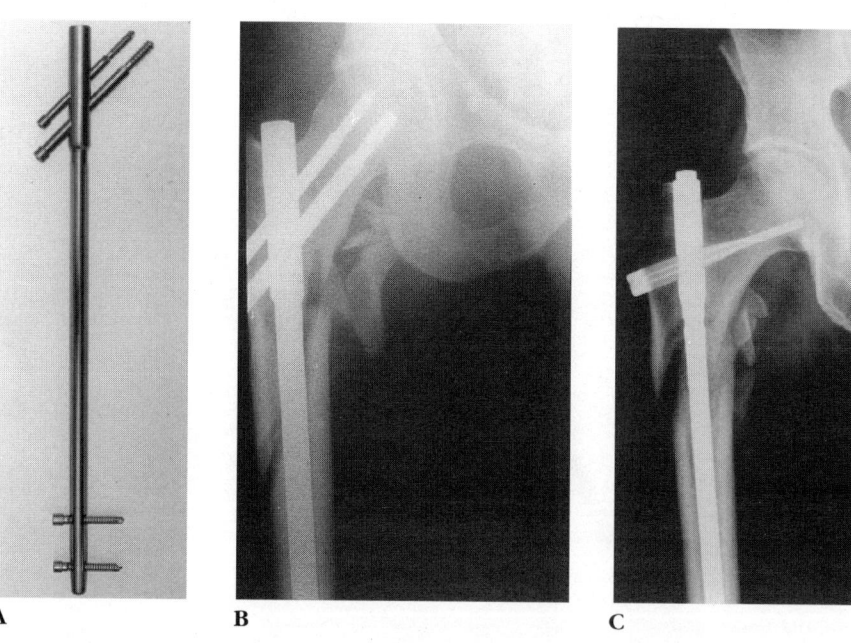

Figure 7.23. Photograph of a cephalomedullary (second-generation) interlocked nail (**A**). Radiograph of a cephalomedullary nail with proximal locking screws (**B**) and one with a spiral blade (**C**).

High rates of union have been reported in large series of subtrochanteric femur fractures stabilized with an interlocked nail.[39–41] Alho et al. reported on a series of 31 subtrochanteric fractures in which the trochanteric area was intact and that were stabilized using a first-generation (centromedullary) interlocked femoral nail.[39] Patient age averaged 24 years (range, 14 to 79 years). Sixteen fractures were comminuted, and 11 were a component of severe multiple injury. All fractures united within 40 weeks, with 16 results graded as excellent, 7 as good, 7 as fair, and 1 as poor. Six fair results were secondary to difficulty aligning the short proximal fragment. One patient with a fair and another with a poor result had excessive shortening of the femur. No infections or other serious complications developed. The authors concluded that locked intramedullary nailing is an appropriate treatment option for subtrochanteric fractures and that static locking is preferable whenever fracture stability is uncertain.

Wu et al. reported on a prospective series of 31 subtrochanteric fractures stabilized with an interlocked nail and followed for a minimum of 1 year.[40] The union rate was 87.1% (27/31); knee range of motion in 28 acute trauma cases averaged 127.5° ± 23.0°. Notable complications included nail breakage (3.2%, 1/31), nonunion without nail breakage (9.7%, 3/31), and malunion (3.2%, 1/31). Wiss and Brien reported the results of 95 subtrochanteric femur fractures stabilized with an interlocked intramedullary nail, of which 89 were treated using a closed insertion technique[41]; the union rate was 95% with an average time to healing of 25 weeks. Like Wu et al., these authors concluded that closed interlocked nailing is the treatment of choice for subtrochanteric fractures.

Slater et al. reported the results of 64 consecutive unstable subtrochanteric fractures treated with the Russell-Taylor reconstruction nail.[42] The majority were the result of a high-energy injury; there were 56 closed and 8 open fractures. Fifty-nine percent of fractures involved loss of the medial femoral cortex or a fracture of the lesser trochanter. Twenty-two percent had fracture extension into the trochanteric mass or piriformis fossa region. Seventy-four percent of the fractures were highly comminuted. In the 12 cases with extension into the piriformis fossa, intraoperative difficulties were high, occasionally requiring open reduction to establish the entry portal. Sixty-one cases were available for follow-up at an average of 11 months; all fractures united without revision surgery, bone grafting, or dynamization. There were no acute infections, but two patients developed late infections at 16 and 18 months postinjury due to sepsis arising from other, new injuries; both responded to implant removal and administration of antibiotics. Taylor et al. reported their experience using the reconstruction nail in five high-energy comminuted subtrochanteric fractures in young paratroopers.[43] Follow-up averaged 22 months, and clinical results were good in that all servicemen were able to return to parachuting.

French and Tornetta reported the results of 45 Russell-Taylor type 1B subtrochanteric femur fractures stabilized using an interlocked cephalomedullary nail (reconstruction nail).[44] The intraoperative complication rate was 13.5%, with the most frequent complication being varus malreduction. The union rate was 100% at an average of 13.5 weeks after surgery; there were no implant failures. Forty-three of 45 patients (96%) regained more than 120° of knee motion.

Recommendations for Implant Use

In treating subtrochanteric fractures, we generally follow the recommendations of Russell and Taylor on the basis of their classification system with use of an interlocked nail whenever possible.[10]

Figure 7.24. Radiograph of a Russell-Taylor type 1A fracture stabilized using a first-generation (centromedullary) interlocked nail.

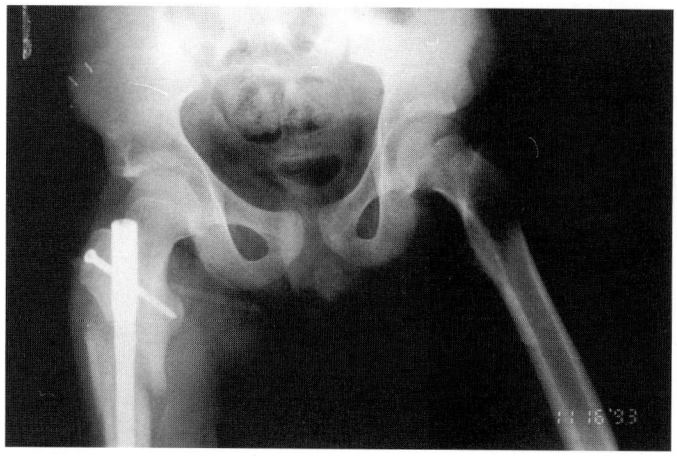

Russell-Taylor type 1A fractures, characterized by an intact piriformis fossa and the lesser trochanter attached to the proximal fragment, are stabilized using a first-generation (centromedullary) interlocked nail (Figure 7.24). Type 1B fractures (intact piriformis fossa, lesser trochanter detached from the proximal fragment) are stabilized using a second-generation (cephalomedullary) interlocked nail (Figure 7.25). Type 2 fractures, characterized by fracture extension into the piriformis fossa, are stabilized using either a 95° fixed-angle plate or a sliding hip screw, depending on the fracture configuration. If the main fracture line is subtrochanteric with minimally displaced fracture extension into the trochanteric region, a 95° fixed-angle device (usually a dynamic condylar screw) is selected for fracture stabilization (Figure 7.26); however, use of the Medoff sliding plate for this fracture has recently yielded excellent results.[31] If the intertrochanteric fracture component is displaced or comminuted, our preference is to use a sliding hip screw or Medoff plate (Figure 7.27).

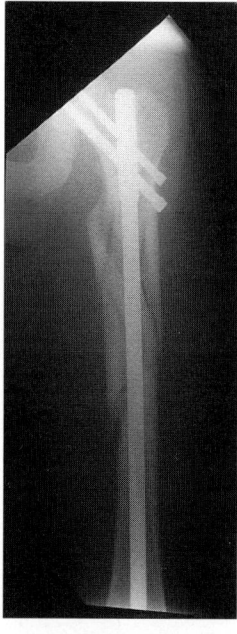

Figure 7.25. Radiograph of a Russell-Taylor type 1B fracture stabilized using a second-generation (cephalomedullary) interlocked nail.

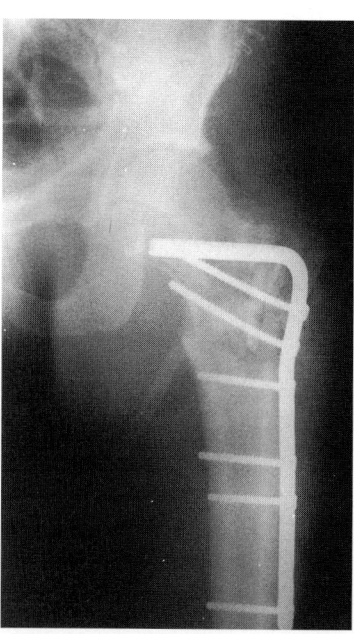

Figure 7.26. Radiograph of a Russell-Taylor type 2 fracture stabilized with a 95° condylar blade plate.

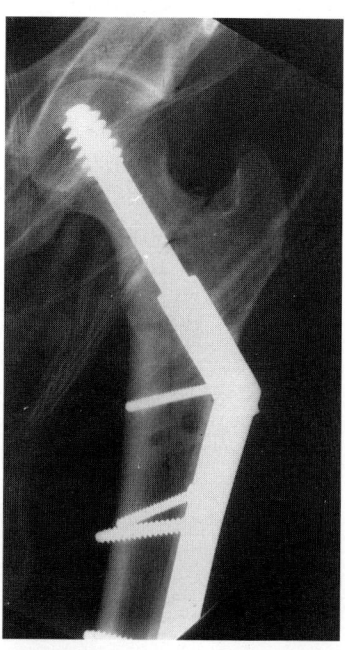

Figure 7.27. Radiograph of a Russell-Taylor type 2 fracture stabilized with a sliding hip screw.

Operative Technique for the 95° Condylar Blade Plate

Preoperative Planning

The exact nature of the fracture should be determined before surgical intervention and all major fracture fragments should be identified; the latter is often facilitated by use of traction radiographs. Radiographs of the contralateral normal extremity can be reversed and serve as templates for preoperative planning. Individual fracture fragments, the implant chosen, and surgical strategy can be drawn on the intact femoral template as a means of helping the surgeon understand the "personality" of the fracture and mentally prepare for the operative procedure (Figure 7.28). Furthermore, with use of a 95° fixed-angle blade plate or condylar screw, preoperative planning allows one to determine optimum placement of the entry point for the blade (or lag screw); this position on the greater trochanter is marked relative to the vastus tubercle. Also noted are the position of the blade (or lag screw) relative to the superior femoral neck and the distance from the tip of the blade plate (or lag screw) to the center of the femoral head. These measurements can serve as a guide to appropriate implant insertion during surgery. The preoperative plan also helps determine the appropriate lengths of the blade and sideplate.

Operative Technique

The patient is placed supine on a radiolucent table or fracture table. Use of a radiolucent operating table allows manipulation of the lower extremity to facilitate fracture reduction and provides adequate fluoroscopic evaluation of the pelvis and femur. Skeletal traction is not necessary with use of a fixed-angle plate; if necessary, intraoperative traction can be applied through use of a femoral distractor or articulating tensioning device. However, visualization of the proximal femur for blade plate insertion is easier when a fracture table is

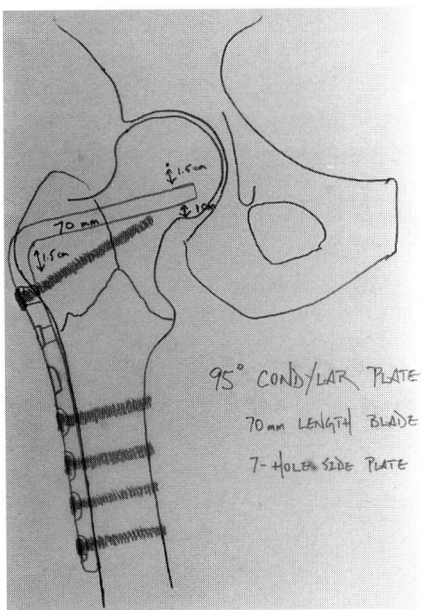

Figure 7.28. Preoperative plan for use of a blade plate to stabilize a subtrochanteric fracture.

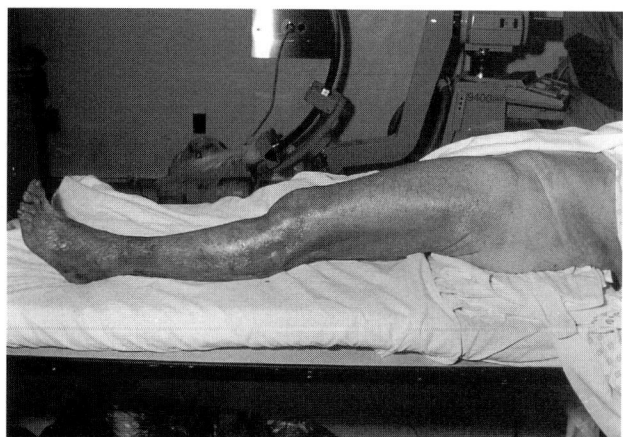

Figure 7.29. Patient positioning on a radiolucent table with a small bolster underneath the buttock on the operative side.

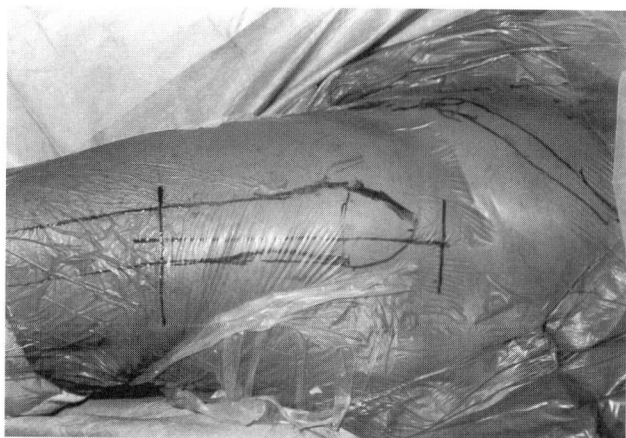

Figure 7.30. The surgical approach is through a straight lateral incision made in the skin along an imaginary line joining the greater trochanter with the lateral femoral condyle.

used. When a radiolucent operating table is used, a small bolster is placed underneath the buttock on the operative side (Figure 7.29); use of a large bolster risks inducing a rotational malalignment. The ipsilateral crest and entire lower extremity are prepared; the leg is draped free, to allow access to the iliac crest for obtaining bone graft and to permit manipulation as needed during surgery.

The surgical approach is through a straight lateral incision made in the skin along an imaginary line joining the greater trochanter with the lateral femoral condyle (Figure 7.30). It should extend from a point above the greater trochanter to approximately a hand's breadth below the fracture. The fascia lata is incised in line with the skin incision. The interval between the tensor fasciae latae muscle and the gluteus medius and gluteus minimus muscles is identified and defined (Figure 7.31). The anterior hip capsule is cleared of soft tissue and incised in line with the femoral neck, exposing the anterior femoral neck. To avoid damage to the blood supply of the femoral head, one should not insert retractors around the superior femoral neck. A blunt retractor is inserted around the inferior aspect of the femoral neck, and a pointed retractor is impacted into the anterior column of the acetabulum.

The vastus lateralis muscle is retracted anteriorly and its origin at the base of the greater trochanter is incised to allow exposure of the lateral femur (Figure 7.32). Rather than a muscle-splitting approach through the vastus lateralis muscle, we prefer to incise the fascia of the vastus lateralis and reflect the muscle from the intermuscular septum. One should take care to identify and ligate the perforators from the profunda femoris artery; otherwise, they may retract posteriorly through the intermuscular septum after being cut and are then difficult to control. The origin of the vastus lateralis muscle on the anterior surface of the intertrochanteric region is also detached, leaving a cuff of tissue for later reattachment.

The blade slot in the proximal fragment is prepared using a seating chisel. One first marks the window for insertion of the seating chisel, located at a given distance from the vastus tubercle as determined by the preoperative plan. This window should lie in the anterior half of the greater trochanter to avoid penetration of the blade through the posterior femoral neck; if the anteroposterior width of the greater trochanter is divided into thirds, the entry window should be at the junction of the anterior and middle thirds (Figure

Treatment

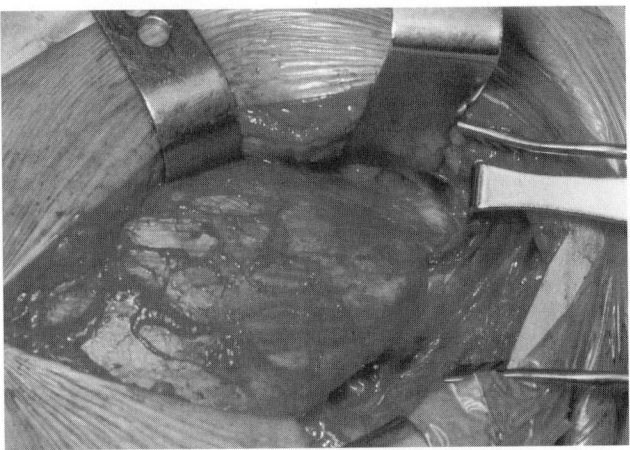

Figure 7.31. The interval between the tensor fasciae latae muscle and the gluteus medius and gluteus minimus muscles is identified and defined.

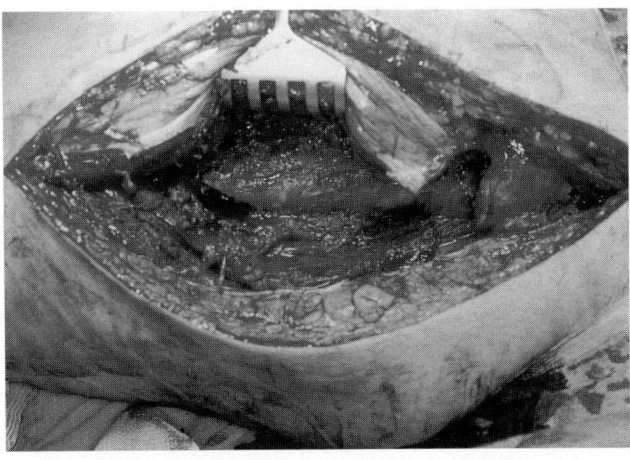

Figure 7.32. Detachment of the vastus lateralis muscle from its origin at the base of the greater trochanter.

7.33). The lateral cortex of proximal femur is opened using 4.5-mm drill bits or an osteotome (Figure 7.34).

The spatial orientation of the seating chisel is determined using Kirschner wires. The first Kirschner guidewire is placed along the anterior femoral neck to mark femoral neck anteversion (Figure 7.35). The second guidewire marks the direction of the seating chisel in the coronal plane. Ideally, it should be inserted at 95° to the anatomic axis of the femur. Placement of this wire can be facilitated by use of the condylar guide placed flush against the lateral cortex of the proximal fragment (Figure 7.36). In a comminuted subtrochanteric fracture that cannot be reduced, one may have to consult the preoperative drawing to establish the direction of this guidewire in relation to such identifiable bone landmarks as the superior cortex of the neck, the center of the femoral head, and the vastus tubercle of the greater trochanter. The second Kirschner wire is driven into the tip of the greater trochanter so as to be out of the way of the seating chisel. It is driven in parallel to the first Kirschner wire, which indicates the anteversion of the femoral neck, and in the same relationship to the superior cortex of the neck and the center of rotation of the femoral head as that marked on the preoperative drawing.

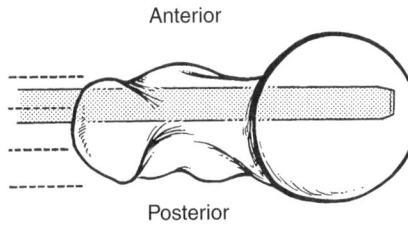

Figure 7.33. The entry site for the condylar blade plate should lie in the anterior half of the greater trochanter to avoid penetration of the blade out the posterior femoral neck If the anteroposterior width of the greater trochanter is divided into thirds, the entry window should lie at the junction of the anterior and middle thirds.

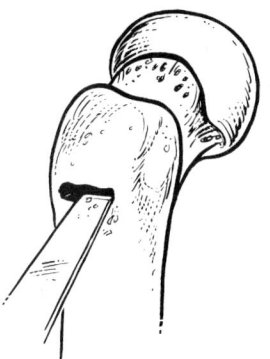

Figure 7.34. Use of an osteotome to open the lateral cortex of the proximal femur.

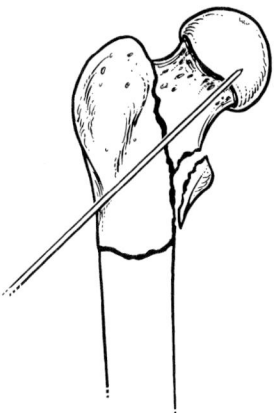

Figure 7.35. The spatial orientation of the seating chisel is determined using Kirschner wires. The first Kirschner guidewire is placed along the anterior femoral neck to mark femoral neck anteversion.

Figure 7.36. Use of the condylar guide to insert the guidewire that marks the direction of the seating chisel in the coronal plane.

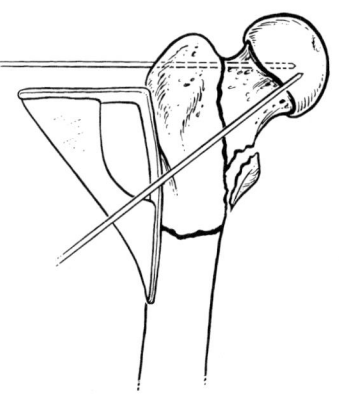

The seating chisel is assembled with its insertion guide; care must be taken to orient the chisel properly on the guide, with the U-shaped seating chisel facing inferiorly. The seating chisel is hammered slowly into the proximal femur, with care taken to keep the blade parallel to the previously placed summation guidewires (Figure 7.37). Flexion and extension of the seating chisel is avoided through use of the seating chisel insertion guide; the flap of the seating chisel insertion guide must be in line with the long axis of the femoral shaft. The seating chisel is slowly advanced into the proximal fragment with alternating forward and backward strokes of the slotted hammer; intermittent disimpaction of the seating chisel from the proximal fragment is important to avoid incarceration of the fully seated chisel in strong cancellous bone. One should carefully monitor the direction of the seating chisel fluoroscopically on both the AP and lateral projections to ensure that it advances within the proximal fragment according to the preoperative plan.

Once the seating chisel has been inserted to the appropriate depth, it is removed and replaced with the condylar blade plate. The appropriate length of the blade is determined by preoperative planning and is verified by direct reading from the calibrated seating chisel (Figure 7.38). Final seating of the blade plate is achieved using an impactor and mallet (Figure 7.39). Occasionally, the plate will not seat flush against the lateral cortex of the proximal fragment. In this situation, osteotomy of the lateral cortex of the proximal fragment distal to the blade with medialization of the blade plate into the proximal fragment will help to improve the plate position (Figure 7.40). Once the plate is fully seated in the proximal fragment, an additional 4.5-mm cortical screw is

Figure 7.37. Insertion of the seating chisel. The seating chisel is hammered slowly into the proximal femur, with care taken to keep the blade parallel to the previously placed summation guidewires (**A**). Flexion and extension of the seating chisel is avoided through use of the seating chisel insertion guide; the flap of the seating chisel insertion guide must be in line with the long axis of the femoral shaft (**B**).

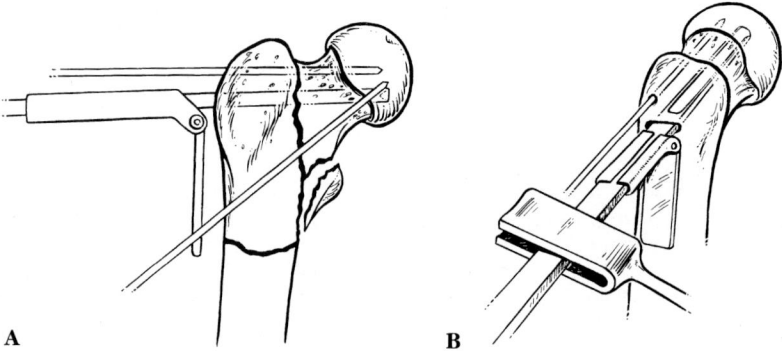

Treatment

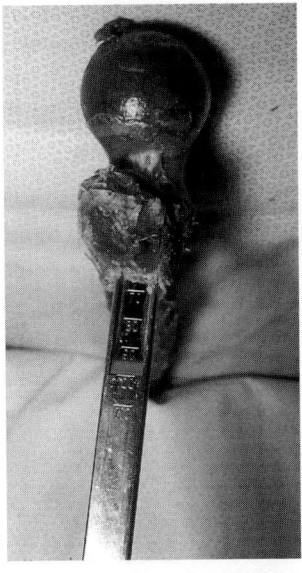

Figure 7.38. Verification of the appropriate blade length by direct reading from the calibrated seating chisel.

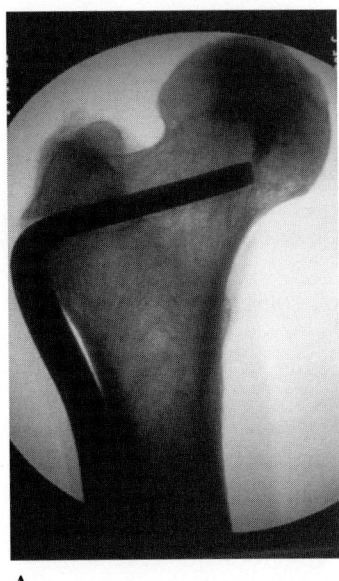
A

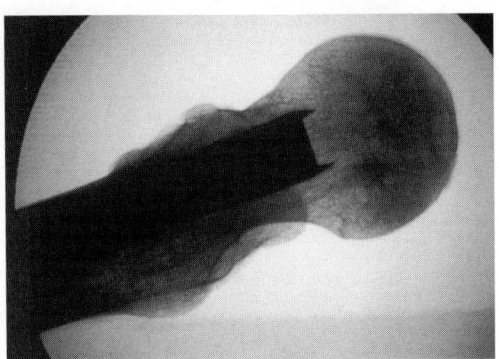
B

Figure 7.39. AP (**A**) and lateral (**B**) radiographs after blade plate insertion.

inserted into the calcar of the proximal fragment through the most proximal hole in the plate (Figure 7.41).

The plate can now be used to effect fracture reduction. To preserve maximum vascularity of the fracture region, no soft tissue dissection or attempts at direct fracture fragment manipulation should be performed. The shaft of the plate is brought to the lateral cortex of the distal fragment, the limb rotation is determined, and the plate is secured with a Verbrugge clamp. Limb length is restored and the fracture fragments are aligned using either an AO/ASIF articulated tensioning device or a femoral distractor. If there is minimal fracture shortening, the articulated tensioning device can be used to distract the fracture fragments, while use of the femoral distractor is reserved for fractures

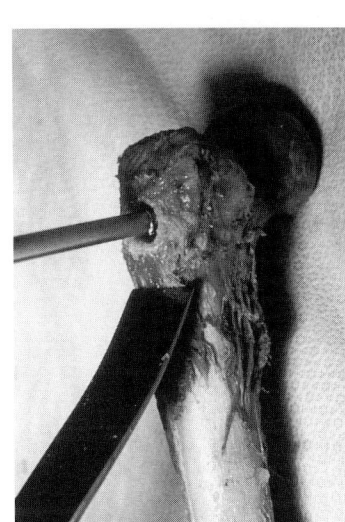

Figure 7.40. If the plate does not seat flush against the lateral cortex of the proximal fragment, osteotomy of the lateral cortex of the proximal femur distal to the blade may help to improve the plate position.

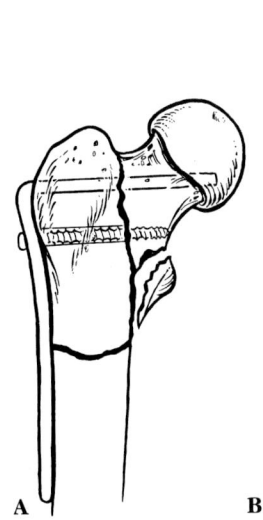
A

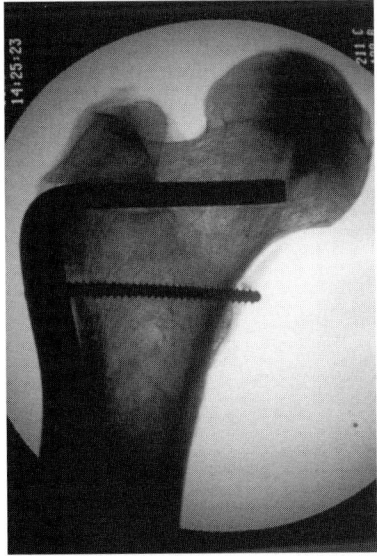
B

Figure 7.41. Placement of an additional 4.5-mm cortical screw into the calcar of the proximal fragment through the most proximal hole in the plate (**A, B**).

with more severe shortening or overlap. Alternatively, one can achieve fracture distraction through use of the fracture table. Use of the articulating tensioning device involves placement of a 4.5-mm cortical screw just distal to the end of the plate. One can use either a unicortical or bicortical screw, depending on bone quality; bicortical fixation is recommended in osteopenic bone. The articulated tensioning device is maximally shortened and assembled onto the cortical screw, the Verbrugge clamp is loosened, and an articulated socket wrench is employed to slowly lengthen the distraction device (Figure 7.42). With appropriate distraction, comminuted medial fragments often reduce spontaneously by their soft tissue attachments (ligamentotaxis). If necessary, displaced medial fragments can be teased into position though the fracture site (Figure 7.43); to avoid soft tissue stripping and osseous devascularization, the fracture fragments should not be manipulated from the medial cortical surface. The goal is anatomic alignment of the femoral shaft, neck, and head, not anatomic reduction of each fracture fragment. If anatomic fracture reduction can be achieved without soft tissue disruption and osseous devascularization, it should be performed; if, however, anatomic fracture reduction would necessitate osseous devascularization, it is better to bridge the fracture site with the plate, leaving the displaced fracture fragments with soft tissue attachments to act as vascularized bone graft.

Once the fracture is aligned and the fracture fragments are reduced, the articulated tensioning device can be used to compress the fracture fragments if the fracture will accept axial compression without loss of reduction (Figure 7.44). Placement of compression across the fracture is important to stabilize the plate–bone construct. Fracture stability can be assessed by determining its ability to sustain a constant level of compression; if the fracture slowly loses its level of compression (as registered by the articulated tensioning device), this is an indication of fracture instability—that is, bone quality and/or fracture pattern are not capable of sustaining osseous compression. If appropriate, the fracture can be further compressed using the self-compressing holes within the blade plate itself and lag screws can be placed across the osseous frag-

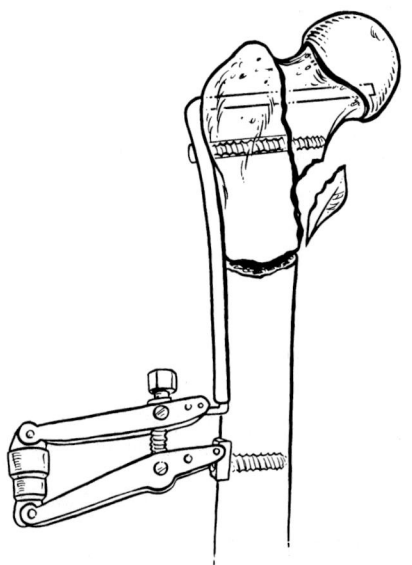

Figure 7.42. Use of an articulated tensioning device to distract the fracture fragments.

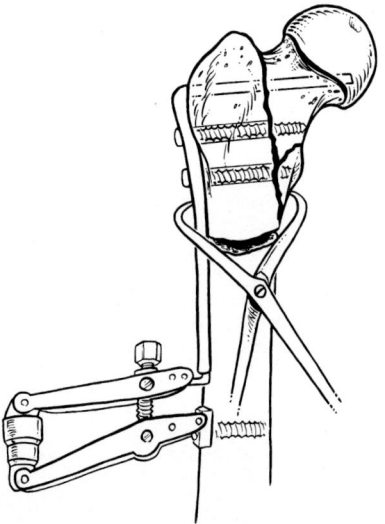

Figure 7.43. Reduction and stabilization of a displaced medial fracture fragment.

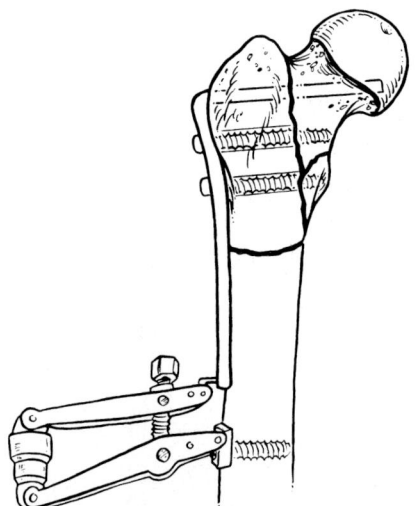

Figure 7.44. Use of the articulated tensioning device to compress the fracture fragments.

Treatment

ments, as determined by the fracture geometry (Figure 7.45). It is not necessary to fill every screw hole in the plate; the number of plate-holding screws required to stabilize a subtrochanteric fracture is dependent on bone quality, fracture pattern, degree of fracture comminution and soft tissue devitalization, amount of osseous compression applied, and plate length. Bone graft is usually not necessary unless soft tissue dissection has resulted in osseous devascularization.[24] If one determines a need for bone graft, it should be inserted through the fracture site, usually before plate application; placement of the bone graft at the end of the procedure usually necessitates further medial soft tissue dissection and osseous devascularization.

In the event of substantial fracture shortening or if additional distraction force is necessary, such as in delayed treatment of a subtrochanteric fracture, the femoral distractor can be used to effect fracture reduction. Placement of the femoral distractor involves placement of a Schanz screw or distractor bolt into the main proximal and distal fracture fragments (Figure 7.46). The proximal screw is optimally placed through one of the proximal plate holes and the distal screw is inserted distal to the plate. Before placement of the screw and bolt, one should ascertain correct limb rotational alignment. The femoral distractor is assembled, secured to the proximal and distal screws and bolts, and used to distract the fracture fragments. Fracture reduction is performed as previously described.

The wound is closed over suction drains after reattachment of the vastus lateralis and fascia lata. The lower extremity is placed in a 90/90 position at the hip and knee; prophylactic perioperative antibiotics are given for 48 hours.

Operative Technique for the 95° Dynamic Condylar Screw

The 95° dynamic condylar screw is a two-piece device with the same basic design as the 95° condylar blade plate except that the blade is replaced by a

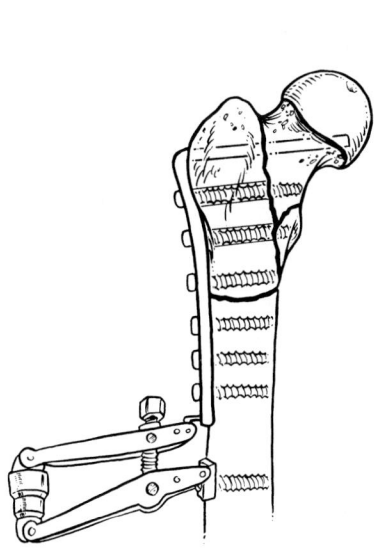

Figure 7.45. Insertion of the remaining plate screws.

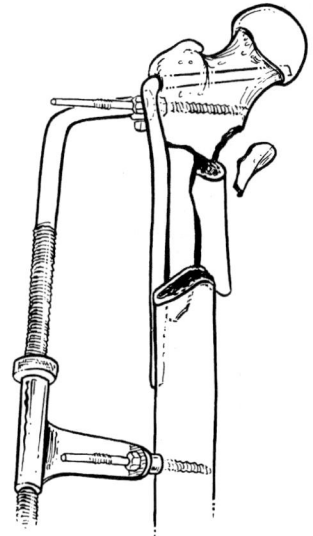

Figure 7.46. Use of a femoral distractor to effect fracture reduction.

large-diameter lag screw. Technically, the 95° dynamic condylar screw is easier to insert than the blade plate; the lag screw is cannulated and is inserted over a guide pin after its channel is reamed and tapped. Varus/valgus malalignment of the guide pin is easily corrected; flexion and extension can be adjusted by rotating the lag screw. The 95° dynamic condylar screw may provide better purchase in osteopenic bone than the condylar blade plate. However, it does not provide as much control of the proximal fragment as does the 95° condylar blade plate, and it requires insertion of an additional screw through the plate into the proximal fragment for rotational stability.

The technique for insertion of the 95° dynamic condylar screw is similar to that described for the 95° condylar blade plate. The surgical approach and entry point for the guide pin (and ultimately the lag screw) are identical; the entry point for the guide pin lies in the anterior half of the greater trochanter, at a position relative to the vastus tubercle determined either by preoperative planning or by use of the condylar guide (Figure 7.47). The spatial orientation of the guide pin is also directed by the anteversion of the femoral neck, which can be determined with use of a guidewire placed over the anterior femoral neck or by direct visualization of the femoral neck after incising the hip capsule. When properly inserted, the guide pin should be no closer than 1 cm from the superior cortex of the femoral neck. Once optimized in both the AP and lateral planes, the guide pin is advanced until its tip is located approximately 1 to 2 cm from the articular surface of the inferior aspect of the femoral head (Figure 7.48). The length of the guide pin is measured (Figure 7.49), and the tract for the lag screw is reamed over that of the guide pin (Figure 7.50). We recommend use of the tap prior to lag screw insertion—regardless of patient age—to minimize the risk of the proximal fragment rotating during placement of the lag screw. The lag screw is then inserted (Figure 7.51) and seated such that the keyed plate can be slid over the screw in line with the femoral shaft (Figure 7.52). The plate is seated against the femoral shaft, the compression screw is inserted, and at least one screw is placed through the plate into the proximal fragment (Figure 7.53); the compression screw prevents disengagement of the lag screw from the barrel, while insertion of a screw through the plate into the proximal fragment prevents the proximal fragment from rotating around the lag screw during the remainder of the fracture reduction. Once the plate is attached to the proximal fragment, the remainder of the fracture reduction is performed as described for use of the 95° condylar blade plate (Figure 7.54).

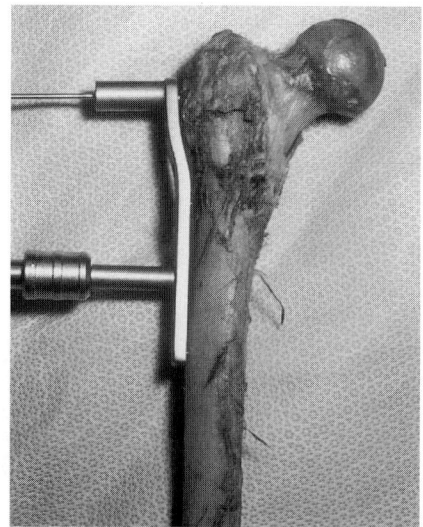

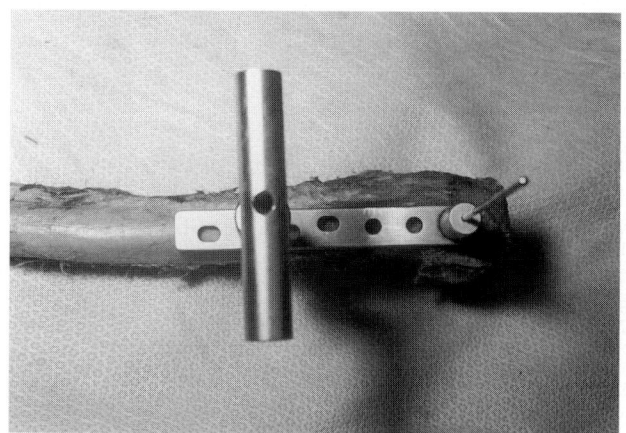

Figure 7.47. Use of the condylar guide from the dynamic condylar screw set to determine the entry point for the guide pin (**A, B**).

A B

Treatment

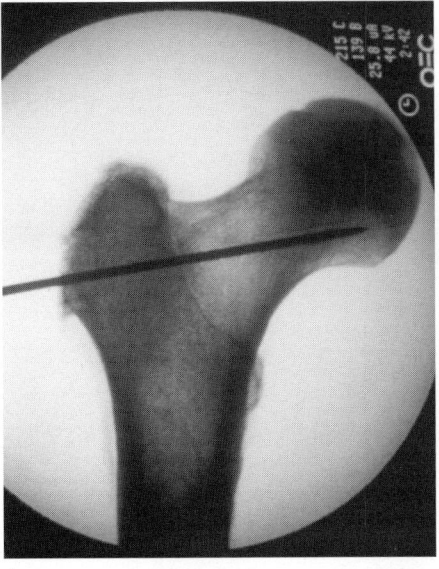

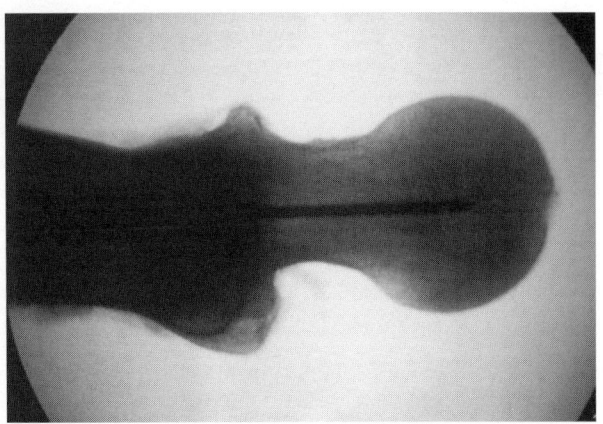

Figure 7.48. Once optimized in both the AP and lateral planes, the guide pin is advanced until its tip is located approximately 1 to 2 cm from the articular surface of the inferior aspect of the femoral head (**A, B**).

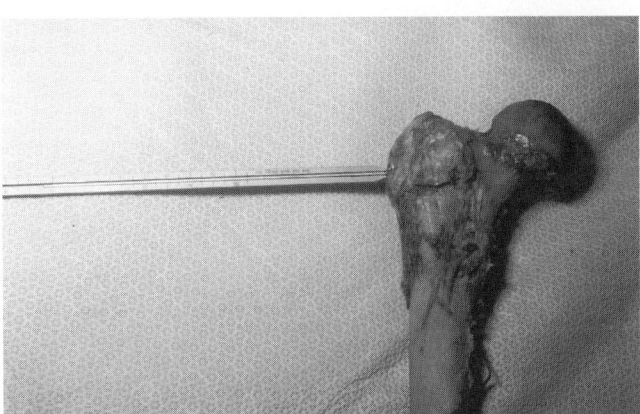

Figure 7.49. Determination of the lag screw length using a cannulated depth gauge.

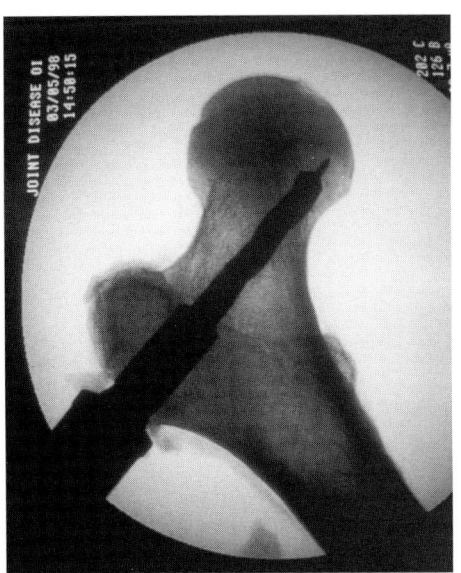

Figure 7.50. Reaming of the proximal femur over the guide pin.

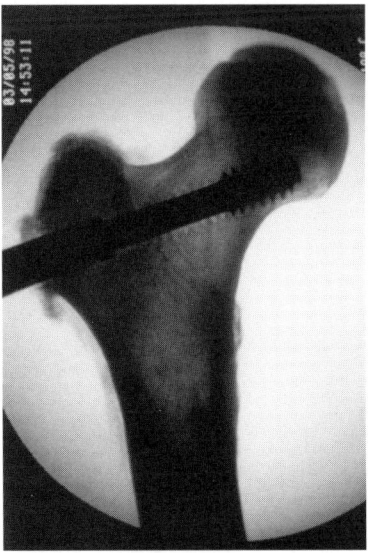

Figure 7.51. Placement of the lag screw.

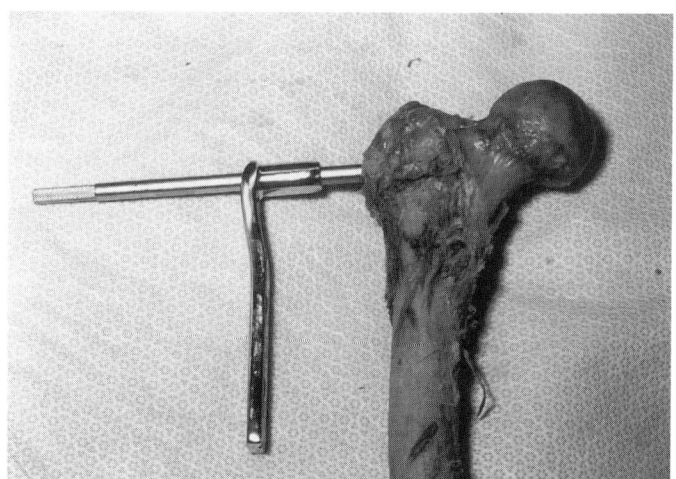
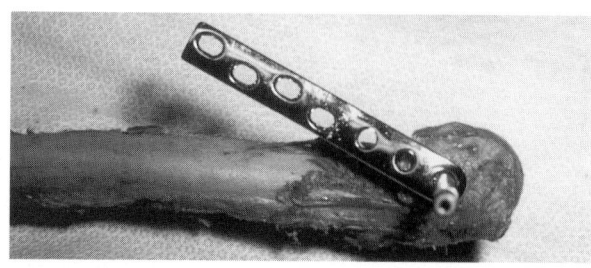
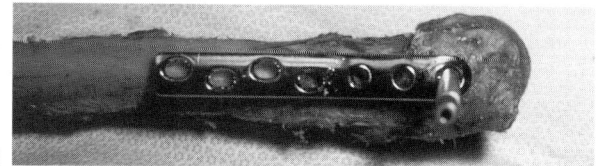

Figure 7.52. Insertion of the 95° plate over the lag screw (**A**). The plate can be rotated (**B**) until it is in line with the femoral shaft (**C**).

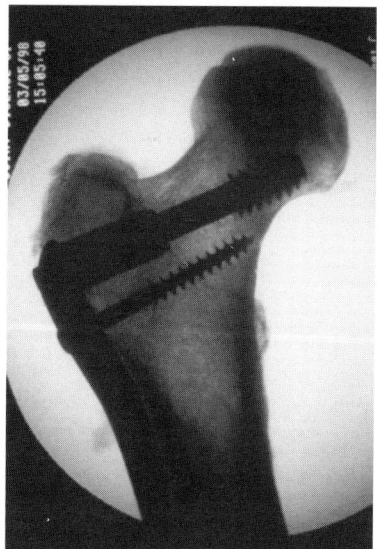

Figure 7.53. The plate is seated against the femoral shaft, the compression screw is inserted, and at least one screw is placed through the plate into the proximal fragment

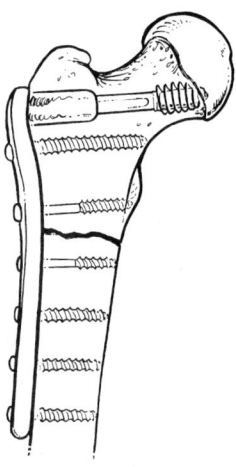

Figure 7.54. Once the plate is attached to the proximal fragment, the remainder of the fracture reduction is performed as described with use of the 95° condylar blade plate.

Operative Technique for the Sliding Hip Screw

The operative technique for achieving subtrochanteric fracture fixation using a sliding hip screw device is similar to that employed for intertrochanteric fractures (Figure 7.55). A fracture table is used, although there is an increased likelihood of posterior sag, which can be corrected by placement of a crutch under the proximal thigh. The operative approach and insertion of the lag screw are performed exactly as described for intertrochanteric fractures; with

Treatment

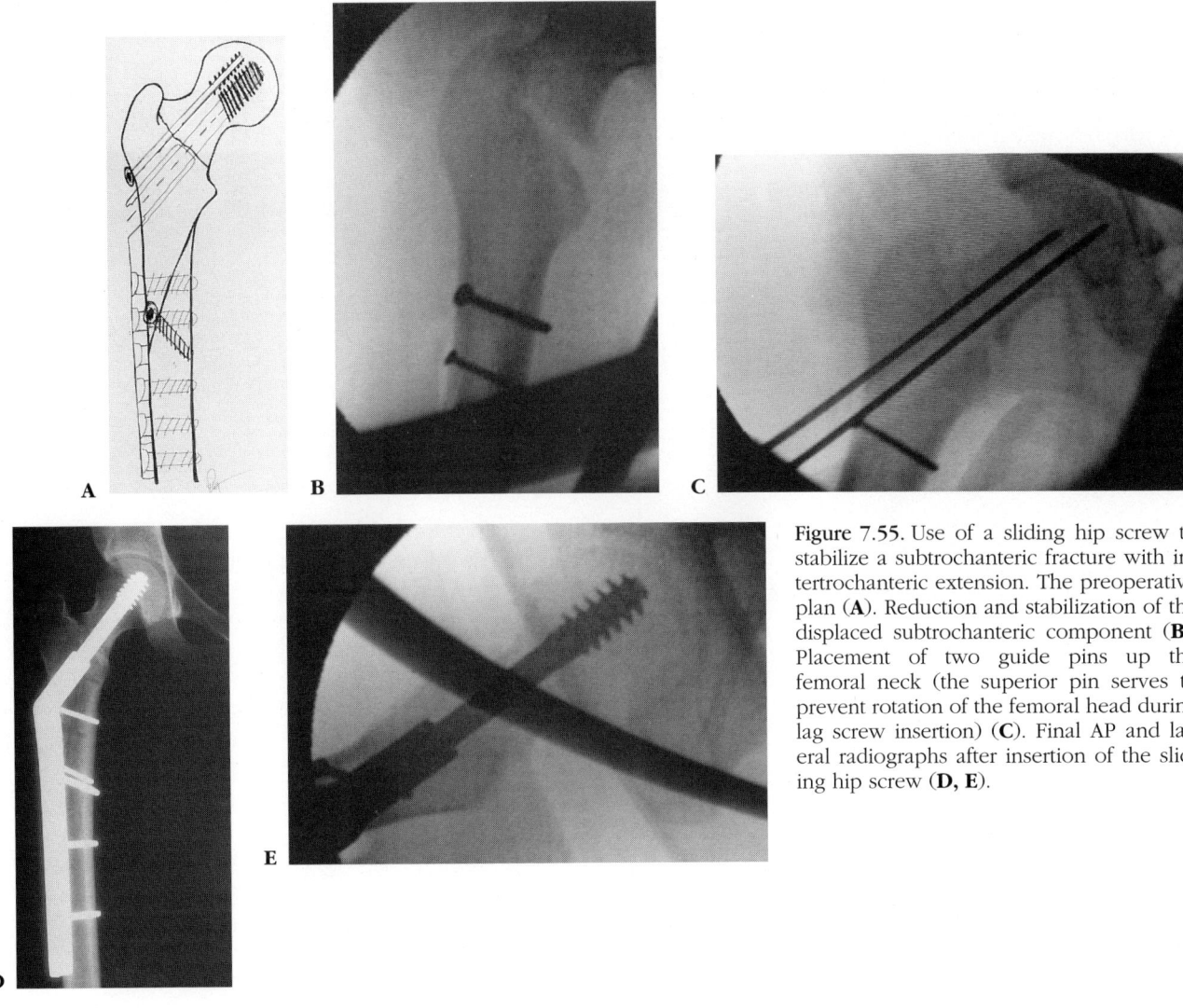

Figure 7.55. Use of a sliding hip screw to stabilize a subtrochanteric fracture with intertrochanteric extension. The preoperative plan (**A**). Reduction and stabilization of the displaced subtrochanteric component (**B**). Placement of two guide pins up the femoral neck (the superior pin serves to prevent rotation of the femoral head during lag screw insertion) (**C**). Final AP and lateral radiographs after insertion of the sliding hip screw (**D, E**).

subtrochanteric fractures, however, it is essential to reconstruct the posteromedial cortical buttress to minimize the risk of varus displacement and implant failure. One can reduce and stabilize the subtrochanteric fracture fragments before insertion of the sliding hip screw by using lag screws or cerclage wire, keeping in mind that injudicious soft tissue stripping increases the risk of delayed union and implant failure. Alternatively, one can insert the lag screw and sideplate and then attempt to reduce and stabilize the posteromedial fracture fragments to the plate. In pure subtrochanteric fractures, one should place an additional screw through the sideplate into the head and neck fragment to prevent rotation of this fragment around the lag screw.

Operative Technique for the Medoff Sliding Plate

Although the surgical technique for the Medoff sliding plate is similar to that described for the standard sliding hip screw, two additional factors must be considered. First, if the fracture line is distal to the entry hole of the lag screw

Figure 7.56. If the fracture line is distal to the entry hole of the lag screw (i.e., pure subtrochanteric fracture), no modification of the lateral cortex is required (**A**). If, however, the fracture line extends into the intertrochanteric region, it is necessary to enlarge the distal aspect of the lag screw entry hole by approximately 2.5 cm to prevent the sideplate barrel from impinging on the lateral cortex of the distal fragment and obstructing dynamic axial slide (**B**).

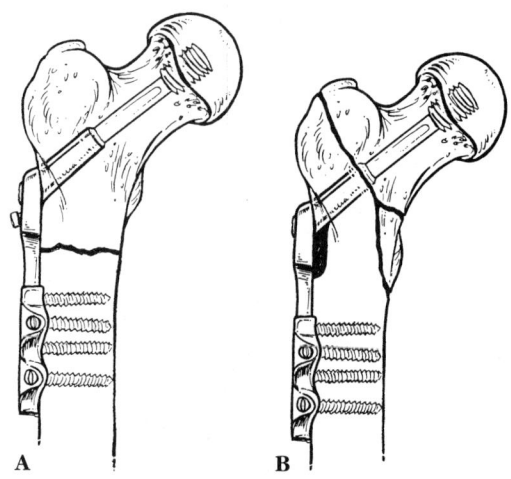

(i.e., pure subtrochanteric fracture), no modification of the lateral cortex is required (Figure 7.56). If, however, the fracture line extends into the intertrochanteric region, it is necessary to enlarge the distal aspect of the lag screw entry hole by approximately 2.5 cm to prevent the sideplate barrel from impinging on the lateral cortex of the distal fragment and obstructing dynamic axial slide (Figure 7.56). The second consideration regards the locking set screw (Figure 7.57): if it is applied to prevent sliding of the lag screw within the barrel, the plate can only slide axially on the femoral shaft (uniaxial dynamization). If, however, one applies the implant without placement of the locking set screw, sliding may occur along both the femoral neck and the femoral shaft (biaxial dynamization).

The patient is positioned supine on a fracture table and the fracture is reduced. Using a lateral approach to the proximal femur, one inserts a standard lag screw guide pin into the center of the femoral head and neck (Figure 7.58). The Medoff plate is currently available only as a 135° device, so the proper angle guide should be used for lag screw insertion. After inserting the guide pin and reaming and tapping (Figure 7.58), one determines whether to enlarge the lag screw entry hole. In pure subtrochanteric fractures, this enlargement is not necessary. In intertrochanteric fractures and subtrochanteric

Figure 7.57. Use of the locking set screw prevents sliding of the lag screw within the Medoff plate barrel; the plate can only slide axially on the femoral shaft (uniaxial dynamization). If, however, one applies the implant without placement of the locking set screw, sliding may occur along both the femoral neck and the femoral shaft (biaxial dynamization).

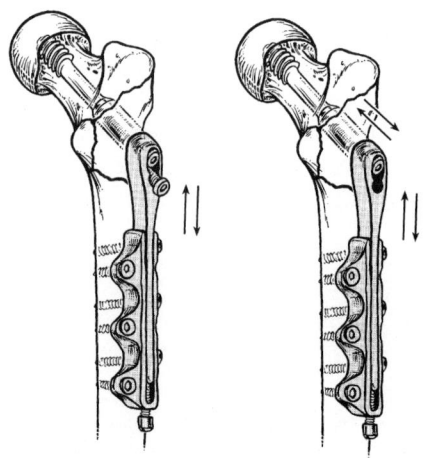

Treatment

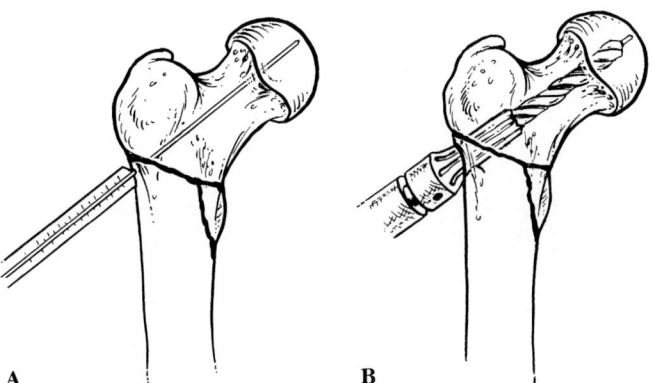

Figure 7.58. Placement of a standard lag screw guide pin into the center of the femoral head and neck (**A**), followed by reaming of the proximal femur (**B**).

fractures with intertrochanteric extension (Russell-Taylor type 2 fractures), the lag screw entry hole is distally slotted approximately 2.5 cm to allow axial slide. The hole can be slotted by placing a second unicortical guide pin through the lateral cortex approximately 1 cm distal to the distal extend of the reamed hole (Figure 7.59). The reamer is then collapsed to its lowest limit, and a second hole is reamed more distally in the lateral cortex (Figure 7.60). A rongeur or burr is used to smooth out the connection between the holes into a slot (Figure 7.61). Alternatively, the slot may be made entirely with a rongeur or burr by removing bone from the lateral cortex distal to the initial reamed hole. Because this distal extension (slot) must be wide enough to allow unimpeded axial plate slide, the slot must be at least as wide as the plate barrel. The lag screw is then inserted (Figure 7.62). The Medoff sideplate is adjusted so that 1.5 to 2.0 cm of plate slide is available; it is then inserted over the lag screw (Figure 7.63). There are two sideplate lengths available: four-hole (for intertrochanteric fractures) and six-hole (for subtrochanteric fractures). The plate is curved to fit around the lateral aspect of the femoral shaft and serves to direct the anterior and posterior plate-holding screws such that they converge at a 30° angle (Figure 7.64). Because of this arrangement, it is easiest to

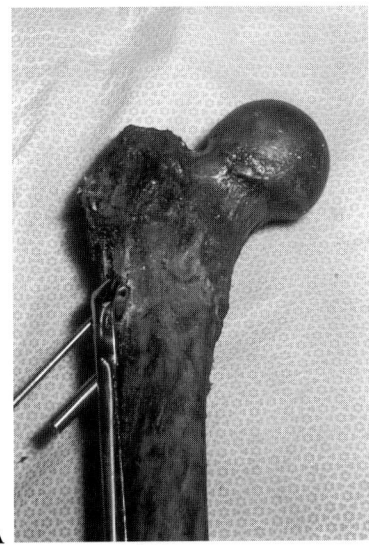

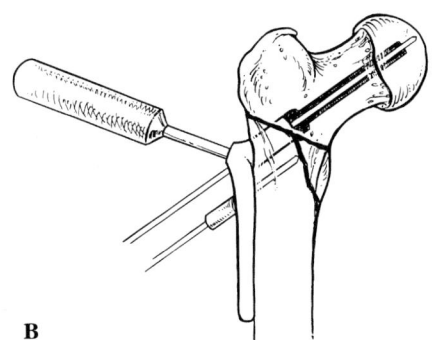

Figure 7.59. Use of a guide to insert a second unicortical guide pin through the lateral cortex approximately 1 cm distal to the distal extend of the reamed hole (**A, B**).

Figure 7.60. The reamer is collapsed to its lowest limit, and a second hole is reamed more distally in the lateral cortex (**A, B**).

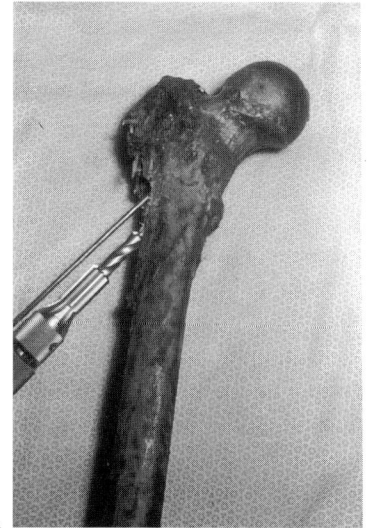
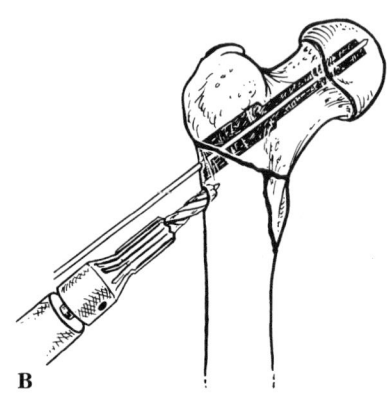

Figure 7.61. A rongeur or burr is used to smooth out the connection between the holes into a slot (**A, B**). Because this distal extension (slot) must be wide enough to allow unimpeded axial plate slide, the slot must be at least as wide as the plate barrel (**C**).

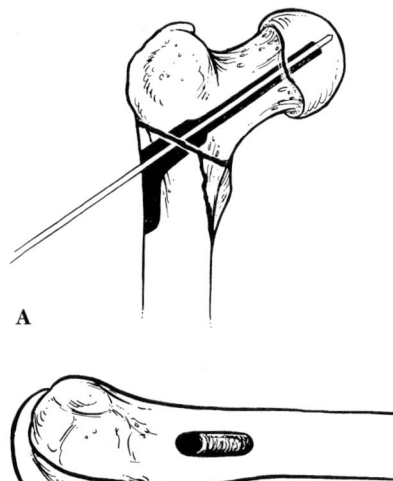
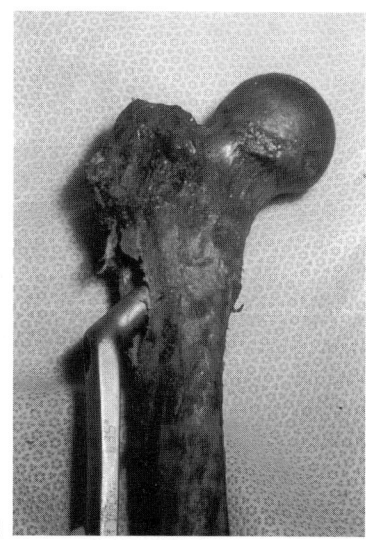

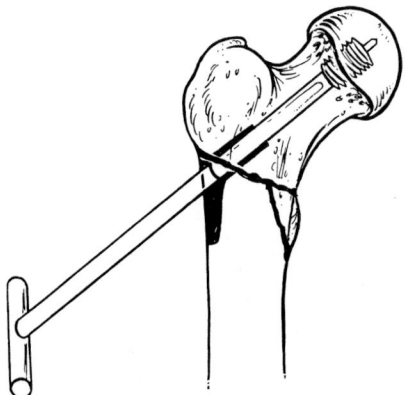

Figure 7.62. Insertion of the lag screw.

Figure 7.63. The Medoff sideplate is adjusted so that 1.5 to 2.0 cm of plate slide is available; it is then inserted over the lag screw. Note the screw that can be used to hold the two plate components together during insertion; this screw is removed after placement of the plate-holding screws.

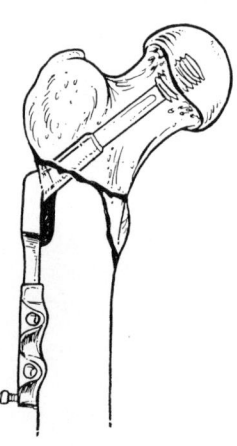

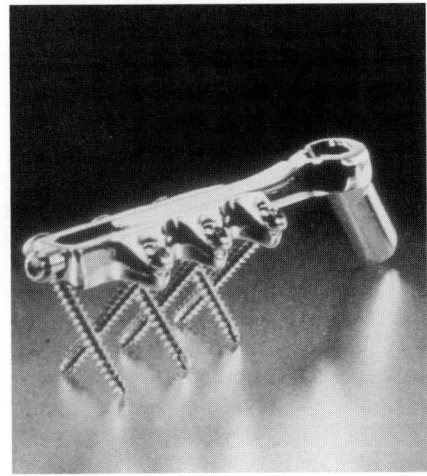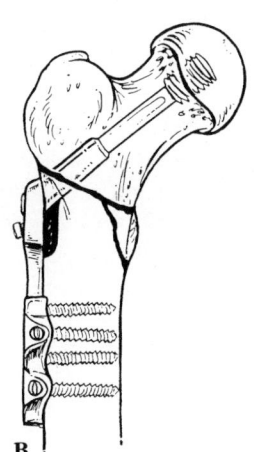

Figure 7.64. The screw holes are designed to direct the anterior and posterior plate-holding screws to converge at a 30° angle (**A**). Insertion of the plate holding screws (**B**).

secure the plate to the femoral shaft by first inserting the anterior screws, internally rotating the lower extremity, and then inserting the posterior screws. One should not attempt to angle the holding screws more than 15° to 30° from the horizontal, or the screws will not fully seat within the plate.

The fracture is next manually impacted after releasing traction from the fracture table. One can insert a set screw to prevent screw-barrel slide along the femoral neck, thus permitting only axial slide along the femoral shaft (uniaxial slide); this configuration, however, is recommended only for pure subtrochanteric fractures (Figure 7.65). For subtrochanteric fractures with intertrochanteric extension, one should allow both axial slide along the femoral shaft and screw-barrel slide along the femoral neck (biaxial slide). As with subtrochanteric fracture fixation using a conventional sliding hip screw, one should attempt to reconstruct the posteromedial cortex to minimize the amount of plate slide and subsequent extremity shortening as well as to decrease the risk of implant failure if the plate utilizes all available slide before fracture impaction.

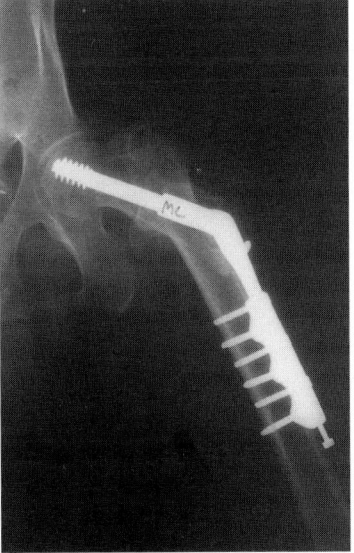

Figure 7.65. Subtrochanteric fracture stabilized with a Medoff sliding plate configured to permit only axial slide along the femoral shaft (uniaxial slide)

Operative Technique for Intramedullary Nail Insertion

Subtrochanteric femur fractures with an intact lesser trochanter and piriformis fossa are best stabilized with a centromedullary (first-generation) interlocked nail. Several studies have reported satisfactory results using reamed interlocked nails for this fracture pattern with either diagonally or transversely oriented proximal interlocking screws, as well as with nails with either an open- or closed-section design.[39–41,45–48] Locked intramedullary nails are available in a range of diameters. The smaller-diameter nails (e.g., Delta nails), which may be inserted without prior reaming, require use of smaller-diameter locking screws, which are at increased risk for fatigue failure. We generally try to place a reamed interlocked nail with a diameter of 11 mm or 12 mm unless the patient has a very small-diameter canal, the subtrochanteric fracture is a high-energy open injury, or the patient has an associated pulmonary contusion as a result of the injury. In these instances, we use either a smaller-diameter interlocked nail inserted without prior reaming or a different type of implant, such as a plate-and-screw device.

Preoperative Planning

Preoperative radiographs should visualize the entire femur, including the femoral head, femoral neck, and knee on both AP and lateral views. Radiographs should be carefully inspected for intraarticular fracture propagation and neoplastic disease. Preoperative radiographs of the uninjured femur may be used to estimate proper nail diameter, anticipated amount of reaming, and nail length for severely comminuted fractures. Radiographic templates for preoperative planning are available from most nail manufacturers. In cases involving a delay from injury to surgery, one should confirm that appropriate femoral length has been obtained with traction; excessive intraoperative traction resulting in pudendal and/or sciatic nerve palsy has been reported after closed antegrade intramedullary nailing.[49]

Choice of nail size depends on the size of the patient and the extent of femoral comminution. Nevertheless, because of a small but consistently reported percentage of complications caused by nail fatigue, it is recommended that, if possible, one try to insert a nail with a diameter of at least 11 or 12 mm.

Operative Technique for an Interlocked Centromedullary Nail (First-Generation Nail)

When an interlocked centromedullary nail is used for subtrochanteric fracture fixation, the patient can be positioned either supine or lateral on a fracture table (Figure 7.66). We prefer to position the patient supine, as this patient positioning is easier to set up than the lateral decubitus position and is better tolerated in patients who have associated pulmonary injury or preexisting lung disease. Use of the lateral decubitus position does, however, facilitate identification and penetration of the nail entry point in the piriformis fossa, which may be the most challenging step in intramedullary nailing of a subtrochanteric fracture. The injured lower extremity is adducted with the hip

Treatment

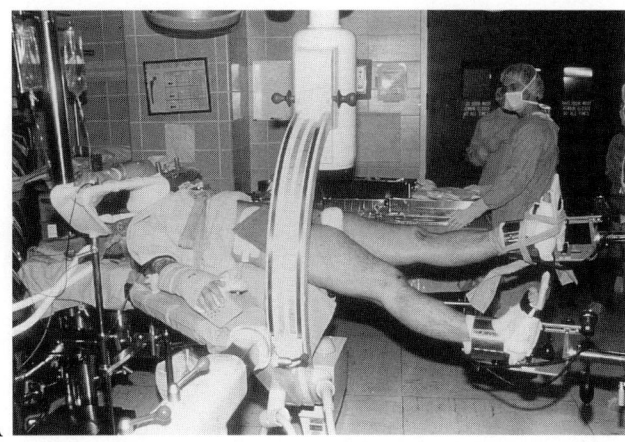

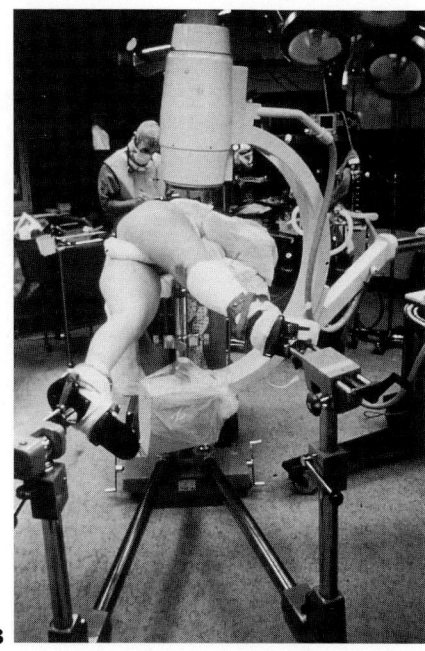

flexed approximately 15°. The contralateral lower extremity is placed into a "heel-to-toe" position, adjacent but inferior to the injured extremity (Figure 7.67). The patient's trunk is adducted away from the operative side to facilitate access to the entry point and nail insertion. Traction is applied through a skeletal pin placed in the anterior aspect of the distal femur (away from the anticipated nail position) or proximal tibia.

Correct rotational alignment can be established using the image intensifier (Figure 7.68). Femoral neck anteversion averages 15° in most adults. The image intensifier is rotated to obtain a perfect cross-table lateral view of the femoral head and neck. The position of the image intensifier is recorded and the unit is moved to the distal femur. The image intensifier beam is rotated 15° to 20° internally and the leg is rotated until a perfect lateral view of the distal femoral condyles and knee is obtained, thus reestablishing the correct anteversion of the femoral neck. Correct rotation of the distal fragment usually

Figure 7.66. Supine (**A**) and lateral (**B**) patient positioning for intramedullary nailing.

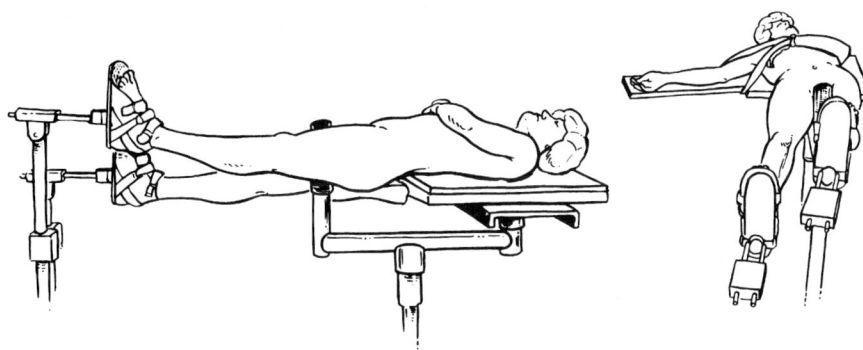

Figure 7.67. The contralateral lower extremity is placed into a "heel-to-toe" position, adjacent but inferior to the injured extremity. The patient's trunk is adducted away from the operative side to facilitate access to the entry point and nail insertion.

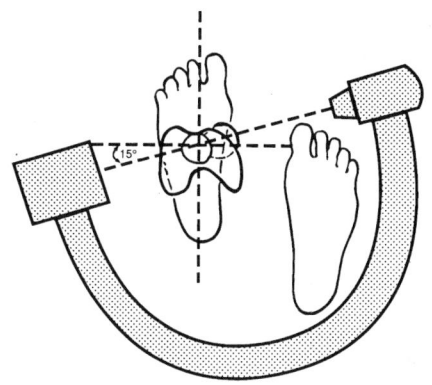

Figure 7.68. Use of the image intensifier to determine correct rotational alignment. The image intensifier is rotated to obtain a perfect cross-table lateral view of the femoral head and neck. The position of the image intensifier is recorded and the unit is moved to the distal femur. The image intensifier beam is rotated 15° to 20° internally and the leg is rotated until a perfect lateral view of the distal femoral condyles and knee is obtained, thus reestablishing the correct anteversion of the femoral neck.

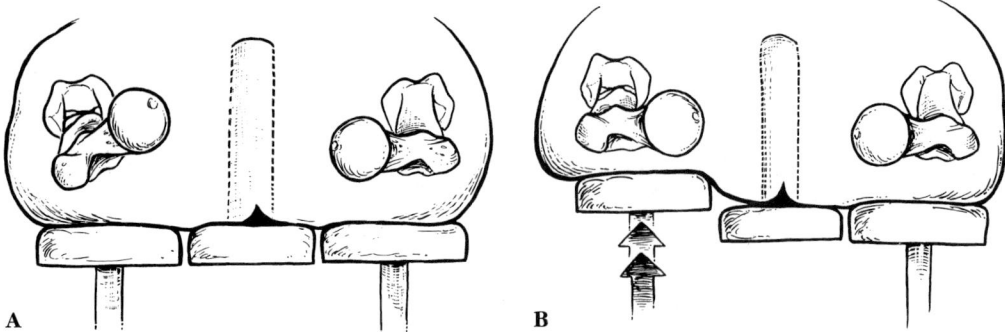

Figure 7.69. Use of a buttock support to internally rotate the proximal fragment (**A, B**).

places the foot in 0° to 15° of external rotation; with the patient placed on the fracture table, however, the proximal fragment may externally rotate as much as 45° to 50°, requiring the foot to be turned out to match this external rotation. Russell and Taylor have described the use of a buttock support to internally rotate the proximal fragment[10] (Figure 7.69); alternatively, a "joystick" can be used to derotate the proximal fragment. Another method of estimating rotation or anteversion of the proximal fragment is to place a small guidewire along the anterior femoral neck. A third method to check rotation is to internally and externally rotate the leg until it can be determined that the skin tension lines are in their most relaxed position.[10]

Once the fracture is reduced, the lower extremity is prepared from the rib cage to an area distal to the tibial tubercle. The operative field is draped using an isolation screen. Alternatively, one can drape the lower extremity, leaving the area from the buttocks and lateral thigh to the popliteal crease exposed, and place a sterile cover over the image intensifier.

An oblique skin incision is made just proximal to the greater trochanter and is extended proximally and posteriorly for approximately 3 to 4 cm (Figure 7.70). The fascia of the gluteus maximus muscle is incised in line with its fibers and the gluteus maximus muscle is bluntly dissected. One should now be able to palpate the piriformis fossa, posterior to the fibers of the gluteus medius muscle.

Determination of the proper entry portal is critical when using an intramedullary nail to stabilize subtrochanteric fractures. For a centromedullary nail, the entry portal should be in the middle of the piriformis fossa, in line with the femoral shaft on both the sagittal and coronal planes (Figure 7.71). A

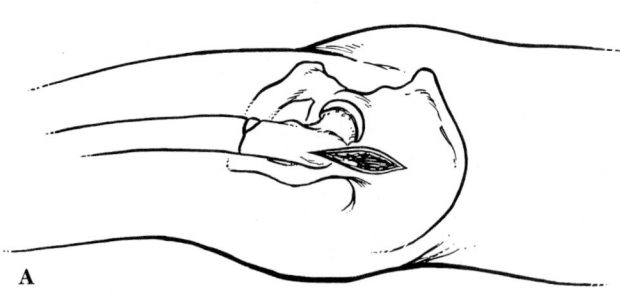

Figure 7.70. An oblique skin incision is made just proximal to the greater trochanter and is extended proximally and posteriorly for approximately 3 to 4 cm (**A, B**).

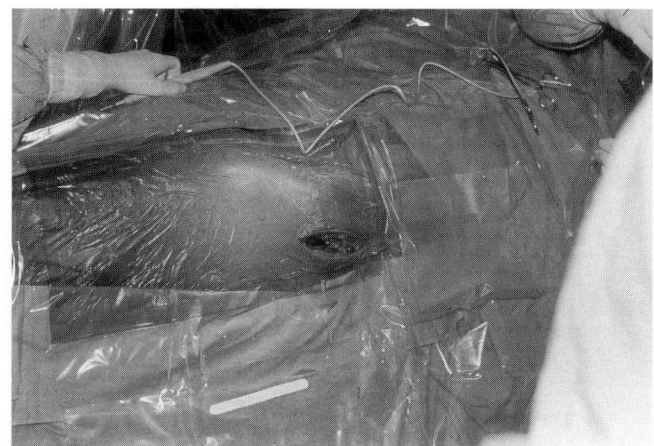

Treatment

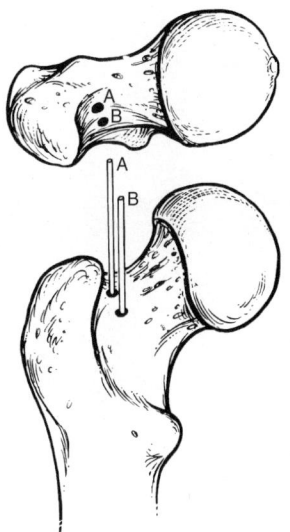

Figure 7.71. For a centromedullary (first-generation) nail, the entry portal should be in the middle of the piriformis fossa, in line with femoral shaft on both the AP and lateral planes (point B). When using a reconstruction (second-generation) nail, the entry portal should be moved anterior to facilitate placement of the proximal locking screws within the femoral neck and head (point A).

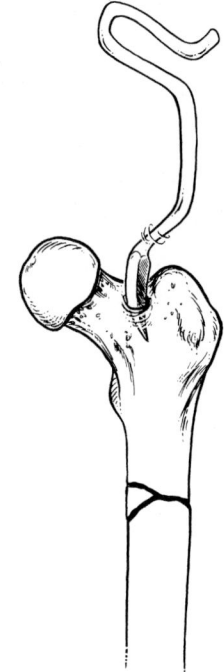

Figure 7.72. Use of a curved awl to create the nail entry hole.

lateral entry portal increases the risk of varus malalignment, whereas a medial entry point increases the risk of iatrogenic femoral neck fracture. When using the reconstruction nail, the entry portal should be moved anteriorly to facilitate placement of the proximal locking screws within the femoral neck and head (Figure 7.71). One can use either a curved awl (Figure 7.72) or a cannulated reamer to create the entry hole. We prefer to use a 3.2-mm guide pin with a threaded tip from the sliding hip screw set (Figure 7.73); once its position is verified on both the AP and lateral views, the entry portal is enlarged with a cannulated reamer (Figure 7.73).

In subtrochanteric fractures, placement of the entry portal is often complicated by the flexed, abducted, and externally rotated position of the proximal fragment. If the proximal femoral fragment is flexed, externally rotated, and abducted to such a degree that an adequate entry portal cannot be created, a joystick can be inserted into or a clamp placed around the proximal fragment to manipulate it into a neutral position (Figure 7.74).

After creation of the entry portal, a ball-tipped guide rod attached to a T-handled chuck is placed down the femoral canal to the fracture (Figure 7.75).

Figure 7.73. Use of a 3.2-mm-tip threaded guide pin from the sliding hip screw set to create the nail entry hole. Once the guide pin is optimally positioned on both the AP (**A**) and lateral (**B**) views, the entry portal is enlarged with a cannulated reamer (**C**).

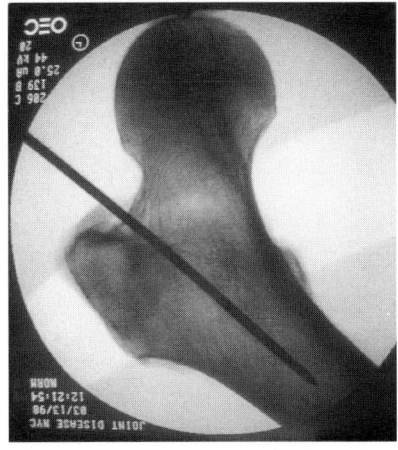
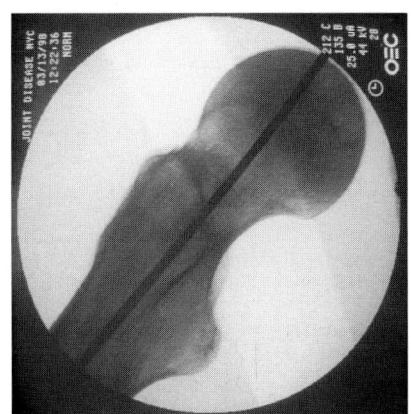
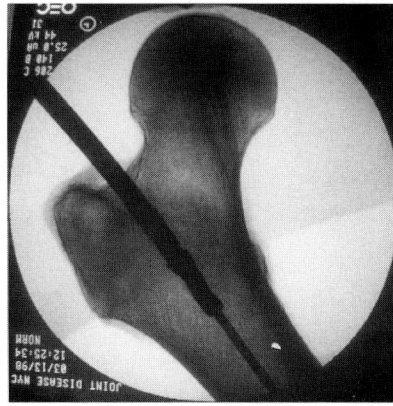

A   B   C

Figure 7.74. Use of a joystick to manipulate a proximal femoral fragment that is flexed, externally rotated, and abducted (**A**) into a neutral position (**B**). Creation of the nail entry portal while the proximal fragment is maintained in the neutral position (**C**).

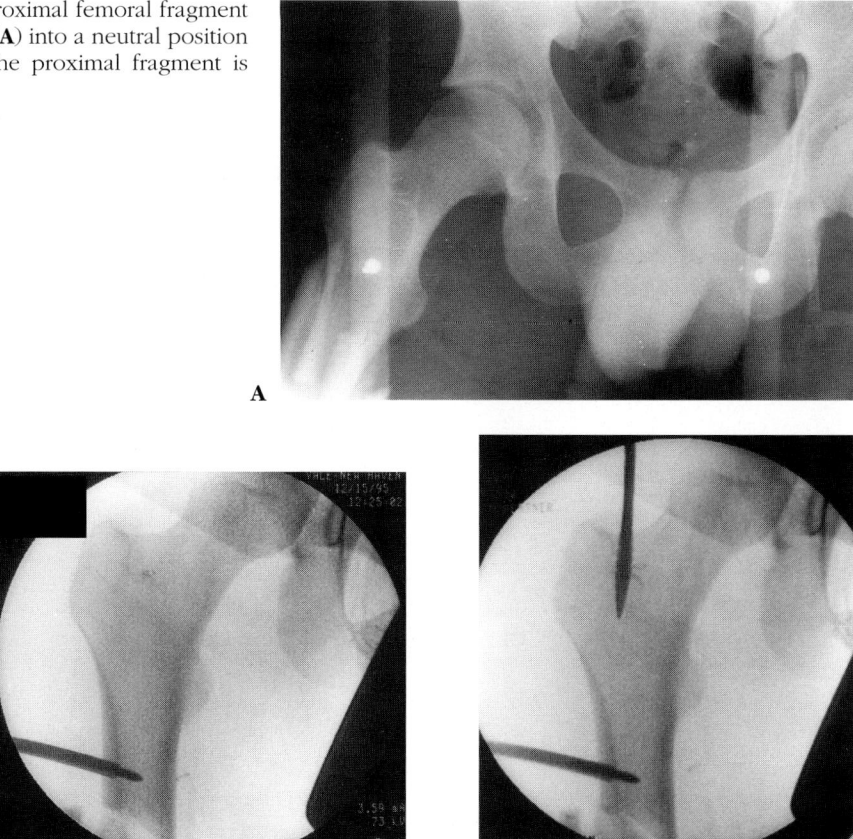

Containment of the guidewire within the femur is confirmed with AP and lateral fluoroscopic views. The fracture is reduced, and the guidewire is advanced down the center of the femoral canal to the epiphyseal scar (Figure 7.76). It is important to centralize the guidewire in both the sagittal and coronal planes; otherwise, an angular malreduction may result when the nail is inserted. If the guidewire can not be successfully advanced across the fracture site, an internal fracture alignment device can be used to reduce the fracture fragments. The proximal fragment is reamed to 10 mm and the internal fracture alignment device is inserted; this cannulated device is used to directly manipulate the proximal fragment. Once the fracture is reduced, the guidewire is

Figure 7.75. Passage of the ball-tipped guidewire down the femoral canal.

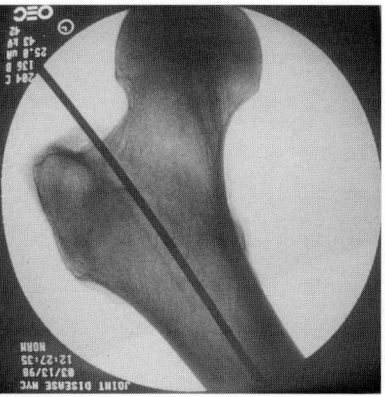

Treatment

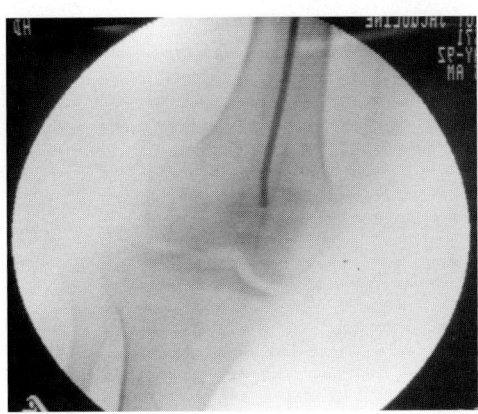
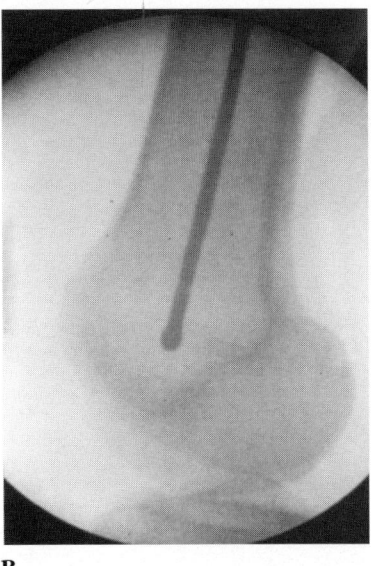

A   **B**

Figure 7.76. Advancement of the guidewire to the epiphyseal scar (**A, B**). It is important to centralize the guidewire in both the AP and lateral planes; otherwise, an angular malreduction may result when the nail is inserted.

advanced through the fracture alignment device into the distal fragment. If reducing the fracture closed proves difficult, one should not hesitate to perform a limited open reduction.

The proper nail length can be determined from preoperative planning and verified using either two guidewires of identical length or a radiolucent ruler (Figure 7.77). In the guidewire method, a second guidewire is overlapped to the portion of the reduction guidewire extending proximally from the femoral entry portal; this distance is subtracted from the total guidewire length to determine nail length. Alternatively, the radiolucent ruler is positioned over the anterior femur and image intensification is used to make a direct reading of the distance from the entry portal to the desired distal nail tip.

The femur is reamed over the ball-tipped guidewire in 0.5-mm increments until the desired canal diameter is achieved (Figure 7.78). We prefer to use a nail with a diameter of 11 or 12 mm and to overream the canal by 1 mm or, in cases of a large anterior femoral bow, 1.5 mm. If the intramedullary canal is small or if significant chatter is encountered during reaming of the femoral canal, a nail of smaller diameter should be selected.

The ball-tipped guidewire is replaced with a straight-tipped guidewire, inserted using the medullary exchange tube to maintain fracture reduction (Figure 7.79). The selected femoral nail is attached to the insertion jig; when properly assembled, the femoral nail should have an anterior bow and the proximal guide should point laterally. It is important to verify that the proximal targeting jig aligns with proximal nail holes before insertion of the nail (Figure 7.80); this can be done by assembling the drill sleeves within the insertion guide and checking that the drill bit smoothly targets the proximal nail screw holes.

The nail is advanced manually down the femoral canal over the guidewire (Figure 7.81). The insertion handle is used to control rotation and direct nail passage. Once the nail will no longer advance manually, a mallet should be used. The mallet should only be used on the insertion driver and not on the proximal drill guide; striking the guide can alter the alignment required for proximal targeting. As the nail is advanced down the femoral canal, one should verify correct nail rotation; the proximal insertion handle should be

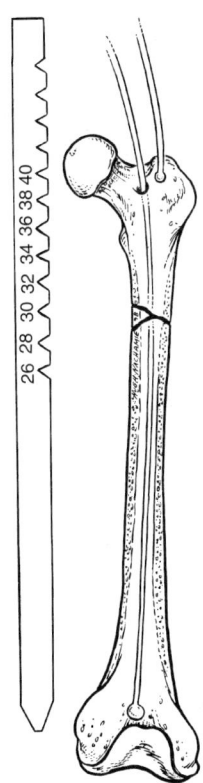

Figure 7.77. Determination of proper nail length can be made from preoperative planning and can be verified by using either two guidewires of identical length or a radiolucent ruler.

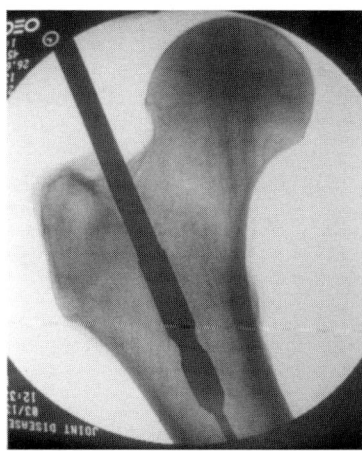

Figure 7.78. Reaming of the femoral canal.

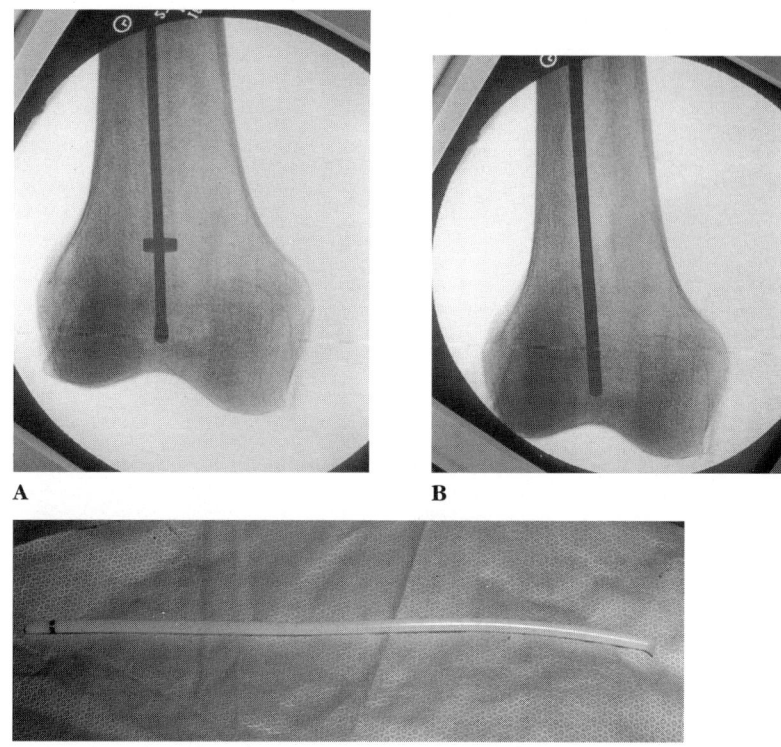

Figure 7.79. Exchange of the ball-tipped guidewire (**A**) with a straight-tipped guidewire (**B**), using the medullary exchange tube (**C**).

parallel to or pointed toward the floor to facilitate insertion of the distal locking screws. With the proximal handle pointed toward the ceiling, it is difficult to place the x-ray beam of many image intensifiers parallel to the distal screw holes, which in turn will complicate insertion of the distal locking screws. To prevent nail incarceration, one should verify that the nail advances with each

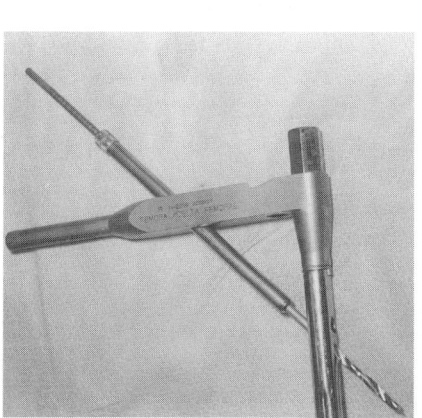

Figure 7.80. Verification that the proximal targeting jig aligns with proximal nail holes before insertion of the nail.

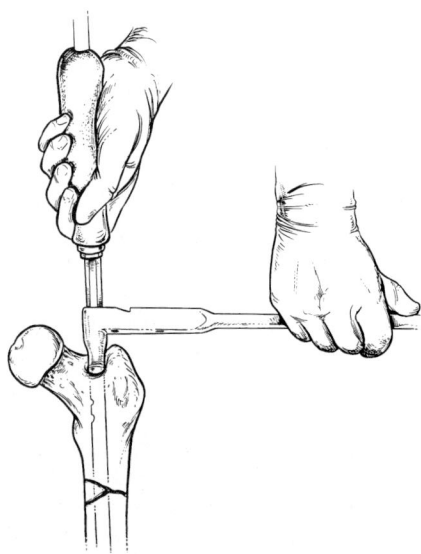

Figure 7.81. Manual insertion of the nail down the femoral canal.

Treatment

mallet blow. During nail insertion, it may be necessary to retighten the bolt(s) of the proximal drill guide assembly before final nail seating.

Once the nail is fully seated and its position verified on both the sagittal and coronal planes, the interlocking screws are inserted. In standard interlocked femoral nails, the proximal locking screws are inserted through the insertion jig and are directed either obliquely or transversely from lateral to medial, depending on the nail manufacturer. The proximal locking screw is bicortical and is inserted after predrilling (Figure 7.82). The positioning of this locking screw is dependent on fracture geometry but is usually at the level of the lesser trochanter. We avoid placing the screw in the inferior femoral neck, which could result in a stress riser effect and consequent femoral neck fracture. The length of the locking screw can be determined directly from the drill bit. We usually measure the length of the drill bit once it contacts the inner aspect of the medial femoral cortex and add 5 mm to this measurement to determine the appropriate length of the proximal locking screw.

Distal locking is routinely advised with use of interlocked nails; a static construct confers stability and is highly unlikely to lose fracture reduction in the postoperative period. Brumback et al. reported a 10.6% loss of reduction when interlocked femoral nails were placed in a dynamically locked mode in fractures without significant fracture comminution.[50] Before insertion of the distal locking screw, the fracture is reassessed to verify correct fracture reduction, femoral length, and rotation. Distal locking screws are inserted using a free-hand technique. There are many ways of placing the distal locking

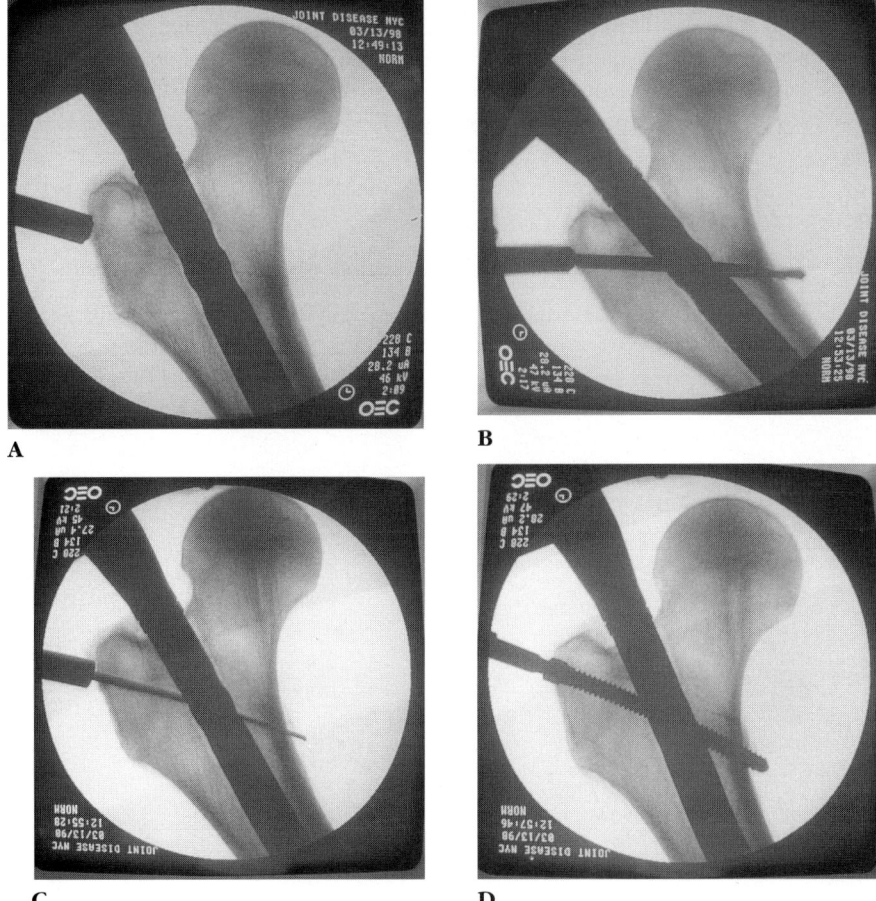

Figure 7.82. After the nail has been inserted to the appropriate depth (**A**), the proximal femur is drilled (**B**), the length of the locking screw is measured (**C**), and the locking screw is inserted (**D**).

Figure 7.83. For insertion of the distal locking screws, the image intensifier is positioned with the beam parallel to the distal locking holes so that the holes appear perfectly round.

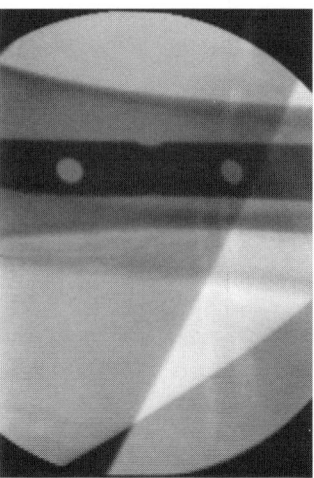

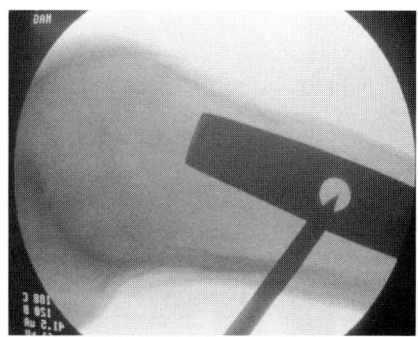

Figure 7.84. The tip of the trocar is positioned in the middle of the locking hole as visualized on the image intensifier.

screws, but all require good image intensification. The image intensifier is positioned with the beam parallel to the distal locking holes; with appropriate adjustment, the holes will appear perfectly round (Figure 7.83). We prefer to use an extra-sharp, pointed trocar to open the lateral cortex of the distal femur. The tip of the trocar is positioned in the middle of the locking hole as visualized on the image intensifier (Figure 7.84). A small skin incision is made at the tip of the trocar and the tissue is dissected down to bone. The tip of the trocar is repositioned in the middle of the locking hole and the trocar is placed on end parallel to the x-ray beam. Once a halo is seen completely surrounding the trocar, it is tapped through the near cortex. Alternatively, one could use a radiolucent targeting device, available from various manufacturers (Figure 7.85). The image intensifier is then positioned in an AP direction and the trocar is drilled across the nail until it engages the opposite cortex (Figure 7.86). Next the image intensifier is positioned laterally so one can verify that the trocar has gone through the nail (Figure 7.87). Once this has been verified, the trocar is advanced through the far cortex (Figure 7.88) and the length of the locking screw is determined. We usually estimate the length of the locking screw based on the AP image intensifier view and the known nail diameter (Figure 7.89). Alternatively, one could use a depth gauge (Figure 7.90) or a second trocar of equal length. The locking screw is then inserted (Figure 7.91).

Figure 7.85. Use of a radiolucent device to target the distal locking holes (**A, B**).

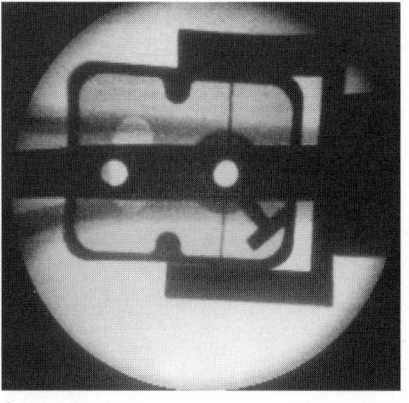

A

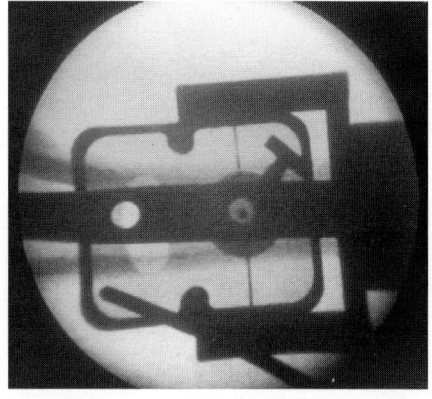

B

Treatment

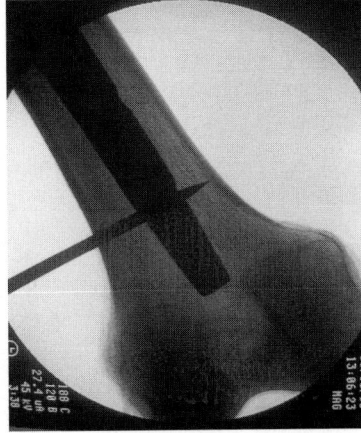

Figure 7.86. The image intensifier is positioned in an AP direction and the trocar is drilled across the nail until it engages the opposite cortex.

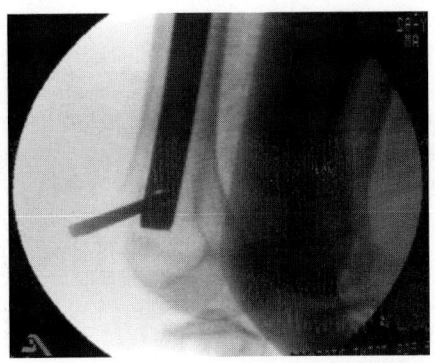

Figure 7.87. Verification that the trocar has gone through the nail.

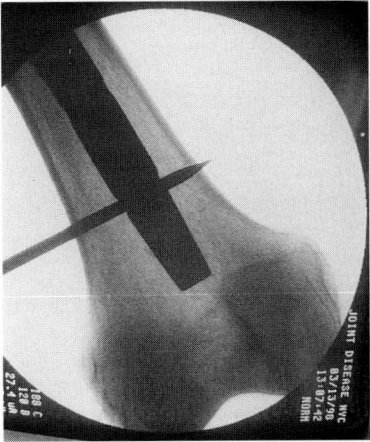

Figure 7.88. The trocar is advanced through the far cortex of the distal femur.

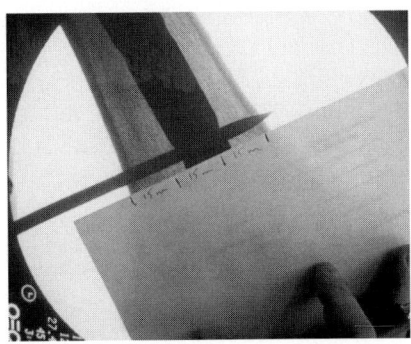

Figure 7.89. Determination of the length of the locking screw based on the AP image intensifier view and the diameter of the inserted intramedullary nail (15 mm in the illustrated case).

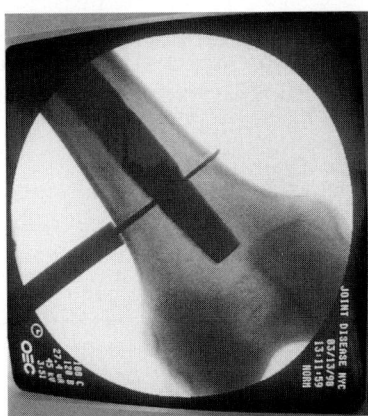

Figure 7.90. Use of a depth gauge to determine the proper length of the locking screw.

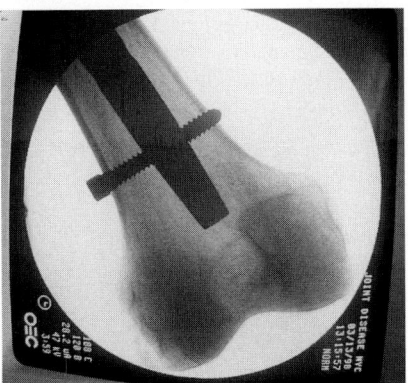

Figure 7.91. Insertion of the locking screw.

A second distal locking screw is inserted in an identical manner. Before closing the wound, fracture reduction and nail position, including all locking screws, are assessed radiographically in the sagittal and coronal planes.

Operative Technique for a Cephalomedullary Nail (Second-Generation Nail)

A cephalomedullary-type (second-generation) interlocking nail is indicated for stabilization of subtrochanteric femur fractures with disruption of the lesser trochanter, pathologic subtrochanteric fractures, and ipsilateral femoral neck and shaft fractures. Although its insertion is technically challenging, this type of nail can also be used to stabilize complex subtrochanteric fractures with

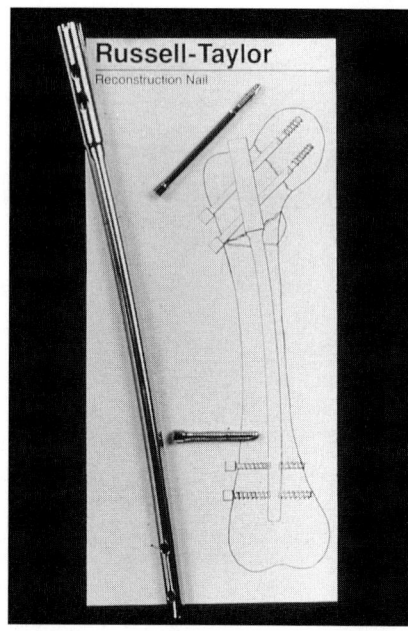

Figure 7.92. Photograph and drawing of reconstruction nail (courtesy of R. A. Calandruccio, The Campbell Clinic Foundation, Memphis, TN).

fracture extension into the piriformis fossa. A cephalomedullary nail should not be considered as a nail of first choice for conventional diaphyseal fractures of the femur, however, because of the complexity of proximal locking screw insertion.

Like centromedullary interlocked nails, cephalomedullary nails are available in a range of diameters. Also, as with centromedullary nails, we try to insert a nail of 11 or 12 mm diameter to optimize nail and locking bolt strength without overwhelming the femur with excessive reaming and vascular destruction. The cephalomedullary nail with which we have the most experience is the reconstruction nail (Smith+Nephew, Memphis, TN) (Figure 7.92). The proximal 8 cm of the reconstruction nail is 15 mm in diameter; its shaft diameters are 12, 13, and 14 mm. In the Delta reconstruction nails, the proximal 8 cm is 13 mm in diameter; its shaft diameters are 10 and 11 mm. Proximal interlocking involves the use of a superior 6.4-mm and an inferior 8.0-mm lag screw with the 12- to 14-mm reconstruction nails and two 6.4 mm screws with the Delta reconstruction nails. The spacing between the two proximal locking screws is 1.3 cm in the reconstruction nail and 1.1 cm in the Delta reconstruction nail. The femoral shaft should be reamed to a diameter 1 mm greater than that of the intended nail, and the proximal 8 cm must be reamed to a diameter of either 13 or 15 mm. Because the reconstruction nail has 8° of anteversion, different nails are required for right and left femurs.

The technique for insertion of the reconstruction nail is similar to that described for centromedullary interlocked nails. The nail entry portal, however, should be moved anteriorly to facilitate placement of the proximal locking screws within the femoral neck and head[51] (Figure 7.93). After fracture reduction, the guidewire is passed to the old epiphyseal scar, the appropriate nail length is determined, and the femoral shaft is reamed.

After the accuracy of its proximal targeting mechanism has been confirmed (Figure 7.94), the reconstruction nail is inserted over a straight-tipped guidewire. The nail must be inserted to the proper depth (determined with the aid of AP image intensification) to optimize proximal screw placement in the

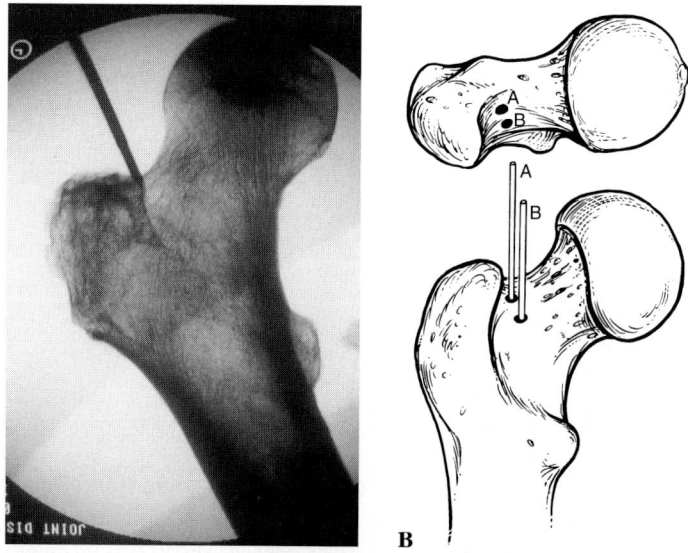

Figure 7.93. The nail entry portal for insertion of the reconstruction nail is anterior to that of conventional centromedullary nails (**A, B**).

Treatment

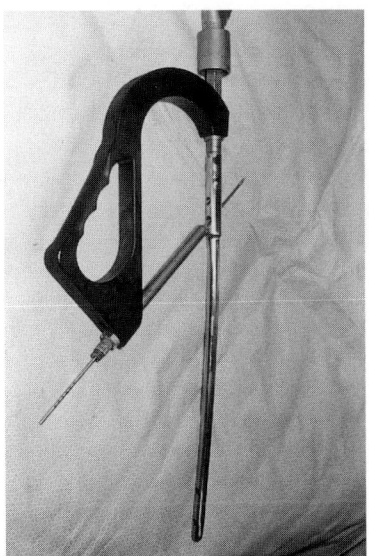

Figure 7.94. Verification of the accuracy of the proximal targeting mechanism before insertion of the reconstruction nail. Note the radiolucent targeting guide.

femoral head. In obese patients, an offset reconstruction nail driver may be attached to the insertion jig. In subtrochanteric fractures with fracture extension into the piriformis fossa, one must carefully assess the nail position during insertion. There is a tendency for the nail to exit posteriorly out of the proximal femur[10] (Figure 7.95); in such an instance, the nail must be lifted anteriorly to permit insertion of the proximal locking screws.

Proximal interlocking involves the use of a superior 6.4-mm and an inferior 8.0-mm lag screw with the 12- to 14-mm reconstruction nails and two 6.4-mm screws with the Delta reconstruction nails. If only one screw is to be used for proximal interlocking, the 8.0-mm lag screw is used; however, a stronger mechanical construct is obtained with both screws inserted. Because the screws are oriented in a 135° angle, when only one screw can be inserted, it is frequently a clue that the fracture may be reduced in varus. Although both cannulated and noncannulated proximal locking screws are available for use with reconstruction nails, we have no experience with the cannulated locking screws. Therefore the technique for insertion of the proximal locking screw that follows applies to use of the noncannulated proximal locking screws.

To determine proper nail insertion depth, the inferior drill sleeves are placed into the proximal drill guide to extrapolate the eventual location of the 8.0-mm inferior locking screw (Figure 7.96). If two proximal locking screws are to be inserted, the nail should be advanced to a level that allows the 8.0-mm inferior locking screw to be placed just superior to the inferior femoral neck. If only one screw is to be used, the nail is inserted to a level that allows the 8.0-mm inferior screw to be centralized in the femoral head.

Once the appropriate nail height is determined, the image intensifier is brought into a lateral position to obtain a true lateral view of the femoral head

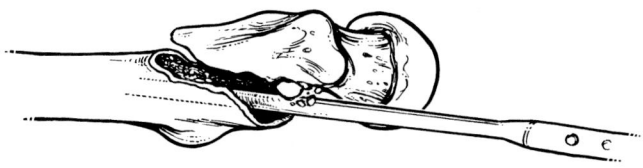

Figure 7.95. With fracture extension into the piriformis fossa, there is a tendency for the nail to exit posteriorly out of the proximal femur; in such an instance, the nail must be lifted anteriorly to permit insertion of the proximal locking screw.

Figure 7.96. To determine proper nail insertion depth, the inferior drill sleeves are placed into the proximal drill guide to extrapolate the eventual location of the 8.0-mm inferior locking screw (**A, B**).

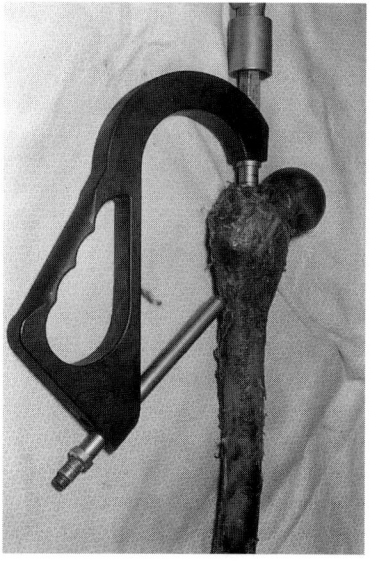
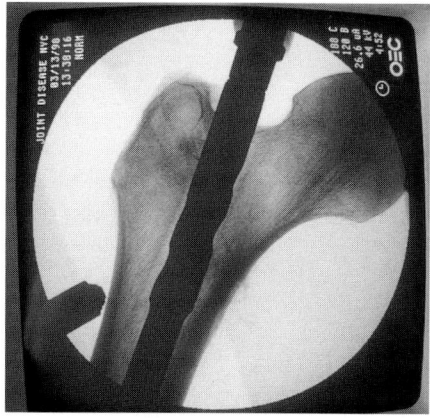

A B

and neck (Figure 7.97). A radiolucent proximal targeting device is available that facilitates centralization of the proximal locking screws in the sagittal plane. In most cases with the patient positioned supine, the femoral head is anterior to the shaft of the femur; therefore, the proximal drill guide is rotated posteriorly to place the screws in the center of the femoral head and neck. The reconstruction nail has 8° anteversion built into the proximal locking holes relative to the distal locking holes to compensate for the anterior offset of the femoral head and neck from the center of the intramedullary canal. Determination of femoral neck anteversion can be facilitated by placement of a guide pin along the anterior femoral neck.

If the proximal targeting guide is radiopaque, the guide is centralized with respect to the femoral head, bisecting the femoral head in the coronal plane on the true cross-table lateral intensifier view[44] (Figure 7.98). The posterior and anterior portions of the femoral head must be seen in relation to the proximal drill guide to ensure that the screws will be contained in the center of the femoral head. Further verification of containment of the proximal locking screws may be obtained with oblique radiographic views.

Once the nail has been optimally positioned in the proximal femur, a skin incision is made at the proximal locking screw insertion level and the under-

Figure 7.97. Once the appropriate nail height is determined, the image intensifier is brought into a lateral position to obtain a true lateral view of the femoral head and neck. A radiolucent proximal targeting device (illustrated here) facilitates visualization of the proximal locking screws in the sagittal plane.

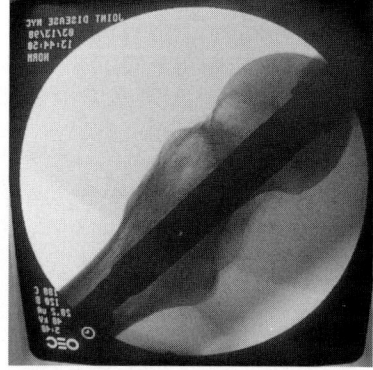

Treatment

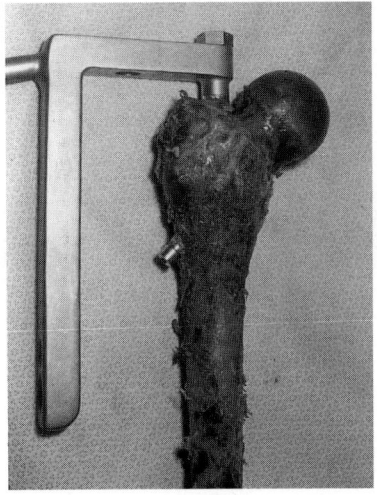

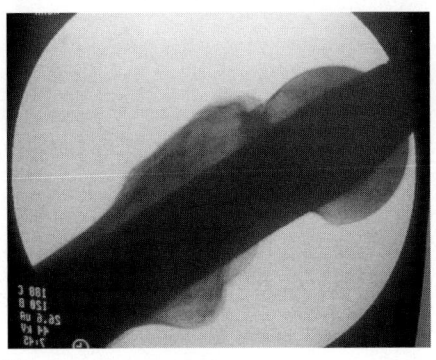

A B

Figure 7.98. If the proximal targeting guide is radiopaque (**A**) the guide is centralized with respect to the femoral head, bisecting the femoral head in the coronal plane on the true cross-table lateral intensifier view (**B**). The posterior and anterior portions of the femoral head must be seen in relation to the proximal drill guide to ensure that the screws will be contained in the center of the femoral head.

lying fascia is incised in line with the skin incision and the anticipated screw path. The stacked drill sleeves (silver, green, blue, and red) are assembled through the inferior locking hole in the drill guide and advanced to bone. A 3.2-mm tip-threaded guide pin is advanced into the femoral head approximately 5 mm superior to the inferior femoral neck to allow for an additional proximal locking screw (Figure 7.99). The guide pin is positioned approximately 5 mm from the subchondral bone of the femoral head. The position of the guide pin within the head must be confirmed on the AP and lateral image intensifier views. If the lateral view is obstructed by the proximal drill guide, one can use oblique projections to infer the position of the guide pin and subsequent screw. Once the position of the inferior guide pin is optimized, a second guide pin is placed though the proximal locking screw hole using the stacked drill sleeves (green, blue, and red) (Figure 7.100).

After the two guide pins are positioned, the inferior guide pin and three innermost drill sleeves are removed and a large-diameter calibrated step drill is used to drill the inferior screw tract through the silver drill sleeve to the appropriate depth (Figure 7.101). The step drill is advanced into the femoral head within 5 mm of the subchondral bone, making sure that the silver drill

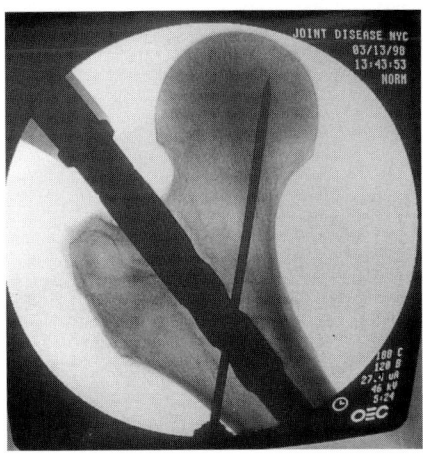

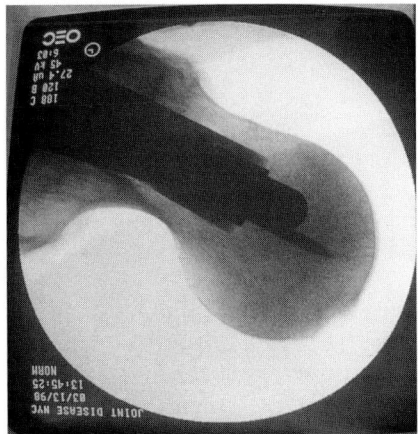

A B

Figure 7.99. A 3.2-mm guide pin is inserted through the stacked drill sleeves into the femoral head approximately 5 mm superior to the inferior femoral neck to allow for an additional proximal locking screw (**A, B**).

Figure 7.100. A second guide pin is placed though the proximal locking screw hole using the stacked drill sleeves (**A, B**).

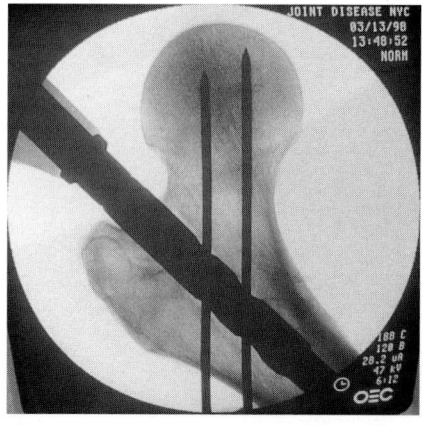
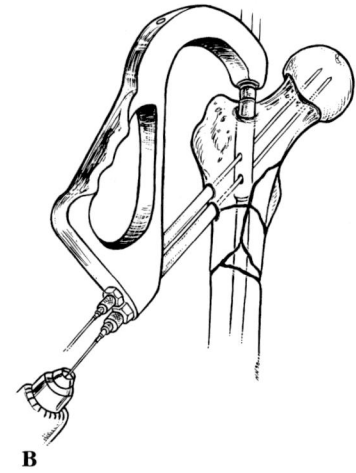

A B

Figure 7.101. After the two guide pins are positioned, the inferior guide pin and three innermost drill sleeves are removed and a large-diameter calibrated step drill is used to drill the inferior screw tract through the silver drill sleeve to the appropriate depth (**A, B**).

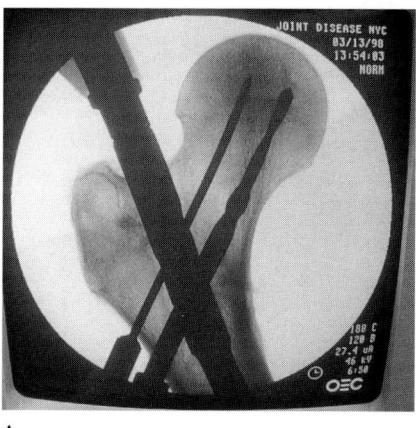
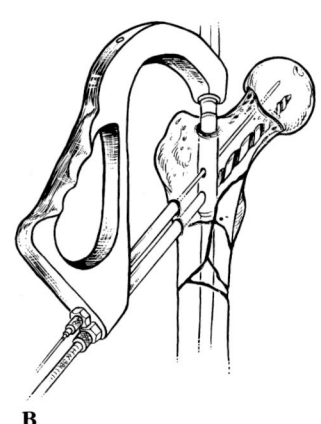

A B

sleeve is against the bone. The surgeon then measures screw length using the drill calibrations, reading the depth against the top of the silver drill sleeve (Figure 7.102). In very dense bone, tapping may be required; the large tap is used through the silver drill sleeve. The 8.0-mm lag screw is then inserted through the silver drill sleeve (Figure 7.103).

The proximal screw is inserted in a similar manner. One removes the guide pin and inserts the smaller-diameter step drill through the green drill sleeve

Figure 7.102. The screw length is determined from the drill calibrations, reading the depth against the top of the silver drill sleeve.

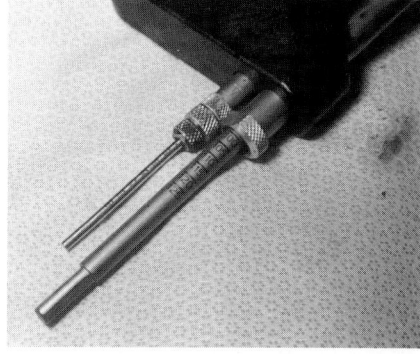

Treatment

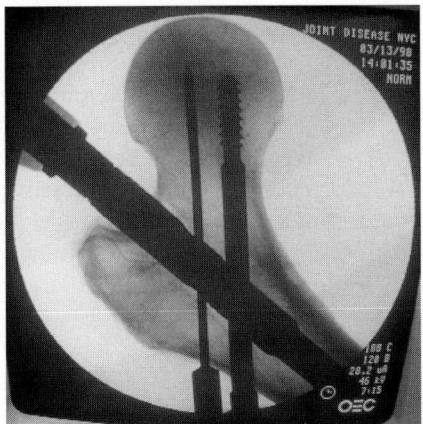

Figure 7.103. Insertion of the 8.0-mm lag screw through the silver drill sleeve.

into the femoral head within 5 mm of subchondral bone, verifying that the drill sleeve is against bone. The screw length is measured using the drill calibrations, and the depth is read against the top of the green drill sleeve. In very dense bone, tapping may be required, using the smaller-diameter tap. After the reamer is removed, the selected 6.4-mm lag screw is inserted into the femoral head through the green drill sleeve. Containment of both screws within the femoral head is confirmed on AP and lateral views (Figure 7.104). Distal locking is performed using the free-handed technique described for centromedullary interlocked nails, after verification of the fracture reduction and limb rotation.

In some patients, one may not be able to insert two locking screws into the femoral head. In this situation, the surgeon should assess for possible varus malreduction, preexisting hip varus, or a femoral neck too narrow for the selected reconstruction nail. Furthermore, the nail must have been inserted to the proper depth. The goal is to place the inferior lag screw just above the medial femoral cortex. If the nail is inserted too deep, the inferior screw will be difficult to insert or will penetrate the inferior cortex. At least 3 to 5 mm should be allowed for spacing of the guide pin proximal to the inferior femoral neck.

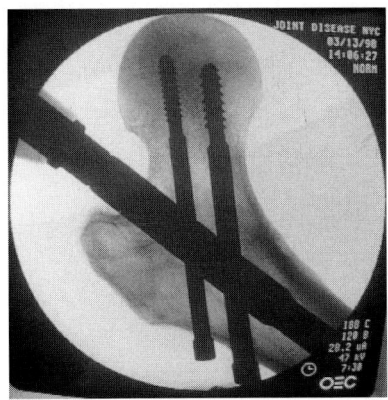

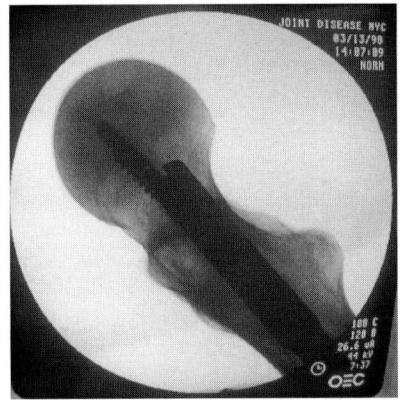

A B

Figure 7.104. Final radiographs after insertion of the proximal locking screws (**A, B**).

Indications for Bone Grafting

The use of autogenous bone graft in the treatment of subtrochanteric fractures has been suggested by numerous authors, especially during revision surgery for internal fixation. Stewart advocated acute autogenous iliac bone grafting of traumatic subtrochanteric fractures in younger individuals, particularly during open reduction of fractures with significant medial comminution.[52] Closed reduction techniques obviate the need for bone grafting, because fracture fragments are not devascularized to the same extent as in open reduction. Kinast et al. reported on a series of 23 subtrochanteric fractures stabilized with a 95° condylar blade plate using indirect reduction techniques without bone grafting[24]; all fractures united, at a mean of 4.2 months. If a bone graft is needed, it should be inserted through the fracture site, usually before plate application; placement of the bone graft at the conclusion of the procedure may necessitate further medial soft tissue dissection and osseous devascularization.

Open Subtrochanteric Fractures

Open subtrochanteric fractures are rare and are almost always associated with either penetrating injury or high-energy trauma from a motor vehicle accident or a fall from a height. The same principles that apply to all open fractures apply as well to open subtrochanteric fractures: immediate surgical débridement to decrease the risk of infection and osseous stabilization to prevent additional soft tissue injury. One should use the minimal amount of fixation necessary to adequately stabilize the subtrochanteric fracture.[10] In the past, this was problematical because most implants available for subtrochanteric fracture fixation involved further tissue dissection and contamination of tissue planes, prompting DeLee et al. to recommend 90–90 traction and cast bracing for open subtrochanteric fractures.[53] Johnson recommended intramedullary fixation of subtrochanteric fractures after adequate débridement and conversion to a clean contaminated wound, either acutely or 10 to 21 days after injury, following delayed primary wound closure.[54]

Russell and Taylor recommended immediate internal fixation of Gustilo type I–IIIA open subtrochanteric fractures after adequate débridement, combined with cephalosporin and aminoglycoside antibiotic coverage[10] (Figure 7.105). They recommended that all wounds be left open, except for surgical extensions, with additional débridement at 24 to 48 hours and as often as necessary until either delayed primary closure or plastic surgical wound coverage was obtained. They suggested external fixation for Gustilo type IIIB or IIIC subtrochanteric fractures when the proximal fragment was large enough to insert pins in a delta configuration and when the fracture was accompanied by vascular injury requiring repair or a clean contaminated wound could not be achieved by initial débridement. With the advent of smaller-diameter cephalomedullary nails, a nonreamed interlocked nail may be used for the treatment of these types of open subtrochanteric fractures. The option of interlocked nail insertion without reaming for the treatment of open subtrochanteric fractures may be beneficial, but studies are so far indeterminate.

Pathologic Fractures

The femur accounts for approximately 60% of all pathologic long bone fractures, with the pertrochanteric area accounting for almost 80% of pathologic

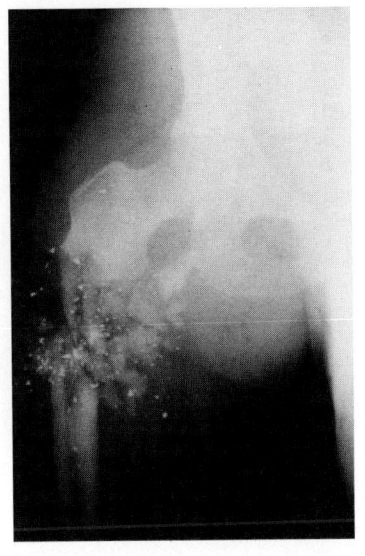
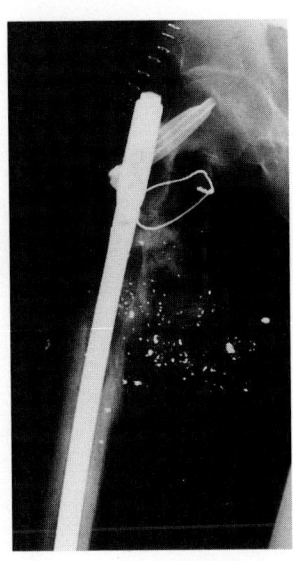

Figure 7.105. Open subtrochanteric fracture (**A**) stabilized with a locked intramedullary nail (**B**) after débridement.

femur fractures.[55] Nonoperative management of pathologic subtrochanteric fractures is difficult, because adequate pain relief is virtually impossible and it is extremely difficult to administer palliative radiation therapy. Furthermore, patients treated nonoperatively are at significant risk for medical complications, including diffuse intravascular coagulopathy and malignant hypercalcemia.[56] For these reasons, nonoperative management is relegated to patients who are in the last phase of their terminal state. Otherwise, pathologic subtrochanteric fractures should be treated surgically whenever possible. Secure internal fixation or prosthetic replacement renders most patients ambulatory or semi-ambulatory and relatively pain free.

Harrington proposed three criteria for choosing operative treatment of pathologic fractures[57]: (1) a life expectancy of at least 1 month and a general condition good enough to tolerate major surgery; (2) the expectation that the procedure will expedite mobilization of the patient and facilitate general care; (3) quality of bone both proximal and distal to the fracture site adequate to support metallic fixation or secure prosthetic seating.

The implant of choice for stabilization of pathologic subtrochanteric fractures is an interlocked nail (Figure 7.106). Although the Zickel nail remains a useful device, we favor the newer-generation reconstruction nails, with their ability for distal locking. Nevertheless, careful attention to detail is required with their use, and stable fixation in the short proximal fragment is mandatory. Supplementary reinforcement with methylmethacrylate is often employed, but this method is more difficult to use because the option of emplacing the device after cement insertion is not practical and placement of cement around a previously inserted device may be less effective and difficult to perform.[55] Occasionally, extensive subtrochanteric and pertrochanteric involvement requires proximal femoral replacement (Figure 7.107).

Barlow and Thomas reported three subtrochanteric fractures, in patients with Paget's disease, stabilized using the Russell-Taylor reconstruction nail.[58] In one patient with severe deformity of the femur, diaphyseal osteotomy was required to allow implant insertion. All fractures (including the osteotomy) united. There were no operative nor long-term complications and no instances of implant failure. Karachalios et al. reported use of a reconstruction

Figure 7.106. Pathologic subtrochanteric fracture (**A**) stabilized with an interlocked nail (**B**).

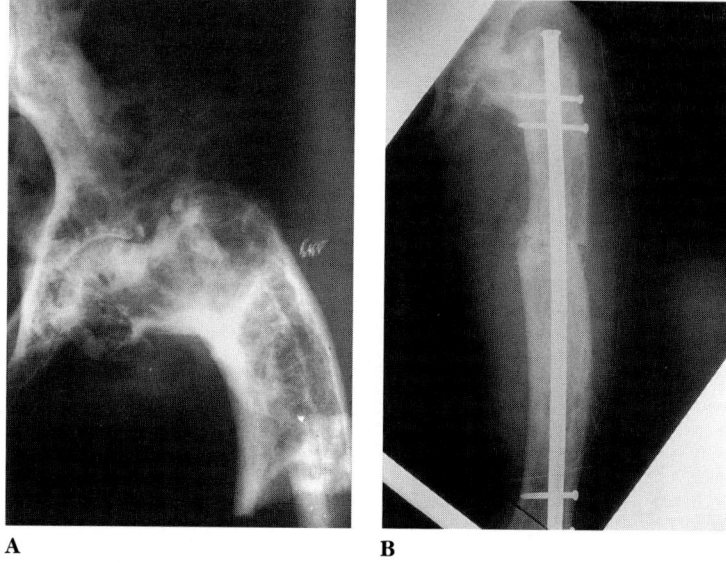

nail for stabilization of 14 pathological subtrochanteric fractures with coexisting metastases in the femoral shaft.[59] After femoral nailing, all patients were pain free and regained functional mobility. Patients were followed up clinically and radiologically until death; there were no instances of mechanical failure, even when a less-than-ideal fracture reduction had been achieved.

Broos et al. reported on a series of 65 patients (53 women and 12 men) with 77 pathological fractures of the femur.[60] Of these, 60 fractures (78%) occurred at the level of the proximal end of the femur; in 29 cases (38%), the fracture was in the subtrochanteric region, and in 6 cases a "prophylactic" osteosynthesis was performed because of an impending fracture. Endoprosthetic surgery was performed in 36 cases (47%). In 41 cases, internal fixation was performed using either plate and screws, a Gamma nail, or an interlocked nail. Forty-six patients (71%) obtained reasonable functional results in that they were able to walk again independently or with the help of a cane or crutches.

Figure 7.107. Pathologic subtrochanteric fracture (**A**) treated with proximal femoral replacement (**B**).

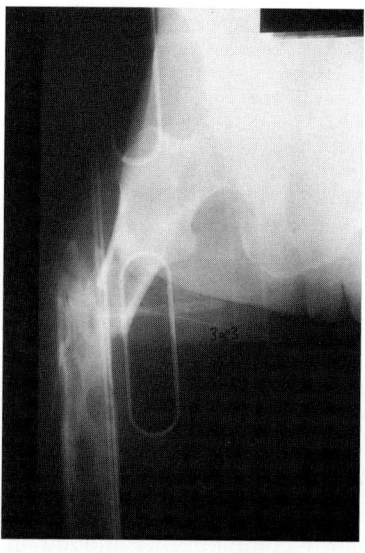 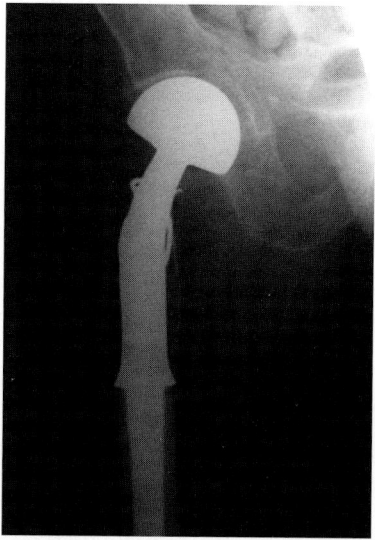

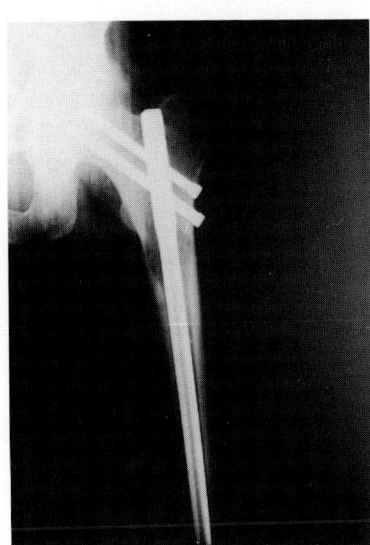

Figure 7.108. Prophylactic stabilization of an impending pathologic subtrochanteric fracture.

Haentjens et al. reported on a series of 28 metastases of the proximal femur, treated by resection and prosthetic replacement using a large femoral component with diaphyseal support.[61] When metastatic involvement of the acetabulum was not evident (17 cases), a bipolar hip prosthesis was used; in the remaining 11 cases, in which metastatic destruction of the acetabulum was evident, total hip arthroplasty was performed. Postoperative pain relief was excellent in 82% and good in 15% of patients. Functional results according to the Merle d'Aubigne rating scale were excellent in 19%, very good in 22%, and good in 22% of patients. The incidence of postoperative dislocation was significantly lower in the bipolar arthroplasty group than in the total hip arthroplasty group.

Controversy remains over the advisability of prophylactic fixation of impending pathologic fractures.[55,56] The relative risk of eventual fracture depends on the fracture location, tumor type, and extent of osseous involvement. Indications for prophylactic fixation of impending subtrochanteric pathologic fractures include cortical destruction greater than 50%, proximal femoral lesion greater than 2.5 cm in diameter, pathologic avulsion of the lesser trochanter, and persistent pain despite adjuvant radiation therapy (Figure 7.108).

Rehabilitation

In the absence of other complicating injuries, patients with subtrochanteric fractures are mobilized on postoperative day 1 from bed to chair; subsequent ambulation training is initiated using a walker or crutches. Weight-bearing status is dependent on the patient's age and bone quality, the fracture pattern, and the type of implant used for fracture stabilization. Older patients have difficulty with partial weight bearing and are allowed to bear weight as tolerated regardless of fracture pattern or implant selection. Younger patients are restricted to foot-flat weight bearing until there is radiographic evidence of healing—unless the fracture was stabilized with an interlocked nail and bone-to-bone contact was achieved at surgery. Hip and knee range-of-motion exercises and straight leg raises are initiated in the early postoperative period. Patients are discharged home when they can ambulate safely with assistive devices and are independent in activities of daily living or sufficient home care can be arranged. A progressive resistance exercise program is prescribed, based on evidence of fracture healing; swimming or stationary bicycling is recommended.

Implant removal is not encouraged and in any case is not considered until mature callus bridging the bone can be visualized on both AP and lateral radiographs. Patients are placed on crutches after implant removal for 2 to 4 weeks. After implant removal, contact sports are avoided for 3 to 6 months or longer, depending on the type of implant removed.

Complications

Complications related to internal fixation (nonunion, malunion, implant failure) have been reported more commonly following subtrochanteric fracture than after intertrochanteric or femoral neck fracture.[62] The incidence of these complications has varied widely, depending on fracture type and fixation technique. It is important to remember that fractures with loss of the posteromedial cortical buttress, especially those in which it cannot be restored, are at greatest risk for healing complications. Symptomatic nonunion with or without implant failure generally requires revision surgery. Unlike femoral neck and intertrochanteric nonunions, prosthetic replacement is not usually an option. Rather, treatment usually consists of implant removal, exposure and curettage of the nonunion site, bone grafting, and revision internal fixation, using an intramedullary device if possible.

Loss of Fixation

With the sliding hip screws in current use, implant failure usually occurs secondary to screw cutout from the femoral head and neck in patients with osteopenic bone.[10] It is important to obtain plate screw purchase of at least eight cortices in the femoral shaft. Fixation failure may be clinically evident as progressive deformity and limb length inequality associated with thigh pain. Loss of fixation with use of interlocked nails is commonly related to failure to statically lock the device, comminution of the entry portal, or use of small-diameter nails (Figure 7.109). Failure of fixation with use of plate and screws involves removal of hardware, revision internal fixation with either plate and screws or an interlocked nail, and bone grafting. Aronoff et al. recommended intramedullary nailing after failure of plate and screws.[63] Stoffelen et al. reported on the use of an endoprosthesis for the treatment of 12 intertrochanteric and subtrochanteric fractures (mean patient age, 79 years; range, 61 to 94 years) following failed internal fixation.[64] Eleven patients were available for clinical and radiographic review at an average of 32 months (range, 4 months to 7 years). Eight patients (72%) were classified as either good, very good, or excellent, whereas three were reported as fair using the Merle d'Aubigne rating system.[65] Nine patients (82%) had no pain at latest follow-up, while two patients complained of occasional discomfort.

Complications

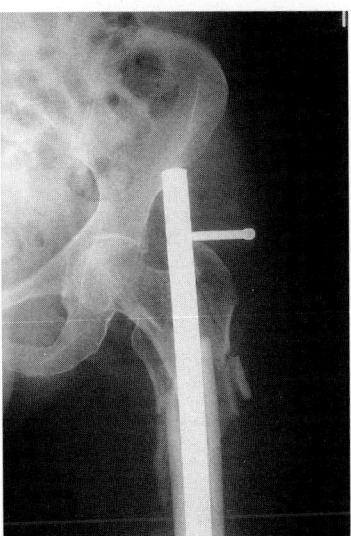

Figure 7.109. Loss of fixation secondary to a "missed" proximal locking screw.

Nonunion

Subtrochanteric nonunion may be evident by a patient's inability to resume full weight bearing within 3 to 6 months.[10] Continued pain about the proximal thigh and pain with attempted weight bearing are clinical indicators of delayed union and nonunion, which may be confirmed by radiographs and/or tomograms.[10] Nonunion usually persists in the femoral shaft portion of the fracture, converting the fracture to a Russell-Taylor type 1 pattern, which is best treated with an interlocked nail (Figure 7.110). If open reduction is performed, autologous iliac bone grafting is indicated. Nonunions that develop after intramedullary nailing can be treated by implant removal followed by further reaming and placement of a larger-diameter intramedullary nail. Our preference is to use a statically locked nail with slotted proximal locking

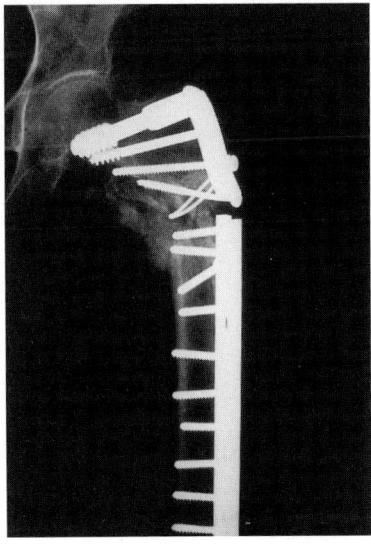
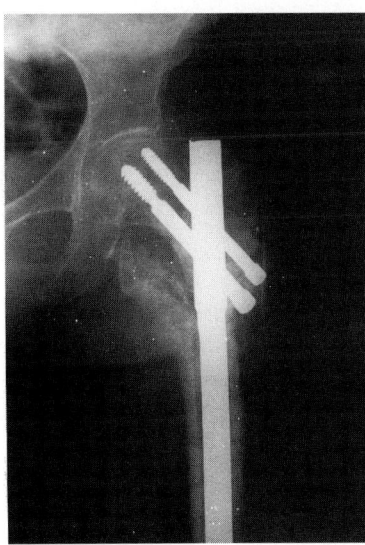

A **B**

Figure 7.110. Subtrochanteric nonunion with plate breakage (**A**) treated with an interlocked nail (**B**).

holes; this resists rotational shear but permits dynamic axial compression with weight bearing. Interlocked femoral nails that have the capacity to place compression across the nonunion site have recently been introduced. Although experience with these nails is limited, they may be useful for the treatment of subtrochanteric nonunions.

Malunion

The patient with a subtrochanteric malunion may complain of a limp, leg length discrepancy, or rotational deformity.[10] The affected leg should be compared to the opposite side for deformity evaluation. Malunions may be related to three aspects of fracture reduction.[10] First, it is imperative that the femoral neck-shaft angle be restored; if not, the patient will have a Trendelenburg gait with abductor weakness secondary to shortening of the abductor muscle group (Figure 7.111). A valgus osteotomy and revision internal fixation with bone grafting is the treatment of choice for a varus malreduction. Varus deformity may occur if an intramedullary nail is used and the entry portal is too lateral in the tip of the greater trochanter (Figure 7.112). Such varus deformity, if less than 10°, is frequently well tolerated by the patient and may not require revision surgery.[10] Second, leg length discrepancy is a complex problem that is more likely to occur following a fracture with extensive femoral shaft comminution stabilized with a dynamically locked rather than a statically locked nail configuration. Because most current lengthening procedures in adults are fraught with complications, avoidance is the best treatment for this complex problem.[10] Careful attention must be paid preoperatively and intraoperatively to restore proper femoral length. Occasionally, with locked intramedullary nailing, the injured limb is stabilized with fracture distraction and unites with excessive femoral length; a closed femoral shortening can subsequently be

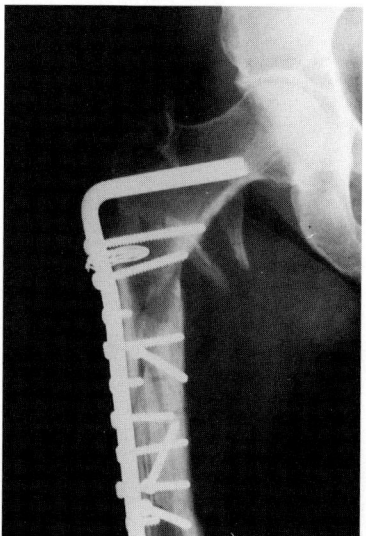

Figure 7.111. Varus malreduction secondary to poor condylar blade plate insertion.

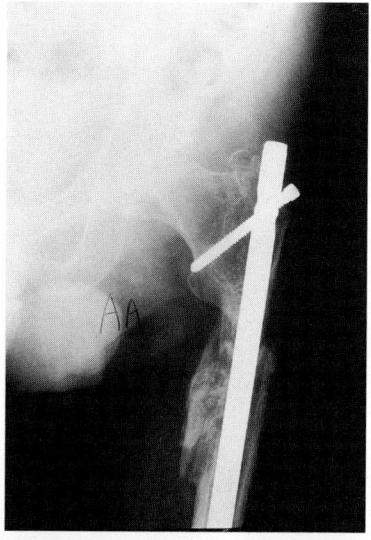

Figure 7.112. Varus malreduction secondary to intramedullary nail insertion through the greater trochanter.

performed to equalize leg lengths. Third, malrotation may occur with use of plate and screws or an intramedullary nail if the surgeon is not alert to this potential complication.[10] Adherence to the guidelines for fracture reduction and confirmation, including radiographic checks and matching of the linea aspera, helps to prevent this complication. It is essential to compare leg lengths and also to confirm rotational alignment by comparing internal and external rotation ranges before awakening the patient after intramedullary nailing. This permits early correction of malalignment. If significant internal or external rotational deformities are detected late, revision surgery with derotation osteotomy may be indicated. After intramedullary nailing, closed derotation osteotomy with a statically interlocked nail is the treatment of choice.

Infection

Acute infection may become evident within the first and second weeks after surgery by increasing pain associated with the usual signs of inflammation.[10] Sterile aspiration of the operative site may be performed to confirm the diagnosis.[10] Late infection may manifest as a nonunion in which sepsis is frequently subclinical. Radionucleotide studies may help to confirm the diagnosis of late infection and can help localize the extent of osseous involvement. Furthermore, when evaluating a nonunion, one should consider performing a biopsy of the nonunion site for anaerobic and aerobic organisms before performing revision surgery. Finally, when any surgical revision is required for subtrochanteric fracture complications, intraoperative cultures for both anaerobic and aerobic organisms should be obtained. Sepsis after subtrochanteric fracture most commonly follows open reduction and internal fixation[10]; with closed intramedullary nailing techniques, the rate of infection is significantly less than with use of plate and screws.[10] The use of prophylactic antibiotics has also significantly decreased the risk of postoperative sepsis.

Acute postoperative infection is best managed by immediate surgery for drainage and débridement of all necrotic material. The wound should be left open for further débridement or closed over antibiotic beads, depending on the extent of infection. If fixation is stable, the implant should be retained until the fracture has united. If the implant is unstable, it should be removed and either traction or external fixation applied. Delayed bone grafting can then be performed to obtain union, or internal fixation can be performed at a later date when the signs and symptoms of infection are absent.

Functional Loss

Functional loss is commonly related to complications about the hip or knee.[10] Heterotopic ossification is a frequent radiographic finding but is rarely symptomatic. Associated lesions of the patella, periarticular knee fracture, and soft tissue injury can all result in functional loss after subtrochanteric fracture.[10] Neurological injuries associated with the subtrochanteric fracture are rare but must be carefully evaluated before intramedullary nailing. Sciatic and pudendal nerve injuries observed postoperatively may be caused by excessive traction required for fracture reduction or by compartment syndrome[10]; these nerve injuries do not always resolve with time and can result in substantial functional morbidity.

References

1. Russell TA, Taylor JC. Subtrochanteric fractures of the femur. In: Browner BD, Jupiter JB, Levine AM, Trafton PG, eds. *Skeletal Trauma*. Philadelphia: WB Saunders, 1992:1485–1524.
2. Boyd HB, Griffin LL. Classifications and treatment of trochanteric fractures. *Arch Surg* 1949; 58:853–866.
3. Michelson JD, Myers A, Jinnah R, et al. Epidemiology of hip fractures among the elderly: risk factors for fracture type. *Clin Orthop* 1995; 311:129–135.
4. Berman AT, Metzger PC, Bosacco SJ, et al. Treatment of the subtrochanteric fracture with the compression hip nail—a review of thirty-eight consecutive cases. *Orthop Trans* 1979; 3:225–256.
5. Robey LR. Intertrochanteric and subtrochanteric fractures of the femur in the Negro. *J Bone Joint Surg Am* 1956; 38:1301–1312.
6. Velasco RU, Comfort T. Analysis of treatment problems in subtrochanteric fractures of the femur. *J Trauma* 1978; 18:513–522.
7. Waddell JP. Subtrochanteric fractures of the femur: a review of 130 patients. *J Trauma* 1979; 19:585–592.
8. Koch JC. The laws of bone architecture. *Am J Anat* 1917; 21:177–298.
9. Frankel VH, Burstein AH. *Orthopaedic Biomechanics. The Application of Engineering to the Musculoskeletal System*. Philadelphia: Lea & Febiger, 1970.
10. Russell TA, Taylor JC. Subtrochanteric fractures of the femur. In: Browner BD, Levine AM, Jupiter JB, Trafton PG, eds. *Skeletal Trauma*. Philadelphia: WB Saunders, 1992:1883–1925.
11. Bergman GD, Winquist RA, Mayo KA, Hansen STJ. Subtrochanteric fracture of the femur: fixation using the Zickel nail. *J Bone Joint Surg Am* 1987; 69:1032–1040.
12. Sangeorzan BJ, Ryan JR, Salciccroli GG. Prophylactic femoral stabilization with the Zickel nail by closed technique. *J Bone Joint Surg Am* 1986; 68:991–999.
13. Jekic M, Jekic I. Primary management and problems with osteosynthesis of subtrochanteric fractures of the femur. *Helv Chir Acta* 1993; 59:553–555.
14. Bone L, Bucholz R. The management of fractures in the patient with multiple trauma. *J Bone Joint Surg Am* 1986; 68:945–949.
15. Johnson KD, Cadambi A, Seibert GB. Incidence of adult respiratory distress syndrome in patients with multiple musculoskeletal injuries: effect of early operative stabilization of fractures. *J Trauma* 1985; 25:375–384.
16. Fielding JW, Magliato HJ. Subtrochanteric fractures. *Surg Gynecol Obstet* 1966; 122:555–560.
17. Seinsheimer F. Subtrochanteric fractures of the femur. *J Bone Joint Surg Am* 1978; 60:300–306.
18. Muller ME, Nazarian S, Koch P, Schatzker J. *The Comprehensive Classifications of Fractures of Long Bones*. Berlin: Springer-Verlag, 1990.
19. Hanson GW, Tullos HS. Subtrochanteric fractures of the femur treated with nail plate devices: a retrospective study. *Clin Orthop* 1978; 131:191–194.
20. Teitge RA. Subtrochanteric fracture of the femur. *J Bone Joint Surg Am* 1976; 58:282.
21. Whatley JR, Garland DE, Whitecloud T, Wickstrom J. Subtrochanteric fractures of the femur: treatment with ASIF blade plate fixation. *South Med J* 1978; 17:1372–1375.
22. Asher MA, Tipper JW, Rockwood CA, Zilber S. Compression fixation of subtrochanteric fractures. *Clin Orthop* 1976; 117:202–208.
23. Van Meeteren M, Van Rief Y, Roukema J, Van der Werken C. Condylar plate fixation of subtrochanteric femoral fractures. *Injury* 1996; 27:715–717.
24. Kinast C, Bolhofner BR, Mast JW, Ganz R. Subtrochanteric fractures of the femur: results of treatment with the 95-degree condylar blade plate. *Clin Orthop* 1989; 238:122–130.
25. Sanders R, Regazzoni P, Routt M. The treatment of subtrochanteric fractures of the femur using the dynamic condylar screw. Paper presented at the annual meeting of the American Academy of Orthopaedic Surgeons, Atlanta, GA, February 1988.
26. Pai C. Dynamic condylar screw for subtrochanteric femur fractures with greater trochanteric extension. *J Orthop Trauma* 1996; 10:317–322.
27. Nungu K, Olerud C, Rehnberg L. Treatment of subtrochanteric fractures with the AO dynamic condylar screw. *Injury* 1993; 24:90–92.
28. Wile PB, Panjabi MM, Southwick WO. Treatment of subtrochanteric fractures with a high-angle compression hip screw. *Clin Orthop* 1983; 175:72–78.

29. Ruff ME, Lubbers LM. Treatment of subtrochanteric fractures with a sliding screw-plate device. *J Trauma* 1986; 26:75–80.
30. Mullaji AB, Thomas TL. Low-energy subtrochanteric fractures in elderly patients: results of fixation with the sliding screw plate. *J Trauma* 1993; 34:56–61.
31. Ceder L, Lunsjo L, Olson O, et al. Different ways to treat subtrochanteric fractures with the Medoff sliding plate. *Clin Orthop* 1998; 348:101–106.
32. Chapman MW. The role of intramedullary nailing in fracture management. In: Browner BD, Edwards CD, eds. *The Science and Practice of Intramedullary Nailing*. Philadelphia: Lea & Febiger, 1987:17–23.
33. Ovadia DN, Chess DN. Intraoperative and postoperative subtrochanteric fracture of the femur associated with removal of the Zickel nail. *J Bone Joint Surg Am* 1988; 70:239–243.
34. Chapman MW, Bowman WE, Csongradi JJ, et al. The use of Enders pins in extracapsular fractures of the hip. *J Bone Joint Surg Am* 1981; 63:14–28.
35. Jensen JS, Sonne-Holm S, Tondevold E. Critical analysis of Ender nailing in the treatment of trochanteric fractures. *Acta Orthop Scand* 1980; 51:817–825.
36. Kuderna H, Bohler N, Collon DJ. Treatment of intertrochanteric and subtrochanteric fractures of the hip by the Ender method. *J Bone Joint Surg Am* 1976; 58:604–611.
37. Lund B, Hogh J, Lucht U. Trochanteric and subtrochanteric fractures. One year follow-up of a prospective study of Ender and McLaughlin osteosynthesis. *Acta Orthop Scand* 1981; 52:645–648.
38. Raugstad TS, Molster A, Haukeland W, et al. Treatment of pertrochanteric and subtrochanteric fractures of the femur by the Ender method. *Clin Orthop* 1979; 138:231–237.
39. Alho A, Ekeland A, Stromsoe KN. Subtrochanteric femoral fractures treated with locked intramedullary nails: experience from 31 cases. *Acta Orthop Scand* 1992; 62:573–576.
40. Wu CC, Shih CH, Lee ZL. Subtrochanteric fractures treated with interlocking nailing. *J Trauma* 1991; 31:326–333.
41. Wiss DA, Brien WW. Subtrochanteric fractures of the femur. Results of treatment by interlocking nailing. *Clin Orthop* 1992; 283:231–236.
42. Slater J, Taylor J, Russell T, Walker B. Intramedullary nailing of complex subtrochanteric fractures of the femur. *Orthop Trans* 1991; 15:774.
43. Taylor D, Erpelding J. Treatment of comminuted subtrochanteric femoral fractures in a young population with a reconstruction nail. *Mil Med* 1996; 161:735–738.
44. French B, Tornetta P. Use of an interlocked cephalomedullary nail for subtrochanteric fracture stabilization. *Clin Orthop* 1998; 348:95–100.
45. Wiss DA, Matta JM, Sima W, Reber L. Subtrochanteric fractures of the femur. *Orthopaedics* 1985; 8:793–800.
46. Wiss DA, Fleming CH, Matta J, Clark D. Commuted and rotationally unstable fractures treated with an interlocking nail. *Clin Orthop* 1986; 212:35–37.
47. Wiss DA, Brien WW, Stetson WB. Interlocked nailing for treatment of segmental fractures of the femur. *J Bone Joint Surg Am* 1990; 72:724–728.
48. Wiss DA, Brien WW, Becker V Jr. Interlocking nailing for the treatment of femoral fractures due to gunshot wounds. *J Bone Joint Surg Am* 1991; 73:598–606.
49. Brumback R, Ellison T, Molligan H, et al. Pudendal nerve palsy complicating intramedullary nailing of the femur. *J Bone Joint Surg Am* 1992; 74:1450–1455.
50. Brumback RJ, Reilly JP, Poka A, et al. Intramedullary nailing of femoral shaft fractures: part I. Decision making errors with interlocking fixation. *J Bone Joint Surg Am* 1988; 70:1441–1452.
51. Ebraheim N, Mekhail A, Checroun A. Entry point of reconstruction nail. *Am J Orthop* 1998; 27:474–476.
52. Stewart MJ. Discussion of paper. Classification, treatment and complications of the adult subtrochanteric fracture. *J Trauma* 1964:481.
53. DeLee JC, Clanton TO, Rockwood CAJ. Closed treatment of subtrochanteric fractures of the femur in a modified cast-brace. *J Bone Joint Surg Am* 1982; 63:773–779.
54. Johnson KD. Current techniques in the treatment of subtrochanteric fractures. *Techniques in Orthopaedics* 1988; 3:14–24.
55. Walling A, Bahner R. Pathological fractures. In: Koval K, Zuckerman J, eds. *Fractures in the Elderly*. Philadelphia: Lippincott-Raven, 1998:247–259.
56. Present D, Shaffer B. Evaluation and management of pathologic fractures. In: Zuckerman J, ed. *Comprehensive Care of Orthopaedic Injuries in the Elderly*. Baltimore: Urban & Schwarzenberg, 1990:513–532.

57. Harrington K. *Orthopaedic Management of Metastatic Bone Disease*. St. Louis: CV Mosby, 1988.
58. Barlow I, Thomas N. Reconstruction nailing for subtrochanteric fractures in the Pagetic femur. *Injury* 1994; 25:426–428.
59. Karachalios T, Atkins R, Sarangi P, et al. Reconstruction nailing for pathological subtrochanteric fractures with coexisting femoral shaft metastases. *J Bone Joint Surg Br* 1993; 75:119–122.
60. Broos P, Reynders P, Van Den Bogert W, Vanderschot P. Surgical treatment of metastatic fracture of the femur: Improvement of quality of life. *Acta Orthop Belg* 1993; 59:52–56.
61. Haentjens P, De Neve W, Casteleyn P, Opdecam P. Massive resection and prosthetic replacement for the treatment of metastases of the trochanteric and subtrochanteric femoral region: bipolar arthroplasty versus total hip arthroplasty. *Acta Orthop Belg* 1993; 59:367–371.
62. Zuckerman JD. *Comprehensive Care of Orthopaedic Injuries in the Elderly*. Baltimore: Urban & Schwarzenberg, 1990.
63. Aronoff PM, Davis PMJ, Wickstrom JK. Intramedullary nail fixation as treatment of subtrochanteric fractures of the femur. *J Trauma* 1971; 11:637–650.
64. Stoffelen D, Haentjens P, Reynders P, et al. Hip arthroplasty for failed internal fixation of intertrochanteric and subtrochanteric fractures in the elderly patient. *Acta Orthop Belg* 1994; 60:135–139.
65. Merle d'Aubigne R. Cotation chiffree de la fonction de la hanche. *Rev Chir Orthop Reparatrice Appar Mot* 1970; 56:481–486.

Chapter Eight
Pitfalls and Their Avoidance

Femoral Neck Fractures

Improper Treatment Selection

Almost all patients who sustain a femoral neck fracture should have operative treatment. Nonoperative treatment of an impacted femoral neck fracture, although advocated by some, is not recommended. Peter et al. reported a fracture displacement rate of 42% in older patients treated nonoperatively after sustaining Garden type I impacted femoral neck fractures[1]; when the fracture resulted in retroversion of the femoral head by more than 40°, loss of reduction occurred in 100% of patients.

There nevertheless remains a role for nonoperative management in certain patients who are nonambulatory and experience minimal discomfort after hip fracture. Another indication for nonoperative management is a patient who is medically unstable and cannot safely be cleared for surgery—for example, a patient who has had a recent myocardial infarction. In this and similar instances, it is better to accept the fracture deformity and perform reconstructive hip surgery at a later time, when the patient is a better surgical candidate.

Although all nondisplaced and many displaced femoral neck fractures should undergo internal fixation, primary hemiarthroplasty is the treatment of choice in certain cases. Elderly patients with a displaced femoral neck fracture and multiple medical comorbidities are best served by a single operation that is associated with a low failure rate (i.e., prosthetic replacement)—particularly when the presence of posterior femoral neck comminution substantially increases the risk for healing complications. Even though no clear relationship has been established between surgical delay and healing complications after displaced femoral neck fracture, we opt for prosthetic replacement in older patients with a displaced femoral neck fracture who present more than 3 days after injury.

Misinterpretation of Fracture Pattern

A common pitfall in the treatment of proximal femur fractures is a failure to properly interpret the fracture pattern. A displaced femoral neck fracture in which the femoral head is posterior to the femoral shaft and the distal fragment is externally rotated can be misinterpreted as a pertrochanteric fracture.

Figure 8.1. A displaced femoral neck fracture in which the femoral head is posterior to the femoral shaft and the distal fragment is externally rotated can be misinterpreted as a pertrochanteric fracture (**A**). A radiograph taken with the extremity internally rotated (**B**) can be used to better delineate the fracture pattern.

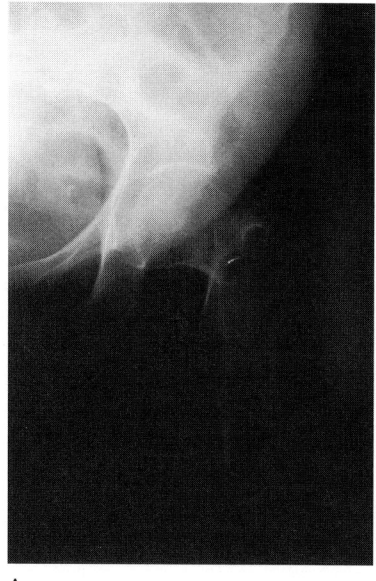
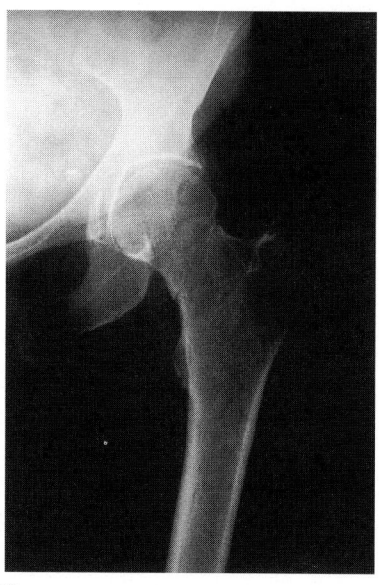

A   B

If the fracture pattern is misinterpreted, it may occur that the femoral neck fracture is properly diagnosed only after the anesthetized patient is placed on a fracture table and traction and internal rotation have been applied. If prosthetic replacement is the preferred procedure, the patient would have to be moved from the fracture table to a flat table. This pitfall can be avoided by the use of both anteroposterior (AP) and cross-table lateral radiographs when evaluating proximal femur fractures. If these radiographs do not clarify the nature of the fracture pattern, a radiograph should be taken with the extremity internally rotated (Figure 8.1).

Pitfalls of Internal Fixation

Improper Patient Positioning and Fracture Visualization

It is important that the patient be positioned on the fracture table with a well-padded fracture post and foot holders. Furthermore, it is imperative that the genital area be inspected before fracture reduction to verify, in men, that the scrotum is not incarcerated against the fracture post and, in women, that the mucosa of the labia is not placed against—or even directed toward—the fracture post (which can result in labial slough) (Figure 8.2).

Although they are usually associated with intramedullary nailing, cases of pudendal nerve palsy secondary to excessive traction and improper patient positioning on the fracture table during hip fracture surgery have been reported.[2,3] In such cases, pudendal nerve palsy results from compression of the patient's perineal region against the fracture post attached to the table. Although the incidence of pudendal nerve injury so induced has not been clearly established (partly because of reluctance among patients to report symptoms of sexual dysfunction), rates as high as 15% have been documented.[4] At least, it is perhaps best to avoid techniques that result in signifi-

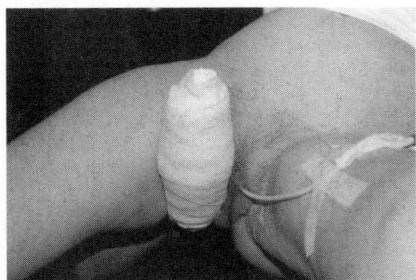

Figure 8.2. One must inspect the genital area before fracture reduction to verify, in men, that the scrotum is not incarcerated against the fracture post and, in women, that the mucosa of the labia is not placed against—or even directed toward—the fracture post.

cant increases in the traction forces. Kruger et al., using a load cell designed and fabricated to work with a standard fracture table, found that adduction of the injured extremity caused significant increases in the traction forces during femoral, tibial, and hip fracture stabilization.[5] Toolan et al., using an instrumented fracture post, reported that adduction of the ipsilateral lower extremity and abduction of the contralateral lower extremity with the hip and knee extended significantly increased the forces exerted on the perineum with use of a fracture table; abduction of the ipsilateral lower extremity and abduction of the contralateral lower extremity with the hip and knee flexed decreased the forces.[6] Because of these studies, we routinely position patients on the fracture table with the ipsilateral lower extremity in neutral abduction/adduction and the contralateral lower extremity abducted with the hip and knee flexed.

To properly assess the fracture reduction and guide implant insertion, one must obtain unobstructed AP and cross-table lateral radiographic images of the entire proximal femur (including the hip joint) before making the skin incision (Figure 8.3). Without visualization of the entire proximal femur, it is difficult to assess the guidewire position as it is advanced into the femoral head. Inappropriate screw length or location may result from inadequate radiographic visualization (Figure 8.4). It may be necessary to alter the positioning of the patient or the image intensifier to obtain an unobstructed cross-table lateral radiograph. In men, placement of the scrotum away from the image beam can help delineate the femoral head on the lateral radiographic view.

Figure 8.3. Positioning of the image intensifier for an AP (**A**) and a cross-table lateral radiograph (**B**).

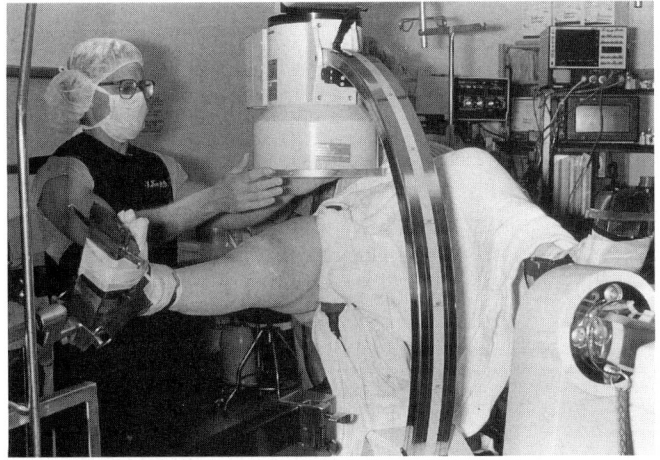

A

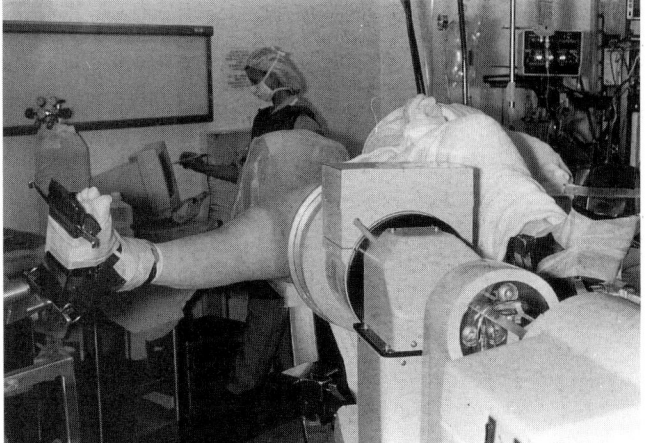

B

Figure 8.4. Improper visualization of the proximal femur (**A**) resulted in intraoperative pin penetration of the femoral head (**B**).

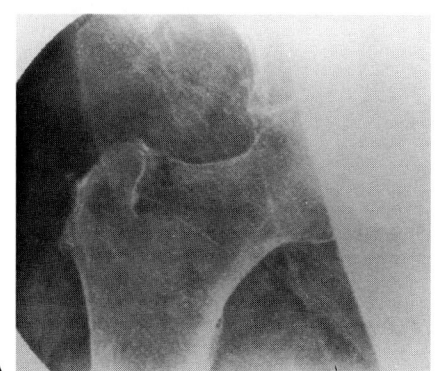
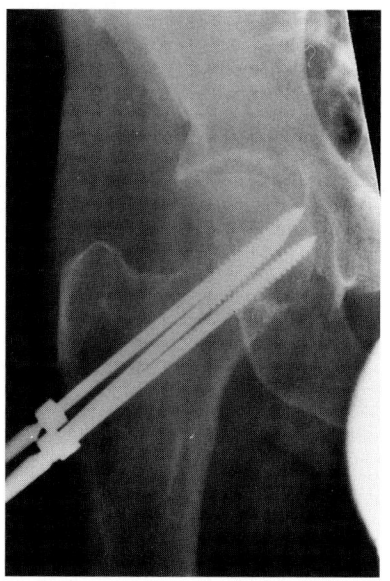

Inadequate Fracture Reduction

The quality of fracture reduction is the key to avoiding healing complications. An acceptable fracture reduction can have up to 15° of valgus angulation and 10° of anterior or posterior angulation. Varus angulation should be absolutely avoided. Excessive valgus angulation increases the risk of osteonecrosis, whereas varus angulation is associated with fracture nonunion. In our experience, fractures with substantial posterior displacement or retroversion of the femoral head are also at increased risk for loss of reduction. One must never judge the quality of fracture reduction or amount of posterior femoral neck comminution on the basis of low-quality fluoroscopic radiographs. If high-quality radiographs cannot be obtained by the image intensifier, hard-copy AP and lateral radiographic views are necessary. It is imprudent to perform repeated attempts at closed reduction; if fracture reduction is not achieved after two or three attempts, one should either perform an open reduction or opt for prosthetic replacement.

Improper Implant Selection

The implant of choice for stabilization of femoral neck fractures is a cancellous lag screw. Several series have confirmed the superiority of fixation with multiple cancellous screws to fixation with a sliding hip screw.[7,8] Large-diameter sliding hip screws, in particular, are associated with displacement of the femoral neck and increased risk of osteonecrosis (Figure 8.5). However, if a sliding hip screw is chosen for stabilization of a femoral neck fracture, a cancellous antirotation screw should be placed within the femoral head before insertion of the lag screw to minimize the risk of fracture displacement.

Improper Implant Insertion

Three or four cancellous lag screws should be inserted in parallel for stabilization of femoral neck fractures. Three screws are used for fractures without

Femoral Neck Fractures

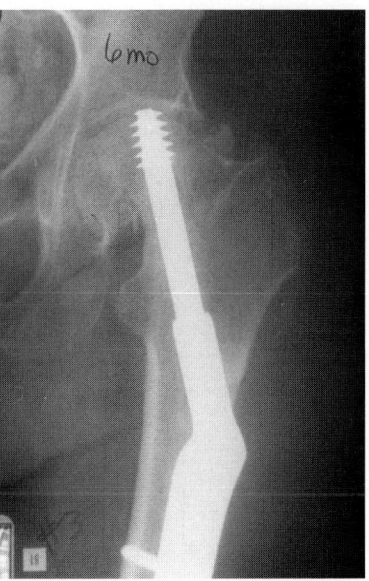

Figure 8.5. Osteonecrosis of the femoral head associated with use of a sliding hip screw to stabilize a femoral neck fracture.

posterior comminution and four are used when posterior femoral neck comminution is present. The three screws should be inserted in an inverted triangular configuration, with two screws superior and one screw inferior in the femoral head and neck[9] (Figure 8.6). Optimally, one screw should be inserted along the inferior femoral neck, one screw along the posterior femoral neck, and one screw sufficiently distanced from the previous two screws to provide a wide-based triangular configuration. A common pitfall during insertion of cancellous lag screws is to place the first guidewire or screw in the middle of the femoral neck and head, making it difficult to insert the remaining screws; this may result in a mechanically weaker configuration in which the screws are too close to one another (Figure 8.7). One should insert all guidewires before placing the screws; we find it easiest to insert the first guidewire in the inferior position, followed by the posterior guidewire, and then the final

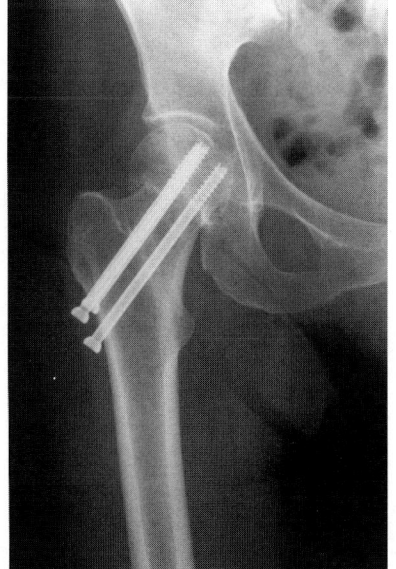

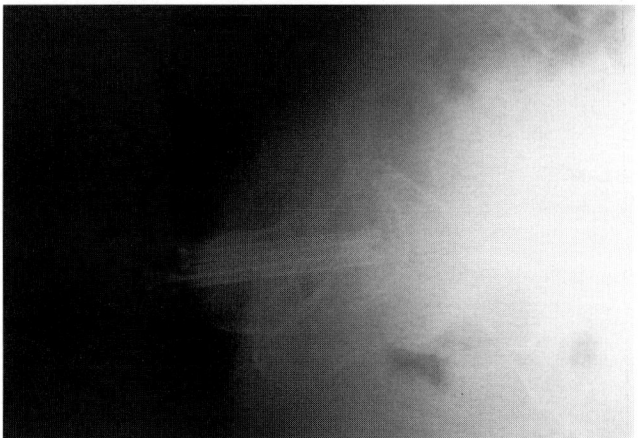

A B

Figure 8.6. Three cancellous lag screws inserted in parallel are used for stabilization of femoral neck fractures without posterior comminution. The three screws are inserted in an inverted triangular configuration, with two screws superior and one screw inferior in the femoral head and neck[9] (**A, B**). Optimally, one screw should be inserted along the inferior femoral neck, one screw along the posterior femoral neck, and one screw sufficiently distanced from the previous two screws to provide a wide-based triangular configuration.

Figure 8.7. Placement of three pins in close proximity to each other resulted in a mechanically weak construct and contributed to early loss of fracture fixation.

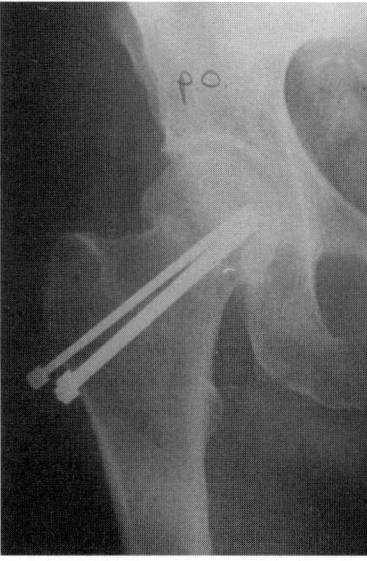
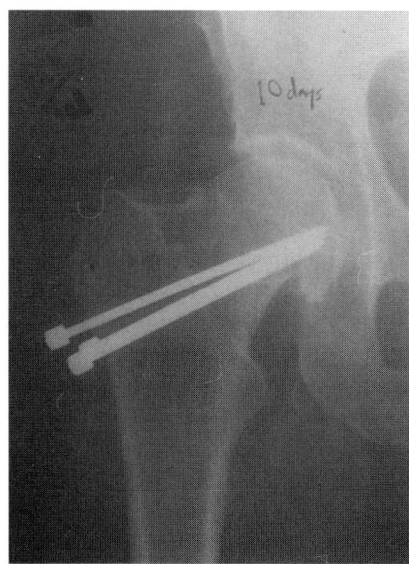

guidewire. The screws should be placed into the dense subchondral bone for improved fixation; short-threaded screws should be used so that the threads completely cross the fracture site.

Another pitfall to avoid is insertion of cancellous screws through the cortical subtrochanteric region; this creates a stress riser effect, increasing the risk for subsequent fracture (Figure 8.8). To minimize the stress riser effect, one should insert the cancellous screws proximal to the lesser trochanter, in the cancellous bone of the metaphyseal region. Finally, one must fluoroscopically assess screw position before closing the wound. It has been demonstrated that femoral head penetration can be missed on AP and cross-table lateral radiographic evaluation.[10] Accurate evaluation of screw position involves rotating the radiographic beam under fluoroscopy. This continuous fluoroscopic evaluation, while the beam is passed from AP to lateral position, is helpful to detect femoral head penetration.

Figure 8.8. Subtrochanteric fracture following stabilization of a femoral neck fracture using multiple pins.

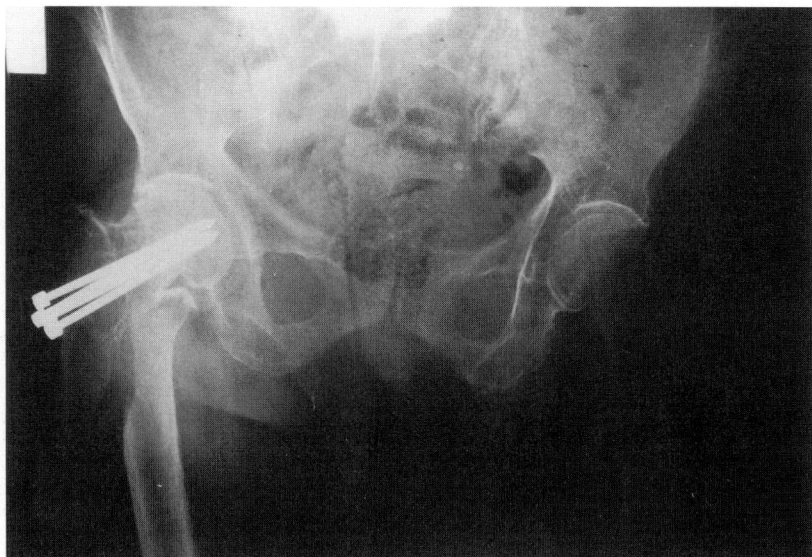

Pitfalls of Prosthetic Replacement

Improper Implant Selection

One-piece noncemented Austin-Moore and cemented Thompson endoprostheses have been associated with increased rates of acetabular erosion and femoral stem loosening[11] and should be used only in older, low-demand individuals. More active elderly patients should receive a cemented modular unipolar or bipolar endoprosthesis. One should not attempt placement of a true press-fit endoprosthesis in an elderly hip fracture patient whose proximal femur has thin cortices; besides representing an unnecessary expenditure for a more costly prosthesis, use of a press-fit prosthesis increases the risk for iatrogenic femur fracture during preparation of the femoral canal and insertion of the prosthesis.

Use of a total hip replacement after displaced femur fracture is associated with a greater incidence of dislocation and loosening (secondary to greater range of hip motion and increased patient demands) than is total hip arthroplasty performed for degenerative hip disease.[11] Primary total hip arthroplasty after acute femoral neck fracture is generally indicated only in patients with preexisting symptomatic acetabular disease.

Mismatch of Femoral Head Size

Placement of a prosthetic femoral head that is smaller in diameter than that removed at surgery will result in asymmetric unequal loads within the acetabulum and an increased risk of acetabular wear and subsequent protrusio acetabuli (Figure 8.9); use of a larger-diameter prosthetic femoral head than that removed at surgery may result in incomplete seating of the femoral head within the acetabulum, increasing the risk of prosthetic dislocation (Figure 8.9). In addition, Johnston et al. reported that patients who had received an oversized femoral head had increased complaints of hip and groin pain.[12] Mismatch can be avoided by carefully sizing the femoral head removed at surgery

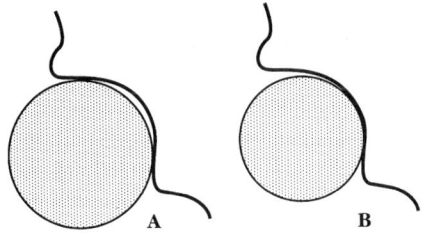
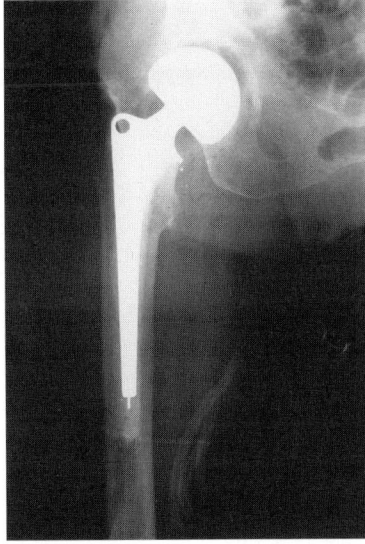

Figure 8.9. Use of a prosthetic femoral head that is larger in diameter than that removed at surgery may result in the prosthetic head not fully seating within the acetabulum, increasing the risk of prosthetic dislocation (**A**); placement of a prosthetic femoral head smaller in diameter than that removed at surgery will result in asymmetric unequal loads within the acetabulum and an increased risk of acetabular wear and subsequent protrusio acetabuli (**B**). AP radiograph demonstrating use of a larger-diameter prosthetic femoral head than that removed at surgery (**C**).

using either calipers or a set of templates provided with many arthroplasty sets. The selected femoral head is then placed within the acetabulum to determine its fit; the trial head should seat fully within the acetabulum, creating a strong suction in reaction to attempted removal. The subtleties of proper femoral head size can be appreciated by choosing the appropriate size based on calipers or templates and attempting to fit the sizes 1 and 2 mm above and below this size. This will allow the surgeon to appreciate the subtle differences between the proper femoral head size and one slightly undersized or oversized.

Inappropriate Femoral Neck Length

An optimum femoral neck length restores leg length equality and provides stability to prevent prosthetic dislocation. Shortening of the limb by excessive femoral neck resection and placement of a short femoral neck component may increase the risk for prosthetic dislocation secondary to soft tissue laxity—specifically the gluteus medius muscle, according to some authors.[13,14] Lengthening of the affected limb is poorly tolerated by patients and may result in increased pressure on the acetabular cartilage, increasing the risk of acetabular erosion.[14] As a general rule, the femoral neck osteotomy should be placed approximately 1 cm proximal to the lesser trochanter. One can estimate the femoral neck length required preoperatively, based on measurement of the uninjured hip and use of prosthetic templates; however, final femoral length, chosen at surgery, must be based on evaluation of hip stability and soft tissue tension. One can assess limb length postoperatively on an AP pelvis radiograph with the lower extremities in a neutral position (Figure 8.10). A line drawn between the inferior aspect of both ischial tuberosities should intersect the same area in both proximal femurs; unequal perpendicular distances from the right and left lesser trochanters to this line indicate a leg length inequality. With the lower extremities in the same neutral position, one should additionally confirm that the tip of the greater trochanter is at the same level with the femoral head bilaterally (Figure 8.10); otherwise, femoral neck lengthening or shortening may be present.

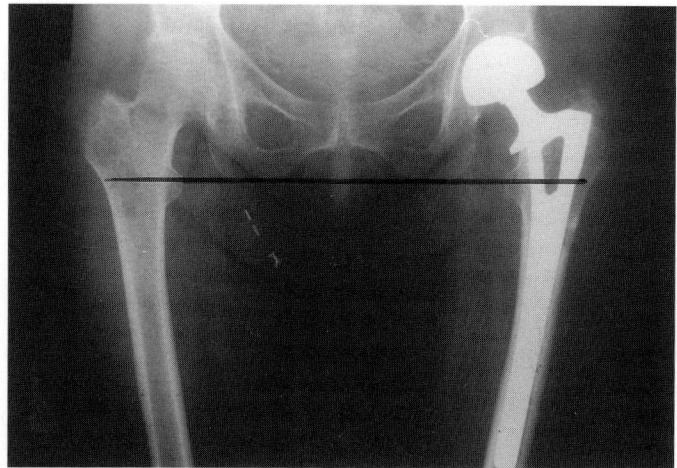
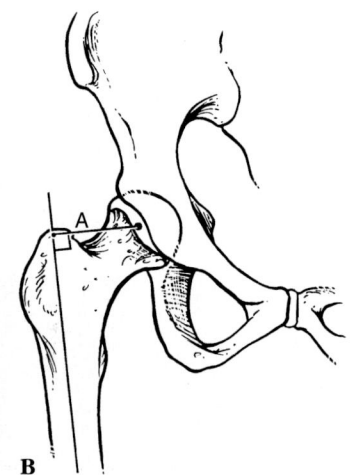

Figure 8.10. One can assess limb length postoperatively on an AP pelvis radiograph with the lower extremities in a neutral position. A line drawn between the inferior aspect of both ischial tuberosities should intersect the same area in both proximal femurs; unequal perpendicular distances from the right and left lesser trochanters to this line indicate a leg length inequality (**A**). With the lower extremities in the same neutral position, one should additionally confirm that the tip of the greater trochanter is at the same level with the femoral head bilaterally (**B**).

Inappropriate Prosthetic Version

The femoral prosthesis should be placed in approximately 10° to 15° anteversion relative to the distal femoral condyles. Excessive anteversion will result in an internal rotation deformity and increase the risk of anterior hip dislocation; retroversion will create an external rotation deformity and increase the risk of posterior dislocation (Figure 8.11). Inappropriate femoral version can be avoided by careful observation of the distal femoral axis during the femoral neck osteotomy, preparation of the femoral canal, and insertion of the femoral prosthesis. With a posterior approach, appropriate femoral neck anteversion can be determined by flexion of the knee and placement of the tibia in a vertical position. Although one can usually place the prosthesis in line with the residual femoral neck, this can result in incorrect prosthetic version if the patient has a developmental anomaly of the proximal femur (e.g., developmental dysplasia of the hip).

Varus Angulation of the Femoral Stem

The femoral prosthesis should be inserted in a neutral varus/valgus position. Although it is not associated with thigh or hip pain, varus positioning of the femoral stem increases the risk of prosthetic loosening.[15] With use of a cemented prosthesis, varus positioning can be avoided through use of a centralizer—a device, sized to the medullary canal, that attaches onto the tip of the femoral stem and positions the tip of the stem centrally within the femoral canal.

Intraoperative Femur Fracture

Intraoperative femur fracture can result during any of several stages of the surgical procedure. It can occur during the reaming process if excessive force is used to assist the hand reaming process. It can also occur if a mechanical reamer is stopped or becomes incarcerated within the femoral canal; the

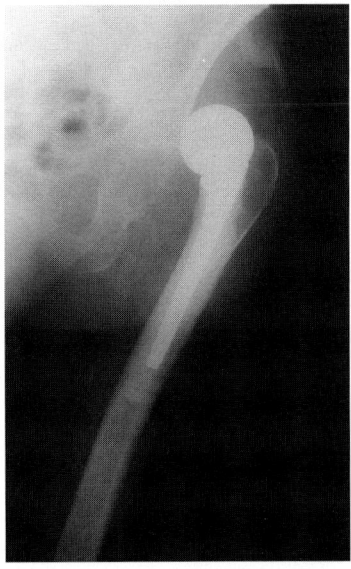

Figure 8.11. Posterior hip dislocation secondary to excess prosthetic retroversion.

torque generated by the mechanical reamer when the reamer is restarted may be sufficient to create an iatrogenic fracture in osteopenic bone. A femur fracture can also result if excessive force is used when attempting to seat the rasp. Rasping should be discontinued once it becomes difficult; at that point, the appropriately sized prosthesis should be inserted. With current metallurgy processes, even small-diameter femoral stems can be expected to withstand breakage over the lifetime of older individuals who sustain a femoral neck fracture.

Intraoperative femur fracture can occur during insertion of the femoral prosthesis. A cemented femoral component should be inserted completely by hand, while the cement is soft; a mallet should not have to be used to insert the cemented femoral prosthesis. Finally, the patient is at risk for iatrogenic femur fracture during the trial or final hip reduction or dislocation. One should direct the femoral head into the acetabulum and avoid excessive force; if the reduction is difficult, one should reassess the femoral neck length and/or capsular tension. During hip dislocation, one should place a bone hook around the femoral neck to pull the femoral head out of the acetabulum; use of excessive torque to dislocate the femoral prosthesis can result in a spiral fracture.

Iatrogenic intraoperative femur fractures must be addressed immediately. Femur fractures that occur during arthroplasty have been classified by Whittaker into three types[16] (Figure 8.12):

- Type I fractures involve the greater trochanter and requires either no treatment or tension band wiring if widely displaced.
- Type II fractures involve the femoral shaft around the prosthesis and require cerclage wiring, cable lock plating, or allograft strut fixation; if a noncemented prosthesis was used or the fracture occurred before insertion of a cemented prosthesis, a longer stem can be used with or without cement fixation.
- Type III fractures occur distal to the tip of the prosthesis and can be treated with either cerclage wiring, cable lock plating, or allograft strut fixation. These fractures are similar to type II fractures in that if a noncemented prosthesis was used or the fracture occurred before insertion of a cemented prosthesis, a longer stem can be used with or without cement fixation.

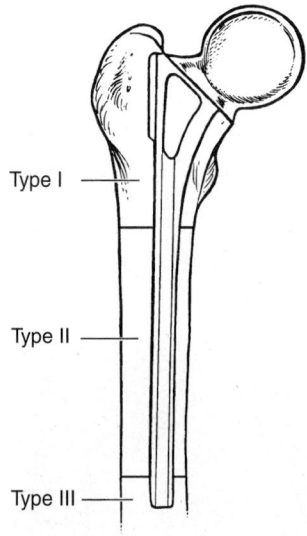

Figure 8.12. The Whittaker classification for periprosthetic femur fractures[16]: type I fractures involve the greater trochanter; type II fractures involve the femoral shaft around the prosthesis; and type III fractures occur distal to the tip of the prosthesis.

Intertrochanteric Fractures

Fracture Reduction

Poor Visualization

The majority of intertrochanteric hip fractures can be reduced closed on a fracture table. Occasionally, however, an open reduction may be necessary to achieve adequate fracture alignment. In either case, it is imperative to adequately assess the fracture reduction and obtain unobstructed anteroposterior and lateral x-ray images of the entire proximal femur, including the hip joint, before making the skin incision. Without visualization of the entire proximal femur, it is difficult to assess the location of the guide pin as it is advanced into the femoral head. In addition, inadequate radiographic visualization can result in inappropriate lag screw length or placement and increases the potential for intraarticular protrusion (Figure 8.13).

Inadequate Fracture Reduction

In the treatment of intertrochanteric hip fractures, it is important to achieve a stable reduction to minimize the risk of postoperative loss of fixation. This can generally be accomplished using one of two methods: anatomic alignment or medial displacement osteotomy. Anatomic alignment differs from anatomic fracture reduction in that the goal is simply to align the head and neck fragment with the shaft rather than to reduce and stabilize all fracture fragments. Biomechanical studies have shown that an anatomic alignment with use of a sliding hip screw results in improved compression across the calcar and lower tensile strain on the sideplate than medial-displacement osteotomy.[17]

Anatomic alignment of an intertrochanteric hip fracture must be critically assessed on the anteroposterior and lateral views. Three common pitfalls leading

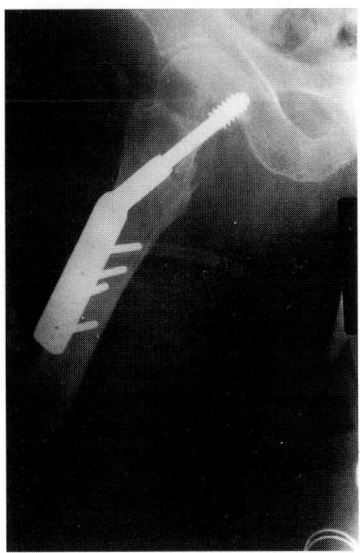

Figure 8.13. Inadequate visualization of the proximal femur resulted in lag screw penetration of the posterior femoral head.

to malreduction include posterior sag, varus angulation, and internal shaft rotation relative to the proximal fragment.[18] Posterior sag involves posterior angulation of the fracture fragments; if this is not recognized and corrected, it may be difficult to insert the implant into the center of the femoral neck and head. With posterior sag, the guide pin and subsequent lag screw will tend to be anterior in the femoral neck and posterior in the femoral head. Manual correction of posterior sag can be accomplished with use of a crutch placed under the thigh at the fracture level or intraoperative use of a periosteal elevator or bone hook (Figure 8.14). Reduction of the posterior sag must be maintained throughout the procedure until the implant is fully inserted; if the crutch, periosteal elevator, or bone hook is removed before insertion of the implant, the sag will recur and the guide pin may bend.

Varus angulation must be corrected before guide pin insertion. If the fracture is stabilized in a varus position, it will also be difficult to insert the implant in the center of the femoral neck and head; the lag screw will tend to be inferior in the femoral neck and superior in the femoral head (Figure 8.15). Varus malreduction results in increased tensile forces on the implant and increases the risk of fixation failure.[18] Furthermore, varus malreduction places the abductor musculature at a mechanical disadvantage and increases the likelihood of a limp secondary to abductor weakness. The use of additional traction to disengage the fracture fragments followed by repeat reduction will often correct this malposition. If varus malpositioning is not corrected with manual traction, one should assess the fracture reduction on the lateral radiographic view, as there may be posterior displacement or sag. One can also consider abducting the leg to correct a varus malposition.

Malrotation deformity is usually associated with an unstable fracture pattern. The femoral shaft fragment may not engage the proximal fragment and manipulation of the leg will not translate to the proximal fragment. Therefore, placement of the leg in internal rotation—as is usual to compensate for the normal anteversion of the femoral neck and facilitate placement of the lag screw in the femoral head—may result in an internal rotation malreduction.[18]

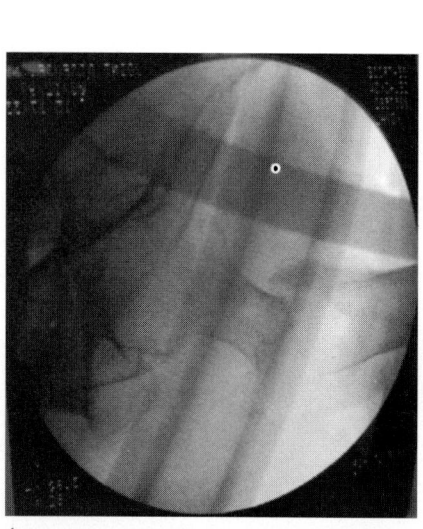

Figure 8.14. Posterior sag involves posterior angulation of the fracture fragments (**A**); if not recognized and corrected, it may be difficult to insert the implant into the center of the femoral neck and head. Manual correction of posterior sag can be accomplished with use of a crutch placed under the thigh at the fracture level (**B, C**) or intraoperative use of a periosteal elevator or bone hook. Reduction of the posterior sag must be maintained throughout the procedure until the implant is fully inserted.

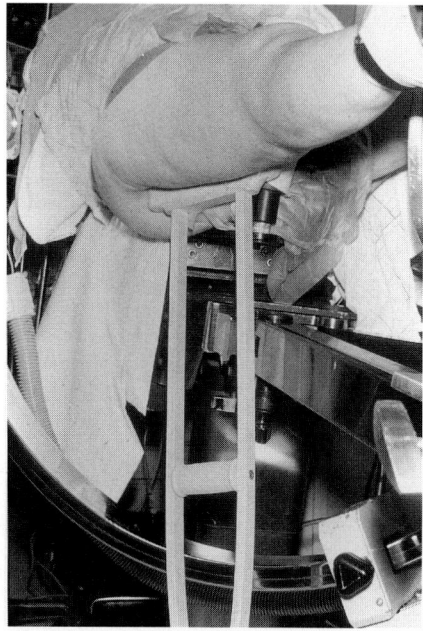

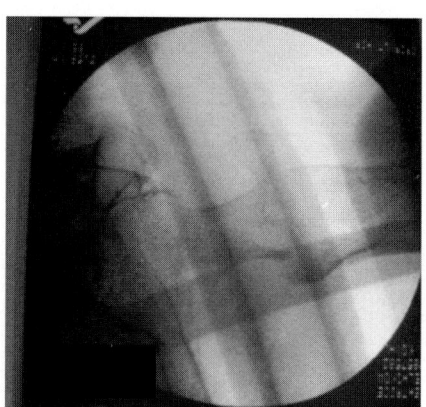

A B C

Intertrochanteric Fractures

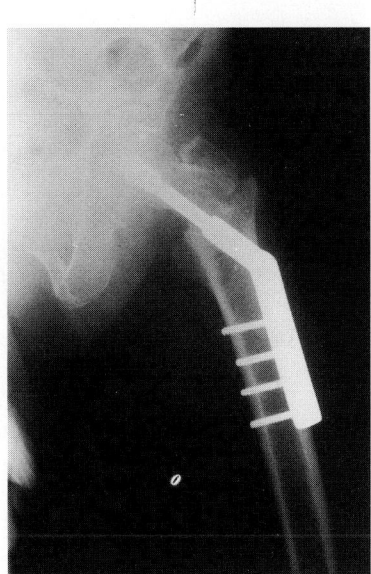

Figure 8.15. With varus angulation, it is difficult to insert the sliding hip screw in the center of the femoral neck and head; the lag screw will tend to be inferior in the femoral neck and superior in the femoral head.

To avoid this, fracture stability should be evaluated fluoroscopically after fracture reduction; if the fracture fragments do not move as a unit, one should place the leg in neutral position or slight external rotation and the insert sliding hip screw in this position.

Sliding Hip Screw

Although a sliding hip screw can be used to stabilize most intertrochanteric fracture types, use of this implant is not indicated for the reverse-obliquity pattern. In this case, fracture impaction results in displacement secondary to the orientation of the fracture line (Figure 8.16). Reverse-obliquity fractures are best stabilized with either a 95° plate or an intramedullary device.

Several pitfalls are related to the use of the sliding hip screw to stabilize intertrochanteric hip fractures.

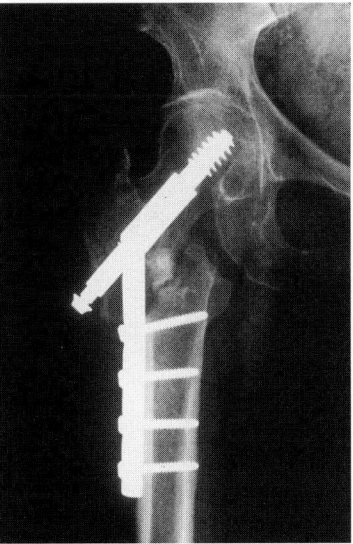

Figure 8.16. Use of a sliding hip screw for stabilization of a reverse-obliquity type intertrochanteric fracture resulted in fracture displacement secondary to the orientation of the fracture line.

Improper Guide Pin Location

The incidence of lag screw cutout is related to the position of the lag screw in the femoral neck and head at the time of insertion.[18] The optimal position of the lag screw is in the center of the femoral head and neck. This center–center position in the AP and lateral planes helps to ensure deep insertion of the lag screw into the femoral head and minimizes the torque on the femoral head during screw insertion. A helpful concept regarding this center–center position is Baumgaertner's *tip–apex distance,* the sum of the distances from the tip of the lag screw to the apex of the femoral head, measured on both the anteroposterior and lateral radiographs (corrected for magnification)[19] (Figure 8.17). To evaluate the ability of this measurement to predict lag screw cutout from the femoral head, Baumgaertner et al. followed 198 pertrochanteric fractures stabilized using a sliding hip screw.[19] Nineteen fractures had loss of fixation, 16 of them secondary to lag screw cutout. The average tip–apex distance was 24 mm for the fractures that united uneventfully and 38 mm for the fractures in which there was lag screw cutout; this difference was statistically significant. No fracture whose tip–apex distance was less than 25 mm had lag screw cutout. When a center–center position is not possible, some authors have suggested a posteroinferior lag screw placement; there is general consensus that an anterosuperior position should be avoided. With superior lag screw placement, the bending and torsional forces transmitted to the implant may lead to cutout during the postoperative period.

Guide Pin Breakage and Penetration

A bent guide pin may bind within the reamer and could subsequently be sheared in two by the reamer blade (Figure 8.18). Bending of the guide pin may be related to failure to maintain correction of posterior sag by removal of the crutch or bone hook once the guide pin is inserted; in this instance, the posterior sag will recur and the guide pin will bend. One should closely monitor the reaming process to detect binding of the guide pin; if it is difficult to advance the reamer over the guide pin, one should stop and reassess the guide pin–reamer relationship. Otherwise, the reamer may score and then cut the guide pin. One method of removing a broken guide pin involves overdrilling the lateral reamer tract with a larger-diameter reamer to the broken

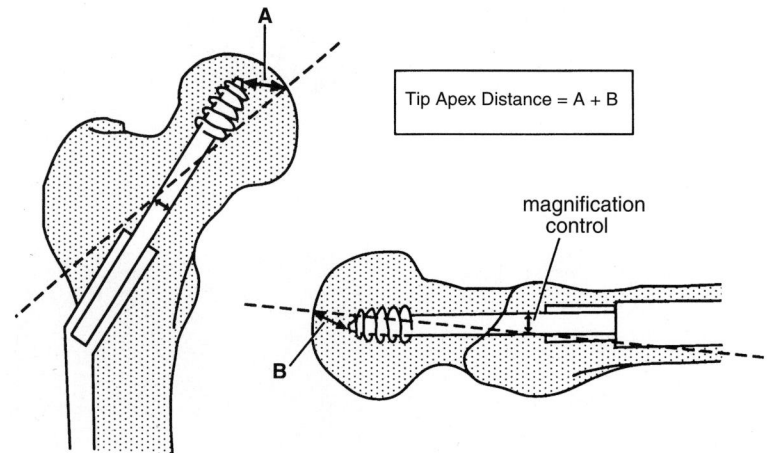

Figure 8.17. The optimal position of the lag screw is in the center of the femoral head and neck. A helpful concept regarding this center-center position is Baumgaertner's *tip–apex distance,* the sum of the distance from the tip of the lag screw to the apex of the femoral head, measured on both the anteroposterior and lateral radiographs (corrected for magnification) Redrawn from Baumgaertner.[19]

Intertrochanteric Fractures

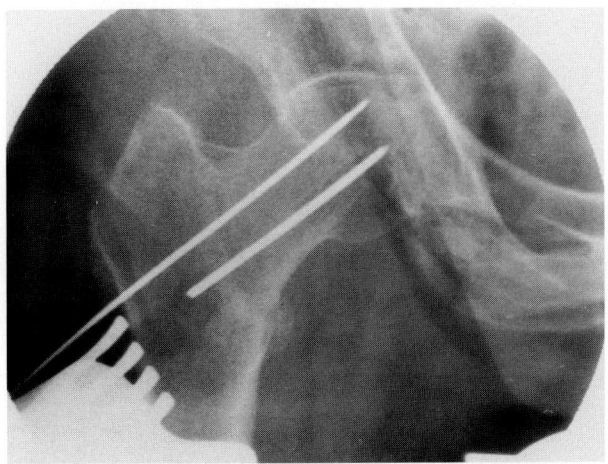

Figure 8.18. A broken guide pin. This guide pin broke during reaming of the proximal femur.

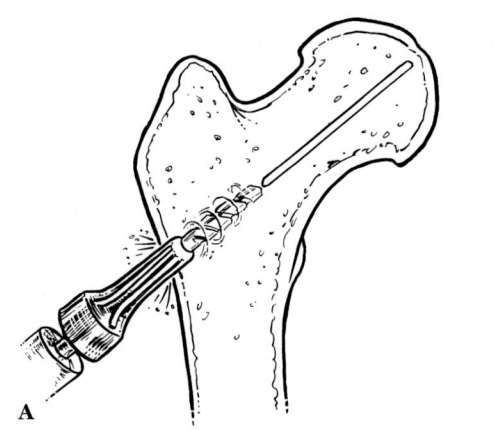
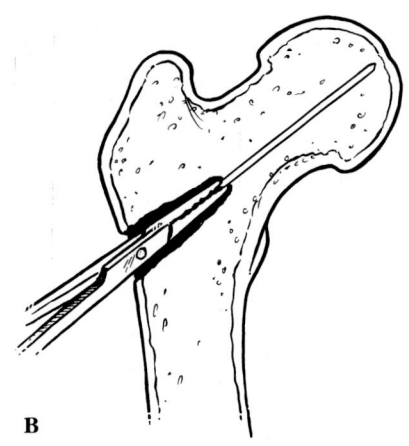

Figure 8.19. One method of removing a broken guide pin involves overdrilling the lateral reamer tract with a larger-diameter reamer to the broken end of the guide pin (**A**) and then removing the broken guide pin with a clamp under fluoroscopic control[18] (**B**).

end of the guide pin and then removing the broken guide pin with a clamp under fluoroscopic control[18] (Figure 8.19).

Binding of the guide pin within the reamer can also lead to guide pin advancement and subsequent intraarticular or intrapelvic penetration[18] (Figure 8.20). This can result in a life-threatening situation. In one case at our hospital, the obturator artery was lacerated, requiring emergent embolization. Several cases of vascular and visceral injury resulting from guide pin or lag screw penetration have been reported.[11]

Loss of Reduction During Lag Screw Insertion

During reaming or lag screw insertion, rotation of the proximal fragment with loss of fracture reduction can occur. This is most commonly encountered in

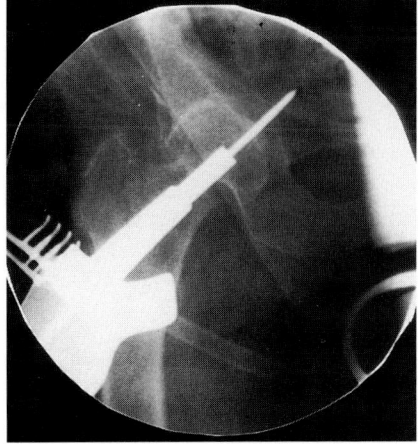

Figure 8.20. Binding of the guide pin within the reamer resulted in guide pin advancement and subsequent intrapelvic penetration.

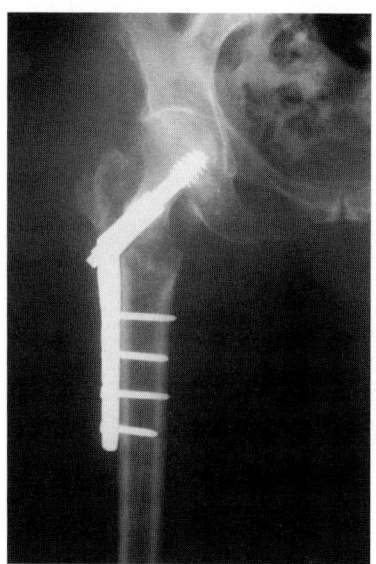

Figure 8.21. Malrotation deformity of the proximal femur that occurred during lag screw insertion. This radiograph provides a lateral view of the proximal fragment and an AP view of the distal fragment. To prevent rotation of the proximal fragment, the femoral head and neck can be tapped before inserting the lag screw. Basicervical fractures lack cancellous interdigitation, which provides rotational stability. To prevent proximal fragment rotation during stabilization of basicervical fractures, a supplemental antirotation wire or screw should be inserted before reaming the femoral head and neck.

cases in which bone density is high (usually in younger patients), in the presence of significant comminution, in basicervical fractures, and with eccentric placement of the lag screw in the femoral head (Figure 8.21). To prevent rotation of the proximal fragment, we routinely tap the femoral head and neck before inserting the lag screws. Basicervical fractures lack cancellous interdigitation, which provides rotational stability. To prevent rotation of the proximal fragment during stabilization of basicervical fractures, a supplemental antirotation wire or screw should be inserted before reaming the femoral head and neck. It is important, however, to place this screw parallel to the lag screw to allow postoperative impaction and to place it sufficiently superior to avoid contact with the lag screw. One may consider removing the anti-rotation screw after fully seating the large-diameter lag screw.

Improper Lag Screw–Plate Barrel Relationship

When a sliding hip screw loses its capacity to slide, it behaves as a fixed-angle device and is at risk for multiple complications: nonunion, lag screw cutout, penetration of the lag screw into the hip joint, sideplate bending or breakage, and loss of reduction (Figure 8.22). Loss of sliding capability may be related to excessive postoperative impaction or "jamming" of the lag screw within the plate barrel. Kyle et al., in a biomechanical study, demonstrated that jamming of the lag screw within the plate barrel will occur when the force of contact between the lag screw and barrel lip is greater than the sliding forces in line with the lag screw.[20] The amount of bending of the lag screw is inversely related to the amount of engagement between the lag screw and the plate barrel; such bending results in impingement of the screw at the barrel junction. Because bending of the lag screw is more likely with use of a short-barrel sideplate, a sideplate with a regular-length barrel is preferred for most intertrochanteric fractures. If a short-barrel sideplate is selected, it is very important to maximize engagement between the screw and barrel to decrease the risk of jamming.

Intertrochanteric Fractures

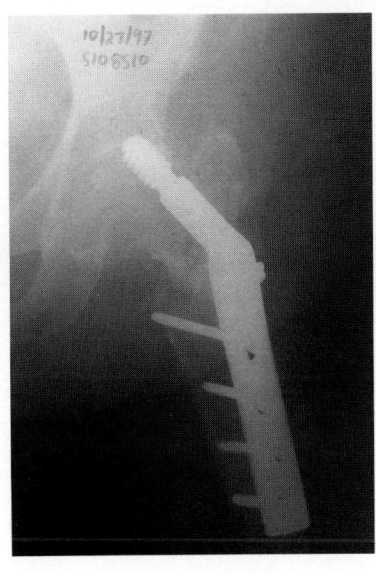 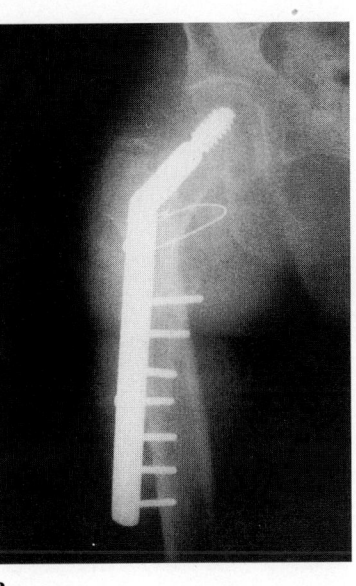

Figure 8.22. When a sliding hip screw loses its capacity to slide, it behaves as a fixed-angle device and is at risk for lag screw cutout (**A**) or sideplate pullout (**B**).

It is important to intraoperatively assess the capacity of the lag screw to slide within the barrel. Gundle et al. reported on a prospective series of 100 consecutive patients who sustained an unstable intertrochanteric fracture that was stabilized using a sliding hip screw.[21] In fractures stabilized with less than 10 mm of available slide, the risk of fixation failure was more than three times greater than in fractures with at least 10 mm of available slide. Based on the specifications for the particular lag screw and sideplate used in this study (DHS, Synthes, Paoli, PA), Gundle et al. advocated use of a short-barrel sideplate when using lag screws of 85 mm or less. Furthermore, one can help prevent the loss of available slide in the postoperative period by impacting the fracture at surgery; the traction on the affected limb should be released while loosely clamping the plate to the femoral shaft and the fracture impacted. The amount of available screw–barrel slide can then be reassessed prior to fixation of the sideplate; if necessary, appropriate changes in the implant can be made.

Disengagement of the lag screw from the barrel is another potential pitfall with use of a sliding hip screw[18] (Figure 8.23). This uncommon complication results from inadequate engagement between the lag screw and plate barrel secondary to use of either a short lag screw or a short-barrel sideplate. Poor lag screw–plate barrel engagement is suggested radiographically by lack of parallelism between the lag screw and the plate barrel. Most cases of lag screw–plate barrel disengagement have been associated with unstable fracture patterns and failure to restore the posteromedial buttress. At surgery, we routinely evaluate the potential for lag screw disengagement by direct visualization of the lag screw within the plate barrel (Figure 8.24); if the screw cannot be visualized, a compression screw is placed, not to generate compression, but to hold the screw and barrel together as a unit.

Improper Sideplate Placement

The plate portion of the sliding hip screw is assembled over the lag screw and is placed in contact with the lateral cortex of the proximal femur. Assembly of the screw and barrel is aided by the use of screw extension devices. The lag

Figure 8.23. Disengagement of the lag screw from the barrel resulting from use of a short-barrel side plate and inadequate lag screw–plate barrel engagement.

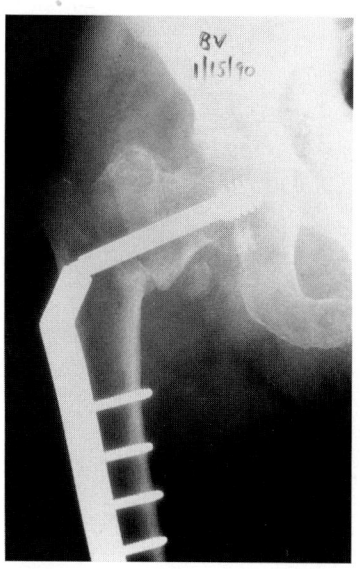

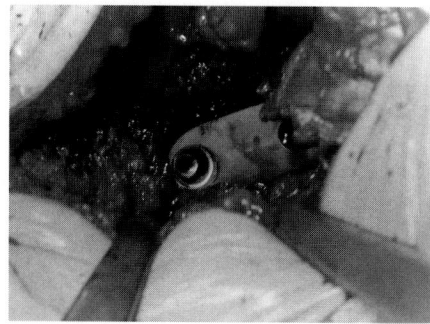

Figure 8.24. At surgery, the potential for lag screw disengagement can be evaluated by direct visualization of the lag screw within the plate barrel; if the lag screw cannot be visualized, a compression screw is placed, not to generate compression, but to hold the screw and barrel together as a unit.

screw and barrel must be properly engaged before the plate is impacted onto the femoral shaft. Otherwise, the lag screw could be driven through the hip joint and into the pelvis. In addition, a prominent lateral cortex may prevent proper placement of the sideplate (Figure 8.25). Removal of a small amount of cortical bone in the region under the plate–barrel junction may be necessary to allow proper plate placement.

Intramedullary Hip Screw

Patient Selection

Although virtually all intertrochanteric fractures can be stabilized with use of a sliding hip screw, such is not the case for an intramedullary hip screw. One

Figure 8.25. Radiograph demonstrating improper sideplate application.

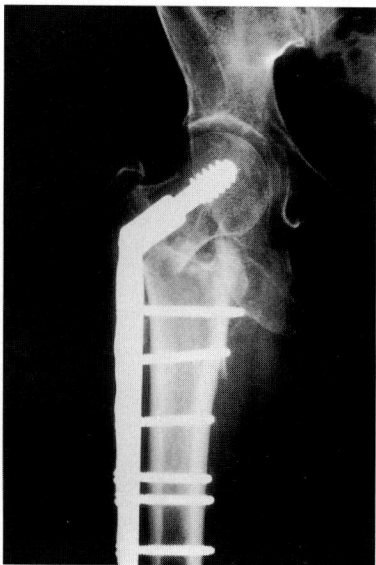

must carefully assess AP and lateral radiographs of the proximal femur for preexisting deformity, including excessive anterior bowing. In the event of obliteration of the medullary canal or excessive bowing of the femoral shaft, placement of an intramedullary device may not be possible. Furthermore, if there is a history of prior infection in the proximal femur, a sliding hip screw is recommended rather than an intramedullary hip screw to minimize the risk of intramedullary osteomyelitis.

Fracture Reduction

Unlike a midshaft femur fracture in which passage of a intramedullary nail will align the fracture fragments, one should not expect an intramedullary hip screw to effect fracture reduction (Figure 8.26). As with a sliding hip screw, one should reduce the fracture before inserting the implant. Unlike a sliding hip screw, however, one cannot place the extremity in abduction to help correct varus positioning. In order to pass an intramedullary nail down the medullary canal and reduce the risk of medial femoral cortex penetration or iatrogenic greater trochanteric fracture, one must ensure that the limb is in neutral alignment or adduction, with the patient's torso "windswept" to the opposite side. As with a sliding hip screw, it is imperative to have unobstructed visualization of the proximal femur, including the hip joint in both AP and lateral planes.

Starting Point

The suggested starting point with use of an intramedullary hip screw is at the tip of the greater trochanter, halfway between its anterior and posterior extent. One must be careful that this point is not too lateral on the greater trochanter. Although there is a built-in lateral bow to the currently available intramedullary hip screws, the nail will not be able to negotiate passage down the femoral canal if the starting point is too lateral. Furthermore, with a lateral starting point, there is an increased likelihood of fracture comminution during

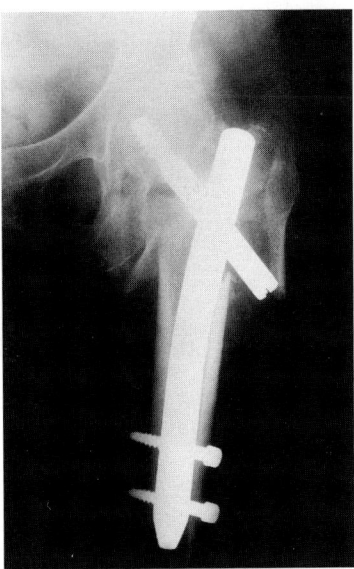

Figure 8.26. Radiograph demonstrating use of an intramedullary hip screw to stabilize a poorly reduced pertrochanteric fracture.

implant insertion. We prefer to err on the side of a medial starting point; we try to place the starting point in line with the anatomic axis of the femur, taking into account the fact that the lag screw should be placed in the center of the femoral head and neck. We use a guide pin from the sliding hip screw set to optimize the starting point on both the AP and lateral planes; once satisfied, we enlarge the entry point using a cannulated reamer from the sliding hip screw set.

Reaming

The entry portal and proximal femur should be reamed before insertion of the nail. In elderly individuals with a wide intramedullary canal, it is usually unnecessary to ream the femoral isthmus. In younger patients, particularly those with subtrochanteric extension, it may be necessary to ream the proximal femoral shaft and isthmus to accommodate the proximal portion of the nail. Reaming of the femoral canal in younger individuals should be performed over a ball-tipped guidewire, using a reamer design with deep flutes and a narrow reamer shaft. Failure to adequately ream the proximal femur may result in fracture comminution, particularly if the entry portal is not in line with the femoral shaft.

Nail Placement

Before nail placement, the insertion handler and driver are attached to the nail. With the intramedullary hip screw (Smith + Nephew, Memphis, TN), there are two intramedullary angle guide attachments, corresponding to the 130° and 135° nails. It is imperative that the angle guide be matched to the chosen nail. If the angle guide attachment and nail are incorrectly matched, it will be impossible to insert the lag screw. After assembly, one should verify that the proximal guide pin and distal locking screws target appropriately through the insertion handle (Figure 8.27). The nail should be inserted by hand through the greater trochanter into the proximal femur. In most cases, the device can be inserted without use of a guidewire. One should avoid use of excessive force, as this may result in comminution of the proximal femoral shaft (Figure 8.28). It is important to carefully follow the progress of the nail as it is inserted, using frequent fluoroscopic evaluation. If the nail does not advance, the surgeon must determine the cause. The tip of the intramedullary

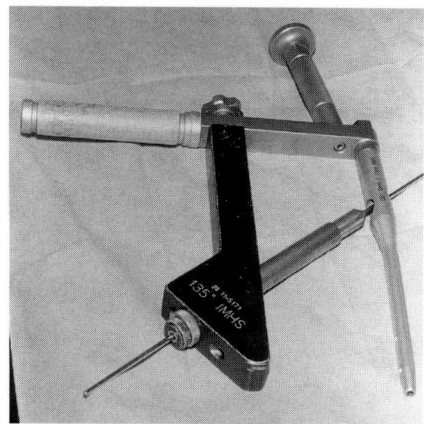

Figure 8.27. After assembly of the intramedullary hip screw and insertion handle, one should verify that the proximal guide pin and distal locking screws target appropriately through the insertion handle.

Intertrochanteric Fractures

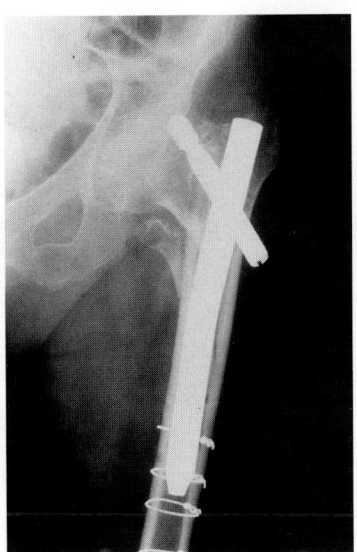

Figure 8.28. Intraoperative femur fracture that resulted from use of excessive force during insertion of the intramedullary hip screw.

nail may impinge on the anterior cortex of the bowed femoral shaft, particularly if the entrance site is too posterior. This can only be appreciated if the lateral fluoroscopic view is carefully examined and adequate visualization is obtained. Treatment involves elevating the insertion handle and readvancing the nail or, if necessary, eccentrically enlarging the anterior aspect of the entrance site.

Lag Screw Placement

The most important aspect of intramedullary hip screw insertion, as with insertion of a sliding hip screw, is placement of the lag screw within the femoral neck and head. The optimal position for the lag screw is the center of the femoral head and neck, within 5 to 10 mm of the subchondral bone. Insertion of the lag screw, however, can be more difficult than with use of a sliding hip screw because placement of the guide pin and lag screw is determined by the position of the intramedullary nail (Figure 8.29). One should take the time to verify that the position of the guide pin is optimized in the center of the femoral head before reaming. As with the sliding hip screw, one should tap the proximal femur to the desired final lag screw position to prevent rotation of the femoral head during lag screw insertion. Once the lag screw is fully seated, its centering sleeve must be appropriately positioned within the nail and held with a set screw inserted into the top of the nail (Figure 8.30); after insertion of the set screw, the lag screw will no longer be able to rotate but will be able to slide.

Distal Locking Screw Insertion

Because essentially all stable fractures and many unstable fracture patterns will move as a unit following the insertion of an intramedullary hip screw, we do not routinely use distal locking screws. If rotational instability or the potential for it exists (as with a large posteromedial fragment), one or two distal interlocking screws should be inserted.[22] Insertion of the distal locking screws is similar to proximal interlocking using conventional interlocked nails: a drill

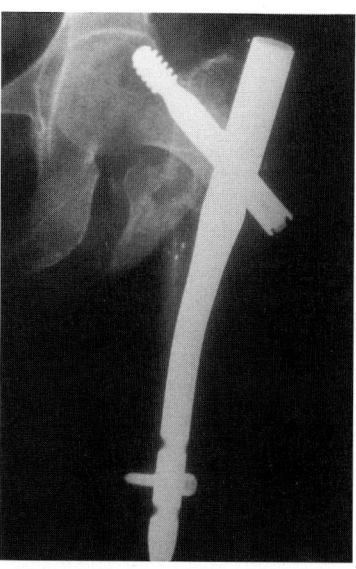

Figure 8.29. Lag screw cutout that resulted from poor lag screw positioning within the femoral head.

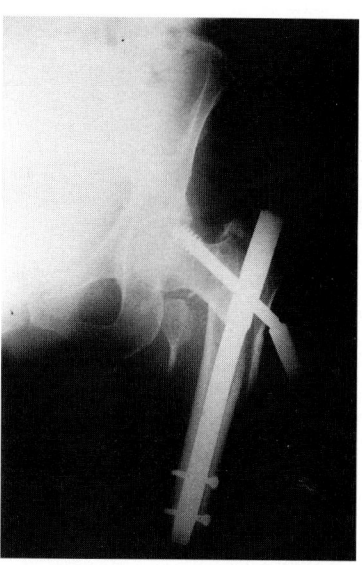

Figure 8.30. Loss of fracture reduction resulting from failure to insert the set screw and stabilize the centering sleeve.

guide is attached to the insertion handle, the drill guide is placed directly on the lateral cortex through a small percutaneous incision, a direct reading for screw length is taken from the drill after drilling is completed, and the screw is inserted through the outer drill sleeve. Because targeting systems are not 100% accurate, one should verify that the distal interlocks have been correctly inserted on both the AP and lateral radiographs before wound closure. The likelihood of the distal interlocks "missing" the nail increases with use of longer nails and when the insertion handle has been deformed during nail insertion (e.g., secondary to driving the nail down the femoral canal by striking the insertion handle with a mallet).

Subtrochanteric Fractures

Implant Selection

Although one can use either a sliding hip screw, a 95° fixed-angle plate, or an interlocked nail to stabilize most subtrochanteric fractures, certain fracture patterns are most amenable to a specific implant type. In this regard, the Russell-Taylor classification can be helpful[23] (Figure 8.31). Type 1A fractures with an intact lesser and greater trochanter behave like a femoral shaft fracture and are best stabilized using a standard (centromedullary) interlocked nail. Type 1B fractures with proximal fracture extension into the lesser trochanter but not the piriformis fossa are amenable to either a cephalomedullary interlocked nail (reconstruction nail) or a plate-and-screw device; in this circumstance, a standard interlocked nail may provide insufficient proximal stability. Type 2A

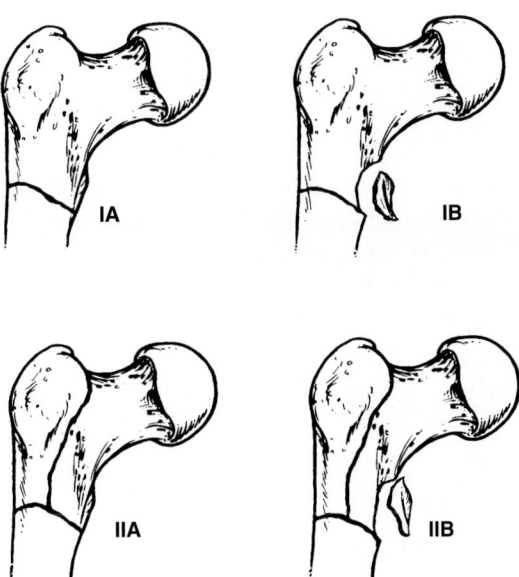

Figure 8.31. The Russell-Taylor classification for subtrochanteric fractures.[23]

fractures with fracture extension into the piriformis fossa are very difficult to stabilize using an intramedullary implant and are more amenable to use of plate and screws; with an intramedullary device, the nail reamers and implant have a tendency to exit posteriorly out of the proximal fragment. Type 2B fractures with comminution of the piriformis fossa, lesser trochanter, and femoral shaft are also very difficult to stabilize with an intramedullary implant and may be best treated with a sliding hip screw or 95° fixed-angle plate using indirect reduction techniques. As with type 2A fractures, an intramedullary nail will tend to exit posteriorly out of the proximal fragment; if a reconstruction nail is selected for fracture stabilization, the nail starting point should be moved anterior to the piriformis fossa with frequent radiographic assessment to verify that the reamer and implant remain within the trochanteric mass.

95° Fixed-Angle Devices

Poor Preoperative Planning

Although the exact nature of the fracture, with identification of all major fracture fragments, should be determined before any surgical intervention, it is essential with use of a 95° fixed-angle device. Preoperative planning helps the surgeon understand the "personality" of the fracture and mentally prepare for the operative procedure; furthermore, it helps to ensure that the proper equipment will be available at surgery. Preoperative planning allows one to determine the entry site of the blade (or lag screw) relative to the vastus tubercle as well as the appropriate lengths of the blade and sideplate (Figure 8.32). Pitfalls associated with poor preoperative planning include poor entry site selection; improper blade plate, condylar screw, or sideplate length; poor fracture reduction; and excessive soft tissue dissection. Without proper preoperative planning, it is possible that the appropriate implant will not be available at surgery.

Figure 8.32. A preoperative plan depicting use of a condylar blade plate to stabilize a subtrochanteric fracture. This plan can help to determine the entry site of the blade relative to the vastus tubercle as well as the appropriate lengths of the blade and side plate.

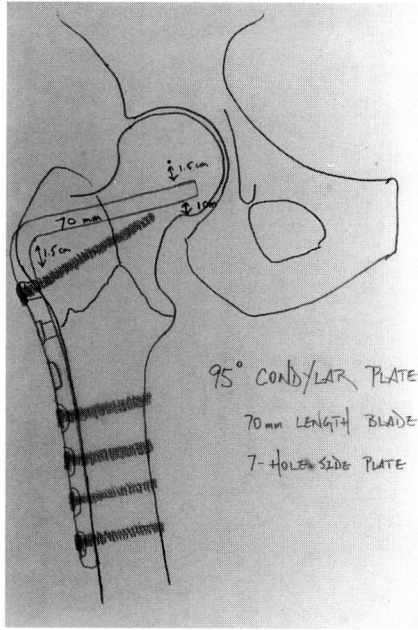

Poor Visualization

Whether the patient is positioned on a fluoroscopic table or a fracture table for subtrochanteric fracture stabilization, it is essential that unobstructed anteroposterior and lateral radiographic images of the entire proximal femur, including the hip joint, be obtained before making the skin incision (Figure 8.33). Although supine positioning on a fluoroscopic table allows free lower-extremity manipulation, it can be difficult to obtain a cross-table or frog lateral; when using a fluoroscopic table and supine patient positioning, we place a bolster under the involved buttock to elevate the proximal femur and adjust the image intensifier to optimize fluoroscopic visualization. Radiographic visualization is facilitated with use of a fracture table.

Figure 8.33. Perforation of the posterior cortex by the condylar blade plate secondary to poor radiographic visualization of the proximal femur.

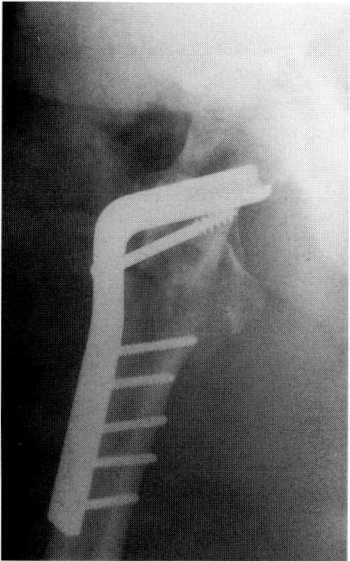

Improper Entry Site

The proper entry site for a 95° fixed-angle plate relative to the vastus tubercle is determined from preoperative planning. This window should lie in the anterior half of the greater trochanter; if the anteroposterior width of the greater trochanter is divided into thirds, the entry window should be at the junction of the anterior third and middle third (Figure 8.34). Placement of the window in the middle of the greater trochanter increases the risk that the blade or condylar screw will penetrate the posterior femoral neck.

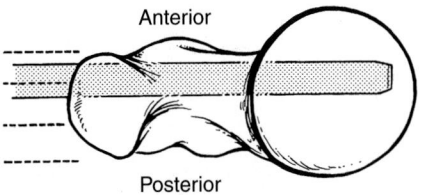

Figure 8.34. Diagram depicting the proper entry site for a 95° fixed-angle device. This entry point should lie in the anterior half of the greater trochanter; if the anteroposterior width of the greater trochanter is divided into thirds, the entry point should be at the junction of the anterior third and the middle third.

Fracture Malreduction

Fracture malreduction can result from improper insertion of a 95° condylar blade plate or screw (Figure 8.35). Since each of these is a fixed-angle device, placement of the blade or lag screw within the proximal fragment determines the fracture reduction. The 95° condylar blade plate is an unforgiving device; correct insertion requires simultaneous positioning in the proximal fragment in three planes. Summation guidewires can be used to determine the spatial orientation of the seating chisel. One guidewire marks the anteversion of the femoral neck; exposure of the anterior femoral neck can be used to further assess the amount of femoral neck anteversion. Another guidewire determines the direction of the seating chisel in the coronal plane; placement of this guidewire can be facilitated through use of the condylar guide, placed flush against the lateral cortex of the proximal fragment (Figure 8.36). If the proximal fragment is too short to allow use of the condylar guide, placement of the second guidewire must be based on the preoperative plan. Because of the complexity of blade–plate insertion, the condylar screw is used more commonly; it is technically easier to insert. The guide pin can be reinserted multiple times until one is satisfied with its position; the channel for the lag screw is then reamed and the lag screw inserted over the guide pin.

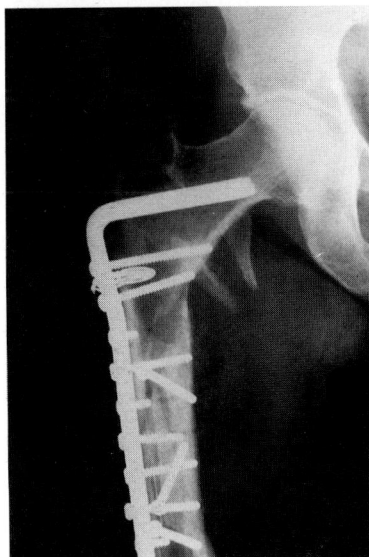

Figure 8.35. Varus malreduction resulting from improper condylar blade plate insertion into the proximal fragment.

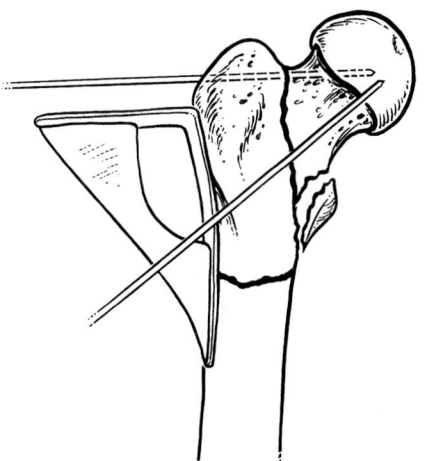

Figure 8.36. Use of summation guidewires to determine the direction of the seating chisel. Placement of the guidewire in the coronal plane can be facilitated through use of the condylar guide, placed flush against the lateral cortex of the proximal fragment.

Improper Assembly of the Condylar Blade Plate Seating Chisel

The seating chisel mirrors the blade portion of the 95° condylar blade plate; it is U-shaped, with the two arms of the U positioned opposite the sideplate. In the proximal femur, the seating chisel must be assembled to its guide with the U-shaped portion facing inferior. If the seating chisel is assembled and inserted in the incorrect reverse position, one will not be able to insert the condylar blade plate. In this instance, the seating chisel would have to be reassembled in the correct position and a new channel prepared in the femoral head and neck.

Incarceration of the Condylar Blade Plate Seating Chisel

One must slowly advance the condylar blade plate seating chisel into the proximal fragment with alternating forward and backward strokes of the slotted hammer; continuous forward advancement of the seating chisel may result in incarceration of the fully seated chisel in strong cancellous bone. We use three to four mallet strokes forward into the proximal fragment and then free the seating chisel with mallet strokes in the opposite direction. It is important to completely free the seating chisel from the surrounding cancellous bone. One must also be careful to replace the seating chisel by hand into the prepared tract so that it does not create multiple tracts in the femoral head and neck.

Excessive Soft Tissue Dissection

The goal of surgery is anatomic fracture alignment with stable fixation, not anatomic reduction of every fracture fragment, which would necessitate extensive soft tissue and osseous dissection. Excessive soft tissue dissection unnecessarily compromises the vascularity of the fracture fragments and thereby extends the time needed for fracture union and increases the risk of healing complications. One should avoid placement of retractors around the medial aspect of the proximal femur so as not to compromise soft tissue attachments to the osseous fragments. Radiographs that show screws inserted from multiple directions are usually an indication of excessive soft tissue dissection (Figure 8.37).

Preoperative planning can help to avoid excessive soft tissue dissection. The 95° condylar blade plate or screw can be used to effect fracture reduction. Once the device is inserted within the proximal fragment, the shaft of the plate is brought to the lateral cortex of the distal fragment, the limb rotation is determined, and the plate is secured with a Verbrugge clamp. The fracture fragments can be reduced using either an AO-ASIF articulated tensioning device or a femoral distractor. With appropriate distraction, comminuted medial fragments often reduce spontaneously as a result of soft tissue attachments (ligamentotaxis). If necessary, displaced medial fragments can be teased into position through the fracture site; to avoid soft tissue stripping and osseous devascularization, the fracture fragments should not be manipulated from the medial cortical surface. If anatomic fracture reduction can be achieved without

Subtrochanteric Fractures

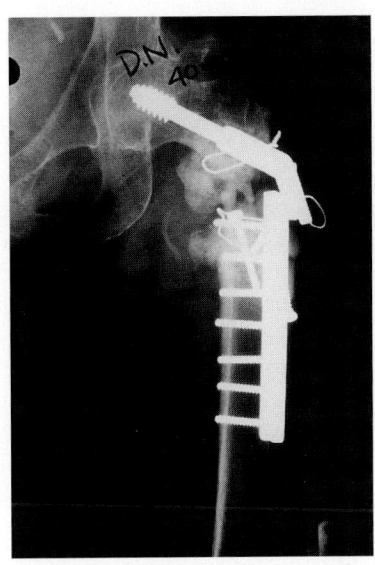

Figure 8.37. Subtrochanteric nonunion with implant failure resulting from excessive soft tissue dissection and osseous devascularization.

soft tissue disruption and osseous devascularization, it should be performed; if anatomic reduction of the fracture fragments would necessitate osseous devascularization, however, it is better to bridge the fracture area with the plate, leaving the displaced comminuted fragments with soft tissue attachments to act as vascularized bone graft (Figure 8.38). Once the fracture is aligned and the fracture fragments teased into position, the articulated tensioning device can be used to compress the fracture fragments if the fracture will accept axial compression without loss of reduction. Bone grafting is usually not necessary unless soft tissue dissection has resulted in osseous devascularization.[24] A bone graft should be inserted through the fracture and should not require further soft tissue dissection.

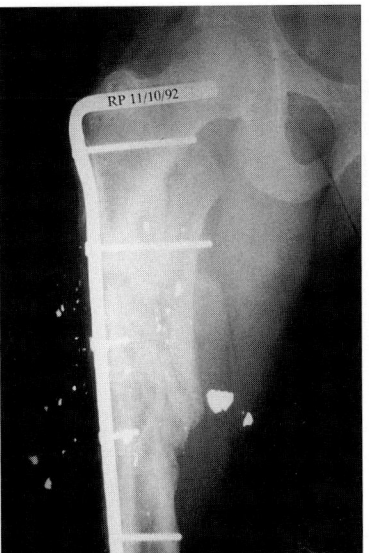

Figure 8.38. Highly comminuted subtrochanteric fracture stabilized with a condylar blade plate using indirect reduction techniques. The implant was used to bridge the area of comminution.

Interlocked Nails

Inappropriate Implant

Subtrochanteric femoral fractures with an intact lesser trochanter and piriformis fossa are best stabilized with a standard (centromedullary) interlocked nail. A cephalomedullary interlocked nail (reconstruction nail) is indicated for the treatment of subtrochanteric femoral fractures with disruption of the lesser trochanter, pathologic subtrochanteric fractures, and ipsilateral femoral neck and shaft fractures. This nail type has also been used to stabilize complex subtrochanteric fractures with fracture extension into the piriformis fossa; however, because the surgery is technically challenging, we believe that plates and screws are better implants for this fracture type. A cephalomedullary nail should not be considered as the device of choice for conventional diaphyseal fractures of the femur.

Poor Visualization

As with use of a 95° fixed-angle device, it is essential that unobstructed anteroposterior and lateral x-ray images of the entire proximal femur, including the hip joint, be obtained before making the skin incision. We perform interlocked nailing on a fracture table to optimize fluoroscopic visualization.

Missed Femoral Neck Fracture

One must always evaluate the status of the femoral neck prior to femoral nailing, since ipsilateral femoral neck and shaft fractures occur in as many as 5% of femoral shaft fractures and are often initially overlooked[25,26] (Figure 8.39). If a nondisplaced femoral neck fracture is diagnosed at surgery before femoral nailing, the femoral neck can be provisionally stabilized using pins or screws followed by definitive fixation of both the femoral neck and subtrochanteric

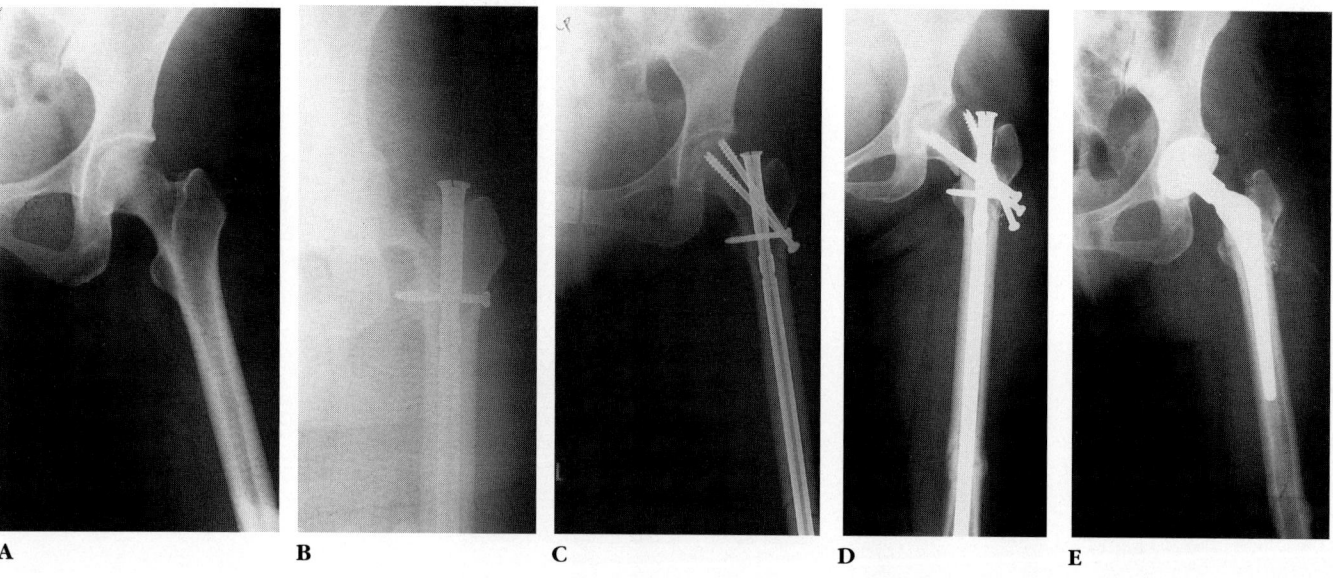

Figure 8.39. Ipsilateral femoral neck and shaft fractures in a 35-year-old woman (**A**). The femoral neck fracture was not recognized until it displaced after femoral nailing (**B**) and was then reduced and stabilized using multiple cancellous screws (**C**). The femoral neck fracture failed to unite (**D**) and eventually required total hip arthroplasty (**E**).

Subtrochanteric Fractures

fractures using a reconstruction nail. Alternatively, if a proximal shaft fracture is present, one may stabilize both fractures using plate and screws. If the femoral neck is displaced, femoral neck fracture reduction should be performed emergently, followed by fracture stabilization.

Improper Insertion Point

Selection of an improper entry point for intramedullary nailing may result in fracture malreduction, iatrogenic femoral neck fracture, or fracture comminution (Figure 8.40). The entry portal should be in the middle of the piriformis fossa, in line with the femoral shaft on both the sagittal and coronal planes. With use of a reconstruction nail, the entry portal should be moved anterior to the piriformis fossa to facilitate placement of the proximal locking screws into the femoral neck and head (Figure 8.41). A lateral entry portal may result in

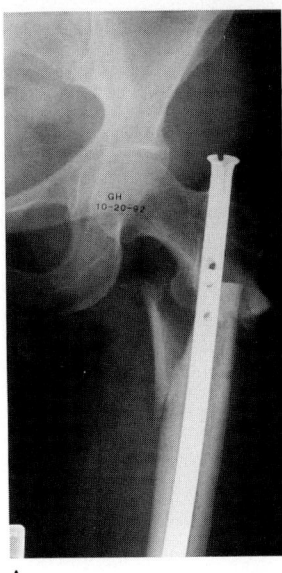
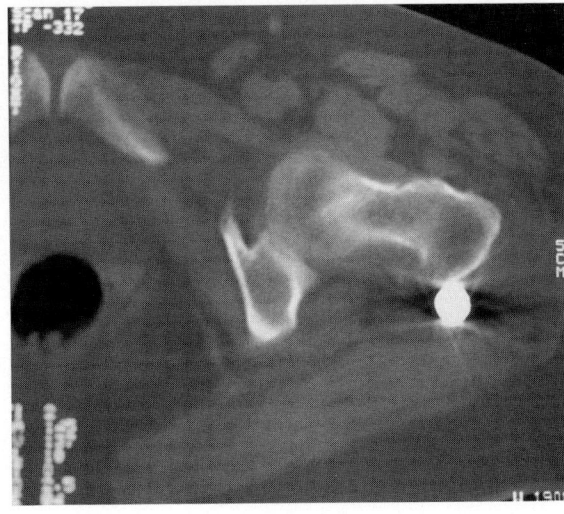

A B

Figure 8.40. Loss of reduction of a subtrochanteric fracture associated with use of an interlocked nail (**A**); computed tomography demonstrated that the intramedullary nail was inserted outside the proximal fragment (**B**).

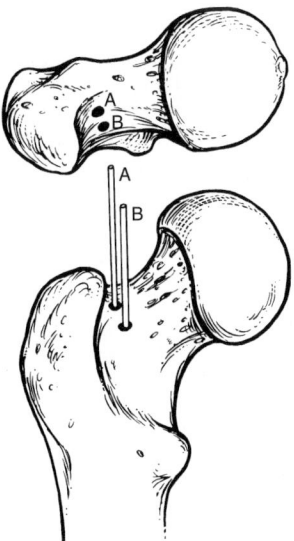

Figure 8.41. The entry portal for intramedullary nailing should be in the middle of the piriformis fossa, in line with femoral shaft on both the sagittal and coronal planes (point B). With use of a reconstruction nail, the entry portal should be moved anterior to the piriformis fossa to facilitate placement of the proximal locking screws into the femoral neck and head (point A).

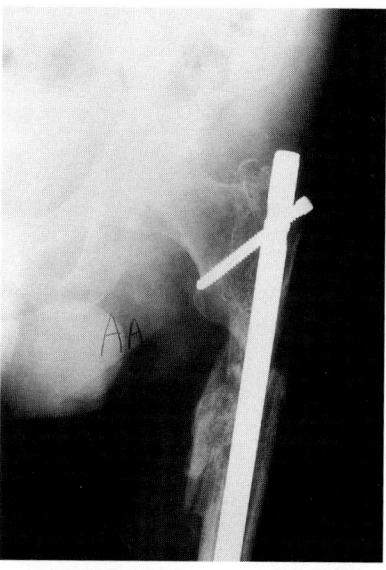

Figure 8.42. Varus fracture reduction resulting from a lateral entry point during intramedullary nailing.

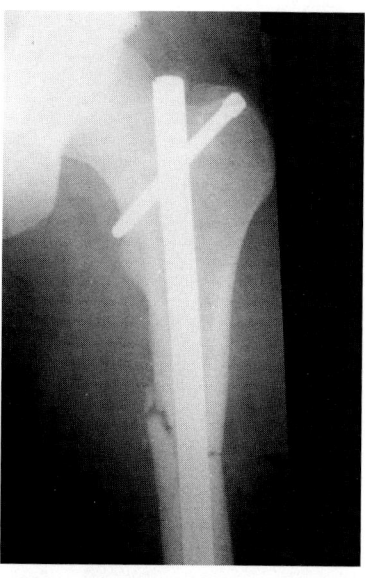

Figure 8.43. AP radiograph demonstrating a medial entry point through the femoral neck.

fracture varus positioning (Figure 8.42), whereas a medial entry portal increases the risk of femoral neck fracture (Figure 8.43). An anterior entry point increases the hoop stresses within the proximal fragment and the risk of comminution of the proximal fragment.[27] With subtrochanteric fractures, creation of the entry portal is often complicated by the flexed, abducted, and externally rotated position of the proximal fragment. In this instance, a pin (joystick) can be inserted into the proximal fragment and used to manipulate the fragment into a neutral position (Figure 8.44).

Fracture Malreduction

One must not depend on the intramedullary nail to effect fracture reduction. The intramedullary nail will follow the guidewire down the femoral canal; if

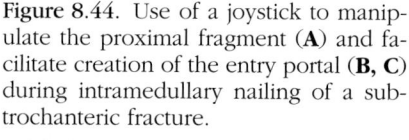

Figure 8.44. Use of a joystick to manipulate the proximal fragment (**A**) and facilitate creation of the entry portal (**B, C**) during intramedullary nailing of a subtrochanteric fracture.

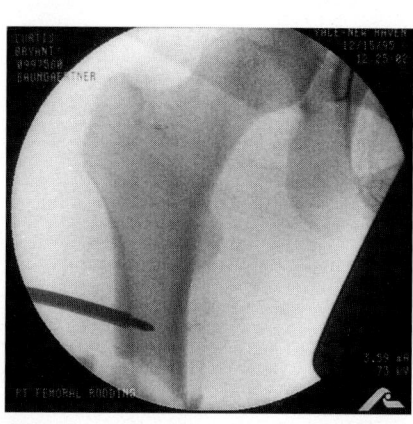

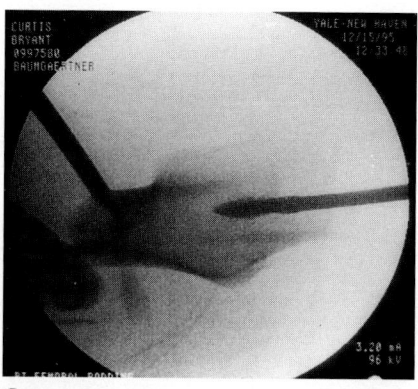

A　　　　　　　　　　　B　　　　　　　　　　　C

Subtrochanteric Fractures

the guidewire is not centralized within the proximal and distal femoral fragments, an angular malreduction will result. Fracture reduction must be achieved prior to guidewire insertion. Fracture reduction can be achieved through ligamentotaxis using the fracture table or femoral distractor or through more direct means by use of an alignment rod or small-diameter nail inserted into the proximal fragment as a joystick. One should verify the fracture reduction during the reaming process to avoid eccentric thinning of the femoral cortex and during nail insertion to avoid iatrogenic fracture comminution.

It is important to verify correct femoral length and rotation before static locking of the intramedullary nail (Figure 8.45). Determination of correct femoral length can be difficult with fracture comminution; preoperative planning using the contralateral side can be used to determine the appropriate nail and limb length. Determination of femoral rotation is facilitated with femoral nailing in the supine position; the risk of rotational deformity is increased with femoral nailing in a lateral position. One can use the normal 10° to 15° anteversion of the femoral neck to help ascertain correct femoral rotation in comminuted fractures. The image intensifier is rotated until a perfect cross-table lateral view of the femoral head and neck without anteversion is obtained; the angular position of the image intensifier is recorded and the distal fragment is rotated until a perfect lateral view of the distal femur is obtained. At this point, the distal fragment is internally rotated 10° to 15° to restore the normal anteversion of the proximal femur. Nailing can then proceed with the fragments in this position.

Locking Screws

All diaphyseal femur fractures should be locked in a static mode. Although a transverse femur fracture in the subtrochanteric area has some inherent stability, Brumback et al. reported a 10.6% complication rate secondary to loss of fixation in a series of dynamically locked reamed femoral nails used to stabilize acute femur fractures.[28] In addition, one must remember to remove the

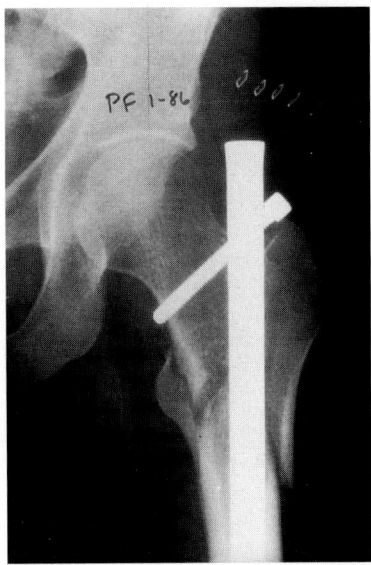

Figure 8.45. Use of a femoral nail of inappropriate length resulted in placement of the locking screw in the medial femoral neck.

guidewire before attempting placement of the proximal or distal locking screws or bolts. We have witnessed several fruitless attempts at nail interlocking without removal of the guidewire; besides being extremely frustrating, it has the potential to cause guidewire breakage, necessitating distal retrieval of the guidewire.

After assembly of the nail and the insertion handle and before nail insertion, one should ascertain that the proximal locking screws target through the nail and insertion handle. The nail should be inserted by hand down the femoral canal, if possible. One should not strike the insertion handle with a mallet, because the handle may deform and misdirect the drill away from the proximal nail locking hole. With use of the reconstruction nail, one must ascertain that the locking screws are completely within the femoral neck and head (Figure 8.46). In subtrochanteric fractures with fracture extension toward the piriformis fossa, there is a risk of the nail exiting posteriorly out of the proximal fragment. If one is not alert to this possibility, the locking screws might be placed posterior to the femoral neck and then enter the femoral head; in this situation, one would have to either elevate the femoral nail before inserting the locking screws or abort the femoral nailing and utilize a different type of implant.

Although radiolucent drill guides are available to assist in distal nail interlocking, we prefer to use a free-hand technique. Regardless of insertion technique, one must verify that the drill has correctly targeted the nail before penetrating the opposite cortex with the drill; suboptimal locking screw purchase may result from multiple penetrations of both the near and far cortices in an attempt to target the nail locking holes. In addition, multiple penetrations increase the potential stress riser effect of the screw holes. Finally, before wound closure, one must radiographically assess the position of all locking screws in both the sagittal and coronal planes (Figure 8.47).

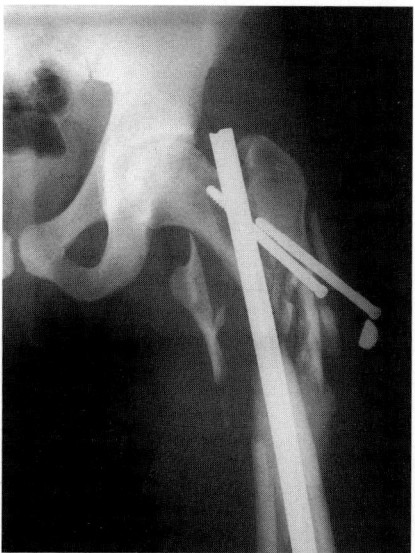

Figure 8.46. Loss of fixation of a subtrochanteric fracture resulting from poor placement of the proximal locking screws.

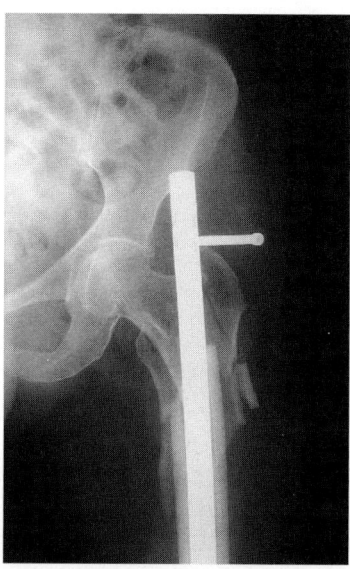

Figure 8.47. Loss of fracture reduction secondary to a "missed" proximal locking screw.

References

1. Peter R, Bedat B, Rossier J, Hoffmeyer P. Impacted Garden I fractures of the femoral neck (31-B1): operative vs. nonoperative treatment? Paper presented at the annual meeting of the Orthopaedic Trauma Association, Louisville, KY, 1997.
2. Hoffman A, Jons R, Schoenvogel R. Pudendal nerve neuropraxia as a result of traction on the fracture table. *J Bone Joint Surg Am* 1982; 64:136–138.
3. Meyers M, Harvey J, Moore T. The muscle pedicle graft in the treatment of displaced fractures of the femoral neck. *Orthop Clin North Am* 1974; 5:779–792.
4. Lyon T, Koval KJ, Kummer F, Zuckerman JD. Pudendal nerve palsy induced by fracture table. *Orthop Rev* 1993; 22:521–525.
5. Kruger D, Kayner D, Hankin F, et al. Traction force profiles associated with the use of a fracture table. *J Orthop Trauma* 1990; 4:283–286.
6. Toolan BC, Koval KJ, Kummer FJ, et al. Effects of supine positioning and fracture post placement on the perineal countertraction force in awake volunteers. *J Orthop Trauma* 1995; 9:164–170.
7. Madsen F, Linde F, Anderson E, et al. Fixation of displaced femoral fractures: a comparison between sliding screw plate and four cancellous bone screws. *Acta Orthop Scand* 1987; 58:212–216.
8. Skinner PW, Powles D. Compression screw fixation for displaced subcapital fracture of the femur: success or failure. *J Bone Joint Surg Br* 1986; 68:78–82.
9. Mizrahi J, Harlon HS, Taylor JK, Solomon L. Investigation of load transfer and optimum pin configuration in the internal fixation by Muller screws of fractured femoral necks. *Med Biol Eng Comput* 1980; 18:319–325.
10. Lehman W, Menche D, Grant A, et al. The problem of evaluating in situ pinning of slipped capital femoral epiphysis: an experimental model and review of 63 consecutive cases. *J Pediatr Orthop* 1984; 4:297–303.
11. Zuckerman JD. *Comprehensive Care of Orthopaedic Injuries in the Elderly*. Baltimore: Urban & Schwarzenberg, 1990.
12. Johnston CE, Ripley LP, Bray CB. Primary endoprosthetic replacement for acute femoral neck fractures. *Clin Orthop* 1982; 167:123–130.
13. Anderson G, Nielson J. Results after arthroplasty of the hip with Moore's prosthesis. *Acta Orthop Scand* 1972; 43:397–410.
14. Salvati EA, Artz T, Aglietti P, Asnis SE. Endoprostheses in the treatment of femoral neck fractures. *Orthop Clin North Am* 1977; 5:757–777.
15. Kwok DC, Cruess RL. A retrospective study of Moore and Thompson hemiarthroplasty. *Clin Orthop* 1982; 169:179–185.
16. Whittaker R, Sotos L, Ralston E. Fractures of the femur about femoral endoprostheses. *J Trauma* 1974; 14:675–694.
17. Chang WS, Zuckerman JD, Kummer FJ, Frankel VH. Biomechanical evaluation of anatomic reduction versus medial displacement osteotomy in unstable intertrochanteric fractures. *Clin Orthop* 1987; 225:141–146.
18. Rokito AS, Koval KJ, Zuckerman JD. Technical pitfalls in the use of the sliding hip screw for fixation of intertrochanteric hip fractures. *Contemp Orthop* 1993; 26:349–356.
19. Baumgaertner MR, Curtin SL, Lindskog DM, Keggi J. The value of the tip-apex distance in predicting failure of fixation of peritrochanteric fractures of the hip. *J Bone Joint Surg Am* 1995; 77:1058–1064.
20. Kyle RF, Wright TM, Burstein AH. Biomechanical analysis of the sliding characteristics of compression hip screws. *J Bone Joint Surg Am* 1980; 62:1308–1314.
21. Gundle R, Gargan MF, Simpson AHRW. How to minimize failures of fixation of unstable intertrochanteric fractures. *Injury* 1995; 26:611–614.
22. Baumgaertner M, Curtin S, Lindskog D. Intramedullary versus extramedullary fixation for the treatment of intertrochanteric hip fractures. *Clin Orthop* 1998; 348:87–94.
23. Russell TA, Taylor JC. Subtrochanteric fractures of the femur. In: Browner BD, Jupiter JB, Levine AM, Trafton PG, eds. *Skeletal Trauma*. Philadelphia: WB Saunders, 1992:1485–1524.
24. Kinast C, Bolhofner BR, Mast JW, Ganz R. Subtrochanteric fractures of the femur: results of treatment with the 95-degree condylar blade plate. *Clin Orthop* 1989; 238:122–130.
25. Riemer B, Butterfield S, Ray R, Daffner R. Clandestine femoral neck fractures with ipsilateral diaphyseal fractures. *J Orthop Trauma* 1993; 7:443–449.

26. Swiontkowski MF. Ipsilateral femoral shaft and hip fractures. *Orthop Clin North Am* 1987; 18:73–84.
27. Johnson KD, Tenscer AF, Sherman MC. Biomechanical factors affecting fracture stability and femoral bursting in closed intramedullary nailing of femoral fractures with illustrative case presentations. *J Orthop Trauma* 1987; 1:1–11.
28. Brumback RJ, Reilly JP, Poka A, et al. Intramedullary nailing of femoral shaft fractures: part I. Decision making errors with interlocking fixation. *J Bone Joint Surg Am* 1988; 70:1441–1452.

Chapter Nine
Rehabilitation

Early mobilization out of bed after hip fracture surgery is important for the general well-being of the patient; it reduces the risks of deep vein thromboembolism, pulmonary complications, skin breakdown, and decline in mental status.[1,2] Mobilization also inspires confidence and encourages the patient on the road to recovery. In addition to early mobilization and ambulation training, treatment goals for the physical therapist include patient training in transfers, improving strength, maintaining balance, and maintaining range of joint motion.

Physical therapy after hip fracture should begin on postoperative day 1. The physical therapist should conduct an acute care evaluation, including review of the patient's diagnosis, surgical procedure, and weight bearing status. He or she should assess the patient's current medical status to be alert to factors that could affect the rehabilitation process. Range of joint motion, muscle strength, and flexibility should be charted, with special attention given to the involved extremity and to the upper extremities if they will be needed for assistive devices; selected neurological, balance, and functional assessments can also be made. The appearance of the patient's surgical wound or dressing should be noted, as should the patient's blood count and the presence of any deformities. The patient's social and living situation should be elicited and evaluated. A physical therapy treatment plan is then formulated based on this initial evaluation and the orthopaedist's physical therapy orders.

At the Hospital for Joint Diseases, the patient is assisted out of bed and into a chair on the first postoperative day (Figure 9.1) (Table 9.1). If the patient is unable to tolerate this transfer, he or she is assisted into a dangling position. The therapist provides instruction in bed mobility, keeping in mind that the operated limb should be kept in proper alignment.[2] The forces exerted across the hip when a patient uses the upper extremities to transfer himself or herself onto a bedpan approach four times body weight.[3] An overhead trapeze helps to reduce this force as well as to facilitate transfers in and out of bed. The physical therapist gradually decreases the amount of assistance given to the patient until he or she can perform transfers independently. Both nursing and physical therapy personnel must use caution when patients indicate that they feel faint, weak, or dizzy. These symptoms are not uncommon in the postoperative geriatric patient and may be exacerbated by inadequate oral intake and poor fluid balance.

Ambulation training is initiated on the first or second postoperative day (Figure 9.2). We believe that the vast majority of patients who have sustained a femoral neck or intertrochanteric fracture and who have been surgically treated with either internal fixation or prosthetic replacement should be allowed to bear weight as tolerated. Elderly patients with decreased upper-extremity

Table 9.1. Hospital for Joint Diseases Rehabilitation Protocol

Day 1	Dangle legs from bed
	Out of bed to chair
	Ambulation training with walker 15 ft (weight bearing as tolerated)
Day 2	Ambulation training 20 ft
Day 3	Ambulation training 40 ft
Day 4	Stair Climbing
Day 5+	Progression of ambulation and stair climbing for endurance and distance with gradual decrease of assistance from therapist

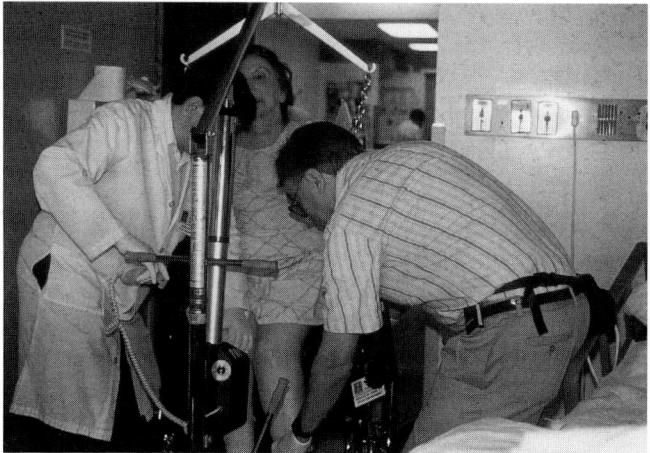

Figure 9.1. Use of a hydraulic lift to assist an elderly patient out of bed on postoperative day 1.

strength, and occasionally those with associated upper-extremity fractures, may find it difficult to comply with a non–weight-bearing or even a partial weight-bearing protocol. Furthermore, it must be kept in mind that even partial weight bearing involves the generation of considerable force across the hip by the lower-extremity musculature.[3] As previously noted, the forces exerted across the hip when a patient uses the upper extremities to transfer himself or herself

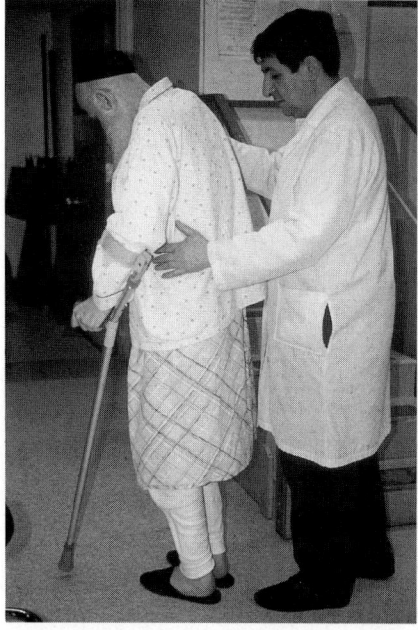

Figure 9.2. Patient ambulation in the early postoperative period with assistance by the physical therapist.

onto a bedpan approach four times body weight. Several studies have demonstrated that unrestricted weight bearing does not increase complication rates following internal fixation or prosthetic replacement after femoral neck or intertrochanteric fracture.[4,5] One such study at our institution prospectively followed 473 patients age 65 years and above with a femoral neck or intertrochanteric fracture who were allowed immediate unrestricted weight bearing after surgery.[6] At 1 year minimum follow-up, 16 patients (3.4%) required additional hip surgery. The revision surgery rate after intertrochanteric fracture secondary to loss of fixation was 2.9%, while that after internal fixation of the femoral neck secondary to loss of fixation or nonunion was 5.3%; for patients followed up for a minimum of 2 years, the osteonecrosis rate after femoral neck fracture was 5.4%. The revision rate after hemiarthroplasty secondary to prosthetic dislocation was 0.6%.

We also utilized gait analysis in a prospective study of 61 patients who sustained a femoral neck or intertrochanteric fracture, underwent surgical treatment, and were allowed to bear weight as tolerated.[7] Computerized gait testing was performed at 1, 2, 3, 6, and 12 weeks after surgery to quantify weight bearing and to determine its relation to treatment technique (Figure 9.3). The maximum load supported by the injured extremity at week 1 was 70% of the maximum load supported by the uninjured extremity; this percentage increased to 77% at week 2, 80% at week 3, 84% at week 6, and 88% at week 12. During the first 3 weeks, patients who underwent internal fixation of an unstable intertrochanteric fracture or a displaced femoral neck fracture placed significantly less weight on the injured extremity than patients who sustained a femoral neck fracture that was treated with prosthetic replacement. By 6 weeks, however, there were no significant differences in weight bearing or other measured parameters between the treatment groups. In all patients who had uneventful union, the amount of weight placed on the injured extremity increased over time.

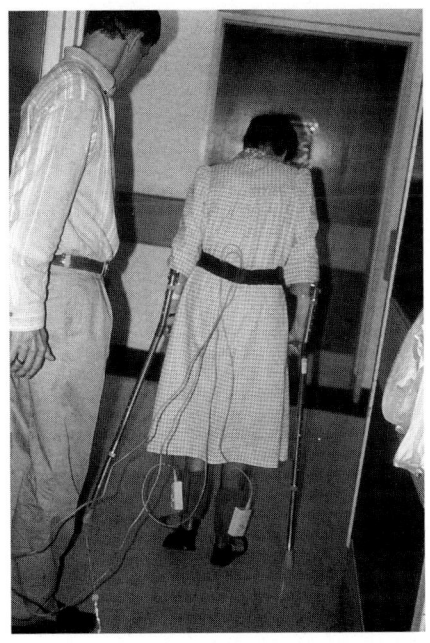
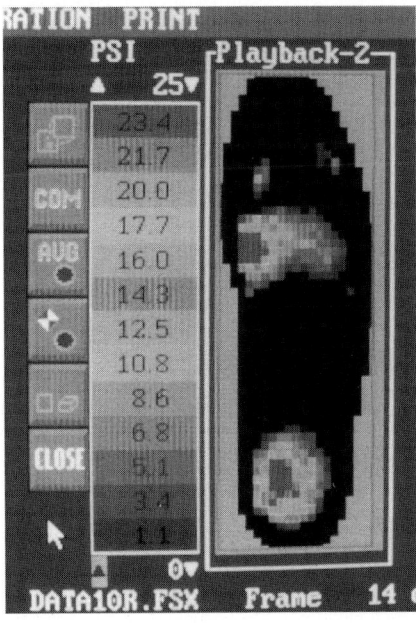
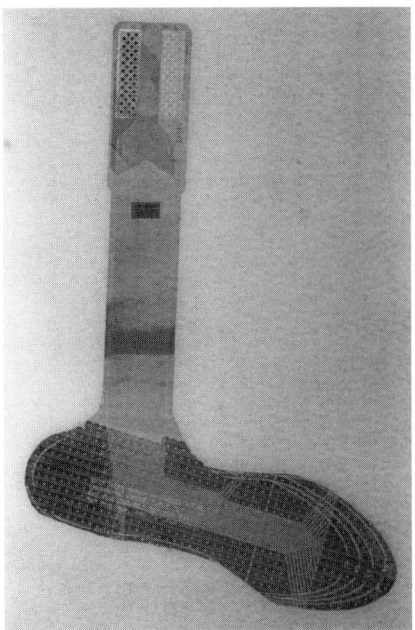

Figure 9.3. Clinical photograph (**A**) and data recording (**B**) during weight bearing and gait analysis. The 900-element-array, flexible flat transducer (**C**) that was inserted between the patient's foot and footwear to measure plantar loads.

A   B   C

The prescription for unrestricted weight bearing might be modified if fixation instability was noted at surgery; we might also consider limited weight bearing in younger patients who sustain a displaced femoral neck or unstable intertrochanteric fracture, although there are no data suggesting that it has a beneficial effect on outcome. Weight-bearing status after subtrochanteric fracture is dependent on the patient's age and bone quality, the fracture pattern, and the type of implant used to stabilize the fracture. Older patients are allowed to bear weight as tolerated regardless of fracture pattern or implant selection. Younger patients are restricted to flat-foot weight bearing until there is radiographic evidence of healing—unless the fracture was stabilized with an interlocked nail and bone-to-bone contact was achieved at surgery.

If there is no orthopaedic contraindication for unrestricted weight bearing, patients' goals are set to ambulate bearing weight as tolerated 15 feet with moderate assistance on postoperative day 1, progressing to 20 feet with minimal assistance on day 2 and 40 feet on day 3. On postoperative day 4, the patient is instructed on stair climbing with maximal supervision. Subsequent patient goals include progression of ambulation to crutches as tolerated and progression of stair climbing with decreased supervision. These goals are to be taken as general guidelines; every patient's rehabilitation program must be tailored to the individual's physical, psychological, and social situation.

While ambulation and transfer training is taking place, the patient is also given instruction in activities of daily living. By helping the patient learn bathing and toileting transfers and skills, as well as how to dress and cook for himself or herself, the occupational therapist greatly contributes to the patient's recovery (Figure 9.4). A visit to the patient's home is ideal, although not always practical; if it is not practical, the rehabilitation and social work team should obtain pertinent information regarding the home environment from the patient, family, and friends. Useful information that can aid in the rehabilitation and training of the patient includes the number and placement of staircases, access to rooms (including kitchen and bathroom), home furnishings, placement of rugs, type of floor surfaces, and resources and support available to the patient at home. Based on this information, the rehabilitation team can devise safety precautions that should be taken to prevent further patient falls and injury and determine specifications for special equipment to help facilitate the patient's independence.

Exercise and strength training is started on the acute care service (Figure 9.5); instruction is given on an exercise program in three positions: supine, sitting,

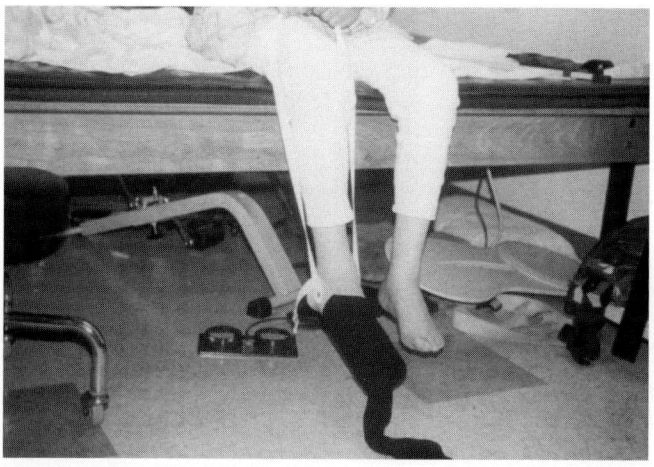

Figure 9.4. Use of a stocking aid to assist the dressing process.

9. Rehabilitation

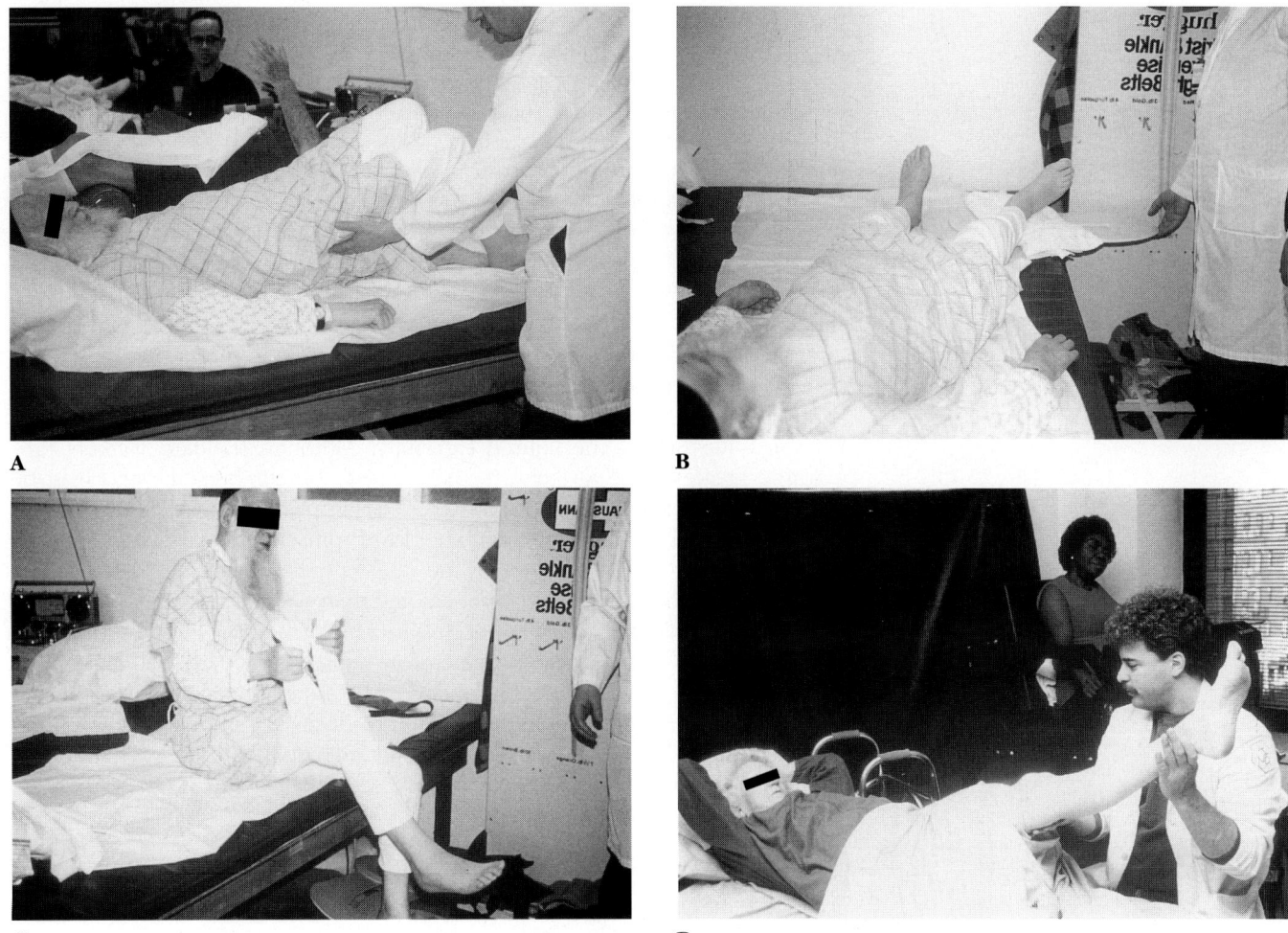

Figure 9.5. Demonstration of hip extension (**A**), abduction (**B**), and flexion (**C**) exercises as well as straight leg raises (**D**).

and standing. The exercises are administered to the patient to tolerance on a daily basis. Supine exercises include quadriceps sets, heel slides, active assisted hip flexion, active assisted straight leg raising, active hip extension and abduction, and ankle pumps. Quadriceps strengthening is important to facilitate independent transfer ability. Barnes and Dunovan found a significant relationship between hip abductor strength and ambulation without supervision.[8] Patients whose fractures were treated with internal fixation have no restriction regarding range of hip motion; patients who had prosthetic replacement, however, are limited to 90° of hip flexion for 6 weeks. In addition, hip adduction and internal rotation are also contraindicated if the prosthetic replacement was performed from a posterior approach; these patients are instructed to keep their legs apart and to place a pillow between their legs when lying on the uninjured side to prevent hip adduction. In a sitting position, exercises start with active knee extension; self-assisted hip flexion with a towel (in patients who had internal fixation) is an effective way to increase the patient's hip flexion strength.

Standing exercises include straight leg raises while the patient holds onto parallel bars, hip abduction, hip flexion, and quarter-knee bends. Standing exercises are performed concentrically with a 5-second isometric hold and then continued eccentrically as the lower extremity is lowered. Exercises progress from active assisted, to active, and then to resistive. Repetitions are increased to enhance the patient's endurance. Patients whose balance is impaired may require contact guarding when performing standing exercises. Balance can be improved by playing ball with the patient and by having patients reach for cones in sitting and standing positions. Deep-breathing exercises and use of an incentive spirometer are encouraged to help prevent pulmonary complications in this vulnerable population.

Adaptive Equipment

Adaptive equipment and assistive devices are routinely prescribed for elderly patients to ease performance of transfers, ambulation, and activities of daily living. Ambulation devices are used to increase stability and lower the weight-bearing forces across the injured extremity. Although standard walkers provide the greatest base of support, they tend to be cumbersome and may be difficult for an elderly patient to advance. Rolling walkers may be moved forward more easily (Figure 9.6), but should be prescribed only for individuals with sufficient coordination to stop the motion when needed. Axillary or Lofstrand crutches tend to be less cumbersome than walkers and may be used to provide unilateral or bilateral support. Canes offer the least degree of stability yet are the least cumbersome and therefore easiest for elderly patients to manipulate. Both "quad" canes with four-pronged support and straight canes are commonly used; either is held in the hand opposite the impaired side.

Wheelchairs should be considered for elderly individuals whose independence in the community is restricted because of an inability to walk long distances. A manual wheelchair, propelled by the individual or a caregiver, may enable such individuals to resume shopping and social activities that would otherwise be precluded by a lack of endurance. In all cases, one should encourage elderly patients to walk whenever possible to maintain their current levels of aerobic conditioning and muscle strength. In individuals with se-

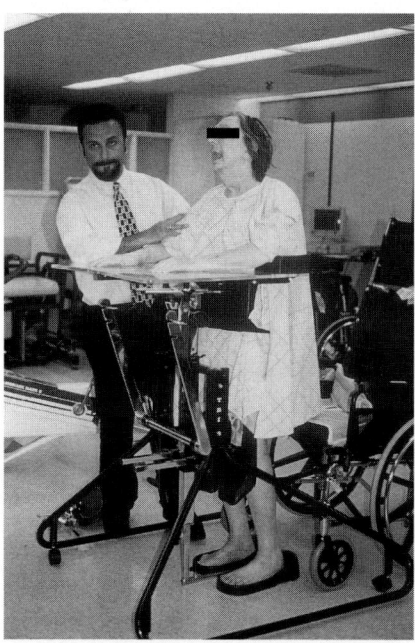

Figure 9.6. Use of a rolling platform walker in a hip fracture patient.

verely compromised neuromuscular, cardiac, or pulmonary status, scooters or motorized wheelchairs may be considered. In such cases, it is necessary to ensure that the individual possesses adequate vision and mental competence to safely operate the device.

Additional devices that can be helpful in the performance of activities of daily living include long-handled reachers and shoe horns, as well as stocking aids and button fasteners that allow individuals with reduced joint range of motion to dress themselves. Shower benches, shower grab bars, and long-handled sponges help elderly patients to bathe in a safe, private manner. In the kitchen, sponge-grip utensils and rimmed plates as well as built-up bottle and can openers can offer assistance with food preparation and consumption.

Discharge Disposition and Rehabilitation Settings

During the early postoperative period, a social worker should meet with the patient and family to assess the patient's needs and resources for hospital discharge. The goal of treatment is to return the patient to his or her preinjury level of independence. Depending on the patient's ambulatory ability, social support network, and financial resources, discharge disposition can range from return to community dwelling, to transfer to an inpatient rehabilitation facility, to placement in a skilled nursing facility. At the Hospital for Joint Diseases, patients who are community dwelling before injury but are slow to progress in rehabilitation are usually transferred to the hospital's inpatient rehabilitation unit.

We recently performed a study to determine the impact of our hospital's rehabilitation service on patient outcome following hip fracture.[9] In January 1990, the hospital initiated an acute rehabilitation program exempt from the financial restrictions of the diagnosis-related group reimbursement model. Patients admitted to this program (after evaluation by a staff physiatrist) receive 2 hours of physical therapy 7 days a week for gait training, stair climbing, transfers, joint range of motion, and upper- and lower-extremity strengthening. They also receive 1 hour of occupational therapy 7 days a week for instruction in activities of daily living. Before 1990 (when no such program existed), 9.0% of patients were discharged to an outside rehabilitation facility. The percentage of patients who were discharged to the hospital's program increased yearly, from 16.8% in 1990 to 64% in 1993 (the increases are statistically significant). Patients' hospital length of stay averaged 21.9 days before 1990; after January 1990, this number was 20.0 days for patients who did not go into the rehabilitation program and 31.4 days for those who did (acute care, 16.1 days; rehabilitation program, 15.6 days). No differences were found in the patients' hospital discharge status, ambulatory ability, place of residence, need for home assistance, or independence in basic or instrumental activities of daily living at 6- and 12-month follow-up between patients treated either before or after initiation of the hospital's rehabilitation program or in patients who were or were not admitted to this program after its inception.

A variety of other settings are available in which elderly patients may receive therapy, each of which should be considered when planning hospital discharge. Skilled nursing facilities offer various degrees of rehabilitation, ranging from little or no therapy to 3 hours of therapy per day. Elderly patients often benefit from less intense rehabilitation programs in skilled nursing facilities or subacute units; patients may be placed in this type of facility either to build up strength before beginning a more intense acute inpatient rehabilitation program or to fine-tune skills learned in an acute rehabilitation program before discharge home.

Day hospitals allow individuals with good social support systems to receive a full day of therapeutic activity in a hospital setting while being able to return home at night. Outpatient facilities generally offer less comprehensive interdisciplinary therapeutic programs than may be provided on an inpatient basis, yet are ideal for individuals requiring limited rehabilitative intervention. Finally, physical and occupational therapy can be provided in the home environment, where individuals have the opportunity to make functional gains in familiar surroundings. In each case, the individual as well as his or her financial resources and social support systems should be considered.

References

1. Allman RM, Laprade CA, Noel LB, et al. Pressure sores amongst hospitalized patients. *Ann Intern Med* 1986; 105:337–342.
2. Parker MJ, Pryor GA. *Hip Fracture Management*. Oxford: Blackwell Scientific Publications, 1993:212–261.
3. Nordin M, Frankel VH. Biomechanics of the hip. In: Nordin M, Frankel VH, eds. *Basic Biomechanics of the Musculoskeletal System*. Malvern, PA: Lea & Febiger, 1989:135–151.
4. Moller BN, Lucht U, Grymer F, Bartholdy NJ. Instability of trochanteric hip fractures following internal fixation. *Acta Orthop Scand* 1984; 55:517–520.
5. Neiman S. Early weightbearing after classical internal fixation of medial fractures of the femoral neck. *Acta Orthop Scand* 1975; 46:782–794.
6. Koval K, Friend K, Aharonoff G, Zuckerman J. Weightbearing after hip fracture: a prospective series of 596 geriatric hip fracture patients. *J Orthop Trauma* 1996; 10:526–530.
7. Koval KJ, Sala DA, Kummer FJ, Zuckerman JD. Postoperative weight-bearing after a fracture of the femoral neck or an intertrochanteric fracture. *J Bone Joint Surg Am* 1998; 80:352–356.
8. Barnes B, Dunovan K. Functional outcomes after hip fracture. *Phys Ther* 1987; 67:1675–1679.
9. Koval KJ, Aharonoff GB, Su ET, Zuckerman JD. Effect of acute inpatient rehabilitation on outcome after fracture of the femoral neck or intertrochanteric fracture. *J Bone Joint Surg Am* 1998; 80:357–364.

Chapter Ten

Outcome Assessment

Measures of Recovery

Practical realization of the long-term goal of fracture treatment—restoration of the patient to preinjury function—requires a reliable method of assessing functional recovery. Such assessment has traditionally focused on physician-defined measures of technical success—fracture union, alignment, and range of joint motion—rather than patient functioning and quality of life. The literature, however, reports weak and inconsistent correlations among improvements in pain, joint motion, functional status, and psychosocial well-being. A patient's quality of life thus does not necessarily reflect the surgeon's clinical evaluation; nor do clinical and radiographic outcomes always equate with functional status, particularly in the elderly.

In recent years, outcome assessment has come to focus on patient-oriented functional outcomes. In this new approach, the patient's broadly defined health status after recovery is a key measure of success. The importance of this approach has only recently been recognized in orthopaedic surgery.

Functional Outcomes

A patient's treatment outcome can fall short of expectations even when he or she has received the most advanced and conscientious care, including the benefits of state-of-the-art operative technique and implant technology. Sometimes, even though surgical management is successful in terms of fracture union, the patient is unable to regain his or her preinjury level of functioning and independence. Evaluation of functional recovery after hip fracture is becoming increasingly important, in recognition of the fact that the true measure of successful medical and surgical management of any injury or disease state is whether the patient has been able to return to his or her premorbid level of functioning. Knowledge of both positive and negative predictors of outcome is needed, as early identification of at-risk patients may have a significant impact on treatment approach, discharge planning, and utilization of health care resources.

Mortality

Mortality is one of the most thoroughly documented and analyzed measurements of outcome. Mortality is discrete and easily measurable; conceptually, it fits well into the medical model of disease.

The reported overall mortality rate in elderly patients 1 year after hip fracture ranges from 14% to 36%.[1-11] Most reports indicate that the highest mortality risk occurs within the first 4 to 6 months after fracture[2,9,12]; after 1 year, the mortality risk returns to that of age- and sex-matched controls.[2,9] The lowest mortality rates are reported among community-dwelling, cognitively intact patients[13]; at our institution, the 1-year mortality rate in this patient population is approximately 12%.[13]

Several studies have attempted to identify the factors predictive of increased mortality in elderly hip fracture patients. These factors can be considered within the context of three phases of patient and fracture management: prefracture patient status, perioperative patient management, and subacute patient care. Factors relating to prefracture patient status include patient age, gender, number of medical comorbidities, prefracture living environment, and prefracture level of functioning. The long-held notion that advancing patient age is associated with increased mortality following fracture of the hip has recently been challenged. Mossey et al. reported no relationship between patient age and mortality in a series of 219 hip fracture patients.[14] In a series of 406 hip fractures, Kenzora et al. found no correlation between mortality and age in patients who had sustained femoral neck fractures, but they did note a positive correlation between these factors in intertrochanteric hip fractures.[8] Furthermore, White et al. found an inverse relationship between mortality and advanced age in a series of 241 hip fractures[11]; mortality rates were highest for those younger than age 70 and lowest for those older than 80 years. At our institution, however, older patient age has consistently been found to be predictive of poorer outcome after hip fracture among community-dwelling elderly patients[13,15,16]; patient age above 85 years was predictive with increased 1-year mortality in a series of 612 hip fracture patients.[13]

Gender has also been reported to be predictive of increased mortality after hip fracture. According to most studies—including those of Clayer et al. and Magaziner et al.—men who sustain a hip fracture have a higher mortality risk than women.[9,17] Recent studies, however, have reported conflicting results. Aharonoff et al., Jensen and Tondevold, and Kenzora et al. reported gender not to be predictive of increased morbidity as an individual factor in multivariate analyses.[6,8,13] In our experience, there is no significant correlation between gender and mortality following hip fracture.[13]

Patients with poorly controlled systemic illnesses (congestive heart failure, atherosclerotic heart disease, diabetes mellitus, chronic obstructive pulmonary disease, and similar serious medical conditions) have increased mortality rates after hip fracture.[1,18,19] Kenzora et al. reported more than a twofold increase in 1-year mortality in patients with four or more medical comorbidities.[8] In this respect, White et al. reported that the best predictor of mortality following hip fracture is the grading system of the American Society of Anesthesiologists (ASA)[11] (Table 10.1). This ASA rating scale categorizes patients according to the following classes: I, normal and healthy; II, having a mild systemic disease; III, having a severe systemic disease that is not incapacitating; IV, having a severe incapacitating systemic disease constituting a constant threat to life; and V, moribund.[11] According to White et al., patients with an ASA grade of I or II had an 8% 1-year mortality rate, while those with ASA grade of III or IV had a 49% 1-year mortality rate. We have also observed that ASA grades III and IV are associated with increased 1-year mortality rates after hip fracture.[13] The number of comorbidities is a reflection of the patient's chronic disease state, whereas the ASA grade is reflective of a patient's acute medical condition.

Table 10.1. American Society of Anesthesiologists (ASA) rating of operative risk

Class	Physical Status
I	Normal, healthy
II	Mild systemic disease
III	Severe systemic disease, not incapacitating
IV	Severe incapacitating systemic disease constituting a constant threat to life
V	Moribund

Acute medical management of preexisting comorbidities performed preoperatively has been shown to have an effect on survival. Often this is reflected by the amount of time from hospital admission until surgery can be performed (surgical delay). Kenzora et al. reported that a surgical delay of less than 1 week to permit stabilization of medical problems did not result in higher 1-year mortality.[8] Sexson and Lehner, however, found that patients with fewer than three comorbid conditions fared better if they underwent surgery within 24 hours[10]; for patients with three or more medical comorbidities, a delay of more than 24 hours was associated with a higher survival rate. A prospective study of 367 geriatric hip fracture patients with multivariate analysis performed at the Hospital for Joint Diseases found that a delay greater than 2 calendar days from hospitalization to surgery resulted in 1-year mortality rate almost double that of patients whose surgery was not delayed so long.[20]

It is generally accepted that institutionalized patients are at increased risk for mortality following hip fracture.[21,22] Holmberg and Thorngren reported a 1-year mortality rate two to three times higher in institutionalized patients than in patients admitted from home.[22] These results are supported by other authors.[23] Prefracture dependency in basic activities of daily living (feeding, bathing, toileting, and dressing) has been shown to be a predictor of 1-year mortality[13]; we reported prefracture dependency in basic activities of daily living to be independently predictive of increased 1-year mortality in a series of 612 ambulatory, community-dwelling hip fracture patients.[13] Jensen and Tondevold measured function as the degree of social dependence and found it to be a strong predictor of increased mortality rate following hip fracture[6]; their study, however, included institutionalized patients as well as community dwellers.

Choice of anesthetic technique has not been shown to have an effect on mortality rate. In a study of 749 community-dwelling hip fracture patients at the Hospital for Joint Diseases, no differences were found in either in-hospital or 1-year mortality rate between patients receiving spinal or general anesthesia.[24] Similar results were reported in randomized prospective studies by Valentin et al. and Davis et al.[25,26]

Development of one or more in-hospital postoperative complications is predictive of increased 1-year mortality rate. This relationship has been documented by numerous authors.[6,8,10] Sexson and Lehner reported that patients who developed an in-hospital postoperative complication had a 1-year mortality rate three times that of control subjects.[10] Both Kenzora et al. and Jensen and Tondevold reported that patients who died prior to hospital discharge were more likely to have had a postoperative complication than those who did not.[6,8] Myers et al. reported that pneumonia and septicemia were associated with increased in-hospital mortality.[27] Furthermore, malnutrition, postoperative decubitus ulcers, and delirium in nondemented patients have been associated with increased mortality rates after hip fracture.[19,28–31] We have also observed that the development of one or more postoperative complications is predictive of increased 1-year mortality rate after hip fracture.[13]

Ambulation

One of the most important goals in the treatment of patients who have sustained a hip fracture is the successful return to prefracture ambulation. Performance of activities of daily living as well as social interaction are dependent on the ability to walk—with or without assistive devices. Ambulatory status in patients after fracture of the hip has major implications for discharge planning; the amount and kind of assistance required for the performance of activities of daily living may direct a patient toward institutionalized living as opposed to home discharge.

Few studies have examined ambulation outcomes prospectively.[12,32–36] Even fewer studies have attempted to categorize and compare prefracture and postfracture ambulatory status.[12,36,37] Ambulatory status is best defined as one of four types:[38] (1) *community ambulators,* who walk indoors and outdoors but may need an assistive device; (2) *household ambulators,* who walk only indoors and generally require an assistive device; (3) *nonfunctional ambulators,* who walk only during physical therapy sessions; and (4) *nonambulators,* who require use of a wheelchair (although they may be able to transfer from bed to chair).

Many studies have attempted to identify factors related to the ability to regain ambulatory ability following hip fracture.[14,32,39–41] A prospective study we performed of 336 community-dwelling ambulatory hip fracture patients at the Hospital for Joint Diseases found that 92% of surviving hip fracture patients remained ambulatory at a minimum of 1 year[15]; 41% regained their prefracture level of ambulation, while 59% lost some degree of ambulatory ability. Multivariate analysis showed that chronological age, ASA classification, fracture type, and preoperative ambulatory status each correlated with ambulatory status at 1 year: patients who were below age 85 years, were ASA class I or II, or had sustained an intertrochanteric fracture were more likely to have regained their prefracture ambulatory status at 1-year follow-up. Interestingly, patients who were relatively limited in their prefracture ambulatory ability were also more likely to regain their prefracture ambulatory status than those who were relatively independent in their prefracture ambulation—possibly because it is easier to return to a lower level of prefracture ambulation than a higher one.

In a study by Miller, a series of 360 hip fracture patients were categorized with respect to prefracture and postfracture ambulation as either independent, ambulatory with aids, or nonambulatory.[42] Fifty-one percent of patients regained independent ambulation and 22% became nonambulatory. Patient age above 60 years and cognitive impairment had a negative impact on ambulatory ability. Magaziner et al. reported that advanced patient age, female sex, the presence of preexisting dementia or postoperative delirium, and rehospitalization were negatively correlated with recovery of ambulatory status at 1 year.[41] In addition, greater contact with one's social network had a positive impact on recovery of walking ability.

The relationship between fracture type and ambulatory ability remains controversial. Some authors report that intertrochanteric fracture type is negatively associated with a return of ambulatory status,[7] whereas others report no difference[32,34] and still others report worse functional results after femoral neck fracture.[15] In our experience, intertrochanteric fracture is a positive predictor for recovery of prefracture ambulatory ability at 1 year.[15]

We studied the effect of anesthetic technique on ambulatory ability in a series of 631 community-dwelling elderly patients at our institution.[16] Ambulatory ability at follow-up was classified according to seven categories: independent community ambulator, community ambulator with a cane, community ambulator with crutches/walker, independent household ambulator, household ambulator with a cane, household ambulator with crutches/walker, and nonfunctional ambulator. Univariate analysis revealed that recovery of ambulatory ability was slightly higher at 6-month follow-up in patients who had undergone general anesthesia. When controlling for potential confounding variables, however, no differences were observed in recovery of ambulatory ability between the two groups at 3, 6, or 12 months following hip fracture.

Discharge Disposition

With increasing economic pressure for early patient discharge from the acute care setting, discharge disposition has become increasingly important as a measure of functional outcome. Studies have identified discharge disposition as an important determinant of social functioning and survival after hip fracture. The proportion of patients who are discharged to their own home varies from 24% to 72%.[9,23,43] Even when patients return home, however, they may require home care services to compensate for loss of function.

Bonar et al. retrospectively studied the need for short-term versus long-term skilled nursing care in 151 previously community-dwelling geriatric patients admitted to a skilled nursing facility after hip fracture.[44] Sixty-four percent of patients were discharged home 6 months after admission to the nursing facility. Factors associated with permanent institutionalization were patient age above 80 years, cognitive dysfunction, need for assistance with activities of daily living, lack of adequate physical therapy, and lack of family involvement.

Early identification of patients at risk for institutionalization may assist in planning a patient's postdischarge living situation. Factors shown to affect discharge disposition include patient age, preinjury functional status, early postoperative ambulatory ability, and the availability of an in-home caregiver.[23,45] In a prospective study performed at the Hospital for Joint Diseases of 516 community-dwelling, ambulatory hip fracture patients who were independent before injury, we found that 76% of patients returned to their prefracture independent living status with no help or part-time help[43]; patients who were below age 85 years, were independent in activities of daily living before fracture, were able to walk independently at the time of hospital discharge, or had three or more medical comorbidities were more likely to regain their independent living status.

Activities of Daily Living

Achieving functional independence is an important measure of functional recovery following hip fracture. To achieve functional independence, one must be able to perform certain activities of daily living (ADLs). These functions are conventionally divided into two groups: basic activities of daily living

(BADLs),[46] which include feeding, bathing, dressing, and toileting, and instrumental activities of daily living (IADLs),[47] which include food shopping, food preparation, banking, laundry, and use of public transportation.

Several studies have attempted to identify factors associated with return to preinjury level of functioning in activities of daily living. In a prospective study by Jette et al., 75 hip fracture patients were assessed at 1-year follow-up for ability to function in BADLs and IADLs[7]; only 33% had regained their prefracture function in BADLs and 21% in IADLs. Patients who had poorer prefracture physical functioning, developed a postsurgical complication, or required nursing home transfer had greater physical disability.

Ceder et al., observing 103 hip fracture patients, reported that the most significant recovery of function in ADLs was achieved within 4 months of surgery and remained constant at 1-year follow-up[33]; only the ability to shop improved after 4 months. These authors emphasized that the role of the caregiver must be weighed into the evaluation of functional recovery in ADLs; caregivers who provide assistance beyond the recovering patient's needs may in fact create greater patient dependencies, particularly in IADLs.

We prospectively observed 338 community-dwelling ambulatory geriatric hip fracture patients to determine which patient and fracture characteristics at the time of hospital admission predicted recovery in basic and instrumental activities of daily living.[48] Before fracture, 84% of patients were independent in BADLs and 54% in IADLs. By 1 year postinjury, 73% had recovered their prefracture BADL status and 48% their IADL status. Patients who were above age 85 years, who had lived alone before fracture, and who had one or more medical comorbidities were at increased risk for delay in recovering or failure to recover BADLs. At 1 year postfracture, only patient age above 85 years was predictive of failure to regain function in IADLs.

Interdisciplinary Hospital Care Programs

The development of in-hospital comprehensive interdisciplinary care programs for elderly hip fracture patients has come about in response to the medical and social complexities associated with this patient population. The concept is one of comprehensive, integrated care provided by a team of health care personnel working in dedicated units. Several studies have documented the efficacy of such a collaborative practice.[45,49,50]

At the Hospital for Joint Diseases, we evaluated the results of an interdisciplinary care program on 431 community-dwelling geriatric hip fracture patients.[50] The multidisciplinary team consisted of an orthopaedic surgeon, a geriatrician, an anesthesiologist, an ophthalmologist, a psychiatrist, a clinical nurse specialist, physical and occupational therapists, a nutritionist, and a social worker. All patients were maintained in a designated patient care area of the hospital; nurses assigned to this area attended staff education sessions that focused on the geriatric hip fracture patient. The results of this program group were compared to those of a matched nonprogram group of 60 patients. Patients in the interdisciplinary program had fewer postoperative complications, fewer intensive care unit transfers, improved ambulatory ability at discharge, fewer nursing home discharges, and shorter length of hospital stay.

Pryor et al. evaluated the effectiveness of a joint hospital and community management approach.[49] Upon hospital admission, each of 200 consecutive hip fracture patients were assessed to determine placement into one of three treatment groups: (1) patients suitable for early discharge with hospital-at-home services who lived in an area where such services were available; (2) patients suitable for early discharge with hospital-at-home services who lived in an area where services were not available; and (3) patients not suitable for early discharge because of medical comorbidities. In the first 10 months of the program, more than half the patients were judged suitable for early discharge. The average length of hospital stay decreased by 35%. The cost of home nursing proved to be considerably less than that of conventional in-hospital care.

References

1. Alffram PA. An epidemiologic study of cervical and trochanteric fractures of the femur in an urban population: analysis of 1,664 cases with special reference to etiologic factors. *Acta Orthop Scand* 1964; 65:9–109.
2. Dahl E. Mortality and life expectancy after hip fractures. *Acta Orthop Scand* 1980; 51:163–170.
3. Gordon PC. The probability of death following fracture of the hip. *Can Med Assoc J* 1971; 105:47–62.
4. Ions GK, Stevens J. Prediction of survival in patients with femoral neck fractures. *J Bone Joint Surg Br* 1987; 69:384–387.
5. Jensen JS, Bagger J. Long term social prognosis after hip fractures. *Acta Orthop Scand* 1982; 53:97–101.
6. Jensen JS, Tondevold E. Mortality after hip fractures. *Acta Orthop Scand* 1979; 50:161–167.
7. Jette AM, Harris BA, Clearly PD. Functional recovery after hip fracture. *Arch Phys Med Rehabil* 1987; 68:735–740.
8. Kenzora JE, McCarthy RE, Lowell JD, Sledge CB. Hip fracture mortality. Relation to age, treatment, preoperative illness, time of surgery, and complications. *Clin Orthop* 1984; 186:45–56.
9. Magaziner J, Simonsick EM, Kashner TM, et al. Survival experience of aged hip fracture patients. *Am J Public Health* 1989; 79:274–278.
10. Sexson SB, Lehner JT. Factors affecting hip fracture mortality. *J Orthop Trauma* 1988; 1:298–305.
11. White BL, Fisher WD, Laurin CA. Rate of mortality for elderly patients after fracture of the hip in the 1980's. *J Bone Joint Surg Am* 1987; 69:1335–1340.
12. Barnes B. Ambulation outcomes after hip fracture. *Phys Ther* 1984; 64:317–321.
13. Aharonoff GB, Koval KJ, Skovron ML, Zuckerman JD. Hip fractures in the elderly: predictors of one year mortality. *J Orthop Trauma* 1997; 11:162–165.
14. Mossey JM, Mutran E, Knott K, Braik R. Determinants of recovery 12 months after hip fracture: the importance of psychosocial factors. *Am J Public Health* 1989; 79:279–286.
15. Koval KJ, Skovron ML, Aharonoff GB, Meadows SE, Zuckerman JD. Ambulatory ability after hip fracture. A prospective study in geriatric patients. *Clin Orthop* 1995; 310:150–159.
16. Koval KJ, Aharonoff GB, Rosenberg AD, et al. Functional outcome after hip fracture. Effect of general versus regional anesthesia. *Clin Orthop* 1998; 348:37–41.
17. Clayer MT, Bauze RJ. Morbidity and mortality following fractures of the femoral neck and trochanteric region. Analysis of risk factors. *J Trauma* 1989; 29:1673–1678.
18. Barnes R, Brown JT, Garden RS, Nicoll EA. Subcapital fractures of the femur. A prospective review. *J Bone Joint Surg Br* 1976; 58:2–24.
19. El-Banna S, Raynal L, Gerbtzop A. Fractures of the hip in the elderly: therapeutic and medico-social considerations. *Arch Gerontol Geriatr* 1984; 3:311–319.
20. Zuckerman JD, Skovron ML, Koval KJ, et al. The effect of surgical delay on postoperative complications and mortality in geriatric hip fracture patients. *J Bone Joint Surg Am* 1995; 77:1551–1556.
21. Elmerson S, Zetterberg C, Anderson GBJ. Ten year survival after fractures of the proximal end of the femur. *Gerontology* 1988; 34:186–191.

22. Holmberg S, Thorngren KG. Statistical analysis of femoral neck fractures based on 3053 cases. *Clin Orthop* 1987; 218:32–41.
23. Broos PLO, Strappaerts KH, Luitten EJT, Gruez JA. Homegoing: prognostic factors concerning the major goal in treatment of elderly hip fracture patients. *Int Surg* 1988; 73:148–150.
24. Koval KJ, Aharonoff GB, Rosenberg AD, et al. Hip fracture in the elderly: the effect of anesthetic technique. *Orthopedics* 1999; 22(1):31–34.
25. Valentin N, Lomholt B, Jensen JS, et al. Spinal or general anesthesia for surgery of the fractured hip? *Br J Anaesth* 1986; 58:284–291.
26. Davis FM, Woolner DF, Frampton C, et al. Prospective, multi-centre trial of mortality following general or spinal anaesthesia for hip fracture surgery in the elderly. *Br J Anaesth* 1987; 59:1080–1088.
27. Myers AH, Robinson EG, Van Natta ML, et al. Hip fractures among the elderly: factors associated with in-hospital mortality. *Am J Epidemiol* 1991; 134:1128–1137.
28. Bastow MD, Rawlings J, Allison SP. Undernutrition, hypothermia, and injury in elderly women with fractured femur: an injury response to altered metabolism? *Lancet* 1983; 1:143–146.
29. Billig N, Ahmed SW, Kenmore PI. Hip fracture, depression and cognitive impairment: a follow up study. *Orthop Rev* 1988; 18:315–320.
30. Dreblow DM, Anderson CF, Moxness CF. Nutritional assessment of orthopedic patients. *Mayo Clinic Proc* 1981; 56:51–54.
31. Jordan MM, Nicol SM, Melrose AC. *Report on the Incidence of Pressure Sores in the Elderly Patients Community of the Borders Health Area on 13th October 1976*. Glasgow: Bioengineering Unit, University of Strathclyde and the Boarders Health Board, 1977.
32. Barnes B, Dunovan K. Functional outcomes after hip fracture. *Phys Ther* 1987; 67:1675–1679.
33. Ceder L, Ekelund L, Inerot S, et al. Rehabilitation after hip fracture in the elderly. *Acta Orthop Scand* 1979; 50:681–688.
34. Cheng CC, Lau S, Hui PW, et al. Prognostic factors and progress for ambulation in elderly patients after hip fracture. *Am J Phys Med Rehabil* 1989; 68:230–233.
35. Dolk T. Influence of treatment factors on the outcome after hip fractures. *Ups J Med Sci* 1989; 94:209–221.
36. Foubister G, Hughes SPF. Fractures of the femoral neck: a retrospective and prospective study. *J R Coll Surg Edinb* 1989; 34:249–252.
37. Elabadien BSZ, Olerud S, Karlstrom G. Ender nailing of peritrochanteric fractures. Results at follow-up evaluation after one year. *Clin Orthop* 1984; 191:53–63.
38. Hoffer MM, Feiwell E, Perry R, et al. Functional ambulation in patients with myelomeningocele. *J Bone Joint Surg Am* 1973; 55:137–148.
39. Cummings SR, Phillips SL, Wheat ME, et al. Recovery of function after hip fracture. The role of social supports. *J Am Geriatr Soc* 1988; 36:801–806.
40. Kauffman TL, Albright L, Wagner C. Rehabilitation outcomes after hip fracture in persons 90 years old and older. *Arch Phys Med Rehabil* 1978; 68:369–371.
41. Magaziner J, Simonsick EM, Kashner TM, et al. Predictors of functional recovery one year following hospital discharge for hip fracture: a prospective study. *J Gerontol* 1990; 45:M101–M107.
42. Miller CW. Survival and ambulation following hip fracture. *J Bone Joint Surg Am* 1978; 60:930–933.
43. Koval KJ, Skovron ML, Polatsch D, et al. Dependency after hip fracture in geriatric patients: a study of predictive factors. *J Orthop Trauma* 1996; 10:531–535.
44. Bonar SK, Tinetti ME, Speechly M, Cooney LM. Factors associated with short versus long term skilled nursing facility placement among community-living hip fracture patients. *J Am Geriatr Soc* 1990; 38:1139–1144.
45. Ceder L, Thorngren KG, Wallden B. Prognostic indicators and early home rehabilitation in elderly patients with hip fractures. *Clin Orthop* 1980; 152:173–184.
46. Katz S, Ford AB, Moskowitz RW, et al. Studies of illness in the aged. The index of ADL. A standardized measure of biological and psychosocial function. *JAMA* 1963; 185:914–919.
47. Lawton M, Brody EM. Assessment of older people: self maintaining and instrumental activities of daily living. *Gerontologist* 1969; 9:179–186.
48. Koval KJ, Skovron ML, Aharonoff GB, Zuckerman JD. Predictors of functional recovery after hip fracture in the elderly. *Clin Orthop* 1998; 348:22–28.
49. Pryor GA, Williams DR, Myles JW, Anand JK. Team management of the elderly patient with hip fracture. *Lancet* 1988; 1:401–403.

Chapter Eleven

Economics of Hip Fracture Treatment

Health care expenditures have risen at an alarming rate worldwide over the past 30 years. The situation is most critical in the United States, which presently spends 12% of its gross domestic product on health care.[1] Between 1950 and 1989, U.S. health-care costs rose from less than $13 billion to over $600 billion.[1] In this context, it is important to recognize that the economic impact of hip fractures extends beyond the individual patient to affect our entire society. In this era of cost-consciousness and the limitations imposed by fiscal constraints, our ability to understand and respond to the economic challenge provided by the increasing number of hip fractures may actually be a prototype for responding to similar health problems in the elderly.

An analysis of the impact of geriatric hip fractures is complicated by its far-reaching ramifications. The overall cost of hip fractures includes not only morbidity and mortality, but also the costs of medical and custodial care, functional limitations, reduced quality of life, loss of independence, inability to work, and other factors that are difficult to assess and quantify—most notably, the indirect impact of the hip fracture on the spouse or family members responsible for care.

Demographics of Hip Fractures

The vast majority of hip fractures follow a fall in men and women with suboptimal bone strength.[2] Only a small minority of hip fractures are due to severe trauma or pathological lesions such as metastatic cancer. The increase in the incidence of hip fractures with age reflects the age-related reduction in bone strength and increased incidence of falling. Among postmenopausal women in the United States, the chances of falling at least once during a given year rises from about one in five for women between 60 and 64 years of age to one in three for those age 80 to 84 years.[3] Bone density of the femoral neck declines by an estimated 58% in women and 39% in men as they grow older; in the intertrochanteric region it declines by approximately 53% and 35% in women and men, respectively.

As the number of elderly persons increases, so will the number of hip fractures. In the United States alone, the number of hip fractures are expected to more than double from 238,000 in 1986 to 512,000 in 2040.[4] The elderly population, however, has been growing even faster than expected; if growth continues at this accelerated pace, the number of people age 65 years and over in the United States could be 22% higher than anticipated and the number of hip fractures by the year 2040 could reach 840,000.[5]

In 1984, the cost of hip fracture care for all age groups in the United States was estimated to be $7.2 billion or an average of $29,800 a fracture.[4] (The components of this figure are discussed in the section that follows.) Assuming a modest 5% rate of inflation and that the average cost of hip fracture care will remain the same, the total annual cost for hip fracture care will reach $62 billion by 2020 and $240 billion by 2040.[4] Considering that the cost of health care services has risen 6% to 11% per year since 1970, these figures may represent gross underestimates.

Between 1950 and 1989, the largest growth in health-care costs was hospital costs, including nursing care, which increased from 32% to 46% of total costs.[6] Hip fractures, which frequently result in prolonged hospitalization and rehabilitative care, are therefore likely to contribute substantially to the health-care burden. Furthermore, as expected, health-care expenditure per capita increases considerably with advancing patient age. Hip fractures, which are predominantly a condition of older individuals, certainly contribute to this expenditure. Health costs per capita for those 65 years of age and older are approximately four times higher than those for the younger population; per capita costs for those under age 65 were $1000, compared to $3600 for those over age 65.[7]

Analysis of information from the Organization for Economic Cooperation and Development (OECD) shows that the mean health-care expenditure in the United States, Canada, Japan, and several European countries has increased linearly from 4% of the gross domestic product (GDP) to over 7% between the 1950s and the 1980s.[1] The rate of increase slowed during the 1980s as a result of cost containment; thus, for example, a mean of 7.6% of the GDP in 1989 was devoted to health care. Cost-containment measures have not yet had an overall impact in the United States, however, where health-care costs absorb 12% of the GDP.[1] Indeed, between 1950 and 1989, U.S. medical costs have increased 50-fold, from $13 billion to over $600 billion. Overall costs were $838 billion in 1992, or over $3000 per person. Another study showed that the cost of health care more than doubled between 1983 and 1993.[8] The projected exponential increase in hip fractures will only exacerbate the already tenuous financial condition of health care in the United States.

Cost Analysis: Methods and Outcomes

Estimates for the cost of hip fracture care in the year after fracture varies widely among researchers, ranging from $19,335 to $41,723.[9] Lost wages and life expectancy are not the primary determinants of cost, because most fractures occur in the elderly; Eiskjaer et al. reported that the 9.2 years of potential life lost per 1000 women secondary to hip fracture was much less than that lost secondary to heart disease, stroke, and breast cancer (73, 29, and 20 per 1000, respectively).[10]

Although researchers use different methods for cost analysis, most studies report that hospitalization accounts for the majority of hip fracture costs. Praemer et al. estimated the total cost of hip fracture care in the United States to be $8.7 billion in 1992.[11] Although many studies use only directs costs to estimate the total cost of hip fracture care, Praemer calculated both the direct and indirect costs. Components of direct cost included hospital inpatient and outpatient services, physician fees, medication, nursing home care, prepayments, and non–health-sector goods and services. Indirect costs included morbidity and mortality, the latter defined as the present value of the patient's lifetime earnings discounted at 4%. The study found that the greatest expenses were incurred by inpatient services (34%), outpatient services (9%), and nursing home care (17%); together these accounted for $5.3 billion, or 61% of the total cost of hip fractures in the year studied.

Beck et al. reported that the average total hospital charges per patient who sustained a hip fracture in the United States in 1994, excluding physician fees, was $16,072 (range, $6,723 to $36,775).[12] Unlike some other authors, who evaluated discrete components of total cost and plugged these figures into an algorithm to derive an "average cost" per patient, Beck simply recorded the total hospital charges per patient from hospital billing data. The average charges for patients treated by hemiarthroplasty was found to be $17,775, compared to $13,412 for those treated with internal fixation. These authors reported that the strongest predictor of total hospital charges was not the type of operative treatment, but the length of hospital stay and the number of in-hospital complications. For hospital stays of 14 days or less, the average cost was $12,984, compared to hospital stays of longer than 14 days, for which the cost rose to $21,957. Patients who experienced no in-hospital complications incurred charges of $13,115; the development of one complication was associated with hospital charges of $17,129; the development of two complications, $22,222.

Brainsky et al., calculating the cost of hip fracture care in 1993 dollars, reported estimates of costs of health services rather than charges as the difference between the sum of the costs in the year after fracture and the annualized costs in the year before fracture.[13] The annualized cost in the year before hip fracture per patient was estimated to be $20,928. The cost in the year after fracture equaled $37,500, of which the average cost of hospitalization, including physician fees, was $11,480, or 30% of the total. Thus the overall cost of a hip fracture was calculated to be $16,322 (the difference between $37,250 and $20,928). These authors reported that although nonmedical services did not add substantially to the cost of hip fracture care, the care provided by family and friends had a profound influence on the patients' lives, including a positive emotional effect that could not be quantified by their study.

French et al. employed the approach of collecting data only on those aspects that dominate the overall costs of care.[14] They found that four categories—acute ward stay, rehabilitation ward stay, operating and recovery room costs, and long-term care (in descending order of magnitude)—accounted for 97% of the total cost of hip fracture care. These authors asserted that the standard "average cost method," which involves multiplying the mean daily orthopaedic bed cost by the mean number of inpatient days, overestimates the cost of hip fracture care by 23% for acute care and as much as 92% for rehabilitation services.

Borgquist et al. in 1991 studied the costs of hip fractures in Sweden and utilized separate calculations for costs in the acute phase (surgery and mobilization in the orthopaedic ward) and in the rehabilitation phase (including three home visits by a physical therapist).[15] Also calculated were visits to the primary health care center, outpatient visits to the orthopaedic department, radiographs, and assistive devices such as canes and crutches. They reported that inpatient services that included acute hospital care accounted for approximately 52% of the total cost of care.

A study by Zethraeus et al. in Sweden estimated direct costs per patient for the first year after fracture to be approximately $ 40,000.[16] They also found that the potential cost savings from preventing a hip fracture was about $22,000, similar to the $21,000 reported by Sernbo and Johnell.[17] This figure was obtained by using the patient as his or her own control subject, as in the study by Brainsky et al., and estimating the cost savings as the difference between direct costs 1 year after and 1 year before hip fracture. Direct costs were compiled for orthopaedic and geriatric services, skilled nursing facilities, homes for the elderly, group living, other acute hospital care, and municipal home help. Geriatric services was the dominant cost item, followed by the total length of stay in the hospital and skilled nursing facilities; together these three constituted 70% of all direct costs. Orthopaedic, geriatric, and other acute hospital care accounted for 59% of the direct cost of hip fracture care, which is comparable to the figures reported by Borgquist et al. (52%). Indirect costs such as outpatient services and relevant societal costs were not included in their analysis. To justify this omission, they cited Borgquist's claim that outpatient cost is a relatively small part (1%) of the direct cost of hip fractures. Costs in this study were calculated as average costs, a source of concern because average costs have been widely criticized by economists as an inaccurate reflection of true resource consumption.

Acute Care Costs

Hospital expenditures represent the single largest component of all medical costs for the treatment of hip fractures: 44% in the United States,[18] 50% in England and Wales,[19] and 52% in Sweden.[15] In the United States, direct inpatient hospital costs following hip fracture were estimated to be $2.8 billion in 1988.[20] In 1992, hip fractures accounted for almost a quarter-million hospitalizations and 3.4 million hospital bed-days.[11]

These figures can be expected to skyrocket as the elderly population continues to grow. Persons age 85 years and older are the fastest-growing segment of the U.S. population, a trend that is likely to continue and that will probably result not only in more hip fractures but in longer hospital stays, especially among women. Sernbo and Johnell reported that mean hospital stay after hip fracture, among individuals admitted from and discharged to home, was less than 15 days for patients under age 65 years and twice as long for patients over 85, probably because elderly patients are more likely to have associated medical comorbidities.[17]

Although health-care costs in the United States constitute a far greater percentage of the GDP than in most other countries, the average inpatient hospital stay for persons who sustain hip fractures is lower in the United States than in every other industrialized country: 14.5 days (1986 figures), compared to, for example, 30 days in both England (1985) and Switzerland (1990).[18] Decreasing length of acute hospital stay has nevertheless become a prime objective in the effort to decrease the cost of care after hip fracture, although the health consequences of shortened stays is controversial. Proponents argue that a shortened hospital stay encourages early patient mobilization and reduces the risk of iatrogenic disease. Critics counter that shorter hospitalizations correlate with inadequate care as well as increases in complications and morbidity.

Examination of the effects of the Medicare Prospective Payment System (PPS), implemented in 1984, on hospital length of stay and functional outcome after hip fracture may prove helpful for the appraisal of the cost-effectiveness of shortened hospitalization. Since introduction of the PPS in October 1984, there has been a significant decline in the length of hospital stay after hip fracture. Under this system, hospitals are reimbursed predetermined amounts for inpatient services based on diagnosis-related groups, thus providing a financial incentive to care for patients in the least costly manner. Predictably, hospitalization stays have become shorter with fewer services provided. Fitzgerald et al. reported that between 1981 (pre-PPS) and 1986 (post-PPS), the mean length of hospitalization after hip fracture decreased from 21.9 to 12.6 days.[21] Kahn et al. reported that the mean length of hospital stay decreased from 20.1 days pre-PPS (1981–1982) to 14.5 days post-PPS (1985–1986).[22] Palmer et al. reported a decrease from 17.0 days pre-PPS to 12.9 days post-PPS.[23]

Fitzgerald et al. reported that following the implementation of the PPS, hip fracture patients have experienced shorter hospital stays, less inpatient therapy, and the need for more frequent and longer-term stays in skilled nursing facilities.[21] The central finding of their study was that nursing home placement one year postfracture increased twofold after the initiation of the PPS. The authors inferred the that overall quality of care had deteriorated as a result of the PPS.

In contrast, Palmer et al. reported that although the average hospital length of stay declined with the initiation of the PPS, the proportion of patients discharged to a skilled nursing facility remained the same and the proportion of patients remaining in a skilled nursing facility 6 months after hospital discharge did not differ significantly.[23] Kahn et al., who found a significant increase in the percentage of patients discharged directly to a nursing home after initiation of the PPS, reported that this did not result in a significant increase in the need for prolonged nursing home stay.[22]

A decade after Fitzgerald, Palmer, and Kahn published their findings, the steadily diminishing length of hospital stay documented by these authors has tapered off, suggesting that successful treatment after hip fracture may not be capable of sustaining further reductions in hospital length of stay. Because hip fracture treatment requires rehabilitation, a certain minimum number of hospital days must be accepted as an assurance of quality so that optimal functional recovery is achieved. It is likely that hospitals in the United States are either approaching or have already reached the threshold beyond which further reduction in hospital length of stay would result in compromised care and unacceptable outcomes.

Cost cutting by reducing length of hospital stay becomes relatively ineffective because the most expensive care occurs in the first few days after admission. Furthermore, any benefits that have so far been accrued from reducing hospital length of stay have been offset by the increasing incidence of hip fractures. Schroder reported that although the average number of hospital days after hip fracture decreased by 48% between 1970 and 1985, the annual number of fractures nearly tripled. Schroder calculated that even if the length of hospitalization could be shortened to less than 12.6 days, the projected increase in age-specific fracture incidence would double the number of hip fractures between 1985 and 2002 and increase hospital utilization by nearly 100%.[24]

Finally, it must be acknowledged that reducing the length of hospital stay, rather than reducing overall costs, may merely shift the economic burden of hip fracture patients to nursing homes and other aftercare facilities. Stromberg et al., analyzing the effect of implementation of a prospective payment system in Sweden, concluded that the decrease in orthopaedic ward stay from 20 to 12 days was achieved by earlier and increased discharge to geriatric wards, where bed-day consumption doubled; the overall total cost of care increased by 12%.[25]

Long-Term Care Costs

One-third of all hip fracture patients may ultimately become totally dependent, and thus the potential for institutionalization is high. One study reported that 10% to 39% of patients admitted from home resided in skilled nursing facilities 6 to 12 months after hip fracture.[26] Another study found that 10% of women who sustained a hip fracture became functionally dependent in activities of daily living[27]; of these, 19% required long-term nursing home care. In the United States, hip fractures result in at least 60,000 nursing home admissions annually in addition to more than 7 million days of restricted activity among noninstitutionalized patients.[28]

One of the strongest predictors of the need for admission to a skilled nursing facility is patient age. With increasing age, it is less likely that a hip fracture patient admitted from home will be discharged back to the home; in some cases this reflects the absence of an able-bodied caregiver at home.[27] Nearly all surviving hip fracture patients admitted from a nursing home are returned to a nursing home. As the elderly population continues to expand, nursing home costs will therefore increase concomitantly.

Since implementation of the Medicare PPS, the number of Medicare-certified, PPS-exempt rehabilitation units has more than doubled to greater than 1000; the total 1993 cost to Medicare was $3.7 billion.[29] Medicare-certified nursing homes have also grown substantially, and by the mid-1990s they numbered more than 12,000, with a total 1994 cost to Medicare of more than $8 billion.[29] Because of the uninterrupted growth of the elderly population, this trend is not anticipated to change in the future.

A substantial proportion of the cost of such aftercare can be attributed to patients who sustain a hip fracture; in the United States in 1986, nursing home costs for hip fracture patients were $2 billion.[20] In Sweden, according to two separate studies, about 40% of the direct costs of hip fracture care went to nursing homes and other types of aftercare facilities.[15,16]

Kramer et al. compared the cost-effectiveness of rehabilitation facilities with that of subacute skilled nursing facilities after hip fracture in the United States.[29] Patients in rehabilitation facilities received significantly more physical, occupational, speech, and recreational therapy. The costs of rehabilitation facility care, however, were significantly higher than those of subacute skilled nursing facility care, despite the fact that there was no difference between the two in terms of either proportion of patients returned to the community or rate of recovery of premorbid function. The authors of the study consequently argued that the higher cost of rehabilitation facilities was not justified by results.

We recently performed a study to determine the impact of our hospital's rehabilitation service on patient outcome following hip fracture.[30] In January 1990, the hospital initiated an acute rehabilitation program exempt from the financial restrictions of the diagnosis-related group (DRG) reimbursement model. Patients admitted to this program (after evaluation by a staff physiatrist) received 2 hours of physical therapy 7 days a week for gait training, stair climbing, transfers, joint range of motion, and upper- and lower-extremity strengthening. They also received 1 hour of occupational therapy 7 days a week for instruction in activities of daily living. Before 1990 (when no such program existed), 9.0% of patients were discharged to an outside rehabilitation facility. The percentage of patients who were discharged to the hospital's program increased yearly, from 16.8% in 1990 to 64% in 1993 (these increases are statistically significant). Patients' hospital length of stay averaged 21.9 days before 1990; after January 1990, this number was 20.0 days for patients who did not go into the rehabilitation program and 31.4 days for those who did (acute care, 16.1 days; rehabilitation program, 15.6 days). No differences were found in the patients' hospital discharge status, ambulatory ability, place of residence, need for home assistance, or independence in basic or instrumental activities of daily living at 6- and 12-month follow-up between patients treated either before or after initiation of the hospital's rehabilitation program or in patients who were or were not admitted to this program after its inception. Since hospital reimbursement by third-party payers for the DRG-exempt rehabilitation unit was approximately $700 per day, patients who were discharged to this program incurred an additional hospital expense of approximately $10,500.

Indirect Costs

Cost analysis is a complex and confounding task. Total costs must reflect not only direct costs such as acute and long-term care, but also indirect costs such as loss of independence, functional limitations, reduced activities of daily living, pain, loss of working days, decreased quality of life, and the socioeconomic and emotional costs to the patient's immediate caregivers. Because of the difficulty in evaluating the "human costs" of hip fracture and the scarcity of this type of data, they are omitted from most cost analyses. How, for example, does one measure economic loss to a patient who severely restricts her activities because of fear of falling? Nevertheless, no study of the socioeconomic impact after hip fracture can be considered complete without examination of these indirect costs.

In a pilot study involving patients who sustained a hip fracture, the impact on quality of life was assessed using five different assessment scales.[6] Compared to age-matched controls, the quality of life in the hip fracture patients was lower on all five assessment scales. Another study, which followed 518 hip fracture patients, found that 2.5 years after surgery deterioration of social function was noted in 31% of patients discharged to home, 45% in those discharged to a skilled nursing facility, and 55% in those discharged to a rehabilitation center.[31] Magaziner et al. reported that a substantial number of geriatric hip fracture patients do not regain preinjury ability to perform activities of daily living 1 year after fracture.[32] Although these studies delineated the social and functional limitations that result from fracture of the hip, the authors were unable to place a dollar value on these indirect costs.

Cost-Reduction Strategies

Cost-effectiveness analyses compare the relative efficiency of interventions in light of their costs. When divided by expense, quality-adjusted life-years (QALYs) yield a measure of cost-effectiveness and help establish priorities for funding.[33] Because most hip fractures occur in the elderly, a widely held perception is that money is being wasted on individuals with very few years to live. In fact, the cost of hip fracture treatment per quality-adjusted life-year compares favorably with the cost of renal transplantation and coronary artery bypass.[34]

This is not to say, however, that the future of hip fracture treatment in the United States looks promising. The growing elderly population will continue to tax the health-care system unless costs are contained. Because further reductions in hospital stay might be detrimental to patient outcome, other approaches to cost containment must be considered. A prospective study in Lund, Sweden, found that better organization of rehabilitation services after early discharge (18 days) yielded a substantial reduction in medical costs and increased the likelihood that patients would be discharged to their homes within 4 months.[15]

Programs that focus on continuity of care and adopt a multidisciplinary approach have been effective in reducing the cost of care after injury. Because of the complexities involved in the management of geriatric hip fracture patients, the success of comprehensive and integrated care provided by teams of health-care personnel working in dedicated units is not unexpected. Farnworth et al. described the efficacy of one such program in Australia, the Fractured Hip Management Programme (FHMP).[35] The aims of this program were to reduce the delay before surgery, provide specialist geriatric medical supervision, improve early postoperative mobility, plan for hospital discharge with rehabilitation in the patient's normal environment, and provide continuity of care by a small number of staff. The team, which worked in conjunction with orthopedic surgeons and geriatric physicians, consisted of a full-time nurse-coordinator, a physiotherapist, a part-time occupational therapist, and a part-time social worker. After implementation of FHMP, hospital length of stay was reduced by 3 days for previously institutionalized individuals and 6 days for community-dwelling individuals; the average cost of hip fracture treatment was reduced by 16% per patient without compromising medical outcomes. Early discharge was achieved without cost shifting onto other agencies.

Integration of a geriatric service working with orthopedic surgeons has been shown to decrease the number of postoperative complications and length of hospital stay.[36] Designated orthopedic-geriatric units can provide effective acute care hospital bed utilization, which can minimize the consumption of limited hospital resources. One British trial reported significantly shorter hospital stays and more frequent discharges to home in hip fracture patients assigned to primary care with geriatric consultation.[37] In the United States, Zuckerman et al. reported that patients who were managed by an interdisciplinary geriatric hip fracture team had fewer postoperative complications, significantly fewer transfers to an intensive care unit, significantly improved ability to walk at the time of discharge, and fewer discharges to nursing homes.[38]

Another novel yet effective approach to cost-effective hip fracture management is the "hospital at home" program implemented in England, which provides nursing care (up to 24 hours a day), social services, and rehabilitation therapists in the patient's home under the supervision of a general practitioner.[39] Patients eligible for the program were discharged after an average hospital stay of 10 days, with an additional 11.5 days under hospital at home supervision. The total direct cost was 13% less for those with access to the program.

Other approaches to reducing costs incurred by extended hospital stays after hip fracture include minimizing technical failures and postoperative complications. Costs can be saved by strict adherence to meticulous surgical technique, early postoperative mobilization, and a high standard of nursing care. One study in Sweden found that the total average cost after hip fracture was 60% lower for patients who did not require revision surgery.[15]

Conclusion

Even when limited to direct medical costs, cost analysis is a complex undertaking. Although the algorithms and methods used to evaluate the total cost of hip fracture care differ from study to study, one conclusion remains the same: the rising costs of hip fracture care must be contained. One strategy seeks to decrease the length of hospitalization after hip fracture. Studies have found that joint orthopedic–geriatric units are effective in decreasing the length of hospital stay while maintaining the quality of care. No realistic decrease in length of hospitalization, however, can offset the costs associated with the projected exponential increase in hip fracture incidence. While more cost-effective treatment and rehabilitation may slow the rise of hip fracture costs, effective prophylaxis offers the only hope of alleviating the enormous socioeconomic burden associated with hip fracture.

References

1. Pinto F. New paradigms for health care. In: Reinhardt U, Pinto F, eds. *New Perspectives in Health Care Economics*. London: MEDIQ Ltd, 1991:108–119.
2. Melton LJ. Epidemiology of fractures. In: Riggs BL, Melton LJ, eds. *Osteoporosis: Etiology, Diagnosis and Management*. New York: Raven Press, 1988:133–154.
3. Cummings S, Nevitt M. Epidemiology of hip fractures and fall. In: Kleere-Koper M, Krane S, eds. *Clinical Disorders of Bone and Mineral Metabolism*. New York: Mary Ann Liebert, Inc, 1989:231–236.
4. Cummings SR, Rubin SM, Black D. The future of hip fractures in the United States: numbers, costs, and potential effects of postmenopausal estrogen. *Clin Orthop* 1990; 252:163–166.
5. Schneider EL, Guralnik JM. The aging of America—impact on health care costs. *JAMA* 1990; 263:2335–2340.
6. Norris RJ. Medical costs of osteoporosis. *Bone* 1992; 13:11–16.
7. McCue J. Cost containment in geriatrics: economics meets reality. In: Reinhardt U, Pinto F, eds. *New Perspectives in Health Care Economics*. London: MEDIQ Ltd, 1991:78–9.
8. Fries JF, Koop CE, Beadle CE, et al. Reducing health care costs by reducing need and demand for medical services. *N Engl J Med* 1993; 329:321–325.
9. Clark AP, Shuttinga JE. Targeted estrogen/progesterone replacement therapy for osteoporosis: calculation of health care costs. *Osteoporos Int* 1992; 2:195–200.
10. Eiskjaer S, Ostgard SE, Jakobsen BW, et al. Years of potential life lost after hip fracture among postmenopausal women. *Acta Orthop Scand* 1992; 63:293–296.
11. Praemer A, Furner S, Rice DP. *Musculoskeletal Conditions in the United States*. Chicago: American Academy of Orthopedic Surgeons, 1992.
12. Beck TS, Brinker MR, Daum WJ. In-hospital charges associated the treatment of adult femoral neck fractures. *Am J Orthop* 1996; 25:608–612.
13. Brainsky A, Glick H, Lydick E, et al. The economic cost of hip fractures in community-dwelling older adults: a prospective study. *J Am Geriatr Soc* 1997; 45:281–287.
14. French FH, Torgerson TJ, Porter RW. Cost analysis of fracture of the neck of the femur. *Age Ageing* 1995; 24:185–189.
15. Borgquist L, Lindelow G, Thorngren KG. Costs of hip fracture: rehabilitation of 180 patients in primary health care. *Acta Orthop Scand* 1991; 62:39–48.

16. Zethraeus N, Stromberg L, Jonsson B, et al. The cost of a hip fracture. Estimates for 1,709 patients in Sweden. *Acta Orthop Scand* 1997; 68:13–17.
17. Sernbo I, Johnell O. Consequences of a hip fracture: a prospective study over 1 year. *Osteoporos Int* 1993; 3:148–153.
18. Barrett-Connor E. The economic and human costs of osteoporotic fracture. *Am J Med* 1995; 98:271–9.
19. Kanis JA. The incidence of hip fractures in Europe. *Osteoporos Int* 1993; 3 (suppl 1):10–15.
20. Phillips S, Fox N, Jacobs J, Wright WE. The direct medical cost of osteoporosis for American men and women aged 45 and older. *Bone* 1988; 9:271–279.
21. Fitzgerald JF, Moore PS, Dittus RS. Changing patterns of hip fracture care before and after implementation of the prospective payment system. *N Engl J Med* 1988; 319:1392–1397.
22. Kahn KL, Keeler EB, Sherwood MJ. Comparing outcomes of care before and after implementation of the DRG-based prospective payment system. *JAMA* 1990; 264:1984–1988.
23. Palmer RM, Saywell RM, Zollinger TW. The impact of the prospective payment system on the treatment of hip fractures in the elderly. *Arch Intern Med* 1989; 149:2237–2241.
24. Schroder H. The cost of hospitalizing hip fracture patients has increased despite shorter hospitalization time. *Injury* 1991; 22:135–138.
25. Stromberg L, Ohlen G, Svensson O. Prospective payment systems and hip fracture treatment costs. *Acta Orthop Scand* 1997; 68:6–12.
26. Cooney LM. Do we understand the true cost of hip fractures? *J Am Geriatr Soc* 1997; 45:382–383.
27. Chrischilles EA, Butler CD, Davis CS, Wallace R. A model of lifetime osteoporosis impact. *Arch Intern Med* 1991; 151:2026–2032.
28. Holbrook TL, Grazier K, Kilsey JL. The frequency, occurrence, impact and cost of selected musculoskeletal conditions in the U.S. Paper presented at the annual meeting of the American Academy of Orthopaedic Surgeons, Chicago, IL, 1984.
29. Kramer AM, Steiner JF, Schlenker RE, et al. Outcomes and cost after hip fracture and stroke. A comparison of rehabilitation settings. *JAMA* 1997; 277:396–404.
30. Koval KJ, Aharonoff GB, Su ET, Zuckerman JD. Effect of acute inpatient rehabilitation on outcome after fracture of the femoral neck or intertrochanteric fracture. *J Bone Joint Surg Am* 1998; 80:357–364.
31. Jensen JS, Bagger J. Long term social prognosis after hip fractures. *Acta Orthop Scand* 1982; 53:97–101.
32. Magaziner J, Simonsick EM, Kashner TM, et al. Predictors of functional recovery one year following hospital discharge for hip fracture: a prospective study. *J Gerontol* 1990; 45:M101–107.
33. La Puma K, Lawlor EF. Quality-adjusted life-years: ethical implications for physicians and policy makers. *JAMA* 1990; 263:2917–2921.
34. Parker MJ, Myles JW, Anand JK, Drewett R. Cost-benefit analysis of hip fracture treatment. *J Bone Joint Surg Br* 1992; 74:261–264.
35. Farnworth MG, Kenny P, Shiell A. The costs and effects of early discharge in the management of fractured hip. *Age Ageing* 1994; 23:190–194.
36. Jensen JS, Tondevold E. A prognostic evaluation of the hospital resources required for the treatment of hip fractures. *Acta Orthop Scand* 1980; 51:515–522.
37. Kennie DC, Reid J, Richardson IR. Effectiveness of geriatric rehabilitative care after fractures of the proximal femur in elderly women: a randomized clinical trial. *BMJ* 1988; 297:1083–1085.
38. Zuckerman JD, Sakales SK, Fabian DR, Frankel VH. Hip fractures in geriatric patients. Results of an interdisciplinary hospital care program. *Clin Orthop* 1992; 274:213–225.
39. Hollingsworth W, Todd C, Parker M, Roberts J, Williams R. Cost analysis of early discharge after hip fracture. *BMJ* 1993; 307:903–906.

Chapter Twelve

Prevention

Prevention of hip fractures involves any or all of three basic measures: fall prevention, prevention and treatment of bone fragility, and the use of external hip protectors. Although none of these approaches is without controversy, as a whole they have substantial potential to conserve health-care resources and maintain the quality of life for many elderly individuals.

Fall Prevention

Efforts at preventing a fall target factors that can be categorized as either *intrinsic* (related to such internal factors as the patient's medical or physical condition) or *extrinsic* (related to external causes, such as environmental hazards or weather conditions) (Table 12.1).

Intrinsic Causes of a Fall

Some intrinsic factors are the result of disease processes, while others occur naturally with aging. It is important to keep in mind that in the elderly, one or more of several affected body systems or conditions may play a contributory role in a fall:

1. *Conditions affecting the eyes.* Problems such as cataracts, glaucoma, macular degeneration, diabetic retinopathy, and improper use of corrective lenses can cause symptoms such as hazy or cloudy vision, altered depth perception, night blindness, and poor peripheral vision. Patients' eyeglasses should be of the appropriate type and adequate power.
2. *Conditions affecting the ears.* A fall can result when an elderly person does not hear such sounds as a car horn or even people approaching on a crowded sidewalk—or hears these sounds too late to react appropriately. Presbycusis, or adult-onset hearing loss, can result in a sense of isolation from others. Complicating these is the fact that many older adults resist the idea of wearing a hearing aid. Furthermore, vestibular dysfunction results from degeneration of the structures of the inner ear and causes poor balance.
3. *Neurological conditions.* Parkinsonism, transient ischemic attacks, residual weakness from stroke, neuropathy, and other neurological disorders may underlie such symptoms as muscle weakness, tremor, balance and gait

Table 12.1. Fall risk factors

Intrinsic	Extrinsic
Visual or hearing disturbance	Indoor or outdoor safety hazards
Neurological, cardiovascular, or psychiatric disease	Environmental conditions
	Innapropriate footwear
Musculoskeletal disorder	Risky behavior
Acute illness	Social isolation
Urinary frequency	
Malnutrition	
Medication	

disorders, dizziness, and sensory disturbances. Associated neurological problems include perceptual impairment as well as diminished reflexes, proprioception, and spatial sense.

4. *Cardiovascular conditions.* Weakness, dizziness, sensory disturbance, and/or fainting arising from hypertension, hypotension, peripheral vascular disease, arrhythmia, and congestive heart failure are typical precursors of a fall.
5. *Psychiatric conditions.* Dementia, depression, psychotic episodes, and substance abuse can cause impaired functional status, poor judgment, social isolation, and hallucinations.
6. *Musculoskeletal conditions.* Osteoarthritis, rheumatoid arthritis, and spinal disorders can lead to a fall as a result of associated deformities, changes in posture, impaired functional status, pain, stiffness, and gait disorders. People who fall often have lower-extremity muscle weakness, particularly involving the hips, knees, and ankles.
7. *Foot Conditions.* Calluses, corns, ingrown toenails, infection, tendon contractures, bunions, and neuromas can result in a fall by causing pain, discomfort, deformity, and skin ulceration.
8. *Acute illness.* A fall is frequently the first indication of an acute illness. Pneumonia, gastrointestinal bleeding, infection, congestive heart failure, and influenza in the elderly often present with weakness, confusion, and a falling incident.
9. *Urinary conditions.* Incontinence, bladder prolapse, and urinary tract infection resulting in urgency and frequency of urination increase the risk of a fall during the rush to reach the bathroom or commode.
10. *Nutritional status.* Malnutrition and dehydration can cause nutrient deficiency or electrolyte imbalance leading to weakness, confusion, dizziness, and syncope.
11. *Medication.* Narcotics, sedatives, and antidepressants can impair balance and gait.

Balance and gait assessment can afford important clues to medical conditions that lead to a fall and thus should be performed early in the examination. Balance and gait abnormalities are typically related to neurological or musculoskeletal disorders. For example, cerebellar disease is characterized by a wide-based, irregular gait; arthritis and pain, by an antalgic gait. Balance disorders can be caused by impairment of vision, vestibular function, postural muscle response, and proprioception.

Balance and gait assessment includes observations of sitting balance, ability to rise from a seated position, and balance while standing still. Baseline performance should be recorded for purposes of future comparison and to determine if further workup or referral to a neurologist is indicated.

Extrinsic Causes of a Fall

Falls arising from extrinsic causes are far easier to prevent by observing simple safety precautions, particularly in the otherwise dangerous home environment. Accidental falls occur when risky behavior occurs in combination with physical changes and environmental hazards. Standing on a chair to change a light bulb, for example, can be dangerous for even a healthy individual; an elderly person with a faulty sense of balance is at even greater risk.

A thorough home assessment should be carried out by a family member or health care worker. Wagner et al. demonstrated in a randomized, controlled trial that intervention consisting of nursing visits to reduce home risk factors for falls resulted in significantly fewer falls in a 1-year period than in a control group.[1] Each room in the home has certain inherent hazards:

1. *Bathroom*. Slippery bathroom surfaces are often responsible for a fall. Safety equipment should include a tub bench and hand-held shower to allow bathing from a seated position. Sturdy handrails positioned next to tub and toilet areas assist in making safe transfers. Rubberized mats or decals should be used inside the tub; bath mats outside the tub should have nonslip backing.
2. *Kitchen*. Many people fall in the kitchen when reaching or bending for stored items. Frequently used items should be stored at waist level. A sturdy step stool with a wide base of support should be used only when necessary.
3. *Bedroom*. Falls in the bedroom frequently occur when a person rises at night to go to the bathroom and encounters an obstacle in the dark. Night lights are a simple and effective remedy. Patients should also be reminded to allow time for their bodies to adjust to an upright position before standing and walking. Bedroom slippers should cover the entire foot and be supportive, with nonslip soles.
4. *Common areas*. The living room, dining room, and hallways should be well lit and free of scatter rugs, torn carpeting, and obstacles. A clear "traffic lane" should exist within and between each room. Telephone and electrical wires should be secured to walls and not strung across the floor.

Outdoor safety hazards include cracked sidewalks, other pedestrians, animals, curbs, crosswalks, and steps. Weather becomes a factor when slippery surfaces result from ice, rain, or snow. It is a good idea for elderly persons to plan ahead and avoid venturing outside in foul weather.

Shoes that are ill-fitting, worn out, or inappropriate for the particular use can lead to a fall both directly and indirectly. For example, tight shoes or high-heeled shoes may not only cause a trip or fall but could also create painful foot conditions. Patients should evaluate their footwear weekly. Shoes should be low-heeled, with either built-in or added support, and have nonslip soles. Boots should have treads sufficient for good traction. Slippers should cover the foot and have nonslip soles.

Psychosocial circumstances are often aggravating factors in an elderly person with a history of falls. Common situations associated with an increased risk of a fall include living alone, inability to afford food and other necessities, and isolation from family and/or community. Poor memory, loneliness, depression, fear of falling, and fear of losing independence compound these factors.

Multidisciplinary programs have been developed that identify risk factors for falling and implement a variety of intervention strategies to reduce the incidence of falls. Intervention consists of medication adjustment, behavioral modification, and exercise programs that serve to mitigate the risk factors for falling. In a controlled study to determine the effects of such a program, Tinetti et al. demonstrated a significantly lower incidence of falls in an intervention group (35%) than in a control group (47%).[2] Sherrington et al.[3] and Rubenstein et al.[4] demonstrated that exercise programs associated with supervised physical therapy significantly increased quadriceps strength and increased walking velocity in the elderly; both of these parameters have been shown to be important risk factors for falls in community-dwelling elderly persons. Mulrow et al.[5] and MacRae et al.,[6] however, reported that physical therapy and supervised exercise sessions had no effect on fall rates. The efficacy of intervention programs in the prevention of falls is therefore controversial and requires additional research.

Prevention and Treatment of Bone Fragility

It is well established that bone mass is related to fracture risk and that bone strength and mass decrease with increasing age.[7,8] Therefore, one approach to hip fracture prevention is to prevent, retard, or perhaps even reverse this process. Substantial literature exists on the effects of a variety of therapeutic agents—including estrogen alone and in combination with progesterone, calcium, vitamin D and vitamin D metabolites, calcitonin, thiazide diuretics, and bisphosphonates—on both osteoporosis and incidence of hip fracture. With few exceptions, the results of studies of the effects of each of these agents have been equivocal. Furthermore, of these agents, only calcium supplementation, calcitonin, estrogen, and bisphosphonates have been approved by the U. S. Food and Drug Administration for the treatment of osteoporosis.

Estrogen is critical in attaining and maintaining a favorable equilibrium between bone resorption and formation; it also helps protect against coronary artery disease. Although the specific interaction between estrogen and bone is not clearly understood, estrogen withdrawal in women is followed by an increase in the rate of bone loss as great as 2% to 3% per year. Hormone replacement therapy, in the form of either combined or unopposed estrogen, has been shown to reduce the hip fracture incidence by 40% to 60% in women between age 65 and 74 years[9]; however, hormone replacement therapy also increases the risk of breast cancer by 30%.[9] Weinstein and Schiff performed a study to determine the costs, risks, and benefits of both combined estrogen/progestin therapy and unopposed estrogen given in 5-, 10-, and 15-year courses[10]; women receiving combined treatment for 10 years or longer had a small net increase in life expectancy. This study, however, which factored in the risk of breast cancer, failed to incorporate the risk of heart disease when calculating life expectancy. Grady et al. reviewed the literature to determine the impact of long-term estrogen replacement and combined estrogen-progesterone therapy on life expectancy in groups of women at risk for osteoporosis, breast cancer, and heart disease.[11] Their study revealed that a 50-year-old woman at increased risk for hip fracture as a result of decreased bone mineral density can expect long-term estrogen therapy to increase her life expectancy by 1 year. Unfortunately, this study also indicated that unopposed estrogen therapy increased the lifetime probability of developing breast cancer from 10.1% to 12.9% and the risk of endometrial cancer from 2.6% to

19.6%. The decision to initiate hormonal replacement as a preventive measure against osteoporosis (and subsequent hip fracture) should be carefully weighed in light of a woman's family history of breast cancer and the status of her uterus. Although combined therapy reduces the risk of hip fracture similar to that of unopposed estrogen, it increases the risk of breast cancer twofold.

The role of calcium supplementation in the prevention of hip fractures is controversial. Studies indicate that increased calcium intake can decrease, increase, or have no effect at all on hip fracture incidence. Matkovic et al. demonstrated an inverse relationship between calcium intake and the incidence of hip fracture in Yugoslavia.[12] Holbrook et al., in a 14-year prospective study of 957 men and women, determined that the risk of hip fracture decreased in response to increased calcium intake when calcium intake was expressed as a function of total caloric intake.[13] On the other hand, a prospective study in 983 individuals conducted by Wickham et al. to determine the effects of dietary calcium and physical activity on the risk of hip fracture found little difference for each of their three calcium intake groups.[14] Cooper et al. similarly concluded that calcium supplementation had little effect on hip fracture incidence.[15] Completing the spectrum of studies dealing with calcium supplementation and hip fracture risk are results that indicate that higher dietary calcium intake not only fails to lower hip fracture incidence but may in fact increase it. Kreiger et al., studying the effect of dietary factors and fracture in postmenopausal women, found that higher dietary calcium intake slightly increased the risk for hip fracture.[16] Studies by Cummings and Klineberg[17] as well as by Freskanich et al.[18] have also indicated that increased dietary calcium intake may be associated with higher hip fracture risk.

The effects of calcium supplementation on femoral neck bone mineral density have also yielded conflicting results. Dawson-Hughes et al. reported that significant reductions in bone loss can be achieved with calcium supplementation in healthy older postmenopausal women with daily calcium doses of less than 400 mg.[19] Aloia et al., however, demonstrated that women on a regimen of calcium supplementation experienced a reduction of bone loss in the femoral neck only.[20] Reid et al. reported no reduction in bone loss in either the femoral neck or intertrochanteric area in women with calcium supplementation.[21]

Several authors have demonstrated the ability of vitamin D supplementation, with or without calcium, to reduce the incidence of hip fracture. In a study of 3270 healthy ambulatory women by Chapuy et al., daily supplements of 800 IU of vitamin D_3 along with 1.2 g of elemental calcium reduced the incidence of hip fracture by 43% compared to a control group ($P < .05$).[22] In a study by Dawson-Hughes et al., 261 postmenopausal women received either 100 or 700 IU/day of vitamin D_3[23]; there was significantly less bone loss from the femoral neck in patients receiving the higher dose. In contrast, a double-blind, placebo-controlled clinical trial was conducted by Lips et al., in which 2578 people (age 70 years or older) were randomly assigned to receive either vitamin D_3 (400 IU/day) or placebo for 3.5 years[24]; no differences were found in the incidence of hip fracture between the two treatment groups. Similarly, Heikinheimo et al., who studied 799 men and women randomized to receive an annual injection containing either 150,000 or 300,000 IU of vitamin D_2 for 2 to 5 years, found no difference in the incidence of hip fracture in patients belonging to either treatment group.[25]

The vitamin D metabolites $1,25(OH)_2D_3$ (calcitriol) and 1α-hydroxyvitamin D_3 (alfacalcidol) may play key roles in prevention of bone loss. Calcitriol improves the intestinal absorption of calcium and inhibits bone turnover. Several studies have shown that vitamin D metabolites can increase bone mass in women with postmenopausal osteoporosis.[26,27] Other authors, however, have reported no such effects on either bone mass or fracture rates.[28]

Calcitonin—a hormone that is secreted by the parafollicular cells of the thyroid gland and that targets bone (as well as the kidneys and intestines) and functions to decrease serum calcium levels—has been the subject of several studies.[29,30] In bone, calcitonin reduces the number and action of osteoclasts. Calcitonin is available as human synthetic calcitonin and salmon calcitonin, the latter injected subcutaneously or intramuscular or applied intranasally or intrarectally; all but the last may have undesirable side effects. Several studies have demonstrated calcitonin to be an effective method to treat postmenopausal osteoporosis,[31,32] although other studies have shown that intranasal and intrarectal salmon calcitonin failed to reduce trabecular bone loss or failed to cause significant changes in mean bone mineral density in the spine or femoral neck.[33] Kanis et al. showed that women over 50 years of age receiving salmon calcitonin had a significantly decreased risk of hip fracture.[34]

Thiazide diuretics, which decrease urinary calcium excretion, have been used to prevent bone loss and subsequent hip fracture. One investigator reported that individuals who used thiazide diuretics had greater bone density than nonusers in the distal radius, distal ulna, proximal radius, proximal ulna, and os calcis.[35] Ray et al. performed a case-controlled study to determine whether long-term thiazide diuretic therapy correlated with a decreased risk of hip fracture[36]; they found increased duration of thiazide usage to be associated with a significant reduction in the risk of hip fracture. In a prospective study of 9518 men and women 65 years of age or older conducted by LaCroix et al., use of thiazide diuretics was associated with a 33% decrease in the risk of hip fracture during a 4-year follow-up period.[37]

Bisphosphonates, synthetic analogues of inorganic pyrophosphate, an endogenous regulator of bone turnover that inhibits bone resorption and mineralization in vitro, have been used to retard osteoporosis in postmenopausal women. Specific inhibitors of osteoclastic bone resorption, bisphosphonates have been shown to increase bone mineral density in the spine, femoral neck, and trochanteric areas in this population.[38] Etidronate is the parent member of the bisphosphonate class of drugs. Studies done by Watts et al.[39] and Storm et al.[40] both demonstrated that cyclical treatment with etidronate increased vertebral bone density and reduced the incidence of new vertebral fractures. On the negative side, to be effective, etidronate must be given at high dosages at which it also blocks mineralization and induces osteomalacia when used continuously. Furthermore, etidronate has not received approval from the U.S. Food and Drug Administration for the treatment of osteoporosis. A recent study by Black et al. (1996) showed that administration of oral alendronate (Fosamax, Merck & Co., Whitehouse Station, NJ), an aminobisphosphonate, reduced the incidence of hip fractures by 50% in postmenopausal women who had previously sustained a vertebral fracture.[41] Lieberman et al. demonstrated that 10 mg/d of oral alendronate increased bone mass in the femoral neck in postmenopausal women with osteoporosis.[38] The effects of bisphosphonates on bone mineral density, however, are not permanent; McClung reported that following cessation of bisphosphonate therapy, bone loss can resume.[42] Although there is a small number of patients who experience esophagitis as a result of alendronate use, these symptoms can usually be managed by encouraging patients to take the medication with at least 8 oz of water and to avoid recumbency for 30 minutes.

From the available studies, it would appear that use of alendronate and estrogen replacement are the most effective methods to halt bone mineral loss and consequently reduce the incidence of hip fracture. Estrogen replacement therapy protects against both hip fracture and coronary heart disease[11]; use of estrogen is inappropriate, however, whenever there is a family history of breast cancer or an increased risk of endometrial cancer. Use of calcitonin is indicated in women who cannot use estrogen and are unable to take alendronate because of malabsorption or gastrointestinal upset. Individuals at risk for hip fracture should receive at least the recommended daily allowances of calcium and vitamin D, since high calcium intake has a positive effect on peak bone mass[12] and vitamin D plays a role in calcium metabolism. Use of thiazide diuretics is most appropriate in patients with elevated urinary calcium levels.

External Protective Devices

Hayes et al. have identified four distinct phases in a fall: (1) instability, causing a loss of balance; (2) a descent phase; (3) an impact phase; and (4) a postimpact phase, when the body comes to rest.[43] According to Cummings and Nevitt, three conditions predispose to hip fracture during a fall[44]: (1) failure of active protective mechanisms; (2) impact near the hip; and (3) insufficient passive energy absorption by local soft tissues. Laboratory tests have determined that the typical impact force generated at the greater trochanter during a fall is 6940 N, while the average force required to fracture the proximal femur of an elderly person is 4170N.[45] Therefore, energy absorption by the local soft tissue is an important factor in determining whether a patient sustains a hip fracture after direct impact onto the greater trochanter. Robinovitch et al. concluded that in a fall involving a direct impact to the hip, fracture cannot be prevented by the force-attenuation properties of trochanteric soft tissues alone.[46]

There has been recent interest in the use of external trochanteric padding to dissipate forces transmitted to the proximal femur after a fall. However, Parkkari et al. demonstrated that the attenuation properties of padding alone are insufficient to reduce impact forces below the fracture threshold and concluded that external padding should also incorporate the principles of energy shunting.[45]

External hip protectors (special underwear designed to dissipate kinetic energy from an impact to the soft tissue and muscle anterior and posterior to the femur) (Figure 12.1) have been shown to protect against hip fracture in individuals needing immediate protection against certain or imminent fall.[44,47,48]

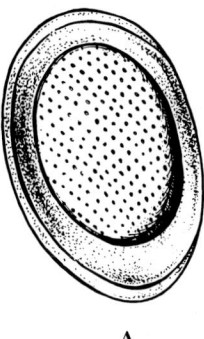 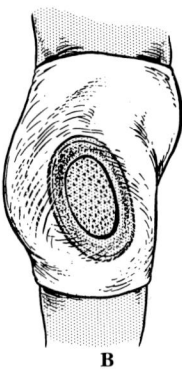

Figure 12.1. Illustrations of an external hip protector (**A**) and a person wearing the specialized underwear (**B**).

Robinovitch et al. utilized the principle of energy shunting in the development of an external hip protector capable of reducing femoral impact force by 65% in vitro.[46] Lauritzen et al. demonstrated that use of an external hip protector prevented hip fractures in nursing home residents[49]; among those who consistently wore external hip protectors, risk of hip fracture was reduced by 53%. The usefulness of the protector, however, is compromised by generally poor patient compliance. To be effective, the device requires 10 cm of padding material, which makes it both awkward to put on and awkward to wear.[50]

Conclusion

The prevention of hip fractures is multifaceted, spanning all ages and both genders, and includes medical, physical, and environmental techniques. Hip fracture prevention can begin in early childhood in the form of a balanced and complete diet along with ample exercise. Active intervention begins in earnest at later ages, with the application of such pharmacological techniques as discussed previously. Upon reaching senescence, one typically requires acute means of hip fracture prevention; external hip protectors are one viable option for preventing fracture in the event of a fall. One can further reduce the risk of hip fracture by eliminating the hazards of the physical environment in which people prone to hip fracture live. Although complete hip fracture prevention is not possible, through these methods it may be possible to significantly reduce their number and severity.

References

1. Wagner E, LaCroix A, Grothaus L, et al. Preventing disability and falls in older adults: a population based randomized trial. *Am J Public Health* 1994; 84:1800–1806.
2. Tinetti ME, Baker DI, McAvay G, et al. A multifactorial intervention to reduce the risk of falling among elderly people living in the community. *N Engl J Med* 1994; 331:821–827.
3. Sherrington C, Lord S. Home exercise to improve strength and walking velocity after hip fracture: a randomized controlled trial. *Arch Phys Med Rehabil* 1997; 78:208–212.
4. Rubenstein L, Robbins A, Josephson K. Effects of an exercise intervention on fall-prone elderly men. *J Am Geriatr Soc* 1994; 41:SA5.
5. Mulrow C, Gerety M, Kanten D. A randomized trial of physical rehabilitation for very frail nursing home residents. *JAMA* 1994; 271:519–524.
6. MacRae P, Feltner M, Reinsch S. A 1-year exercise program for older women: effects on falls, injuries, and physical performance. *Journal of Aging and Physical Activity* 1994; 2:127–142.
7. Cummings S, Black D, Nevitt M. Bone density at various sites for prediction of hip fracture. *Lancet* 1993; 341:72–75.
8. Lips P. Vitamin D deficiency and osteoporosis: the role of vitamin D deficiency and treatment with vitamin D and analogues in the prevention of osteoporosis related fractures. *Eur J Clin Invest* 1996; 26:436–442.
9. Henderson B, Ross R, Lobo R, et al. Re-evaluating the role of progesterone therapy after the menopause. *Fertil Steril* 1988; 49:9S–15S.
10. Weinstein M, Schiff I. Cost-effectiveness of hormone replacement therapy in the menopause. *Obstet Gynecol Surg* 1982; 38:445–455.
11. Grady D, Rubin SM, Petitti DB, et al. Hormone therapy to prevent disease and prolong life in post-menopausal women. *Ann Intern Med* 1992; 117:1016–1037.

12. Matkovic V, Kostiac K, Simonvic I, et al. Bone status and fracture rates in two regions in Yugoslavia. *Am J Clin Nutr* 1979; 32:540–549.
13. Holbrook T, Barrett-Connor E, Wingard DL. Dietary calcium and risk of hip fracture: fourteen-year prospective population study. *Lancet* 1988; 2:1046–1049.
14. Wickham C, Walsh K, Cooper C, et al. Dietary calcium, physical activity, and risk of hip fracture: a prospective study. *BMJ* 1989; 299:889–892.
15. Cooper C, Barker D, Wickham C. Physical activity, muscle strength and calcium intake in fractures of the proximal femur in Britain. *BMJ* 1988; 297:1443–1446.
16. Kreiger N, Gross A, Hunter G. Dietary factors and fracture in postmenopausal women: a case-control study. *Int J Epidemiol* 1992; 21:953–958.
17. Cummings R, Klineberg R. Case control study of dairy product consumption and risk of hip fracture. *Am J Epidemiol* 1994; 139:S2.
18. Feskanich D, Colditz G, Stampfer M, Willett W. Dietary calcium and bone fractures in middle aged women. *Am J Epidemiol* 1994; 139:S55.
19. Dawson-Hughes B, Dallal GE, Krall EA, et al. A controlled trial of the effect of calcium supplementation on bone density in postmenopausal women. *N Engl J Med* 1990; 323:878–883.
20. Aloia J, Vaswani A, Yeh J, et al. Calcium supplementation with and without hormone replacement therapy to prevent postmenopausal bone loss. *Ann Intern Med* 1994; 120:97–103.
21. Reid I, Ames R, Evans M, et al. Effect of calcium supplementation on bone loss in postmenopausal women. *N Engl J Med* 1993; 328:460–464.
22. Chapuy M, Arlot M, Duboeuf F, et al. Vitamin D3 and calcium to prevent hip fracture in elderly women. *N Engl J Med* 1992; 327:1637–1642.
23. Dawson-Hughes B, Harris S, Krall E. Rates of bone loss in postmenopausal women randomly assigned to one of two dosages of vitamin D. *Am J Clin Nutr* 1995; 61:1140–1145.
24. Lips P, Graafmans W, Ooms M, et al. Vitamin D supplementation and fracture incidence in elderly persons. A randomized placebo-controlled clinical trial. *Ann Intern Med* 1996; 124:400–406.
25. Heikinheimo R, Inkovaara J, Harju E. Annual injection of vitamin D and fractures of aged bone. *Calcif Tissue Int* 1992; 51:105–110.
26. Aloia J. Role of calcitriol in the treatment of postmenopausal osteoporosis. *Metabolism* 1990; 39:35–38.
27. Caniggia A, Nuti R, Martini G, et al. Long term treatment with calcitriol in post menopausal osteoporosis. *Metabolism* 1990; 39:43–49.
28. Ott S, Chestnut C. Calcitriol treatment is not effective in postmenopausal osteoporosis. *Ann Intern Med* 1989; 110:267–274.
29. Kallis D, Garant P, Minkin C. Ultrastructural effects of calcitonin on osteoclasts in tissue culture. *J Ultrastruct Res* 1972; 39:205–216.
30. Chambers T, Dunn C. Pharmacological control of osteoclast mobility. *Calcif Tissue Int* 1983; 35:566–579.
31. Gruber H, Ivey J, Baylink D, et al. Long term calcitonin therapy in postmenopausal osteoporosis. *Metabolism* 1984; 33:295–303.
32. Mazzuoli G, Passeri M, Gennari C, et al. Effects of salmon calcitonin in postmenopausal osteoporosis: a controlled double-blind clinical study. *Calcif Tissue Int* 1986; 38:3–8.
33. Kollerup G, Herman A, Brixen E, Lindblad B, Mosekilde L, Sorensen O. Effects of salmon calcitonin suppositories on bone mass and turnover in established osteoporosis. *Calcif Tissue Int* 1994; 54:12–15.
34. Kanis J, Johnell O, Gullberg B, et al. Evidence for efficacy of drugs affecting bone metabolism in preventing hip fractures. *BMJ* 1992; 305:1124–1128.
35. Wasnich RD, Benfante RJ, Yano K, et al. Thiazide effect on the mineral content of bone. *N Engl J Med* 1983; 304:344–347.
36. Ray W, Griffin M, Downey W, Melton LD. Long-term use of thiazide diuretics and risk of hip fracture. *Lancet* 1989; 1:687–690.
37. LaCroix A, Wienpahl J, White L, et al. Thiazide diuretic agents and the incidence of hip fractures. *N Engl J Med* 1990; 322:286–290.
38. Lieberman UA, Weiss SR, Broll J, et al. Effect of oral alendronate on bone mineral density and the incidence of fractures in postmenopausal osteoporosis. *N Engl J Med* 1995; 333:1437–1443.
39. Watts N, Harris H, Genant H, et al. Intermittent cyclical etidronate treatment on postmenopausal osteoporosis. *N Engl J Med* 1990; 323:73–79.

40. Storm T, Thamsborg G, Steiniche T, et al. Effect of intermittent cyclical etidronate therapy on bone mass and fracture rate in women with postmenopausal osteoporosis. *N Engl J Med* 1990; 322:1265–1271.
41. Black DM, Cummings SR, Karpf DB, et al. Randomized trial of effect of alendronate on risk of fracture in women with existing vertebral fractures. *Lancet* 1996; 348:1535–1541.
42. McClung M. Current mineral density data on bisphosphonates in postmenopausal osteoporosis. *Bone* 1996; 19:195S–198S.
43. Hayes WC, Meyers ER, Morris JN, et al. Impact near the hip dominates fracture risk in elderly nursing home residents who fall. *Calcif Tissue Int* 1993; 52:192–198.
44. Cummings SR, Nevitt MC. A hypothesis: the causes of hip fractures. *J Gerontol* 1989; 44:107–111.
45. Parkkari J, Kannus P, Heikkila J, et al. Energy shunting external hip protector attenuates the peak femoral impact force below the theoretical fracture threshold: an in-vitro biomechanical study under falling conditions of the elderly. *J Bone Miner Res* 1995; 10:1437–1442.
46. Robinovitch S, McMahon T, Hayes W. Force attenuation in trochanteric soft tissues during impact from a fall. *J Orthop Res* 1995; 13:965–962.
47. Lauritzen JB, Askegaard V. Protection against hip fractures by energy absorption. *Dan Med Bull* 1992; 39:91–93.
48. Hayes W, Myers E, Maitland L. Relative risk for fall severity, body habitus and bone density in hip fracture among the elderly. *Transactions of the Orthopaedic Research Society* 1991; 16:139.
49. Lauritzen JB, Peterson MM, Lund B. Effect of external hip protectors on hip fractures. *Lancet* 1993; 341:11–13.
50. Parkkari J, Kannus P, Poutala J, Vuori I. Force attenuation properties of various trochanteric padding materials under typical falling conditions of the elderly. *J Bone Miner Res* 1994; 9:1391–1396.

Index

A

Accessory obturator nerve, 5
Acetabular erosion, 78, 114, 259
Acetabulum, 3, *4*
Activities of daily living (ADLs)
   and ambulation, 298
   and assistive devices, 293
   basic (BADLs), 299–300
   instrumental (IADLs), 300
   and outcomes, 297
   postoperative, 290
   rehabilitation, 299–300
Acute care, costs of, 306–308
Acute illnesses, and falls, 314
Adaptive equipment, 292–293
Addisonian crisis, 35
Adductor longus muscles, 5, *6*
Adductor magnus muscles, 5
Age
   and femoral neck stress fracture, 118
   and fracture type, 18
   and hip fracture, 10, 17
   mortality rates, 296
   and muscle mass, 20
   and postoperative weight bearing, 290
   and postsurgical ambulation, 298
   and risk of thrombosis, 39
   and skilled nursing facility care, 308
Albumin levels, 34
Alcohol consumption, 15
Alendronate, 318–319
Alignment index, 71
Alta expandable dome plunger, 137, *138*
Aluminum, 100
Alzheimer's disease, 28
Ambulation. *See also* Mobilization
   postoperative, 290
   and rehabilitation, 298–299
   use of devices, 292–293
Ambulation training, 133, 287–288
Ambulatory status
   types of, 29, 298
American College of Cardiology, 32
American Heart Association, 32
American Society of Anesthesiologists (ASA)
   mortality rates, 296
   operative risk, 28, *297*
γ-Amino transferase, 34
Ancef, 45
Anemia, 33–34
Anesthetics
   considerations, 38–39
   and LMWHs, 42
   techniques and ambulation, 299
   techniques and outcomes, 297
Angina, 32
Anterolateral approach, 74–77
Anteroposterior (AP) radiographs
   assessment of limb length, 260
   diagnosis of hip fracture, 29
   and fracture patterns, 254
   and the Garden classification, 49, 51
   pelvis, *30*
   use in templating, 85
Antibiotics
   perioperative prophylaxis, 108–109
   prophylactic use of, 44–45
   and wound infection, 183
Anticoagulation, 40–43, 108
Anticonvulsants, 13–14
Antidepressants, 13–14
Antihypertensives, 13–14
Antipsychotic agents, 13–14
Antithrombin III, 41
AO/ASIF classifications
   intertrochanteric fractures, 131, *132*
   long bone fractures, 50–51, *52*
   subtrochanteric fractures, 195–196, *196*
AO/ASIF screws, 61, 110
Apatite, osteoconductive carbonated, 177
Arbeitsgemeinschaft für Osteosynthesefragen/Association for the study of Internal Fixation. *See* AO/ASIF
Arrhythmias, cardiac, 32
Arthritis, 12, 101–102
Articular cartilage, 1
Asnis screws, 61, *61*
Aspirin, 42–43
Assistive devices, 292–293
Austin-Moore prostheses, 79
   and acetabular erosion, 259
   design of, 78
   insertion of, 97–98
   radiograph, *82*
Awls, curved, 229

B

Balance, 292, 314
Basicervical fractures, 49, 171–172, 268
Bateman endoprostheses, 80
Bathrooms, falls in, 315
Bed-days. *See* Lengths of stay
Bedrooms, falls in, 315
Benzodiazepines, 13–14
Biceps femoris muscles, 5, 6
Bilirubin levels, 34
Biomechanical studies, 146
Biomechanics
   bedpan approach forces, 287, 289
   femoral neck stress fractures, 116–117
   and fixation techniques, 172
   impact forces, 319
   mechanical stresses, 20–21
   and sliding hip screw angles, 146
   subtrochanteric region stresses, 3, 191, *192*
Bisphosphonates, 316, 318
Blood counts, 32
Blood gas analysis, 32
Blood pressures, 32–33
Blood transfusions, allogenic, 34
Blood urea nitrogen (BUN), 32, 34–35
Body habitus, and hip fractures, 13–14
Body mass index, 14
Bone cement. *See also* Methylmethacrylate
   and acetabular erosion, 80
Bone density
   and fracture risk, 316
   and hip fractures, 13–14, 303
   and postoperative weight bearing, 290
Bone fragility, 316–319
Bone grafting, 242, 279
Bone hooks, use of, 77
Bone ingrowth prostheses
   femoral stem fixation, 82, 83
   insertion, 96

Bone loss, 12
Bone scans
　diagnosis of osteonecrosis, 112
　evaluation of blood flow, 53–54
　and femoral neck stress fractures, 117, 118
Box osteotome, *91*
Boyd and Griffin classifications, *130*
Broaching, *92,* 93
Buck's skin traction, 37, 199
Burrs, use of, *224*
Buttock supports, *228*
Buttress plates, *161, 162*

C

Calcar femorale, 2–3, *3*
Calcar planer, 93, *93*
Calcar replacement prosthesis, *174*
Calcitonin, 316, 317–318
Calcitrol, 317–318
Calcium
　excretion of, 318
　and fracture risk, 14, 316
Cancellous bone
　in the femoral head, 1
　radiograph, *2*
Cancellous lag screws. *See also* Lag screws
　backout of, *110*
　and femoral neck fractures, 256–257
　insertion, 61, *61, 67*
　ipsilateral femoral fractures, 106
　placement of, *73*
　stabilization with, *62*
Canes, 292, 305
Cannulated depth gauge, *219*
Cannulated impactor, *170*
Cannulation, of screws, 58–59, 62
Capsular artery, 7
Capsular pressures, 53
Capsulotomies, 73, 84
Cardiac arrhythmias, postoperative, 108
Cardiac diseases, 12, 32–33
Cardiopulmonary disease, 27–28
Cardiovascular conditions, 314
C-Curves, 71–72, *72*
Cefadroxil, 44–45
Cefazolin, 45
Centromedullary interlocked nails. *See also* Intramedullary nails
　description of, 205
　entry portal, *281*
　first generation, *208*
　　entry portal, *229*
　　insertion, *232*
　　operative technique for, 226–235
　fracture malreduction, 282–283
　implant selection pitfalls, 280
　insertion point pitfalls, 281–282
　measurement of, *232*
　missed femoral neck fractures, 280–281
　second generation, 208–209
　　entry portal, *236*
　　insertion depth, 237, *238*
　　operative technique, 235–241
　　for pathological fractures, 243
　subtrochanteric fractures, 280–283
　visualization pitfalls, 280
Cephalomedullary interlocked nails. *See also* Intramedullary nails
　description of, 205
　diameter choice, 236
　for pathologic fractures, 178
　second generation, *208*
Cephalosporin, 45
Cerebrovascular diseases, 12
Chronic obstructive pulmonary disease (COPD), 33
Climate, and hip fractures, 16
Common areas, falls in, 315
Community ambulators, 29, 298
Comorbidities
　and falls, 314
　and hip fractures, 12
　mortality rates, 296
　and outcomes, 297
Compartment syndrome, 249
Complications. *See also specific complications*
　and outcomes, 297
　prediction of, 31
Compression screws, *159,* 165
Compression ultrasonography, 42
Computed tomography, 53–54, 105, 112
Condylar blade plate, 95°
　entry site for, *213*
　operative technique for, 211–217
　operative technique for insertion, *220*
　preoperative planning, 211
　seating chisel pitfalls, 278
　for subtrochanteric fractures, 199–201, *200*
Condylar screws, 95°, *201,* 202, 217–219
Condylocephalic nails, 205. *See also* Intramedullary nails
Congestive heart failure, postoperative, 108
Continuity of care, 310
Core decompression, 112
Corticosteroids, 13–14, 35
Cost analysis
　acute care costs, 306–308
　cost reduction strategies, 309–311
　demographics of fractures, 303–304
　indirect costs, 309
　long-term care costs, 308–309
　methods and outcomes, 304–306
Creatinine, 32, 34–35
Cruciate anastomoses, 6
Crutches, 290, 292, 305
Cultures, obtaining samples for, 109, 182–183
Cushing's disease, 12

D

Day hospitals, 294
Decubitus ulcers
　after hip fractures, 183–184
　in hip fractures, 29
　and outcomes, 297
　postoperative, 108
Dehydration, 12
Dextran, 42
Dextran 70, 41
Deyerle pin plate, *60*
Diabetes, 12, 33
Diagnosis
　of hip fractures, 27–36
Diameters, of screws, 62
Diet
　and falls, 314
　and hip fractures, 14
　malnutrition, 15
　and outcomes, 297
Dimon-Hughston osteotomy. *See* Medial-displacement osteotomies
Dipyridamole thallium stress test, 32
Discharge disposition, 293–294, 299, 310
Dislocation, 114
Distal locking screw, 273–274
Dobutamine echocardiogram stress tests, 32
Drains, Hemovac, 96

E

Ecchymosis, 29
Economics, of treatment, 303–312
Egger's plates, 136
Elastic stockings, 43
Electrolyte levels, 32, 108
Ender nails, 137, *138,* 139, 205, 206–207
Endoprostheses
　and acetabular erosion, 259
　bipolar, *80,* 80–81, 175
　design, 80–81
　femoral, 79–80, *97*
　inappropriate version, 261
　loosening, 114
　pitfalls of replacement, 259–262
　replacement, 67–68
　unipolar, *81*

Index   **325**

Entry portals
  centromedullary interlocked nails, 281–282
  determination, 228
  intramedullary hip screws, 272
  for intramedullary nailing, 281
Epilepsy, 12
Epiphyseal scars, 231
Estrogens, 316, 318–319
Etidronate, 318–319
Evaluation of Gamma nails, 141–142
Evans classifications, 130
Exercise programs
  and falls, 316
  postoperative, 290–291
Eyesight, and falls, 313

F
Factor IIa, 41
Factor Xa, 41
Falls
  epidemiology of, 19
  external protective devices, 319–320
  extrinsic causes of, 315–316
  incidence of hip fractures, 20
  intrinsic causes of, 313–314
  phases of, 319
  prevention of, 313–316
  risk factors, 314
Fat embolization, 193
Fatigue fractures, 20–21, 114. See also Stress fractures
Femoral artery, 6, 6
Femoral canal, 91, 91
Femoral distractor, 217
Femoral fractures
  intraoperative, 261–262
  Whittaker classifications, 262
Femoral head, 1
  assessment of viability, 31, 69–70
  compressive forces on, 116
  description, 1
  extraction, 91
  sclerosis, 19
  size mismatch, 259–260
  sizing, 91
Femoral neck, 1, 2
  cancellous bone, 2
  exposure, 76
  inappropriate lengths, 260
  osteotomy, 90, 90
  regions, 49
Femoral neck fractures, 49–127
  anterolateral approach, 74–77
  and arthritis, 101–102
  biomechanics and stress, 116–117
  classification, 49–52

  complications following, 108–119
  displaced, 67–78, 73
  effect on vascular supply, 52–54
  epidemiology, 17–19
  evolution of surgical techniques, 55–63
  incisions, 65
  internal fixation, 70–74
  interpretation of fracture pattern, 253–254
  ipsilateral, 104–108
  nondisplaced, treatment of, 63–67
  nonoperative treatment, 54–55
  nonunion, 110–111
  osteonecrosis following, 111–113
  overlooked, 280–283
  Paget's disease, 99–100
  Parkinson's disease, 99
  pathologic fractures, 102–103
  pitfalls of internal fixation, 254–258
  prediction of, 18
  rehabilitation, 103–108
  spastic hemiplegia, 99–100
  stress, 114–119
  total hip arthroplasty for, 98
  treatment selection, 253
Femoral nerve, 5, 6
Femoral shaft fractures, ipsilateral, 104–108
Femoral stem
  types of fixation, 82–83
  varus angulation of, 261
Femoral triangle, 6, 6
Femoral vein, 6
Femur. See Specific regions
125I-Fibrinogen scanning, 41
Fielding and Magliato classification, 194, 194
Fixation failure, 109–110, 110
  after subtrochanteric fractures, 246, 247
  and Ender nails, 206, 207
  following intertrochanteric fracture, 180–181
  subtrochanteric fracture, 284
Fixed-angle devices, 95°, 275–279. See also Condylar blade plates
Flexibility, assessment of, 287
Fluoridated water, 15
Fluoroscopic radiographs, 256
Fluoroscopic tables, 276
Foot conditions, and falls, 314
Foot pumps, 43
Fractured Hip Management Program (FHMP), 310
Fracture patterns
  interpretation of, 253–254
  and postoperative weight bearing, 290
  sliding hip screw use, 265–270

Fracture post, 255
Fullerton and Snowdy classification, 116
Functional status, 28–29, 244, 249, 295

G
Gait analysis, 289, 314
Gamma nail, 141, 165, 166. See also Lag screws
Garden classification, 49–51, 51
Garden screws, 61, 61
Gemelius inferior muscle, 5
Gemelius superior muscle, 5
Gender
  and ambulation, 298
  and hip fractures, 10, 17–19
  mortality rates, 296
  risk of stress fractures, 115
Genital area, 255
Geometry, and fractures, 12–13
Gilberty endoprostheses, 80
Glomerular filtration rate (GFR), 34–35
Gluteus maximus muscle, 5, 88
Gluteus medius muscle, 5
  function, 5–6
  insertion sites, 2
  laxity, 260
  and load distribution, 116
Gluteus minimus muscle, 5
  function, 6
  insertion sites, 2
  and load distribution, 116
Gouffon pins, 59
Gracilis muscles, 5, 6
Greater trochanter, 5, 173, 185
Guide pins
  bending in reamers, 267
  breakage and penetration, 266–267
  broken, 267
  confirmation of positioning, 239, 240
  improper location of, 266
  insertion, 152
  and reaming, 154
  repositioner, 155
Guidewires
  ball-tipped, 230, 232
  and fracture reduction, 230–231
  insertion, 66, 213, 214
  placement into femoral neck, 66
  straight-tipped, 232
  summation, 277

H
Hagie pins, 59
Hansson hook pins, 59, 59–60
Health status, and fracture type, 18
Hearing, and falls, 313
Heel slide, 291

Height, and hip fracture, 13–14
Hemarthrosis, 53–54
Hematoma, 53, 109, 182
Hemiarthroplasty. *See also* Total hip arthroplasty
  cemented bipolar, *83*
  costs of, 305
  functional recovery, 82
  modular unipolar, 87–98
Hemoglobin levels, 18, 34
Heparin
  low-molecular weight (LMWH), 41–42
  and risk of thrombosis, 40–41
  unfractionated (UFH), 41
Hepatitis, viral, 34
Heterotopic ossification, 249
Hip capsule
  attachment of, 4
  exposure of, 76
  T-type incision, *89*
Hip fracture. *See also specific regions*
  demographics, 303–304
  diagnosis, 27–36
  economics of treatment, 303–312
  epidemiology, 17–19
  incidence, *9,* 9–10
  laboratory indices, 32
  mechanisms of injury, 19–21
  mortality rates, 296
  prevention, 313–322
  risk factors, 10–17
  treatment principles, 37–48
Hip
  anatomy overview, 1–8
  dislocations, *261*
  extension exercises, *291*
  external protectors, *319*
  flexion, 291
  views, *5*
Histories
  of accident, 27
  medical, 27–28
  of medications, 28
Hohmann retractors, *66,* 151
Holt nails, 135
Home, discharge to, 299
Home visits, postoperative, 290
Hormone replacement therapy, 316–317
Hospital at home programs, 310
Hospital costs, growth of, 304. *See also* Cost analysis
Hospitalizations, and hip fractures, 11
Household ambulators, 29, 298
Hunter's canal, 7
Hydraulic lifts, *288*
Hyperglycemia, 33
Hyperparathyroidism, 12, 100
Hypertension, 32

Hyperthyroidism, 12
Hypothermia, 16
Hypovolemia, 35

I
Iatrogenic fractures, 261–262
Iliac crest, *5*
Iliofemoral ligament, 4, *5*
Iliopsoas muscle, 2, *5, 6, 6*
Iliotibial band division, *65*
Image intensifiers, 233
  for AP radiographs, 71
  positioning of, *64, 148, 255*
  use of, 227
Immunosuppression, 34
Impact forces, 319
Impedance plethysmography, 41
Implants
  choice of, 142, 209–210
  improper insertion, 256–258
  improper selection, 256
  pattern of screws, 62
  removal for infections, 114
  stabilization, *145*
Incentive spirometry, 33
Incisions
  centromedullary interlocked nail insertion, *228*
  closing after IMHS insertion, *171*
  femoral neck fractures, *65*
  for hemiarthroplasty, 87, *88*
  insertion of IMHS, 166
  sliding hip screw insertion, *151*
  T-type, *89*
Infections
  after prosthetic replacement, 113–114
  after subtrochanteric fracture, 249
  diagnosis, 113, 183
  following surgery, 108–109
  intertrochanteric fractures, 182–183
  postoperative, 183, 249
  prophylactic antibiotics, 44–45
  radionucleotide studies, 249
Inferior gemelli muscle, 6
Inguinal ligaments, *6*
Institutionalization
  and hip fractures, 11
  as outcome, 299
  and outcomes, 297
Insufficiency fractures, 114, 115
Insulin, 33
Interdisciplinary hospital care programs, 300–301
Interference fit, 82, 83
Intermittent pneumatic compression, 43
Internal fixation
  complications following, 108–113
  operative technique, 70–74

pitfalls in femoral neck fractures, 254–258
Intertrochanteric crest, *1*
Intertrochanteric fractures, 129–190
  Boyd and Griffin classification, *130*
  classifications, 129–132
  complications, 180–184
  displaced, *29*
  epidemiology of, 17–19
  Evans classification, *130*
  evolution of surgical techniques, 134–142
  fixation failure, 180–181
  infection, 182–183
  Jensen and Michaelsen classification, *130*
  Kyle classification, *131*
  malrotation deformity, 182
  nonoperative treatment, 133–134
  nonunion, 181–182
  operative treatment, 134–179
  pathological, 177–178
  pitfalls, 263–286
  prediction of, 18
  primary prosthetic replacement, 174–176
  reduction, *147,* 149
  reduction techniques, 142–145
  rehabilitation, 179
  with subtrochanteric extension, 172–173
  wound drainage, 182–183
Intertrochanteric line, *1*
Intertrochanteric region, 2
Intertrochanteric-supracondylar distal femur fractures, 179
Intracapsular fractures, 4
Intracapsular hematoma, 53
Intracapsular pressure, 53–54
Intramedullary hip screw (IMHS)
  distal locking screw insertion, 273–274
  entry portal, 272
  fracture reduction, 271
  insertion, 166–171
  for intertrochanteric fractures, 141
  lag screw placement, 273
  nail placement, 272–273
  patient selection, 270–271
  pitfalls in use, 270–274
  reaming, 272
  Smith+Nephew, *140, 166*
  starting points, 271–272
  use of, 165–171
Intramedullary nails, *138*
  categories, 205
  flexible, 137
  operative insertion techniques, 226
  size choice, 226

for subtrochanteric fractures, 204–209
Intramedullary screws. *See also* Sliding hip screws
Ischial tuberosity, *5*
Ischiofemoral ligament, 4, *5*
Isolation screen, 64, 150

J
Johansson nail, *56*

K
Kabi 2165, 41
Ken-Pugh nail, 135
Kidneys, chronic renal failure, 100
Kitchen, falls in, 315
Knowles pins, *59*, 110
Kyle classification, *131*

L
Labia major, 147
Labrum, 3, *4*
Lag screw-plate barrel relationship, 268–269
Lag screws. *See also* Cancellous lag screws
  assembly and insertion, *155*
  bending of, 268
  cutout, 180
  disengagement, *270*
  guide placement, *223*
  insertion of, 218, *224*
  insertion of sideplate, *156*
  lagging, 156
  length, *154, 169, 219*
  and loss of reduction, 267–268
  methylmethacrylate enhancement, 177
  optimal position, *266*
  placement, *170*
  placement pitfalls, 273
  positions, 155
  prediction of backout, 153
  separation from sideplates, 184
Lateral decubitus position, *87*
Lateral-displacement osteotomy, 142, 143
Lateral epiphyseal artery, 52–53, *53*
Lateral femoral circumflex artery, 6, *6*
Lateral radiographs, 30
Laxity, assessment of, *94*
Lengths of stay
  for hip fractures, 306
  and multidisciplinary management, 301
  and quality of care, 306–307
  and rehabilitation programs, 293
Lesser trochanteric fracture, 185
Life expectancy, 304
Ligaments, 4–5
Limb lengths, 199, 248, 260, *260*
Liver function, 34

Loading
  repetitive, 20–21
  and stress fractures, 116–117
Locking screws
  inappropriate length, *283*
  pitfalls, 283–284
Locking set screws, *162*, 203, *204, 222*
Long-bone injuries, 193
Long-term care costs, 308–309
Loss of fixation. *See* Fixation failure
Lovenox, 42

M
Magnetic resonance imaging (MRI)
  diagnosis of hip fractures, 30
  diagnosis of osteonecrosis, 112
  intertrochanteric fracture, *31*
Malnutrition. *See also* Diet
  and alcohol consumption, 15
  and hip fracture, 14
  and outcomes, 297
Malrotation deformities
  and Ender nails, 206
  intertrochanteric fractures, 182
  and lag screw insertion, *268*
  and posterior sag, 264
Malunion, 248–249. *See also* Nonunion
Massie sliding nail, *57*, 135
Mechanisms of injury
  determination of, 27
  hip fractures, 19–21
  subtrochanteric region, 192–193
Medial-displacement osteotomy, 142, *142,* 142–143, 144
Medial femoral circumflex artery, 6, *7,* 89
Medicare Prospective Payment System (PPS), 307, 308
Medications
  and falls, 314, 316
  and fracture type, 18
  and hip fractures, 13
  history, 28
Medoff plate, 136, *137,* 161–165, *162*
Medoff sideplate, *224*
Medoff sliding plate, *203*
  operative technique for, 221–225
  for subtrochanteric fracture, 203, 204
Medullary canal, opening of, *167*
Mental status
  and ambulation, 298
  and hip fracture, 12
  and outcomes, 297
  postoperative, 38
Methylmethacrylate. *See also* Bone cement; Polymethylmethacrylate cement
  adjunctive use, *176*
  composite fixation, 176–177

insertion of plugs, *95*
Microcracks, 116
Microfracture, 117
Mobilization. *See also* Ambulation
  after subtrochanteric fracture, 245
  after surgery, 103
  early, 287
  and length of stay, 306
Moore pins, *58*
Morse taper junctions, 84
Mortality rates, 38, 295–298
Multidisciplinary care, 300–301, 310
Muscle pedicle bone graft, 77–78, *78*
Muscles
  assessment of strength, 287
  fatigue and falls, 21
  fatigue and load distribution, 117
  views of, *5*
Musculoskeletal conditions, and falls, 314
Myocardial infarction, 108
Myocardial ischemia, 32

N
Nail backout, and Ender nails, 206, *207*
Nailing, history of, 55–57
Nail length, preoperative planning, 231
Neurological conditions, and falls, 313
Neurovascular injuries, 29
Nonambulator, 29, 298
Nonfunctional ambulator, 29, 298
Nonunion. *See also* Malunion
  after subtrochanteric fracture, *247,* 247–248
  femoral neck fracture, 110–111
  following intertrochanteric fracture, 181–182
  and intracapsular fracture, 49
  subtrochanteric fracture, *279*
  and surgical delay, 69
Nursing homes, 11
Nursing personnel, 287, 300–301
Nutritional status, and falls, 314. *See also* Diet
Nutritionists, 300–301

O
Obturator artery, *184*
Obturator externus muscles, 6
Obturator internus muscle, *5*
Obturator nerve, 5
Occult fracture, 31
Occupational therapists, 300–301
Occupational therapy, 290, 308–309
Open reduction, 108–113
Operating tables, 63, *64*
  fluoroscopic, 276
  radiolucent, 212
Operative risk, ASA rating, *297*

Org 10172, 41
Organization for Economic cooperation and Development (OECD), 304
Orthopaedic-geriatric units, 310
Osseous devascularization, 278–279
Osteoarthritis, 19, 101–102
Osteoconductive carbonated apatite, 177
Osteodystrophy, 100
Osteomalacia
  and bone fatigue, 21
  and climate, 16
  and hip fracture, 17
  and renal failure, 100
Osteomyelitis, intramedullary, 273
Osteonecrosis
  early diagnosis, 112
  and femoral neck fracture, 52
  following femoral neck fracture, 111–113
  intertrochanteric fracture, 184
  and intracapsular fracture, 49
  prediction, 31, 69–70
  reduction of risk, 53
  and sliding hip screw, 257
  and surgical delay, 69
  treatment, 112
  and valgus angulation, 258
Osteopenia, 17, 109, 176
Osteoporosis
  and alcohol consumption, 15
  and bisphosphonates, 318
  and bone fatigue, 20–21
  FDA-approved treatments for, 316
  and fracture type, 18–19
  and hip fracture, 17
  total hip arthroplasty, 175
Osteotomes, *91*, *213*
Osteotomies
  Dimon-Hughston, 142, *143*
  femoral neck, 90, *90*
  medial-displacement, 142, *142*
Outcomes
  assessment of, 295–302
  cost analysis, 304–306
Outdoor safety hazards, 315
Outpatient facilities, 294

P
Paget's disease, 99–100, 243
Pain
  after prosthetic replacement, 114
  and femoral neck stress fracture, 117
  pathologic subtrochanteric fracture, 243
  postoperative relief, 245
Parkinson's disease, 12, 28, 99
Partial prothrombin time, 32
Patellar lesions, 249
Pathological fracture, 102–103, 177–178

Patient management. *See also* Cost analysis
  initial, 37
  surgical timing, 37–38
Patient positioning
  on a fluoroscopic table, 276
  on fracture table, 63
  for hemiarthroplasty, 87, *87–88*
  improper, 254–255
  insertion of 95° condylar blade plate, 211
  insertion of IMHS, 166
  intramedullary nailing, *227*
  sliding hip screw insertion, 146–149
Pauwels classification, 49–50, *50*
Pectineus muscle, *5, 6*
Penicillin, 45
Perineal post, 146, *147*
Periprosthetic femur fracture, *262*
Pertrochanteric fracture, 139, 140–141
Petrochanteric fracture, 139–140
Phlebography, 41
Physical examination, 29
Physical therapist, 300–301
Physical therapy
  and falls, 316
  role of, 287
  treatment plan, 287
Physician fees, 305
Pinning, 58–61
Piriformis fossa, 237
Piriformis muscle, *5, 6*
Plantar venous plexus, 43
Platelets, and aspirin, 42–43
Pneumonia, 108, 297
Polymethylmethacrylate cement, 82, 83. *See also* Methylmethacrylate
Polypharmacy, 28
Popliteal artery, 7
Popliteal vein, 39
Posterior sag, 150, *150*, 167, 220, 264, *264*
Posteromedial buttress, 157, *159*
Posteromedial fragment, 160, *160*
Postoperative wound infection. *See* Infections
Preoperative planning
  condylar blade plates, 211
  fixed-angle devices, 275, *276*
  nail length, 231
Prevention of hip fracture, 313–322
Primary prosthetic replacement, 78–85, 78–98, 113–114, 174–176
Profunda femoris artery, *6*, 151, *151*
Progesterone, 316
Prostheses. *See* Endoprostheses
Protective devices, external, 319–320
Prothrombin time, 32

Protrusio acetabuli, 78, 83, *259*
Proximal femur
  muscle insertion sites, *3*
  views of, *1*
Proximal femur fracture
  clinical deformity in, 29
  pathological, 177–178
  thromboprophylaxis, 39–44
Proximal targeting guides, *239*
Psychiatric conditions, 314
Psychiatrists, 300–301
Psychosocial circumstances, and falls, 315
Pubofemoral ligament, 4–5, *5*
Pudendal nerve, 249, 254
Pugh sliding nail, 57
Pulmonary disease, 33
Pulmonary embolism, 39

Q
Quadratus femoris muscle, *5*
  function of, 6
  pedical graft, 77–78
  release of, 88
Quadriceps strengthening, 291
Quality-adjusted life years, 309–310
Quality of life assessments, 309

R
Race
  and hip fracture, 11, 17–19
  hip geometry, 12–13
Radiographs. *See also* Anteroposterior (AP) radiographs
  diagnosis of hip fracture, 30–31
  diagnosis of ipsilateral femoral fracture, 105
  femoral neck alignment, 71–72
Radiolucent operating tables, 212
Radiolucent proximal targeting devices, *237*, *238*
Radiolucent ruler, 231
Range-of-motion
  assessment of, 29, 287
  exercises, 103, 246
Reamers
  bending of the guide pin, 267
  binding of guide pin in, 184
  blunt T-handled, *92*
  cannulated, 168
  collapse of, *224*
Reaming
  of the femoral canal, 91, *92, 232*
  femoral neck, 154, *154*
  of the femur, 231
  and intramedullary hip screws, 272
  and intraoperative fracture, 261–262
  proximal femur, *163, 169, 219*
Reconstruction nails, 178

Delta, 236
Russell-Taylor, 205, 209
Smith+Nephew, 178, 236
Recovery, measures of, 295–300. *See also* Outcomes
Rectus femoris muscle, 5
Reductions
   and 95° fixed-angle devices, 277
   inadequate, 256, 263–265
   intertrochanteric fracture, 142–145, 263–265
   and intramedullary hip screws, 273
   intramedullary nail pitfalls, 282–283
   loss in a subtrochanteric fracture, *284*
   loss of, 267–268, *281*
   open, 108–113
Rehabilitation
   activities of daily living, 299–300
   acute, 308
   after hip fracture, 287–294
   discharge disposition, 299
   femoral neck fracture, 103–108
   interdisciplinary hospital care programs, 300–301
   intertrochanteric fracture, 179
   postoperative teams, 290
   protocols, *288*
   settings for, 293–294
   subtrochanteric fracture, 245–246
Renal diseases, 34–35, 100
Retinacular vessels, 7, *7*, 52
Revascularization, 52
Reverse-obliquity pattern, 265
Rheumatoid arthritis, 101–102
Running, load distribution, 116
Rural residence, and fracture, 16
Russell-Taylor classification
   and implant choice, 209–210
   subtrochanteric fracture, 196–197, *197, 275*

S

Sacrum, 5
Sarmiento osteotomy. *See* Valgus osteotomy
Sartorius muscle, 5
Sciatic nerve, 88, 249
Sclerotic bone, 100
Screws. *See also* Specific screw types
   backout of, *110*
   design concepts, 62–63
   for femoral neck fracture, 62–63
   lengths of, *67*
   plate-holding, *158*
   prediction of backout, 153
   self-tapping, 62
Scrotum, 255, *255*
S-Curves, 71–72, *72*

Seating chisel
   improper assembly of, 278
   incarceration of, 278
   use of, *213*, 214, *214*
Seinheimer's classification, 194–195, *195*
Semimembranosus muscle, *5*, 6
Semitendinosus muscle, *5*, 6
Sepsis, 249
Septicemia, 297
Serosanguinous drainage, 109
Serum glucose level, 33
Shoes, and falls, 315
Sideplates, improper placement, 269–270
Skilled nursing facilities, 293
   discharge to, 299, 307
   prediction of need for, 308
Sliding hip screws, 57, 136, 202. *See also* Intramedullary screws
   basicervical fracture, *172*
   femoral hip fracture, *257*
   implant stabilization, *145*, 145–161
   insertion in stable fracture, 151–157
   insertion in unstable fracture, 157–161
   insertion of, 146–150, *161*
   intertrochanteric fracture, 141, *144*, 265–270
   introchanteric fracture fixation, 135–136
   "keyed," 155, *156*
   and loss of fixation, 109
   and loss of slide, 268–269
   operative technique for insertion, 220–221
   petrochanteric fracture, 139
   stabilization of osteotomies, *143*
   subtrochanteric fracture, 202–203, *221*
Sliding nail-plate device, 135
Sliding plates, design of, 161
Smith-Petersen nails, 55, *56*
Smoking, 15, 33
Social functioning, 309
Social workers, 293–294, 300–301
Soft tissue
   excessive dissection of, 278–279
   laxity of, 260
Spastic hemiplegia, 99–100
Speed of sound (SOS), 118
Spinal hematomas, 42, 43
Spiral fracture, subtrochanteric, 192
SRS, 177
Stability testing, 93, *94*
Stair climbing, 290
Staphylococcus areus, 44–45
Strain-gauge studies, 116
Strength training, 290–291
Stresses. *See* Biomechanics
Stress fracture
   compression, 116
   displaced femoral neck, 116

   femoral neck, 114–119
   hip, 21
   tension, 115
Stress tests, 32
Subcapital fracture, 49
Subsynovial intracapsular arterial ring, 7
Subtrochanteric fracture, 191–252
   classifications, 194–196, *275*
   complications, 246–249
   evolution of surgical techniques, 199–209
   fixation failure, *284*
   95° fixed-angle devices, 275–279
   implant choice pitfalls, 274–275
   implant choices, 204, 209–210
   interlocked nail pitfalls, 280–283
   intramedullary nails, 204
   loss of reduction, *284*
   nonoperative treatment, 197–198
   nonunion, *279*
   open, 242
   operative treatments, 199–245
   pathological, 177–178, 242–245
   pitfalls, 274–284
   rehabilitation, 245–246
   stabilization, *221*
Subtrochanteric region
   associated injuries, 193
   definition, *191*
   description, 3
   mechanisms of injury, 192–193
   stresses, *3*, 192
Superficial femoral artery, 7, 184
Superior gemelli muscle, 6
Surgical delay, 297
Sutures, interrupted, 96

T

Technetium bone scan
   diagnosis of hip fracture, 30
   femoral head viability, 69
   intertrochanteric fracture, *31*
Technetium 99m medronate disodium scintimetry, 70
Templating, in hemiarthroplasty, 85–87
Tensioning devices, 216, *216*
Tensor fasciae latae muscle, *5*, 6, 151
Tetracycline labeling, 70
Thiazide diuretics, 316, 318
Third-party payers, 309
Thompson prostheses, 78, *79*, 259
Thornton nail, *56*
Thread, of screws, 62
Thrombin. *See* Factor IIa
Thromboembolism, 108
Thrombophlebitis, 108
Thromboprophylaxis, 39–40
Thrombosis, 43

Timing
  of injury, 27
  of surgery, 37–38, 69
Tip-apex distance (TAD), 152–153, 266
Total hip arthroplasty, 175. *See also* Hemi-arthroplasty
  after displaced femur fracture, 259
  and arthritic hip, 102
  for osteonecrosis, 112
  primary, 98
Trabecular bone, 1
Traction, 133, 197–198
Transaminase levels, 34
Transcervical fracture, 49
Trapezes, 287
Trauma
  high energy, 192
  low energy, 192–193
  polytrauma patients, 178–179
Trendelenburg gait, 248
Trocar positioning, *234*
Trochanteric fracture, 185

U

Ultrasonography
  and diagnosis of stress fracture, 118
  evaluation of blood flow, 53–54
Uppsala screws, 61
Urban residence, and fracture, 16
Urinary conditions, 314
Urinary tract infection, 108
U.S. Food and Drug Administration (FDA), 316

V

Valgus angulation, 258
Valgus-impacted fracture. *See* Garden classifications
Valgus osteotomy, 110, 111, 142, 143
Vancomycin, 45
Varus angulation, 258
  correction of, 264
  of the femoral stem, 261
  sliding hip screw insertion, *265*
Varus fracture, reduction of, *282*
Varus malreduction, 248, *248*
Varus osteotomy, 248
Vastus lateralis muscle, *75*, *76*, 151, *151*, *213*
Verbrugge clamp, 160, 216
Visualization, inadequate, 263–265
Vitamin D
  and alcohol consumption, 15
  and climate, 16
  and fracture risk, 316
  and hip fracture, 13–14
  and renal failure, 100
Vitamin D metabolites, 316, 317–318
Vitamin K, 14
Von Bahr screws, 61

W

Waddell's classification, 194, *194*
Wages lost, 304
Walkers, 292
Walking, loads distribution, 116
Watson-Jones approach, 74–77
Wayne County osteotomy. *See* Lateral-displacement osteotomy
Weight bearing
  after subtrochanteric fracture, 245, 247
  and outcomes, 103–104
  postoperative, 289, 290
Wheelchairs, 292
Whittaker classification, 262
Wound drainage, 182–183

Z

Zickel nail, 205–206, *206*, 243
Zona orbicularis, 5, *5*